Interstitial Cystitis

Interstitial Cystitis

Editor

Grannum R. Sant, M.D.
Professor and Acting Chair
Department of Urology
Tufts University School of Medicine
New England Medical Center
Boston, Massachusetts

Lippincott - Raven
PUBLISHERS
Philadelphia • New York

Acquisitions Editor: R. Craig Percy
Developmental Editor: Ellen DiFrancesco
Manufacturing Manager: Dennis Teston
Production Manager: Maxine Langweil
Production Editor: Rita Madrigal
Cover Designer: Kevin Kall
Indexer: Linda Van Pelt
Compositor: Lippincott–Raven Electronic Production
Printer: Maple Press

Printed in the United States of America

9 8 7 6 5 4 3 2 1

Library of Congress Cataloging-in-Publication Data

Interstitial cystitis / Grannum R. Sant.
p. cm.
Includes bibliographical references and index.
ISBN 0–397–51695–9
1. Interstitial cystitis. I. Sant, Grannum R.
[DNLM: 1. Cystitis, Interstitial. WJ 500 I6146 1997]
RC921.C9I573 1997
616.6′23—dc21
DNLM/DLC
For Library of Congress 97–10327
CIP

To my wife, Kathleen and my children, Justin and Sinead,
for their unfailing support and encouragement.

To all my interstitial cystitis patients,
who have made me a better physician.

Contents

Contributing Authors

Said A. Awad, M.B., B.Ch.
Professor of Urology
Department of Urology
QEII Health Sciences Centre
Dalhousie University
1278 Tower Road
Halifax, Nova Scotia B3H 2Y9
Canada

Tamara G. Bavendam, M.D.
Associate Professor of Urology
Department of Urology
University of Washington
Box 356510
1959 Pacific Avenue N.E.
Seattle, WA 98195

Richard E. Berger, M.D.
Professor of Urology
Department of Urology
University of Washington
Box 356510
1959 Pacific Avenue N.E.
Seattle, WA 98195

Dale E. Bjorling, D.V.M.
Professor and Chair
Department of Surgical Sciences
University of Wisconsin
School of Veterinary Medicine
2015 Linden Drive West
Madison, WI 53706

Daniel Brookoff, M.D., Ph.D.
Clinical Associate Professor, Preventive Medicine
Department of Medical Education
University of Tennessee, Memphis
Methodist Hospital
1265 Union Avenue
Memphis, TN 38104

C.A. Tony Buffington, D.V.M., Ph.D.
Professor of Clinical Nutrition
Department of Veterinary Clinical Sciences
The Ohio State University Veterinary Hospital
601 Vernon L. Tharp Street
Columbus, OH 43210-1089

Arnold D. Bullock, M.D.
Instructor of Surgery
Division of Urologic Surgery
Washington University School of Medicine
216 N. Kingshighway
Suite 3304
St. Louis, MO 63110

Dennis J. Chew, D.V.M.
Professor, Internal Medicine
Department of Veterinary Clinical Sciences
The Ohio State University
College of Veterinary Medicine
601 Vernon L. Tharp Street
Columbus, OH 43210-1089

Timothy J. Christmas, M.D.
Consultant Urological Surgeon
Department of Urology
Charing Cross Hospital
Fulham Palace Road
London W6 8RF, England
United Kingdom

Carol Dalton, R.N., N.P.
Registered Nurse Clinician
Wellspring for Women, PC
900 28th Street #201
Boulder, CO 80303

Stephen P. DiBartola, D.V.M.
Professor of Medicine
Department of Veterinary Clinical Sciences
The Ohio State University
College of Veterinary Medicine
601 Vernon L. Tharp Street
Columbus, OH 43210-1089

Gerald J. Domingue, Ph.D.
Professor of Urology, Microbiology, and Immunology
Department of Urology and Microbiology-Immunology
Tulane University School of Medicine and Graduate School
1430 Tulane Avenue
New Orleans, LA 70112-2699

Deborah R. Erickson, M.D.
Assistant Professor of Surgery
Department of Surgery
Division of Urology
Pennsylvania State University College of Medicine
500 University Drive
Hershey, PA 17033-0850

Magnus Fall, M.D., Ph.D.
Associate Professor and Chief Urologist
Department of Surgery
Division of Urology
Sahlgrenska University Hospital
University of Göteborg
Göteborg
Sweden

Jerzy B. Gajewski, M.D.
Associate Professor of Urology
Department of Urology
QEII Health Sciences Centre
Dalhousie University
New Halifax Infirmary Site
1225B-1796 Summer Street
Halifax, Nova Scotia B3H 3A7
Canada

Niall T. Galloway, M.B.Ch.B.
Associate Professor of Surgery/Urology
Department of Surgery/Urology
Emory University School of Medicine
1364 Clifton Road N.E.
Atlanta, GA 30322

Gamal M. Ghoniem, M.D.
Associate Professor of Urology and Gynecology
Department of Urology
Tulane University School of Medicine
1430 Tulane Avenue, SL-42
New Orleans, LA 70112

Larrian M. Gillespie, M.D.
Associate Clinical Professor of Urology and Urogynecology
Western University of Health Sciences
505 South Beverly Drive
Suite 1233
Beverly Hills, CA 90212

Christian Hampel, M.D.
Clinical Instructor
Department of Urology
University of Mainz
Langenbeckstrasse 1
55131 Mainz
Germany

Philip M. Hanno, M.D.
Professor and Chairman
Department of Urology
Temple University School of Medicine
3401 North Broad Street
Philadelphia, PA 19140

Ngoc Ho, M.B.S.
Department of Epidemiology
University of Washington
Seattle, WA 98103

Markus Hohenfellner, M.D.
Associate Professor of Urology
Department of Urology
University of Mainz
Langenbeckstrasse 1
55131 Mainz
Germany

Gero Hohlbrugger, M.D.
Professor of Urology
Department of Urology
University of Innsbruck
Anichstrasse 35
6020 Innsbruck
Austria

Robert E. Hurst, Ph.D.
Professor of Urology
Department of Urology
Oklahoma University Health Sciences Center
920 S.L. Young Boulevard
Oklahoma City, OK 73104

Paul P. Irwin, M.Ch.
Lecturer in Urology and Honorary Senior Registrar
Department of Urology
University of Manchester
Manchester Royal Infirmary
Oxford Road
Manchester M13 9WL, England
United Kingdom

Sonny L. Johansson, M.D., Ph.D.
Professor of Pathology
Department of Pathology and Microbiology
University of Nebraska Medical Center
600 South 42nd Street
Omaha, NE 68198-3135

Mickey M. Karram, M.D.
Associate Professor
Department of Obstetrics and Gynecology
University of Cincinnati
Good Samaritan Hospital
375 Dixmyth Avenue
Cincinnati, OH 45220

Ingegerd M. Keith, Med. Kand., Ph.D.
Professor of Neuroendocrine Physiology and Neurochemistry
Department of Comparative Biosciences
University of Wisconsin
School of Veterinary Medicine
2015 Linden Drive West
Madison, WI 53706

Carl G. Klutke, M.D.
Associate Professor
Department of Surgery
Division of Urology
Washington University School of Medicine
4960 Children's Place
St. Louis, MO 63110

Neeraj Kohli, M.D.
Division of Urogynecology and Reconstructive Pelvic Surgery
Good Samaritan Hospital
375 Dixmyth Avenue
Cincinnati, OH 45220

James A. Koziol, Ph.D.
Professor of Biomathematics
Department of Molecular and Experimental Medicine
The Scripps Research Institute
10666 N. Torrey Pines Road
La Jolla, CA 92037

J. Richard Landis, Ph.D.
Professor of Biostatistics
Center for Biostatistics and Epidemiology
Pennsylvania State University College of Medicine
500 University Drive
Hershey, PA 17033-0850

Dennis R. La Rock, M.D.
Department of Urology and Interstitial Cystitis Clinic
New England Medical Center
750 Washington Street, Box 142
Boston, MA 02111

Monica Liebert, Ph.D.
Department of Urology
University of Texas
M.D. Anderson Cancer Center
Box 110
1515 Holcombe Boulevard
Houston, TX 77030

Jürgen F. Linn, M.D.
Department of Urology
University of Mainz
Langenbeckstrasse 1
55131 Mainz
Germany

Terrence R. Malloy, M.D.
Clinical Professor of Urology
Department of Urology
University of Pennsylvania
Pennsylvania Hospital
299 South 8th Street
Philadelphia, PA 19106

Rita M. Martel, R.N., A.N.P.
Director of Continence, Nonsurgical
Department of Obstetrics and Gynecology
University of Colorado Health Sciences Center
4200 E. 9th Avenue, Box B198
Denver, CO 80262

Naomi B. McCormick, Ph.D.
Visiting Scholar
Family Studies and Psychology
University of Northern Iowa
Latham Hall
Cedar Falls, IA 50614-0332

Francine Mendelowitz, M.S.W.
Department of Urology
Long Island Jewish Medical Center
270-05 76th Avenue
Oncology Building, Rm. 4005
New Hyde Park, NY 11042

Jane L. Miller, M.D.
Assistant Professor
Department of Urology
University of Washington
1959 Pacific Avenue N.E.
Seattle, WA 98195

Robert Moldwin, M.D.
Assistant Professor of Urology
Albert Einstein College of Medicine
Director, Interstitial Cystitis Center
Department of Urology
Long Island Jewish Medical Center
270-05 76th Avenue
Oncology Building, 4th Floor
New Hyde Park, NY 11042

Denise A. Nigro, M.D.
Physician, Scientist Fellow
Division of Urology
University of Pennsylvania Medical Center
First Floor Rhoads Pavilion
3400 Spruce Street
Philadelphia, PA 19104

Leroy M. Nyberg, M.D., Ph.D.
Director, Urology Programs
NIH/NIDDK
Natcher Building, Room 6A.S.13G
45 Center DR MSC 6600
Bethesda, MD 20892-6600

Robert L. Ochs, Ph.D.
Assistant Professor
Department of Molecular and Experimental Medicine
The Scripps Research Institute
10550 N. Torrey Pines Road
La Jolla, CA 92037

Kumiko Ogawa, M.D., Ph.D.
Department of Pathology and Microbiology
The Eppley Institute for Research in Cancer and Allied Diseases
University of Nebraska Medical Center
600 South 42nd Street
Omaha, NE 68198-3135

Michael P. O'Leary, M.D., M.P.H.
Assistant Professor of Surgery
Harvard Medical School
Brigham and Women's Hospital
Division of Urology
45 Francis Street
Boston, MA 02115

C. Lowell Parsons, M.D.
Professor of Surgery/Urology
Division of Urology
University of California
San Diego Medical Center
200 W. Arbor Drive
San Diego, CA 92103-8897

Michel A. Pontari, M.D.
Assistant Professor
Department of Urology
Temple University School of Medicine
3401 North Broad Street
Philadelphia, PA 19140

Timothy L. Ratliff, Ph.D.
Associate Professor and Director of Urologic Research
Department of Surgery
Division of Urology
Washington University School of Medicine
4960 Children's Place
St. Louis, MO 63110

Vicki Ratner, M.D.
President, Interstitial Cystitis Association
P.O. Box 1553
Madison Square Station
New York, NY 10159

Johnny B. Roy, M.D.
Professor of Urology
University of Oklahoma College of Medicine
Oklahoma City
105 S. Bryant, Suite 401
Edmond, OK 73034

Ricardo Saban, D.V.M., Ph.D.
Associate Scientist
Department of Surgical Sciences
University of Wisconsin
School of Veterinary Medicine
2015 Linden Drive West
Madison, WI 53706

Grannum R. Sant, M.D.
Professor and Acting Chair
Department of Urology
Tufts University School of Medicine
New England Medical Center
750 Washington Street, Box 142
Boston, MA 02111

Allan M. Shanberg, M.D.
Professor of Clinical Surgery-Urology
Department of Surgery/Urology
University of California, Irvine
101 The City Drive
Route 81
Orange, CA 92868

Carolyn C. Shea, B.S.N., R.N.
Department of Urology
Interstitial Cystitis Clinic
New England Medical Center
750 Washington Street, Box 142
Boston, MA 02111

Laura J. Simon, M.A.
Instructor
Department of Statistics
Pennsylvania State University
326 Thomas Building
University Park, PA 16802

Debra K. A. Slade, M.A., B.A.(Oxon)
Executive Director
Interstitial Cystitis Association
279 Mamanasco Road
Ridgefield, CT 06877

William D. Steers, M.D.
Chairman and J.Y. Gillenwater Professor of Urology
Department of Urology
University of Virginia Hospital
Box 422
Charlottesville, VA 22902

Eddie H.M. Sze, M.D.
Assistant Professor of Obstetrics and Gynecology
Director of Undergraduate Medical Education
Mercer University School of Medicine
Medical Center of Central Georgia
729 Pine Street
Macon, GA 31201

Eng M. Tan, M.D.
W.M. Keck Autoimmune Disease Center
Department of Molecular and Experimental Medicine
The Scripps Research Institute
10550 N. Torrey Pines Road
La Jolla, CA 92037

Theoharis C. Theoharides, M.D., Ph.D.
Clinical Pharmacologist
Massachusetts Drug Formulary Commission
Professor of Pharmacology and Medicine
Department of Pharmacology and Experimental Therapeutics
Tufts University School of Medicine
136 Harrison Avenue
Boston, MA 02111

Joachim W. Thüroff, M.D.
Professor of Urology
Department of Urology
University of Mainz
Langenbeckstrasse 1
55131 Mainz
Germany

John E. Tomaszewski, M.D.
Professor of Pathology and Laboratory Medicine
Department of Pathology and Laboratory Medicine
University of Pennsylvania Medical Center
3400 Spruce Street
Founders 6
Philadelphia, PA 19104-4283

Jeremy B. Tuttle, Ph.D.
Associate Professor of Urology and Neuroscience
Department of Urology
University of Virginia Health Sciences Center
Cobb Hall 3014, Box 230
Charlottesville, VA 22908

Philip E.V. Van Kerrebroeck, M.D., Ph.D.
Professor of Urology
Department of Urology
University Hospital Maastricht
Box 5800
N1 6202 AZ Maastricht
The Netherlands

Anita K. Wagner, Pharm.D.
Assistant Clinical Professor
Department of Neurology
Tufts University School of Medicine
Senior Project Director
The Health Institute
New England Medical Center
750 Washington Street, Box 345
Boston, MA 02111

Denise C. Webster, R.N., M.S.N., Ph.D., C.S.
Professor of Nursing
School of Nursing
University of Colorado Health Sciences Center
4200 East Ninth Avenue
Denver, CO 80262

Alan J. Wein, M.D.
Professor and Chair
Chief of Urology
Division of Urology
University of Pennsylvania Medical Center
First Floor Rhoads Pavilion
3400 Spruce Street
Philadelphia, PA 19104

Bruce E. Woodworth, M.D.
Clinical Assistant Professor
Department of Surgery
The Ohio State University
3555 Olentangy River Road
Suite 2050
Columbus, OH 43214

Preface

In the early 1980s, interstitial cystitis (IC) was a female urologic disorder of unknown etiology that was infrequently diagnosed, poorly treated, and incompletely understood. Persistent prodding from the Interstitial Cystitis Association (ICA), a patient advocacy group, resulted in the convening of a National Institutes of Health (NIH-NIDDK) International Conference on Interstitial Cystitis in 1987. This conference promulgated consensus-criteria for diagnosis, identified areas for future research, and established a cadre of investigators, clinicians and researchers interested in IC. Over the last 10 years, a significant body of literature dealing with IC has developed, and the diagnosis and treatment of IC, as well as research into IC, have been brought into the urologic mainstream. This book attempts to summate the current state of knowledge regarding IC. Hopefully, it will also act as a stimulus for clinicians and researchers to advance our understanding and treatment of this syndrome.

The authors who have contributed to the text are all recognized experts in the field of IC. They all gave generously of their time, and for this, I am very grateful. Interstitial cystitis has protean manifestations—gynecologic, urologic, and pain—and the chapter authorship reflects this by including urologists, gynecologists, and pain experts. The symptoms of IC significantly affect patients' quality of life, and the holistic approach to treatment of IC is represented by chapters dealing with psychological issues, pain management, nursing care caveats, and quality-of-life issues.

Advances in treatment for any disease, particularly one as enigmatic as IC, depend on elucidation of its etiology, pathogenesis, and pathophysiology. Basic research studies into IC have flourished over the last decade, and the chapters dealing with these areas present state-of-the-art knowledge. The symbiotic efforts and interests of clinicians and basic scientists are amply reflected in the authorship of many of these chapters. The commendable efforts of the Interstitial Cystitis Association in the dissemination of knowledge about IC, patient education, fostering of research, and political advocacy at the federal level is also recognized.

I hope that this book meets the needs of its intended readership: urologists, gynecologists, basic researchers, pain clinic specialists, nurses, and patients. The book outlines the current approach to the diagnosis and treatment of IC and provides an up-to-date summation of current research into the etiology and pathogenesis of the disease. Researchers entering the field of IC research, and those contemplating same, should find this text a useful compendium.

Grannum R. Sant, M.D.
Boston, Massachusetts
April, 1997

Acknowledgments

My initial interest in interstitial cystitis was kindled during my residency training by Edwin M. Meares, Jr., M.D., who continued to be my mentor until his retirement in 1996. This interest was further nurtured by the advice, scientific exactitude and encouragement of other urologists, including Thomas Stamey, M.D., Edward Messing, M.D., and Jay Gillenwater, M.D., to name a few. The constant support of the Interstitial Cystitis Association, particularly Vicki Ratner, M.D. and Debra Slade has been an immense source of inspiration and encouragement.

Over the years, the nursing, secretarial, and support staff at the New England Medical Center have been instrumental in the establishment and growth of our Interstitial Cystitis Clinic and its recognition as a patient-centered facility for clinical and research studies of interstitial cystitis. Carolyn Shea, R.N. has been a "Rock of Gibraltar" in the clinic and Susan Mayo, my long-serving secretary and administrative assistant, has performed over and above the call of duty. Susan contributed her abundant word-processing and editorial skills during the long period of preparation, revisions, and corrections of the manuscripts.

To Craig Percy, medical editor "extraordinaire," I am indebted for his initial enthusiasm for this book and his detailed suggestions and advice during the gestation and birth of this text.

To all of these individuals, I am most grateful.

Interstitial Cystitis, edited by Grannum R. Sant.
Lippincott–Raven Publishers, Philadelphia ©1997.

CHAPTER 1

Historical Aspects of Interstitial Cystitis

Timothy J. Christmas

Historically, interstitial cystitis (IC) has been a relatively poorly recognized condition; its etiology has remained obscure at least partly because of a lack of research into the disorder. One of the problems in drawing conclusions regarding IC has been the precise definition and diagnosis of the disease. Large series of IC cases have been reported from the United States, whereas the condition appears to be rare in Europe and almost unknown in developing countries. This trans-Atlantic disparity in epidemiologic data appears to relate to the adoption of different diagnostic criteria.

Fortunately, there are now internationally recognized diagnostic criteria (1) that permit a more scientific approach to research and therapeutic developments in IC. The history of IC between 1836 and 1960 is outlined below. More modern aspects of IC are described in later specialized chapters.

HISTORICAL REVIEW

The first written reference to what was almost certainly IC described a case of spontaneous rupture of the urinary bladder secondary to ulceration (2). This is a most unusual occurrence in contemporary experience, but the clinical history of the case is otherwise typical of IC. In 1870, Lawson Tait described two cases of perforating bladder ulcer in young women under the care of Sir James Simpson (Fig. 1) at the Royal London Hospital (then the London Hospital). Both presented with bladder pain, dysuria, and urinary frequency, and one had been symptomatically relieved by intravesical instillation of silver nitrate under chloroform anesthesia. Tait advocated formation of a vesicovaginal fistula to allow healing of the ulcer, and this maneuver relieved the symptoms in the two cases that he described. The fistulas were later successfully closed after the ulcers had healed, without recurrence of symptoms. Tait pointed out the similarity between these ulcers and those of the stomach with particular reference to involvement and perforation of the deep muscle layers. This initial description of surgical intervention for the relief of symptoms of IC introduced the now well-recognized concept that urinary diversion may alleviate the symptoms of IC (3).

The descriptive term *interstitial cystitis* was first coined by Skene in a book on diseases of the female urethra and bladder (4). In 1896, E. Hurry Fenwick (Fig. 2) gave a lecture on *the simple solitary bladder ulcer,* and this was subsequently published. He described solitary painful trigonal ulcers presenting with hemorrhage in two young men and one young woman without a history of tuberculosis or venereal infection. He advocated scraping the ulcer slough at the time of cystoscopy (5).

Nitze later described a condition of the bladder in which frequency of micturition, pain, and mucosal ulceration were features and referred to this as *cystitis parenchymatosa* (6). In most of the early reports, no clear distinction was drawn between chronic infective cystitis and chronic idiopathic cystitis.

The ulcer that still bears his name was first described by Guy Hunner (Fig. 3) in 1914, although he acknowledged the previous descriptions by Tait and Fenwick, which he felt were separate pathologic conditions. Hunner's ulcer differed from Fenwick's in its predominant incidence in women, its location within the dome or lateral walls of the bladder (rather than the trigone), and its presentation with pain rather than hematuria. Hunner also described associated areas of mucosal congestion adjacent to the ulcers, hemorrhage following cystodistension, and resistance to established treatment regimens. Hunner advocated surgical excision of the ulcer as the best treatment and described a satisfactory outcome in four of five cases. The bladder was irrigated daily with silver nitrate for 10 to 14 days postoperatively. Histologic examination of the excised ulcers showed absence of surface epithe-

T.J. Christmas: Department of Urological Surgery, Charing Cross Hospital, London W6 8RF, United Kingdom.

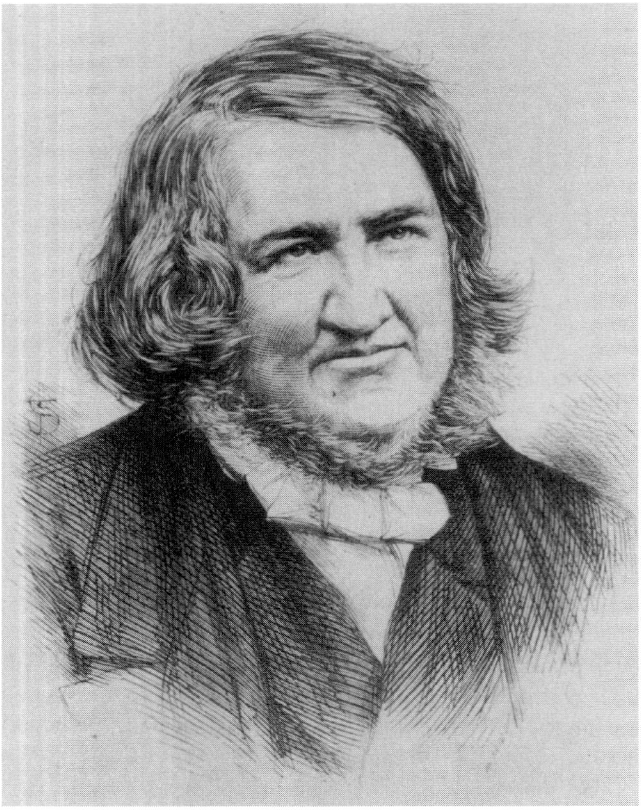

FIG. 1. Sir James Simpson, Surgeon to the London Hospital.

lium, an increase in the size and number of capillaries, and infiltration of the submucosa and muscle layers by leukocytes and lymphoid cells (7). A subsequent review of 25 cases treated by surgical ulcer excision revealed symptom recurrence in six (8).

It later became apparent that Hunner's ulcer was not the only feature of the condition with which it was usually associated, and new descriptive terms appeared. Keene referred to the condition as *panmural ulcerative cystitis* (9).

THEORIES OF CAUSATION

In the 1920s, most inflammatory disorders were thought to arise from bacterial infection, and it was therefore not surprising that bacteria should be implicated as the cause of IC. A series of 15 cases of *submucous ulcer* were reported from the Mayo Clinic, and two of these were the first men to be described with classical Hunner's ulcer. It was also postulated that ulceration resulted from spread of bacteria from dental abscesses, and this theory was reinforced by the finding that injection of bacteria from patients' dental abscesses into experimental animals led to bladder ulceration (10).

In two papers on Hunner's or elusive ulcer, Kretschmer agreed with the suggested etiology of septic foci, particularly those harboring streptococci, and, with Kreutzmann, was the first to report symptomatic relief after fulguration of ulcerated areas under general anesthetic (11,12). Bladder biopsies from two cases of IC grew "fine *Streptococcus*" on banana medium, and it was therefore suggested that this was the causative organism of the condition (13). It was later proposed that distant foci of sepsis should be eradicated before localized cystitis with submucous fibrosis or Hunner's ulceration is treated (14).

Hunner did not propose an etiology for the *elusive ulcer* in his earlier papers but later suggested that blood-borne spread of infection from tonsillitis led to the condition. He also reported the results of 48 ulcer excision operations: one death and 26 (42%) recurrences. As a result of these disappointing results, he no longer recommended this procedure (15). Bumpus suggested that the condition was more common in women because of spread of infection from the closely situated cervix and reported that animals developed a similar bladder condition after inoculation with bacteria from cervical swabs (16). The

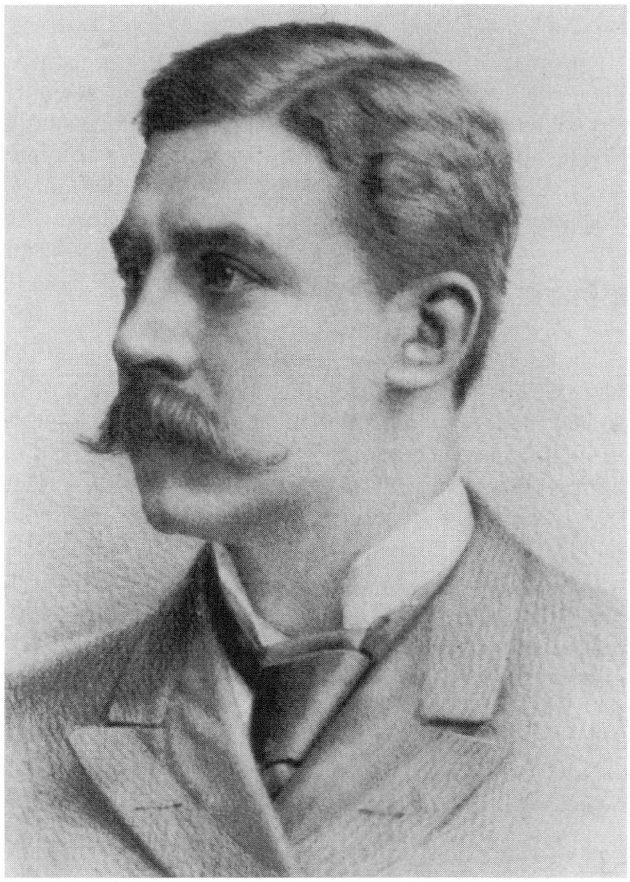

FIG. 2. Hurry Fenwick, Surgeon to the London Hospital.

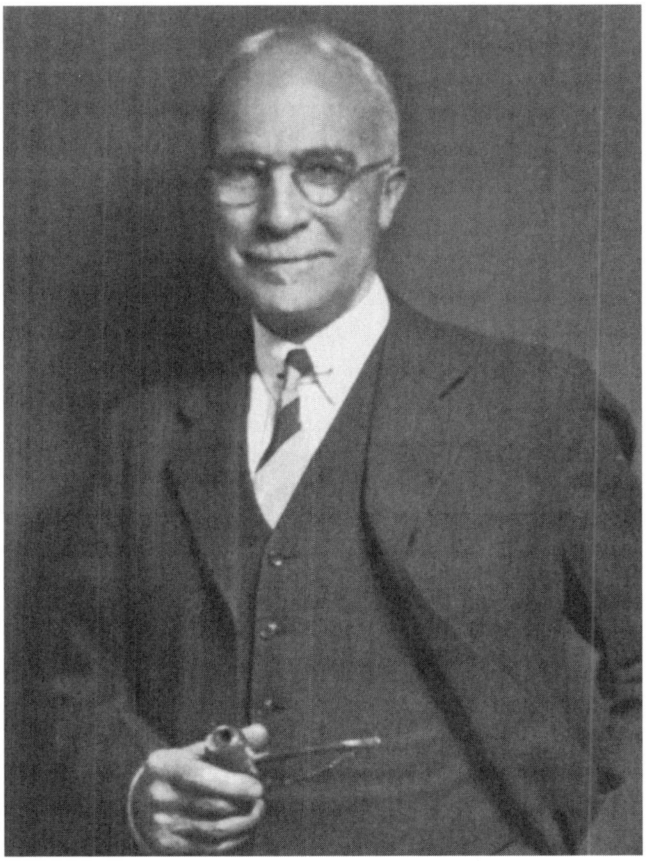

FIG. 3. Guy Hunner, who described Hunner's ulcer.

belief that IC and Hunner's ulceration resulted from bacterial infection persisted throughout the 1930s, and it was suggested that infection reached the bladder via the bloodstream or by local spread. Winsbury-White described lymphatic connections between the cervix uteri and the bladder, and his work was cited to support the theory that bacteria from the cervix spread locally to induce IC (17). A further theory for the etiology of IC was presented when two women with Hunner's ulcer were found to have associated idiopathic hypochromic anemia, and an analogy was drawn between IC and buccopharyngeal changes in anemia. A hypothesis that IC results from some form of nutritional deficiency was also expounded (18).

A study of the lymphatic supply of the bladder in female cadavers and the finding that obstruction of pelvic lymphatics in dogs caused bladder ulceration led to the theory that Hunner's ulcer was secondary to lymphatic occlusion, but no other studies have been able to substantiate these findings (19).

In an experimental study in dogs, bone spicules contaminated with *Streptococcus viridans* were surgically placed behind the bladder to induce *paracystitis*, which had cystoscopic and histologic features in common with IC. The findings of bladder wall thickening and chronic inflammatory cell infiltrate were even more pronounced when blood vessels of the vertex and posterior wall of the bladder were ligated. The conclusion was that IC resulted from extrinsic pelvic infection exacerbated by local ischemia (20).

Emotional and psychiatric disturbances had previously been reported in women with severe IC, but in most cases this was thought to be a phenomenon secondary to the distressing symptoms. However, a paper from Newark, New Jersey describes a long psychiatric and medical case history from childhood to 29 years of age of a woman with severe IC. A psychosomatic etiology was suggested, in particular "repressed hostility towards parental figures handled masochistically via bladder symptoms since infancy" and "polysurgery leading to worsening of the bladder pathology" (21). No prior reports upheld this etiologic hypothesis, although Gil-Vernet and colleagues later agreed with this psychosomatic theory but proposed that the treatment of choice was extensive partial cystectomy and colocystoplasty rather than psychotherapy (22).

THERAPEUTIC APPROACHES TO IC

It has been said that the number of suggested treatments for a condition is inversely related to the amount known about its etiology. This concept seems to apply to IC, and from the 1930s onward a large number of treatment modalities were described. These are described below along with the underlying rationales for their modes of action.

In an important paper, Bumpus reported the finding that the disease not only involved submucosal tissues below the ulcer but was more extensive than had previously been appreciated and, in fact, involved most of the bladder. He therefore suggested that the descriptive term *submucous ulcer* was no longer appropriate and should be replaced by *interstitial cystitis*. Bumpus upheld the view that because of extensive bladder involvement, local ulcer excision was inappropriate, and he reported successful relief of symptoms in more than 100 cases by cystodistention at a pressure of 120 mm Hg under general anesthesia (16).

Pain is a chronic and distressing feature of IC, and hence, attention has been paid to the treatment of this symptom. In 1926, Pieri, an Italian, was the first surgeon to perform presacral neurectomy as a treatment for pain in IC and also treated tuberculous cystitis in the same way (23). Later, Foulds showed that presacral neurectomy alone would not completely ablate painful sensations from the bladder and suggested that this procedure should be performed only as a last resort (24).

The first reference to augmentation enterocystoplasty in the treatment of IC came from the Mayo Clinic. Initial experimentation with dogs showed that bladder capacity could be increased by anastomosis of an isolated segment of small intestine to the dome of the bladder. The same operation was shown to successfully relieve symptoms of bladder contracture secondary to chronic infection and IC in humans (25).

Local bacterial infection, rather than hematogenous spread of bacteria, was suggested as an etiologic factor in IC, and just as untreated urethritis may lead to stricture formation, neglected bacterial cystitis was proposed as the cause of IC. Attention to foci of infection such as dental abscesses and tonsillitis failed to improve 12 cases of IC. Histologic examination of bladder biopsies showed thickening of vascular walls in two of the 12 cases. A single severe case had bilateral vesicoureteric reflux. Local resection and ureteral transplantation were recommended as treatment for severe cases (26).

A further neurosurgical treatment approach was advocated by Douglass, who felt that many patients with IC suffer from overactivity of the sympathetic system, leading to internal sphincter spasticity and on occasion urinary retention. He therefore recommended surgical excision of the superior hypogastric plexus and reported six cases in whom a satisfactory result was achieved (27). In a later study, this concept was extended so that the superior hypogastric plexus, fibers accompanying the distal inferior mesenteric and superior hemorrhoidal arteries, and sympathetic branches coming directly from the sacral chain were divided, leading to relief of bladder pain (28).

In 1935, Young reviewed the Cleveland Clinic experience with 45 cases of IC, 90% of whom were female, with a peak incidence in the fifth decade (29). He agreed with earlier suggestions that the condition was secondary to focal infection outside the urinary tract and recommended treatment of such foci before other therapy. The mean bladder capacity in his series was only 135 ml, and all had frank ulceration. Young recommended conservative treatment and surgical ulcer excision only as a last resort. Cystoscopic treatment by local ulcer resection, fulguration, or concentrated phenol application was recommended, and good results were reported in 11 of the 12 patients treated by the latter technique (30).

Chronic inflammation is known to predispose to malignant transformation, and it is not surprising, therefore, that Hunner's ulcer may rarely develop into carcinoma. The first report of carcinoma developing in IC was in an elderly patient with a 4-year history of Hunner's ulcer (31).

In a lecture at the American Urological Association, Fister compared IC and cutaneous lupus erythematosus (LE) and noted similarities such as the age of onset, female predominance, chronicity, and histologic appearance (32). This was the first publication to suggest a similarity between IC and connective tissue disorders, although at that time LE and IC were both thought to result from dissemination of bacteria and their toxins. Fister did not describe any cases with both IC and LE but did report symptomatic relief after intramuscular injection of sodium gold thiosulfate therapy and bismuth ethylcamphorate in IC.

Transvesical alcohol injection was shown to relieve symptoms in seven cases without side effects (33). Tait was the first surgeon to realize the benefit of urinary diversion as a treatment for IC, and Counsellor used this concept when he introduced bilateral ureterosigmoidostomy as a treatment for severe IC; however, his success at relieving bladder symptoms was overshadowed by a 23% operative mortality rate (34).

A single case of severe intractable IC was treated by simultaneous bilateral ureterosigmoidostomy with satisfactory outcome and complete relief of bladder pain. This operation was recommended as appropriate treatment for IC that had failed to respond to other treatments in spite of earlier reports of a high postoperative mortality rate (35).

A more radical surgical approach to severe cases of IC was recommended following experiments in dogs that had undergone subtotal cystectomy and subsequently regenerated their bladders. A series of eight women underwent similar subtotal cystectomy, leaving only the trigone of the bladder; the reported results were apparently good, with only one case requiring subsequent urinary diversion, and a good neobladder capacity was achieved in the others. Two cases developed bilateral vesicoureteric reflux after the procedure (36).

In the first half of this century, x-ray therapy was regarded as a panacea for conditions ranging from acne, scalp ringworm, and tonsillitis to benign and malignant tumors. Interstitial cystitis was not excluded from such blanket therapy; five women and one man treated with a dose of 1,200 to 4,200 Gray were reported to achieve temporary (7 to 12 months) symptomatic improvement in half, but in no case was there a permanent cure (37).

Cystodistention and fulguration of inflamed and ulcerated areas persisted as the most popular conservative treatment regimen in the 1940s. However, local application or intravesical instillation of caustic chemical agents began to gain popularity. Aniline dyes such as methyl violet, gentian violet, and crystal violet at dilutions of 1:10 to 1:20,000 were used in 16 cases in whom an initial reaction was followed by temporary relief (mean 5.5 months) and then relapse in at least nine (38). Instillation of 4% argyrol or 16% gomenol led to symptomatic relief in four patients, and local direct irradiation with ultraviolet light from a quartz tube conductor led to questionable improvement in two cases (39). Local silver nitrate therapy was also advocated, and in a series of 74 cases, 89% had a good immediate response, and 31% experienced no further symptoms after a single treatment (40).

Interstitial cystitis and Hunner's ulceration are both predominantly diseases of women, and it was not until 1944 that attention was drawn to its presence in men. A review of 78 cases of IC in men concluded that the incidence was low but significant and that IC was often inappropriately confused with symptoms of outflow obstruction (41).

A series of 223 cases of IC from Portland, OR showed a female-to-male ratio of 11:1, and the disease was graded from 1 to 3 according to cystoscopic findings (42). An association with allergic reactions, previous pelvic surgery, *nonsurgical thyroid disease*, and *nonsurgical gallbladder disease* was reported, and a single case developed carcinoma of the bladder in an area of ulceration. Histologic examination of a cystectomy case showed transmural fibrosis; submucosal accumulations of monocytes, young fibroblasts, and lymphocytes; and thickening of arteriolar walls suggesting vasculitis. A striking abundance of unmyelinated nervous tissue in the subepithelial layer and infiltration of nerve sheaths by leukocytes were also described. It was concluded that IC might result from neurogenic influences (42).

In 1951, Bourque reported the results of selective neurectomy procedures designed to relieve bladder pain in six cases of chronic IC. Selective presacral, hypogastric, and erector neurectomy was performed with complete relief of pain in three, partial relief in two, and no relief in one (43).

Smith reviewed the potential treatments for IC and Hunner's ulceration in 1952 and concluded from his experience of 64 cases that fulguration of affected areas and bladder dilation at least once a month was the best form of management. He also reported complete cure in 13 women (44).

Interstitial cystitis was first described in children in 1953, when a series of six children (all girls) aged 3 to 10 years were reported with the condition. They presented with nocturnal and diurnal incontinence and urgency. They were treated by fulguration and cystodistension (45).

Just as radiotherapy was used to treat many conditions earlier in the century, corticosteroids and adrenocorticotropic hormone (ACTH) became the vogue later, and IC, as an inflammatory condition, was thought to be suitable for such treatment. Hoyt treated four cases of IC (although one was subsequently found to have bladder carcinoma) with oral cortisone at a dose of 300 mg on the first day, 200 mg on the second day, and 100 mg per day thereafter. Three of the four (the fourth having bladder carcinoma) had partial symptomatic relief (46). The same therapeutic principle was applied when five cases of Hunner's ulcer were treated with ACTH over 3 weeks and the therapeutic response was monitored. Three of the five were partially relieved of pain, although the results were generally disappointing (47). Soon after, a report from Liverpool of the injection of Hunner's ulcers with hydrocortisone at cystoscopy described a symptomatic improvement in all three cases (48).

A study of 59 cases of IC from the Karolinska Institute, Sweden, collected over the period 1940 to 1956 was reported in 1957 (49). Associated colitis was present in 11, gastritis in seven, arthralgia in 12, allergic skin diseases in five, a history of rheumatic fever in two, asthma in one, and lupus erythematosus in one. Histologic studies of 21 of the cases revealed evidence of eosinophilia within the bladder wall in nine and periarteritis in seven. The distal ureters and proximal urethras were also shown to be involved in the disease process, with chronic inflammatory cell infiltrate, mucosal ulceration, and fibrinoid degeneration all present. Sacral root (S_{1-3}) posterior rhizotomy was performed in eight cases, and histologic examination of the nerve roots revealed round-cell infiltration and myelin sheath degeneration. Hematologic examination demonstrated elevation of the γ-globulin level in ten of 17 cases and LE cells in one of 12 tested (not the case with LE). It was suggested that IC might result from infectious or allergic factors. Good results were achieved by cystodistention, local resection, ileocystoplasty, antibiotics, cortisone, ACTH, or sacral rhizotomy (49). A separate review of the eight cases from this series who underwent sacral posterior rhizotomy (S_{2-3}) reported a reduction in the frequency of micturition and bladder pain but no change in the bladder volume or mucosal lesions (50).

Sacral root neurectomy (excision of a root segment to prevent regeneration) at the S_3 level was reported to bring about relief of symptoms and mucosal healing in four cases of severe IC and symptomatic improvement but incomplete mucosal resolution in a single case of severe IC that had previously undergone partial cystectomy (51).

Following the discovery of an increase in the numbers of mast cells within the bladder wall in IC, antihistamine agents such as pyribenzamine were used and shown to improve symptoms (52) (see Chapter 12).

In 1958, a series of 187 cases of IC from St. Louis, MO was reported; two cases died of bowel carcinoma, and one from bladder carcinoma (53). The first British review of a series of IC series did not appear until 1958, when the experiences of St. Peter's and St. Paul's Hospitals was published (54). Hunner's ulcer was found to be a rare condition, constituting only 0.23% of the cases treated at the above institutions between 1947 and 1956. Hunner's ulcer was initially misdiagnosed in five cases: the true diagnosis was bladder carcinoma in one, simple infective ulcer in three, and healed tuberculous bladder in one. Ureterosigmoidostomy was performed in ten, with two resultant deaths; ileocystoplasty helped three, and the results of this procedure were better when it was performed with extensive partial cystectomy. The etiology was thought to be unrelated to infection, but hormonal influences were postulated, as were psychosomatic influences (54).

Two reports of IC in a total of 52 children again showed a female predominance (46 women, one man), and most presented with diurnal enuresis. A therapeutic response to cystodistension was described, but caution

TABLE 1. *Historical review of etiologic hypotheses for IC*

Etiological theory	Reference
Ectopic bacterial spread from dental abscesses	Bumpus, 1920 (16)
Streptococcal infection	Bidgood, 1928 (13)
Ectopic spread of bacteria from tonsillitis	Hunner, 1930 (15)
Local spread of bacteria from the cervix	Bumpus, 1930 (16)
Chronic bacterial cystitis	Meads, 1934 (26)
Nutritional deficiency	Robb, 1941 (18)
Perivesical lymphatic occlusion	Powell, 1945 (19)
Neurogenic influences	Hand, 1949 (42)
Extrinsic pelvic infection and local ischaemia	Baumrucker, 1955 (20)
Allergy and infection	Franksson, 1957 (49)
Psychosomatic masochism	Bowers et al., 1958 (21)
Hormonal influences	Smith, 1958 (44)
Mast cells	Simmons and Bunce, 1958 (52)
Collagen disease	Shipton, 1965 (57)
Organ-specific anti-bladder antibodies	Silk, 1970 (58)
Neuro-vegetative-vascular disturbance	Skoluda et al., 1974 (59)
Antibodies to microfibrils in vascular wall	Mattila et al., 1983 (60)
Leaking urothelium, defective tight junctions	Eldrup et al., 1983 (61)
Defective surface glycosaminoglycans layer	Parsons et al., 1983 (62)
Antibiotics—Nitrofuantoin or Tetracyclines	Gillespie et al., 1985 (63)
Epstein–Barr virus infection	Gillespie and Jones, 1986 (64)
Angioneogenesis and related factors	Witherow et al., 1989 (65)
Fastidious bacteria—Gardnerella sp., Lactobacillus sp.	Wilkins et al., (66)
Aberrant urothelial HLA-DR expression	Christmas et al., 1992 (67)

was recommended because bladder rupture occurred in three and marked hemorrhage in four cases following this procedure (55,56).

SUMMARY

During the 125 years following the first description of IC, few major advances took place. Skene was the first to name the condition interstitial cystitis in 1887, and Hunner described the ulcer that is sometimes a feature of the disease in 1914. These were perhaps the most significant milestones. Over 15 different names for IC or associated Hunner's ulcer were suggested, including, perhaps most appropriately, submucous ulcer and panmural cystitis. Such variety is nothing compared to the multitude of proposed etiologies, which range from the bizarre and obscure to the positively ridiculous. The most unlikely etiologies include ectopic spread of infection from dental abscesses (16), pelvic lymphatic occlusion (19), and masochistic psychosomatic disease (21).

Much of the early experimental studies of the etiology of IC added little to our knowledge of the disease. A review of etiologic theories is shown in Table 1, and further details appear in later chapters (57–67). The poten-

TABLE 2. *Overview of intravesical pharmacotherapy*

Silver nitrate	Tait, 1980 (3)
Phenol	Sears, 1936 (30)
Aniline dyes	Davis, 1941 (38)
4% Argyrol	Davis, 1941 (38)
16% Gomenol	Davis, 1941 (38)
Dimethyl sulphoxide (DMSO)	Stewart et al., 1972 (68)
Sodium oxychlorosene	Messing and Stamey, 1978 (69)
Orgotein	Mayer and Schilling, 1983 (70)
Sodium cromoglycate	Edwards et al., 1986 (71)
DMSO and steroids	Witherow et al., 1989 (65)
Doxorubicin	Khanna and Loose, 1990 (72)
Heparin	Perez-Marrero et al., 1993 (73)
Hyaluronic acid	Morales and Emerson, 1995 (74)
Interferon	Benson et al., 1995 (75)

TABLE 3. *Overview of systemic pharmacotherapy*

Sodium gold thiosulphate	Fister, 1938 (32)
Bismuth ethyl camphorate	Fister, 1938 (32)
α-Tocopherol	van Duzen et al., 1951 (76)
Corticosteroids	Hoyt, 1952 (46)
ACTH	Burke and Vernon, 1952 (47)
Pyribenzamine	Simmons and Bunce, 1958 (52)
Heparin	Weaver et al., 1963 (77)
Oxyphenbutazone	Guerrier et al., (78)
Chloroquine	Oravisto and Alfthan, 1976 (79)
Azathioprine	Oravisto and Alfthan, 1976 (79)
Carbenoxolone	Mooreville et al., 1983 (80)
Angiosone	Gillespie, 1988 (81)
Sodium pentosanpolysulfate	Parsons et al., 1983 (62)
Amitriptyline	Hanno et al., 1989 (82)
Nalmefene	Stone, 1994 (83)
Nifedipine	Fleischmann, 1994 (84)

TABLE 4. *Review of surgical treatments for IC*

Surgical treatment	Reference
Formation of vesico-vaginal fistula	Tait, 1870 (3)
Local debridement	Fenwick, 1896 (5)
Local excision of ulcers	Hunner, 1915 (7)
Fulguration of ulcers	Kreutzmann, 1922 (12)
Dental extraction	Frontz, 1928 (14)
Cystodistension under general anaesthesia	Bumpus, 1930 (16)
Presacral neurectomy	Pieri, 1930 (23)
Cordotomy	Grant, 1931 (85)
Augmentation enterocystoplasty	Sebening, 1932 (25)
Excision of superior hypogastric plexus	Douglass, 1934 (27)
Cystoscopic ulcer resection	Sears, 1936 (30)
Transvesical alcohol injection	Folsom and O'Brien, 1937 (22)
Bilateral ureterosigmoidostomy	Counsellor, 1937 (34)
Sensory denervation by local sympathectomy	Scott and Schroeder, 1938 (28)
Subtotal cystectomy and substitution enterocystoplasty	Folsom et al., 1940 (36)
Cystoscopic hydrocortisone infiltration	Johnston, 1956 (48)
Sacral (S_{1-3}) root rhizotomy	Franksson, 1957 (50)
Sacral (S_{2-3}) root rhizotomy	Bohn and Franksson, 1957 (50)
Sacral (S_3) root neurectomy	Milner and Garlick, 1957 (51)
Subtotal cystectomy and colocystoplasty	Gil-Vernet et al., 1960 (22)
Cystocystoplasty	Warwick and Ashken, 1967 (86)
Cystolysis	Worth and Warwick, 1973 (87)
Total cystectomy and ileal conduit diversion	Jacobo et al., 1974 (88)
Neodymium YAG-laser therapy	Shanberg et al., 1985 (89)
Laparoscopic laser destruction of nerve plexus	Gillespie, 1994 (90)
Total bladder replacement by ileocolic segment	Bejany and Politano, 1995 (91)
Total bladder replacement by Kock pouch	Christmas et al., 1995 (92)

tial treatments can be classified as local medical, systemic medical (68–84), or surgical (85–92), and they are summarized in Tables 2, 3, and 4. Reviews of the literature pertinent to aspects of IC from 1961 onward are described in detail elsewhere in this book.

REFERENCES

1. Gillenwater JY, Wein AJ. Summary of the National Institute of Arthritis, Diabetes and Kidney Diseases workshop on interstitial cystitis, National Institutes of Health, Bethesda, MD. *J Urol* 1988;140:203–205.
2. Mercier LA. Mémoire sur certaines perforations spontanées de la vessie non décrites jusqu'a ce jour. *Gaz Méd Paris* 1836;4:257–263.
3. Tait L. Cure of the chronic perforating ulcer of the bladder by the formation of an artificial vesico-vaginal fistula. *Lancet* 1870;2:738.
4. Skene AJC. *Diseases of Bladder and Urethra in Women.* New York: Wm Wood, 1887;167.
5. Fenwick EH. The clinical significance of the simple solitary ulcer of the urinary bladder. *Br Med J* 1896;1:1133–1135.
6. Nitze M. *Lehrbuch de Kystoskopie: Ihre Technik und Klinische Bedeutung.* Berlin: JE Bergman, 1907;410.
7. Hunner GL. A rare type of bladder ulcer in women: report of cases. *Trans South Surg Gynecol Assoc* 1915;27:247–292.
8. Hunner GL. Elusive ulcer of the bladder: further notes on a rare type of bladder ulcer with a report of twenty-five cases. *Am J Obstet Dis Child* 1918;78:3–8.
9. Keene FE. Circumscribed pan-mural ulcerative cystitis. *Ann Surg* 1920; 71:479–485.
10. Meisser JG, Bumpus HC. Focal infections in relation to submucous ulcer of the bladder and to cystitis. *J Urol* 1921;6:285–298.
11. Kretschmer HL. Elusive ulcer of the bladder, a further report. *Surg Gynecol Obstet* 1922;35:759–765.
12. Kreutzmann HAR. The treatment of Hunner's ulcer of the bladder by fulguration. *Cal State Med J* 1922;20:128–130.
13. Bidgood CY. Tissue cultures in two cases of interstitial cystitis. *Am J Surg* 1928;4:140–142.
14. Frontz WA. Observations on the pathology, clinical diagnosis and treatment of submucous fibrosis (localised cystitis). *South Med J* 1928; 21:899–903.
15. Hunner GL. Neurosis of the bladder. *J Urol* 1930;24:567–585.
16. Bumpus HC. Interstitial cystitis: its treatment by over-distension of the bladder. *Med Clin North Am* 1930;13:1495–1498.
17. Winsbury-White H. Spread of infection from cervix to urinary tract. *Br J Urol* 1933;5:248–252.
18. Robb D. Two cases of Hunner's ulcer of the bladder or interstitial cystitis in the presence of idiopathic hypochromic anaemia. *Aust NZ J Surg* 1941;10:393–397.
19. Powell TO. Studies on the aetiology of Hunner ulcer. *J Urol* 1945; 53:823–835.
20. Baumrucker GO. An experimental study of the elusive bladder ulcer of Hunner. *J Int Coll Surg* 1955;23:221–225.
21. Bowers JE, Schwarz BE, Leon MJ. Masochism and interstitial cystitis. *Psychosom Med* 1958;20:296–302.
22. Gil-Vernet JM, González V, Fernández E. Etiopathogénie y traitement de la cystite interstitielle. *Acta Urol Belg* 1960;28:425–440.
23. Pieri G. Clinical contributions on the surgery of the sympathetic nervous system. The treatment of tuberculous cystitis. *Arch Ital Chir* 1930;27:454–482.
24. Foulds GS. Resection of presacral nerve in genitourinary cases. *Br J Surg* 1932;143:143–146.
25. Sebening W. The use of an isolated intestinal loop to enlarge the capacity of the bladder. Clinical and experimental study. *Proc Staff Meet Mayo Clin* 1932;7:123–124.
26. Meads AM. "Hunner's ulcer." *Urol Cutan Rev* 1934;38:631–634.
27. Douglass HL. Excision of the superior hypogastric plexus in the treatment of intractable interstitial cystitis, report of five cases. *Am J Surg* 1934;25:249–257.
28. Scott WJM, Schroeder CF. Denervation of the bladder for relief of intractable pain. *Ann Surg* 1938;108:730–740.
29. Young JE. Hunner ulcer of the bladder; a report of 45 cases. *Cleve Clin Q* 1935;2:51–54.

30. Sears NP. Elusive ulcer of the bladder with special reference to its treatment with phenol. *NY State J Med* 1936;36:724–728.
31. Hagner FR. Malignancy of bladder occurring in a Hunner ulcer. *Trans Am Assoc Genito-Urinary Surg* 1937;30:197–199.
32. Fister GM. Similarity of interstitial cystitis (Hunner ulcer) to lupus erythematosus. *J Urol* 1938;40:37–51.
33. Folsom AI, O'Brien HA. Transvesical alcoholic injection for elusive ulcer of the bladder—preliminary report. *J Urol* 1937;37:808–815.
34. Counsellor VS. Bilateral transplantation of the ureters in the female. *Am J Obstet Gynecol* 1937;33:234–249.
35. Lower WE, Schlumberger FC. Bilateral simultaneous uretero-sigmoidostomy for chronic interstitial cystitis. *Cleve Clin Q* 1939;6:181–184.
36. Folsom AI, O'Brien HA, Caldwell GT. Subtotal cystectomy in the treatment of Hunner ulcer. *J Urol* 1940;44:650–666.
37. Kreutzmann HAR. The treatment of Hunner's ulcer with deep x-ray therapy. *J Urol* 1941;46:907–912.
38. Davis E. Aniline (triphenylmethane) dyes in the treatment of Hunner ulcer. *J Urol* 1941;46:899–906.
39. Higgins CC. Hunner ulcer of the bladder (review of 100 cases). *Ann Intern Med* 1941;15:708–715.
40. Pool TL, Rives HF. Interstitial cystitis: treatment with silver nitrate. *J Urol* 1944;51:520–525.
41. Cristol DS, Greene LF, Thompson GJ. Interstitial cystitis of men, a review of seventy-eight cases. *JAMA* 1944;126:825–828.
42. Hand JR. Interstitial cystitis: report of 223 cases (204 women and 19 men). *J Urol* 1949;61:291–310.
43. Bourque JP. Surgical management of the painful bladder. *J Urol* 1951; 65:25–35.
44. Smith GG. Interstitial cystitis. *J Urol* 1952;67:903–915.
45. McDonald HP, Upchurch WE, Sturdevant CE. Interstitial cystitis in children. *J Urol* 1953;70:890–893.
46. Hoyt HS. Cortisone in urological conditions with a report of a trial in interstitial cystitis. *J Urol* 1952;67:899–902.
47. Burke J, Vernon HK. Effects of ACTH on Hunner's ulcer of the urinary bladder. *Br Med J* 1952;2:477.
48. Johnston JH. Local hydrocortisone for Hunner's ulcer of the bladder. *Br Med J* 1956;35:698–699.
49. Franksson C. Interstitial cystitis: a clinical study of fifty-nine cases. *Acta Chir Scand* 1957;113:51–62.
50. Bohm E, Franksson C. Interstitial cystitis and sacral rhizotomy. *Acta Chir Scand* 1957;113:63–67.
51. Milner WA, Garlick WB. Selective sacral neurectomy in interstitial cystitis. *J Urol* 1957;78:600–604.
52. Simmons JL, Bunce PL. On the use of an anti-histamine in the treatment of interstitial cystitis. *Am Surg* 1958;24:664–667.
53. Burford EH, Burford CE. Hunner ulcer of the bladder: a report of 187 cases. *J Urol* 1958;79:952–955.
54. Kinder CH, Smith RD. Hunner's ulcer. *Br J Urol* 1958;30:338–343.
55. McDonald HP, Upchurch WE, Artime M. Bladder dysfunction in children caused by interstitial cystitis. *J Urol* 1958;80:354–356.
56. Chenoweth CV, Clawater EW. Interstitial cystitis in children. *J Urol* 1960;83:150–152.
57. Shipton EA. Hunner's ulcer (chronic interstitial cystitis), a manifestation of collagen disease. *Br J Urol* 1965;37:443–449.
58. Silk MR. Bladder antibodies in interstitial cystitis. *J Urol* 1970;103: 307–309.
59. Skoluda D, Wegner K, Lemmel EM. Kritische Benerkungen zur Immunopathogenese der interstitiellen cystitis. *Urologe A* 1974;13: 15–23.
60. Mattila J, Pitkänen R, Vaalasti T, Seppänen J. Fine structural evidence for vascular injury in patients with interstitial cystitis. *Virchows Arch [A]* 1983;398:347–355.
61. Eldrup J, Thorup J, Nielsen SL, Hald T, Hainau B. Permeability and ultrastructure of human bladder epithelium. *Br J Urol* 1983;55:488–492.
62. Parsons CL, Schmidt JD, Pollen JJ. Successful treatment of interstitial cystitis with sodium pentosanpolysulfate. *J Urol* 1983;130:51–53.
63. Gillespie LM, Said J, Cain D, van der Veld R. Antibiotic-induced interstitial cystitis: a model for cell membrane instability. In: *Proceedings of the International Continence Society Annual Meeting.* London: ICS, 1985;254.
64. Gillespie LM, Jones JF. Epstein–Barr virus infection and interstitial cystitis: the rosetta stone of inflammatory disease? *J Urol* 1986;135: 271A.
65. Witherow RO'N, Gillespie L, McMullen L, Goldin RD, Walker MM. Painful bladder syndrome—a clinical and immunopathological study. *Br J Urol* 1989;64:158–161.
66. Wilkins EGL, Payne SR, Pead PJ, Moss ST, Maskell RM. Interstitial cystitis and the urethral syndrome: a possible answer. *Br J Urol* 1989;64:39–44.
67. Christmas TJ, Bottazzo GF. Abnormal urothelial HLA-DR expression in interstitial cystitis. *Clin Exp Immunol* 1992;87:450–454.
68. Stewart BH, Shirley SW. Further experience with intravesical dimethyl sulfoxide in the treatment of interstitial cystitis. *J Urol* 1976;116: 36–38.
69. Messing EM, Stamey TA. Interstitial cystitis early diagnosis, pathology and treatment. *Urology* 1978;12:381–392.
70. Mayer P, Schilling A. *Medikamentöse rehabilitation der interstitiellen cystitis mit orgotein.* Paper presented at proceedings of 25th congress of the North German Urological Association, 1983.
71. Edwards L, Bucknall TE, Makin C. Interstitial cystitis: possible cause and clinical study of sodium cromoglycate. *Br J Urol* 1986;58:95–96.
72. Khanna OM, Loose JH. Interstitial cystitis treated with intravesical doxorubicin. *Urology* 1990;36:139–142.
73. Perez-Marrero R, Emerson L, Maharajah DO, et al. Prolongation of response to DMSO by heparin maintenance. *Urology* 1993;41(Suppl): 64.
74. Morales A, Emerson L. Treatment of refractory interstitial cystitis with intra-vesical hyaluronic acid. *J Urol* 1995;153:288A.
75. Benson RC, Knoll LD, Furlow WL, Bilhartz DL, McLaren RH. Intravesical interferon for the treatment of interstitial cystitis. *J Urol* 1995; 153:288A.
76. van Duzen RE, Mustain R. Alpha-tocopherol in treatment of interstitial cystitis: preliminary report. *J Urol* 1951;65:1033–1040.
77. Weaver RG, Dougherty TF, Natoli CA. Recent concepts of interstitial cystitis. *J Urol* 1963;89:377–383.
78. Guerrier HP, Roberts JBM, Slade N. Anti-inflammatory agents in the management of interstitial cystitis. *Br J Urol* 1965;137:88–92.
79. Oravisto KJ, Alfthan OS. Treatment of interstitial cystitis with immunosuppression and chloroquine derivatives. *Eur Urol* 1976;2:82–84.
80. Mooreville M, Fritz RW, Mulholland SG. Enhancement of the bladder defense mechanism by an exogenous agent. *J Urol* 1983;130:607–609.
81. Gillespie L. Angiosone inhibits angioneogenesis in interstitial cystitis. *Br J Urol* 1988;62:481–482.
82. Hanno PM, Buehler J, Wein AJ. Use of amitriptyline in the treatment of interstitial cystitis. *J Urol* 1989;141:846–848.
83. Stone NN. Nalmefene in the treatment of interstitial cystitis. *Urol Clin North Am* 1994;21:101–111.
84. Fleischmann JD, Huntley HN, Shingleton WB. Clinical and immunological response to nifedipine for the treatment of interstitial cystitis. *J Urol* 1991;146:1235–1239.
85. Grant FC. Cordotomy for relief of pain in the genito-urinary tract. *J Urol* 1931;25:551–558.
86. Turner-Warwick RT, Handley Ashken M. The functional results of partial, subtotal and total cystoplasty with special reference to ureterocaecocystoplasty, selective sphincterotomy and cystocystoplasty. *Br J Urol* 1967;39:3–12.
87. Worth PHL, Turner-Warwick RT. The treatment of interstitial cystitis by cystolysis with observations on cystoplasty. *Br J Urol* 1973;45:65–71.
88. Jacobo E, Stamler FW, Culp DA. Interstitial cystitis followed by total cystectomy. *Urology* 1974;3:481–485.
89. Shanberg AM, Baghdassarian R, Tansey LA. Treatment of interstitial cystitis with the neodymium-YAG laser. *J Urol* 1985;134:885–888.
90. Gillespie L. Destruction of the vesicoureteric plexus for the treatment of hypersensitive bladder disorders. *Br J Urol* 1994;74:40–43.
91. Bejany DE, Politano VA. Ileocolic neobladder in the woman with interstitial cystitis and a small contracted bladder. *J Urol* 1995;153: 42–43.
92. Christmas TJ, Holmes SAV, Hendry WF. Bladder replacement by rescystoplasty: the final treatment for interstitial cystitis. *Br J Urol* 1996;78:69–73.

Interstitial Cystitis, edited by Grannum R. Sant.
Lippincott–Raven Publishers, Philadelphia ©1997.

CHAPTER 2

Epidemiology of Interstitial Cystitis

Ngoc Ho, James A. Koziol, and C. Lowell Parsons

Interstitial cystitis (IC) is a syndrome characterized by variable motor and sensory dysfunctions of the bladder. Diagnosis is usually based on patient's symptomatology, urologic evaluation including cystoscopy, and the exclusion of other recognizable bladder diseases. The most prevalent symptoms of IC are urinary frequency, urgency, and suprapubic, pelvic, or perineal pain.

Interstitial cystitis can be classified into the two categories of Hunner's ulcer (classic) and nonulcer (early), based on cystoscopic findings. The cystoscopic appearance of the ulcerative or "classic" type described by Johansson and Fall (1) is as follows:

> It displays single or multiple patches of reddened bladder mucosa. The redness, on careful examination, is shown to be caused by erythema of the mucosa with small vessels radiating to a central, pale scar, fibrin deposit or coagulum. Central rupture at this site occurs during bladder distension with the patient under general or spinal anesthesia, at a hydrostatic pressure of 70 to 80 cm water. After mucosal rupture, oozing of blood from the mucosal margins and the ulcer bottom occurs, and this is the so-called elusive ulcer of Hunner. After a second distension petechial hemorrhages frequently are seen in areas next to the ulcer but also frequently in areas distant from the ulcer. Another characteristic, postdistension finding is mild or occasionally marked bullous swelling.

Another distinction is that granulation tissue was present in 94% of the ulcerative cases. The remaining 6% had moderate symptoms, and only limited biopsy tissues were available for examination. In contrast, no granulation tissue was found in nonulcerative IC patients (1).

The nonulcerative or "early" type of IC does not display any circumscript lesions, only strawberry-like hemorrhages that are commonly referred to as glomerulations. This occasionally is seen during the first filling but usually appears throughout the vesical mucosa on redistention. Occasionally, stellate scars that crack and bleed, or mucosal fissures, may be seen (1–3).

Koziol et al. (4) investigated whether the classification of 565 IC cases into ulcer and nonulcer categories from cystoscopic findings could be correlated with epidemiologic data relating to demographics, risk factors, symptoms, pain, and psychosocial factors. From univariate analyses, ten nonivasive variables (hematuria, pain centered at right lower abdomen, standing relieves pain, sharp pain, weight change or eating disorder, irritable bowel syndrome, dull aching pain, dyspareunia, and efficacy of urination) were significantly associated with the presence of Hunner's ulcers. However, none of the variables could individually discriminate ulcer from nonulcer patients with a high degree of accuracy. On the other hand, reasonable accuracy in classifying ulcer and nonulcer patients was obtainable from linear discriminant analysis, logistic regression, and recursive partitioning, three statistical methodologies that combine the ten variables into multivariate classification rules. These findings suggest the two categories of IC might well represent different manifestations of underlying disease pathophysiology.

Koziol et al. (5–7) recently reported that 10% to 20% of IC patients suffer from the classic type. This is more than a previous estimate by Sant (8) of 5% to 10%. It should be noted, however, that the cohort of IC patients studied by Koziol et al. is likely more representative of moderate to severe IC, with very few early-onset patients.

The bladder capacity is found to be more reduced in the classic type of IC. Messing and Stamey (3) reported cystoscopy findings in 16 patients (nine early and seven classic) under anesthesia. They found all but one patient to have bladder capacity less than 450 ml in the classic IC type, and all of the early IC type to have capacity greater than 450 ml. Johansson and Fall (1) found the mean capacity to be 453 ml (range 75 to 1,100 ml) in patients with classical IC, compared to 816 ml (range 450 to 1,250 ml) in patients with early IC. Another revealing dis-

N. Ho and J. A. Koziol: Department of Molecular and Experimental Medicine, The Scripps Research Institute, La Jolla, California 92037.

C. L. Parsons: Division of Urology, Department of Surgery, University of California San Diego, La Jolla, California 92093.

tinction between the two types is the concentration of mononuclear cells present in the mucosa. Of the patients with classic IC, 91% had an extensive inflammatory response (++ or +++), which was in stark contrast to the early IC patients, of whom only 20% had + or ++ degree of mononuclear inflammatory infiltrate (1). Erickson et al. (9) found that patients with severe inflammation (100 or more mononuclear cells per high-power field or lymphoid aggregates) experienced better symptom relief after cystoscopy with bladder distention under anesthesia than patients with milder inflammation (<100 mononuclear cells per high-power field). A host of plausible hypotheses exist for the etiology of IC (10,11). Among these, autoimmunity, dysfunctional bladder epithelium, and mast cells are currently areas of extensive research activity relating to causative factors of IC.

ETIOLOGY

Autoimmunity

Autoimmune disorders caused by antibodies and immune cells reacting against components are either organ-specific or non-organ-specific. Various bladder injuries may cause cellular destruction and may release or alter antigens, which brings forth antibody production. This causes more damage within the bladder. Consequently, normal bladder antigens or some nonbladder antigen, through an inappropriate immune response, may begin antibody production; the antibody then causes symptoms of IC (12).

Silk (13) compared the sera of 20 patients with IC, ten normal volunteers, 15 patients with acute and chronic bacterial cystitis, and ten samples from a bank of sera from patients with known thyroid, adrenal, and gastric antibodies for the presence of bladder antibodies. He was unable to demonstrate bladder antibodies in controls, patients with acute and chronic cystitis, or patients with known gastric, thyroid, or adrenal antibodies. On the other hand, nine of the 20 patients with IC had bladder antibodies. This observation lent support to the conjecture that IC may in part be an autoimmune disease.

Jokinen et al. (14) investigated the sera from 33 female patients with IC for the presence of antitissue antibodies. They found elevated serum levels of antinuclear antibodies in 85% of IC patients. They also found that 21% of their IC patients had antinuclear antibodies of titer 1:160 to 1:1,280, with fine speckled nuclear staining the most common pattern. However, after nonspecific antibodies had been removed from sera positive with antinuclear antibodies by an absorption procedure, they were unable to show that the antibodies were bladder-specific and could not confirm the earlier finding of Silk (13) that such antibodies were present in 45% of IC patients. (Silk did not undertake a similar absorption method.) Jokinen et al. concluded that IC belongs to the group of autoimmune diseases that waivers between being organ-specific and non-organ-specific. The disease is confined to one organ, but the tissue antibodies are nonspecific.

Anderson et al. (12) studied 26 patients with interstitial cystitis with mean duration 5 years along with a control group of similar age and sex but with other urologic complaints. They performed a standard autoimmune profile and searched for specific antibodies to normal human bladder in the serum. Specific antibladder antibodies were found in the sera of patients with IC in up to 75% of cases and in 40% of controls. Statistically, there was no significant difference between the presence of these antibodies in patients and that in controls. The antibladder antibodies found in the control group reflected a lack of specificity for IC. Furthermore, they found fixed immunoglobulin in the bladder wall in only 29% of patients with IC, whereas up to 50% of patients with other urologic disorders had a similar immunoglobulin deposition. So, although IC patients demonstrated a nonspecific increase in antibody formation, this was not significantly different from a similar group of patients with other urologic syndromes. This lack of specificity makes this immunologic response more likely to be a secondary phenomenon associated with inflammatory damage to the bladder rather than the primary cause of the disease.

Ochs et al. (15) found antinuclear antibodies in 35 of 96 IC patients (36%). The most common patterns of antinuclear antibodies observed were dense, fine nuclear speckles (69%) and nucleolar (20%) staining in indirect immunofluorescence. None of the patients had bladder-tissue-specific autoantibodies. Thirty-one of the 35 antinuclear-antibody-positive sera were exclusively of the IgG class, two had IgG with IgM, and two had IgG with IgA. The autoimmune correlates of IC are fully described in Chapter 6.

Dysfunctional Bladder Epithelium

The bladder mucosa is lined by a layer of sulfonated glycosaminoglycans (GAGs): hyaluronic acid, heparin, chondroitin sulfates, dermatin sulfate, and keratin sulfate. Lilly and Parsons (16) suggested that the bladder surface GAG maintains the epithelial permeability barrier between the bladder wall and urine. Bladder surface GAGs contain negatively charged sulfated polysaccharide groups that have a high affinity for binding water molecules. This hydrated surface layer forms an underlying barrier between the bladder wall tissues and the urine, which prevents urinary solutes (such as urea and calcium) from damaging bladder cells. A defective GAG layer would subject bladder cells to harmful solutes.

Lilly and Parsons (16) examined the ability of surface GAG to prevent a small molecule, urea, from moving across the human bladder epithelium. They conducted a three-stage study: stage 1, urea instillation; stage 2, treatment of the bladder with protamine sulfate, 5 mg/ml (100 ml total volume), for 15 min followed by urea; and stage 3, 2,000 units/ml (100 ml total volume) of heparin for 15 min, followed by urea. At the end of each stage, the urea content was measured. A control group of 27 normal volunteers had 100 ml of a 200 g/liter urea solution placed into their bladders for 45 min. The net flow of urea from the bladder lumen was 5.1%. From this initial group, 19 individuals who were capable of completing the study proceeded to stage 2 of the study. These volunteers had protamine sulfate (5 mg/ml) instilled in the bladder for 15 min and then removed, and a second urea analysis done. Urea loss was significantly higher at 22% ($p < 0.02$ by Student's t test). In stage 3, a solution of heparin (1,000 units/ml) was instilled for 15 min, followed by a third urea analysis; urea loss was reversed to 9%. All volunteers experienced significant urinary urgency and discomfort after protamine treatment. These symptoms were relieved by the instillation of heparin. This study suggests that the most important permeability defense mechanism of the epithelium is the surface GAG, which prevents the small molecule urea from leaking across it. This defense mechanism can be impaired by a quaternary amine, such as protamine sulfate, and can be restored by a sulfated polysaccharide (heparin) instilled into the bladder. This in turn suggests that the polysaccharide on the surface of the bladder is an effective permeability barrier. A deficiency of this layer, either by poor quality or quantity or by the presence of urinary quaternary amines (similar to protamine), may be an important initiator of the disease. The overall importance of understanding the role of urinary GAG is further illustrated by the therapeutic value of using exogenous polysaccharide to treat urinary tract disease, a therapy based on the augmentation of natural defense mechanisms or the inactivation of urinary polysaccharide.

Chelsky et al. (17) argued that the "epithelial leak" theory may not be valid. They determined bladder permeability in a more direct fashion by measuring the actual transvesical migration of the radioisotope technetium-99m-diethylenetriaminepentaacetic acid (^{99m}Tc-DTPA) into the systemic circulation in ten IC patients and nine gender-matched normal controls. The ^{99m}Tc-DTPA is somewhat larger in size than urea [a test compound that is often used by Parsons et al. (5,18)] but is still a relatively small molecule as evidenced by its ability to undergo glomerular filtration. Presumably, the permeability of ^{99m}Tc-DTPA should be similar to that of urea. Considerable variability in the absorption of this acid occurred within the IC of patients and controls; the differences were not statistically significant. This implies that although some IC patients have a more permeable bladder than others, the same is true for normal, symptom-free volunteers. Thus, the concept of increased bladder permeability in IC was not supported by this examination of bladder permeability using ^{99m}Tc-DTPA as a test compound.

Nevertheless, the many reports of the success of synthetic polysaccharides in the treatment of IC cannot be discounted. Such successes support the concept that some patients with the IC syndrome do indeed have a leaky epithelium.

In a clinical 1987 study of IC, Parsons et al. (19) used a dose of 100 mg of sodium pentosanpolysulfate (PPS) three times daily for a minimum of 4 months, which was continued for longer than 18 months in some individuals. A total of 62 IC patients were evaluated at two different medical centers. Subjective improvements were greater in all parameters when the drug was compared to placebo therapy, with significant improvement in pain, urgency, frequency, and nocturia. Objective improvement in average voided volumes was greater with the drug than with placebo ($p = 0.009$).

In 1993, Parsons et al. (20) conducted a randomized, prospective, double-blind, placebo-controlled study at seven clinical centers on 148 IC patients. Patients received either 100 mg PPS or a placebo three times daily orally. Of the patients on PPS, 32% showed significant improvement compared to 16% of those on placebo ($p = 0.01$). Patients on drug therapy experienced a significant diminution in pain and urgency ($p = 0.04$ and 0.01, respectively) on visual analog scales; in addition, more drug patients showed an average increment of more than 20 ml in voided volume than did placebo patients ($p = 0.02$). In 1994, Parsons et al. (21) reported that in over half of a cohort of 48 IC patients, intravesical heparin controlled the symptoms of IC, with continued improvement even after 1 year of therapy.

Mulholland et al. (22) compared PPS with placebo for the symptomatic therapy of IC in a double-blind, multicenter study. A total of 110 patients were enrolled and treated for 3 months. Overall improvement of greater than 25% was reported by 28% of the PPS-treated patients and by only 13% of the placebo-treated patients ($p = 0.03$). The investigators' overall evaluation provided similar results, 26% versus 11% in favor of PPS ($p = 0.07$).

Fritjofsson et al. (23) studied 87 patients with IC symptoms in a 2-year protocol at 17 centers in Finland and Sweden. The medication (400 mg of PPS daily in two oral doses) was discontinued after 6 months. Most patients responded favorably, many experiencing a decrease in pain as early as 4 weeks from the start of treatment. Pain reduction was typically sustained.

Kalota et al. (24) demonstrated in two *in vivo* models and an *in vitro* model the ability of PPS to reduce toxic effects of acrolein (the active metabolite of cyclophosphamide, capable of damaging the transitional epithelium of the bladder). *In vivo* (adult female rats), PPS improves the functional properties of the GAG layer of the intact bladder (relative to adherence and permeability). Although pentosanpolysulfate does not appear to have a complete protective effect against acrolein-induced tissue damage, it does prevent a significant amount of damage from cyclophosphamide's metabolite acrolein when given intravesically for 15 min before the instillation of acrolein. In the *in vitro* model, there was an increased survival of cell tissues following the use of PPS pretreatment with various concentrations of acrolein.

Koziol et al. (7) examined the effect of sulfated polysaccharide therapy in IC patients classified into three severity levels of IC, mild, moderate, and severe, based on symptoms, in particular, pain, urgency, and nocturia scores. They found no apparent improvement in symptoms during polysaccharide therapy among those patients in the mild group, a slight improvement among the moderate group, and a dramatic improvement among those patients in the severe group. In general, pain and urgency scores tended to decline throughout the therapeutic interval, whereas nocturia seemed to plateau after 12 to 24 months on therapy. Pain and urgency seemed relatively more affected by polysaccharide therapy than was nocturia.

On the basis of these findings, it is plausible that a defect or absence of the surface GAG layer is involved in the pathogenesis of IC. It is suggested that this mucous barrier functions abnormally in a subset of individuals with IC. Hence, synthetic polysaccharide will help only these individuals. It is estimated that more than 50% of IC patients will benefit from this treatment regimen (16,19–22,24,25). The role of glycosaminoglycans in IC is considered in detail in Chapter 11.

Mast Cells

The mast cell is a potential pathogenetic effector mechanism in IC (see Chapter 12). Mast cells contain water-soluble metachromatic staining cytoplasmic granules. Simmons (26) reported mast cells in the wall of the normal bladder, with these cells secreting histamines. West and Riley (27) found the amount of histamine in various tissues to be proportional to the mast cell content. Histamine release causes pain, fibrosis, and hyperemia, notable features of IC. Simmons (26) observed a small series of IC patients treated with an antihistamine, tripelennamine (Pyribenzamine), 50 mg three times daily: this resulted in the improvement of symptoms, but with variable duration. Antihistamine works by blocking the response of the end organ to the histamine; it does not alter the production or release of histamine. One might conjecture that many of the pathologic changes in the bladder wall occurring in IC may be secondary to the presence of mast cells and the local release of histamine.

Some investigators have attempted to quantify the presence of mast cells with respect to symptoms. Holm-Bentzen et al. (28) attempted to elucidate differences in symptoms and in cystoscopy and cystometric findings in 115 patients with a painful bladder with and without detrusor mastocytosis. Based on mast cell counts in the bladder biopsies of the detrusor muscle, the patients were divided into two groups: those with more than 28 and those with fewer than 28 mast cells per square millimeter. Patients with more than 28 mast cells/mm^2 had hematuria more often than the other patients (23% versus 13%). The former had a significantly more damaged bladder than the other painful bladder patients, in that half of these patients had redness, scarring, and increased vascularization of the bladder mucosa at cystoscopy before bladder distension. The bladder capacity also was significantly reduced in these patients. Petechial bleeding was found in 60% to 75% of the patients in both groups, not a significant difference. The patients without detrusor mastocytosis had a vulnerable mucosa after bladder distension (petechial bleeding), but there was no chronic contracted bladder. Holm-Bentzen et al. concluded that if patients with chronic abacterial cystitis of unknown etiology are divided into two groups on the basis of fewer or more than 28 mast cells/mm^2, certain differences in the clinical findings between the groups can be ruled out. However, because the groups largely overlapped, mast cells cannot be the only factor responsible for the symptoms.

Johansson and Fall (1) suggested that only patients with classic IC have elevated mast cells counts. They conducted a detailed histopathologic analysis of the lesions seen in patients with classic and early IC. Mast cell counts were determined in 47 classic and 30 early IC patients and in 14 controls. The data showed that mast cells were significantly increased in the patients with the classic syndrome only; in particular, mast cells were increased in the lamina propria as well as in the detrusor muscle. The mucosal mast cells were seen in the urothelium of all patients except two with the classic syndrome, but they were not detected in any patients with the early syndrome. Mast cell density was markedly increased in patients with classic IC, especially in the lamina propria. There was no significant difference in mast cell numbers in the detrusor muscle or lamina propria between the early IC patients and the controls, but numbers differed significantly between these two groups and the classic IC patients ($p < 0.05$).

Hanno et al. (29) evaluated 55 patients with IC and compared them to a control group of 21 patients who had voiding dysfunction conclusively proved to be other than IC on evaluation. The latter group included patients being screened for bladder and prostate cancer and those with hyperactive bladder dysfunction and voiding dysfunctions other than IC. Of the patients diagnosed as having IC, 64% had detrusor mastocytosis, compared to 80% of non-IC patients. Mean detrusor mast cell counts were not statistically different between the two groups.

From these various findings, it is apparent that although detrusor mastocytosis might be an important mediator of the disease, it cannot be used to confirm the diagnosis of IC.

Summary

Interstitial cystitis is a condition in which few specific diagnostic criteria have been established. From this brief review of autoimmunity, dysfunctional bladder epithelium, and mast cell correlates of IC, it is reasonable to conclude that the etiology of IC is multifactorial.

An elevated level of autoantibodies found in the majority of patients with IC suggests that IC is an autoimmune syndrome. However, a comparable increase is also present in other urologic patients. Because of this lack of specificity, it is unlikely that this immunologic response is the primary cause of IC.

A subset of IC patients may have a "leaky" epithelium, and their symptoms could be alleviated by synthetic polysaccharide therapy in over 50% of IC patients (16, 21–23,25).

Mast cells are often found in increased numbers in IC patients relative to normal controls. There is a significant increase of mast cells in patients with classic IC compared to early IC, but no difference in mast cell level between early IC patients and a group of normal control (1). Hence, mastocytosis may be an important mediator in patients with classic IC, but it cannot be used to confirm the diagnosis of IC.

No single treatment prescribed in accordance with a hypothesized etiology will benefit all patients with IC. Each treatment, nonetheless, will likely benefit a select subset of IC patients. If, in fact, the etiology of IC is multifactorial, it is critical to identify distinct subgroups of these patients: such subdivision of this ill-defined syndrome will allow for more effective treatment programs by identifying a treatment of choice appropriate for each particular subgroup.

PREVALENCE

Oravisto (30) in 1975 estimated the prevalence of IC for Helsinki, Finland and in the surrounding area to be 10.6 patients per 100,000 inhabitants for the total population. The female prevalence was 18.1 per 100,000 women of all ages.

A 1987 epidemiology study by Held et al. (31) used three methods to estimate the prevalence of IC in the United States from information supplied in a random survey of 127 board-certified urologists. The three estimated values were 16.3 per 100,000, 25.1 per 100,000, and 76.3 per 100,000, and the average was 36.6 per 100,000.

Bade et al. (32), on the basis of a urologist-based questionnaire study, estimated the prevalence of IC in The Netherlands to be 8 to 16 cases per 100,000 female patients, in close agreement with Oravisto's estimate. On the other hand, a recent population based survey (18) suggested that the prevalence of IC in the United States might well exceed 0.51% among adults, an order of magnitude higher than any previous finding (although the methodology of Jones et al. has yet to be validated).

INCIDENCE

Between 1962 and 1972, Oravisto (30) observed a minimal annual incidence rate of 0.66 cases of IC per 100,000 inhabitants in the city of Helsinki and surrounding area. The yearly estimated female incidence rate during the same period was 1.2 cases per 100,000 women. In a 1987 epidemiology study by Held et al. (31), the incidence rate for the United States was estimated to be 2.6 per 100,000, a figure four times higher than the estimate reported by Oravisto.

Several possibilities for the incongruities in incidence and prevalence rates between the two studies were postulated by Held et al. (31): (a) extrapolation of Oravisto's estimates from Finland in 1975 and the United States in 1987 may not be valid; (b) there may be a nonresponse bias from the 1987 survey because the response rate from urologists asked to participate in the survey was only 26%; (c) the population may not be the same for these two studies because no uniform or established diagnostic criteria for IC were applied in both studies.

EPIDEMIOLOGIC FACTORS

Koziol (6) examined epidemiologic evidence relating to (a) demography, (b) medical history, (c) type and severity of symptoms, (d) location, frequency, and intensity of pain, (e) duration of symptoms, (f) behaviors that exacerbate or curtail symptoms, and (g) psychosocial factors in 565 IC patients. Patients were classified into three severity groups based on treatment histories and physiological findings relating to IC. This classification scheme was used subsequently to ascertain whether variables such as risk factors, duration of disease, symptoms, and psychosocial factors were related to disease history and severity. Category 3 included 111 patients (19.7%) with severe symptoms and Hunner's ulcers (classic IC). Category 2 included 403 patients (71.3%) with severe symptoms who had documented abnormal bladder biopsies and urodynamic and endoscopic findings excluding neurologic causes of frequency or urgency. Category 1 included 51 patients (9.0%) with severe symptoms who had documented abnormal bladder biopsies but lacked reports of other supportive endoscopic and urodynamic findings. Patients were also classified into four subgroups with respect to the number of years with symptoms, the purpose here being to ascertain whether any survey response variables tend to increase or decrease among patients as the number of years with symptoms increases. A brief discussion of these findings follows.

Demography

Patients were primarily Caucasian (94.3%) and female (88.8%). Patients suffering from the classic syndrome were significantly older than other IC patients. The mean age reported for these patients was 57.9 years; the mean age reported for early IC patients was 50.1 years. It was also noted that patients suffering from the classic syndrome experienced first symptoms at a later date than early IC patients. Oravisto (33) reported that the symptoms associated with IC generally progress rapidly to a final state, with little worsening thereafter. Koziol noted similarly that symptoms typically plateau within 5 years of onset and that onset of IC is not homogeneous over time. Overall, patients with symptoms for longer periods of time tended to be older than patients with symptoms for shorter periods.

Risk Factors

Sixty-four percent of patients with IC and only 23% of controls had one or more risk factors among the group: abdominal cramping, irritable bowel syndrome, spastic colon, and a cluster of factors with a possible psychosomatic component ($p < 0.00001$). Overall, 72% of patients and 50% of controls had one or more risk factors from the group consisting of sensitivity or allergic reaction to medication, rheumatoid arthritis, sinusitis, food allergy, hay fever, asthma, and a cluster of immunopathologic abnormalities associated with an autoimmune component ($p < 0.00001$). Other investigators have also reported a high frequency of allergy among IC patients: Messing et al. (3), 25%; Oravisto et al. (33), 26%; Holm-Bentzen (28), 34%; and Hand (34), 15% in IC patients versus 8.5% in controls.

Because a large number of IC patients undergo surgical, gynecologic, and obstetric procedures, Hollander (35) suggested that an allergy to silk sutures remaining in the urogenital region might cause the symptoms of IC in some susceptible individuals. Silk had also been reported to cause symptoms of pneumonitis, pulmonary fibrosis, postoperative "pyoderma gangrenosum," and asthma. (In contrast, Koziol found no significant relation between asthma and symptoms of IC; $p = 0.153$.) Oravisto et al. (33) observed that in two of their patients, symptoms began abruptly after a gynecologic operation.

Few studies have investigated any genetic or ethnic associations with IC. Oravisto (36) reported IC developing in a set of monozygotic twins and in a mother and daughter. From the sample obtained by Koziol (6), two sets of sisters, including one set of monozygotic twins, were found with formally diagnosed IC. One cannot therefore dismiss a genetic component to the origin of IC. Held et al. (31) had reported 14% (126 of 902) of one sample of IC patients to be of Jewish origin, compared with 3% (three of 119) of a general population sample. In comparison, 15.3% (20 of 131) of the sample in Koziol's study are of Jewish origin, a higher-than-expected proportion under a nonassociation model. This suggestion of an excess risk of IC among individuals of Jewish origin would not be unique to IC: for example, ulcerative colitis is two to four times more frequent in individuals of Jewish origin than in non-Jews.

Symptoms of IC

Substantial proportions of patients reported symptoms of urgency (91.9%), frequency (91.2%), pelvic pain (69.9%), pelvic pressure (63.3%), dysuria (60.5%), pain during intercourse (55.2%), burning (55.1%), being awakened at night by pain (50.8%), pain for days after intercourse (36.7%), and hematuria (21.6%). In addition, patients with bladder ulcers tended to report greater frequency (increased number of voids per 24-hr period, shorter interval between nighttime voids) than other IC patients; they also reported blood in their urine more often and were more likely to be awakened at night by IC pain. Frequency, bladder spasms, and efficacy of urinating were found to increase significantly as duration of symptoms increased.

Pain

Over 55% of patients reported daily or constant pain, and nearly 57% characterized their pain as severe or excruciating. Frequency and intensity did not vary across severity groups, nor did frequency, intensity, and type of pain vary with duration of symptoms. Patients with the classic syndrome tended to report less dull, aching pain but more spasms and sharp or hot, stabbing pain in the right lower abdomen than do other IC patients. Urinating was quite effective in relieving IC pain, particularly for Hunner's ulcer patients. Medication was also somewhat effective, but behaviors such as hot baths, heating pad, activity, diversion from the pain, lying down (stretched out), lying down (curled up), sitting, and standing seemed ineffective. Stress increased IC pain in more than 61% of patients. Pain during sexual intercourse was reported by 50% of respondents. Acidic, alcoholic, or carbonated beverages and spicy foods tended to increase IC pain for more patients with the classic syndrome than with other IC patients. Patients tended to become increasingly intolerant of the beverage and food types listed as the number of years with symptoms increased, although the trends were not statistically significant.

Psychosocial Factors

Overall, a substantial number of patients reported psychological or related symptoms such as inability to enjoy usual activities, 68% (only 5.7% of patients found travel not to be difficult or impossible, 10.3% leisure activities, and 11.6% sleep); tiredness, 63.6%; depression, 56.4%; inability to concentrate, 50%; insomnia or excessive daytime sleepiness, 49.7%; weight change or eating disorder, 36.4%; feelings of worthlessness, 30.8%; phobias, anxiety, or panic attacks, 27.3%; nervous breakdown or need for psychiatric care, 16.7%. There were insignificant differences in the prevalence of symptoms when patients were classified by either severity or duration. Difficulties in performing everyday tasks were experienced at equivalent rates by patients in each severity group regardless of duration of symptoms, with the exception that there was less job satisfaction in terms of positions matching qualifications among the longer-term (10 years or more with symptoms) IC patients than among those with less than 10 years with symptoms. Family relationships and responsibilities were adversely affected in 70% of the patients.

SOCIAL AND ECONOMIC COSTS OF IC

The economic costs of IC can be profound. Held and colleagues provided economic findings from a 1987 epidemiologic investigation of IC (these estimates might be viewed as provisional, since few details concerning the conduct, reliability, or validity of this study were provided).

Held et al. (31) divided the costs of IC into two components: (a) medical care, which includes the cost of hospitals, doctors, and therapy, and (b) losses related to the inability to work or to emotional and physical suffering.

In 1987, the average annual medical cost per IC patient was estimated to be $3,870. This leads to a total estimated annual cost in the United States to be $170.3 million (estimated prevalence in 1987 is 44,000 female IC patients). However, this estimate includes medical costs in the absence of IC. The estimated incremental medical cost attributable to IC is $116.6 million per year.

In terms of indirect costs, Held et al. (31) estimated that 24.9% of female IC patients were less likely to be working full time compared with a normal female population (matched for age, sex, and education). This loss in income was partially compensated by a 4.1% increase in part-time work, again compared with a matched sample. The IC patients were also reported to receive, on the average, $3.41 less per hour than did a matched sample. From the national average wage rate for all women, the lost income per year would amount to $4,039 per patient, not including any wage reduction for those IC patients who did work. The inclusion of the IC wage reduction would increase the amount to $7,084 per year. The total lost incomes in 1987 would amount to $177.7 million or $311.7 million with the wage reduction (31).

COMMENTS

Since Hunner's seminal report in 1915 on "a rare type of bladder cancer" (37), the complex of symptoms and cystoscopic findings recognized as IC has become the increasing focus of clinical and basic research. Nevertheless, there are still no definitive answers to such pertinent issues as the etiology, the efficacy of therapeutic options, prevalence, incidence, risk factors, and social and economic costs of IC. Substantive and updated information concerning these issues would be most welcome to practitioners and patients alike.

REFERENCES

1. Johansson SL, Fall M. Clinical features, and spectrum of light microscopic changes in interstitial cystitis. *J Urol* 1989;143:1118–1124.
2. Hanno PM, Wein AJ. Lesson 10: Interstitial cystitis, part II. *AUA Update Ser* 1987;6:2–7.
3. Messing EM, Stamey TA. Interstitial cystitis, early diagnosis, pathology, and treatment. *Urology* 1978;12:381–392.
4. Koziol JA, Adams HP, Frutos A. Discrimination between the ulcerous and the nonulcerous forms of interstitial cystitis by noninvasive findings. *J Urol* 1995;155:87–90.
5. Koziol JA, Clark DC, Gittes RF, Tan EM. The natural history of interstitial cystitis—a survey of 374 patients. *J Urol* 1993;149:465–469.
6. Koziol JA. Epidemiology of interstitial cystitis. *Urol Clin North Am* 1994;21:7–20.
7. Koziol JA, Frutos A, Ho N, Parsons CL. Epidemiology of interstitial cystitis (submitted).
8. Sant GR. Interstitial cystitis. *Monogr Urol* 1991;12:37–63.
9. Erickson DR, Simon LJ, Belchis DA. Relationships between bladder inflammation and other clinical features in interstitial cystitis. *Urology* 1994;44:655–659.
10. Hanno PM, Wein AJ. Lesson 9: Interstitial cystitis, part I. *AUA Update Ser* 1987;9:3–7.
11. Messing EM. Interstitial cystitis and related syndromes. In: Walsh PC, Gittes RF, Perlmutter AD, Stamey TA, eds. *Campbell's Urology,* 5th ed. Philadelphia: WB Saunders, 1985;1070–1086.
12. Anderson JB, Parivar F, Lee G, Wallington TB, MacIver AG, Bradbrook RA, Gingell JC. The enigma of interstitial cystitis, an autoimmune disease. *Br J Urol* 1989;63:58–63.
13. Silk MR. Bladder antibodies in interstitial cystitis. *J Urol* 1970;103: 307–309.
14. Jokinen EJ, Alfthan O, Oravisto KJ. Antitissue antibodies in interstitial cystitis. *Clin Exp Immunol* 1972;11:333–339.
15. Ochs RL, Stein TW Jr, Peebles CL, Gittes RF, Tan EM. Autoantibodies in interstitial cystitis. *J Urol* 1994;151:587–592.
16. Lilly JD, Parsons CL. Bladder surface glycosaminoglycans is a human epithelial permeability barrier. *Surg Gynecol Obstet* 1990;171:143–145.
17. Chelsky MJ, Rosen SI, Knight LC, Maurer AH, Hanno PM, Ruggieri MR. Bladder permeability in interstitial cystitis is similar to that of normal volunteers—direct measurement by transvesical absorption of ^{99m}technetium-diethylenetriaminepentaaccetic acid. *J Urol* 1994;151: 346–349.
18. Jones CA, Harris M, Nyberg L. Prevalence of interstitial cystitis in the United States. *J Urol* 1994;151:423A.
19. Parsons CL, Mulholland SG. Successful therapy of interstitial cystitis with pentosanpolysulfate. *J Urol* 1987;138:513–515.
20. Parsons CL, Benson G, Childs SJ, Hanno P, Sant GR, Webster G. A quantitatively controlled method to study prospectively interstitial cystitis and demonstrate the efficacy of pentosanpolysulfate. *J Urol* 1993; 150:845–848.
21. Parsons CL, Housley JD, Schmidt JD, Lebow D. Treatment of interstitial cystitis with intravesical heparin. *Br J Urol* 1994;73:504–507.
22. Mulholland SG, Hanno P, Parsons CL, Sant GR, Staskin DR. pentosan polysulfate sodium for therapy of interstitial cystitis. *Urology* 1990; 35(6):552–558.
23. Fritjofsson A, Fall M, Juhlin R, Persson E, Ruutu M. Treatment of ulcer and nonulcer interstitial cystitis with sodium pentosanpolysulfate—a multicenter trial. *J Urol* 1987;138:508–512.
24. Kalota SJ, Stein PC, Parsons CL. Prevention of acrolein-induced bladder injury by pentosanpolysulfate. *J Urol* 1992;148:163–166.
25. Parsons CL, Lilly JD, Stein P. Epithelial dysfunction in nonbacterial cystitis (interstitial cystitis). *J Urol* 1991;145:732–735.

26. Simmons JL, Bunce PL. On the use of an antihistamine in the treatment of interstitial cystitis. *Am Surg* 1958;24:664–667.
27. Riley JF, West GB. The presence of histamine in tissue mast cells. *J Physiol* 1953;120:528–533.
28. Holm-Bentzen M, Jacobsen F, Nerstrom B, Lose G, Kristensen JK, Pedersen RH, Krarup T, Feggetter J, Bates P, Barnard R, Larsen S, Hald T. Painful bladder disease—clinical and pathoanatomical differences in 115 patients. *J Urol* 1987;138:500–502.
29. Hanno PM, Levin RM, Monson FC, Teuscher C, Zhou ZZ, Ruggieri M, Whitmore K, Wein AJ. Diagnosis of interstitial cystitis. *J Urol* 1990; 143:278–281.
30. Oravisto KJ. Epidemiology of interstitial cystitis. *Ann Chir Gynaecol Fenn* 1975;64:75–77.
31. Held PJ, Hanno PM, Wein AJ, Pauly MV, Cann MA. Epidemiology of interstitial cystitis 2. In: Hanno PM, Staskin DR, Krane RJ, Wein AJ, eds. *Interstitial Cystitis.* New York: Springer-Verlag, 1990; 29–48.
32. Bade JJ, Rijcken B, Mensink HJA. Interstitial cystitis in the Netherlands. Prevalence, diagnostic criteria and therapeutic preferences. *J Urol* 1995;154:2035–2038.
33. Oravisto KJ, Alfthan OS, Jokinen EJ. Interstitial cystitis. *Scand J Urol Nephrol* 1970;4:37–42.
34. Hand JR. Interstitial cystitis, report of 223 cases (204 women and 19 men). *J Urol* 1949;61:291–310.
35. Hollander DH. Interstitial cystitis and silk allergy. *Med Hypotheses* 1994;43:155–156.
36. Oravisto KJ. Interstitial cystitis as an autoimmune disease (a review). *Eur Urol* 1980;6:10–13.
37. Hunner GL. A rare type of bladder ulcer in women; report of cases. *Boston Med Surg J* 1915;172(18):660–665.

Interstitial Cystitis, edited by Grannum R. Sant.
Lippincott–Raven Publishers, Philadelphia ©1997.

CHAPTER 3

The Interstitial Cystitis Data Base Study

Laura J. Simon, J. Richard Landis, John E. Tomaszewski, Leroy M. Nyberg, and the ICDB Study Group

In recent years, much research has been done to conquer the elusive painful bladder disease known as interstitial cystitis (IC). Despite the testing of many different scientific hypotheses, to date, research has been inconclusive about the etiology, pathology, epidemiology, and treatment of IC (1–9). Much remains unknown. Several factors have inhibited advances in the understanding of IC, such as the lack of specific diagnostic criteria, the lack of specific histopathologic changes, the unpredictable fluctuation in symptoms, and the extreme variability among patients in terms of symptoms, objective findings, and treatment responses.

In an effort to advance knowledge of IC and better determine its treated history, the National Institute of Diabetes and Digestive and Kidney Diseases (NIDDK), in early 1991, invited cooperative agreement applications from investigators to design and implement a data base of IC patients. The *Request for Application* led to the identification of the Interstitial Cystitis Data Base (ICDB) Study Group, comprised of five clinical centers (in nine locations), a data coordinating center, and an anatomic pathology laboratory (Table 1).

THE ICDB STUDY OBJECTIVES

The overriding goal of the ICDB Study is to develop and maintain a centralized, standardized registry containing data on a large group of patients with symptomatology consistent with IC. Data collected on patients, at base line and longitudinally, include demographic and diagnostic information, dietary effects, patient and family medical history, symptoms, and treatments and their outcomes. In addition, bladder tissue specimens are obtained on a subset of patients and stored in a central repository for future use.

Before developing the study, the investigators identified five primary scientific objectives:

- Characterizing the age, race, sex, and other demographic factors of patients with symptomatology consistent with IC.
- Developing a symptom index that discriminates among patients with various presentations of IC symptoms.
- Determining the treated history of IC for selected subgroups.
- Developing and maintaining a central repository of bladder biopsy specimens from IC patients.
- Providing other qualified investigators with data and specimens for their own epidemiologic and clinical research.

These five objectives have driven all aspects of the design and implementation of the ICDB Study.

STUDY ORGANIZATION AND OPERATIONS

The ICDB Study Group is organized functionally by the main operational centers, namely the five clinical centers, the data coordinating center, the anatomic pathology laboratory, and the NIDDK. The Group is directed by three scientific governing bodies, a Steering Committee, an External Advisory Committee, and the NIDDK Project Scientist. Each operational center and governing body serves a unique function.

Clinical Centers

The clinical centers have primary responsibility for all activities involving patient care, data collection, and spec-

L. J. Simon and J. R. Landis: Center for Biostatistics and Epidemiology, Penn State University College of Medicine, Hershey, Pennsylvania 17033-0850.

J. E. Tomaszewski: Surgical Pathology, Department of Pathology and Laboratory Medicine, University of Pennsylvania, Philadelphia, Pennsylvania 19104.

L. M. Nyberg: Urology Programs, NIDDK, National Institutes of Health, Bethesda, Maryland 20892-6600.

TABLE 1. *Interstitial Cystitis Data Base (ICDB) study group*

Clinical centers	Locations	Investigator
Philadelphia	U. of Pennsylvania	Alan J. Wein, MD[a]
	Temple University	Philip M. Hanno, MD
	Graduate Hospital	Kristene E. Whitmore, MD
Chicago/Madison	Northwestern University	Anthony J. Schaeffer, MD[a]
	U. of Wisconsin	David T. Uehling, MD[c]
		Edward M. Messing, MD[d]
Detroit	William Beaumont Hospital	Ananias C. Diokno, MD[a]
	Henry Ford Hospital	Aaron K. Kirkemo, MD
San Diego	U. of California at San Diego	Lowell C. Parsons, MD[a]
Oklahoma	U. of Oklahoma	Daniel J. Culkin, MD[a,c]
		Johnny B. Roy, MD[a,d]
Coordinating Centers	**Locations**	**Investigator**
Data	Penn State College of Medicine	J. Richard Landis, PhD[a]
Biopsy specimens	U. of Pennsylvania	John E. Tomaszewski, MD[b]
Funding agency	**Location**	**Project Scientist**
National Institute of Diabetes & Digestive & Kidney Diseases	Bethesda,MD	Leroy M. Nyberg, PhD, MD

[a]Principal Investigator.
[b]Director, Anatomic Pathology Laboratory (subcontracted under Data Coordinating Center).
[c]Current Investigator
[d]Original Investigator

imen acquisition and shipment. Patient-related responsibilities include recruiting and retaining compliant patients, evaluating whether patients meet study eligibility criteria, treating and counseling patients, and following patients throughout the duration of the study. Data-related responsibilities include completing patient-interview data forms, reviewing patient-completed data forms, submitting data forms in a timely manner to the data coordinating center, and interacting with the data coordinating center to resolve problem data. Specimen-related activities include collecting, processing, and shipping of bladder biopsy specimens and slides to the anatomic pathology laboratory. In performing all activities, each clinical center is responsible for adhering to the study protocol and operation procedures.

Each of the five clinical centers is staffed by the Principal Investigator, a coinvestigator, and at least one dedicated research coordinator. The Principal Investigator and coinvestigator provide the clinical center with its scientific direction, and the Research Coordinator performs all of the day-to-day operations of the clinical center. Each of the five clinical center Principal Investigators is a urologist. Four of the seven Research Coordinators are nurses, one is an international medical graduate, one is a medical lab technician, and one is a data manager.

Data Coordinating Center

The data coordinating center (DCC) provides leadership and coordinates all activities pertaining to forms development, forms production, forms distribution, database development, data entry, data management, protocol monitoring, data quality assurance, data reporting, and statistical analysis. Specifically, in collaboration with the Steering Committee, the DCC wrote the study protocol and manual of operations; designed and developed the data collection forms; trained the research nurse coordinators in the proper execution and completion of study procedures and data forms; developed a database management system with several quality assurance modules, such as a validation module that flags missing data fields, out-of-range values, and data conflicts; developed data- and specimen-tracking systems; developed accrual and quality assurance monitoring reports; participated in on-site clinical center data audits; and developed the operations protocol for the review of bladder biopsy specimens.

On an ongoing basis, the DCC coordinates meetings and phone conferences of the Steering Committee and Research Coordinators; monitors clinical center adherence to the study protocol; fields questions from clinical center staff on execution of the study protocol; disseminates relevant information to the ICDB Study Group; runs and disseminates accrual and data quality reports; and collaborates with ICDB investigators in the analysis and publication of study results.

Anatomic Pathology Laboratory

The anatomic pathology laboratory (APL) has primary responsibility for receiving, tracking, evaluating, processing, and banking ICDB bladder biopsy specimens and slides. The APL also has primary responsibility for coordinating the activities of the pathology reading group, comprised of three pathologists, in the review and classification of stained slides.

Steering Committee

The Steering Committee, which is the primary governing body of the ICDB Study, is comprised of the NIDDK Project Scientist, the five clinical center Principal Investigators, and the data coordinating center Principal Investigator. Each member of the Committee has one vote. The Steering Committee is responsible for making all major scientific decisions governing the conduct of the ICDB Study, such as formalizing the scientific study design, developing the study protocol and operating procedures, and monitoring overall study quality. In August 1992, the Steering Committee selected Alan J. Wein, M.D., to serve as its chairman. During the development of the study protocol, the Steering Committee met on a bimonthly basis. Currently, during the main study, the Steering Committee meets biannually; otherwise, phone conferences are held as necessary.

External Advisory Committee

The External Advisory Committee is an independent advisory group composed of 11 experts in relevant medical, statistical, and bioethical fields. The primary responsibility of the External Advisory Committee is to periodically review the progress of the ICDB Study and to provide advice to the NIDDK Project Scientist regarding the scientific merit of the study. The External Advisory Committee met in Bethesda, MD, in November 1992 to review the ICDB Study protocol before its finalization.

NIDDK Project Scientist

The NIDDK Project Scientist, Leroy M. Nyberg, Ph.D., M.D., provides the Steering Committee with scientific and administrative direction in all aspects of the ICDB Study, including protocol development, quality control, interim data monitoring, final data analysis and interpretation, preparation of publications, and performance monitoring.

THE ICDB STUDY DESIGN

The ICDB Study is an observational, longitudinal study. Patients enrolled in the study are treated by their physician according to usual clinical care, in the absence of a protocol-specific treatment intervention. The study population was defined and the sample size requirements determined so that statistically valid comparisons could be made between various subgroups of patients.

Study Population

The study population of interest comprised patients with symptomatology consistent with IC. Any patient at least 18 years of age presenting with symptoms of urinary urgency, frequency, or pain of unknown cause that has persisted for at least 6 months is considered a candidate for enrollment into the study. However, a patient must meet all of the eligibility criteria outlined in Table 2. In order to capture a broader range of patients, such as patients with newly developing IC, the eligibility criteria are slightly less restrictive than the criteria established at the National Institutes of Health workshop in August 1987 for the diagnosis of IC (10). For example, patients with symptoms for less than 12 months but longer than 6 months are permitted to enter the study.

TABLE 2. *Interstitial Cystitis Data Base (ICDB) study eligibility criteria*

- Providing informed consent to participate in the study
- Willing to undergo a cystoscopy under general or regional anesthesia, when indicated, during the course of the study
- At least 18 years of age
- Having symptoms of urinary urgency, frequency, or pain for more than 6 months
- Urinating at least seven times per day or having some urgency or pain (measured on linear analog scales)
- No history or current genitourinary tuberculosis
- No history of urethral cancer
- No history or current bladder malignancy, high-grade dysplasia, or carcinoma *in situ*
- Men: no history or current prostate cancer
- Women: no history of ovarian, vaginal, or cervical cancer
- Women: no vaginitis, clue cell, trichomonas, and yeast infections
- No bacterial cystitis in previous 3 months
- No active herpes in previous 3 months
- No antimicrobials for urinary tract infections in previous 3 months
- Never having been treated with cyclophosphamide (Cytoxan)
- No radiation cystitis
- No neurogenic bladder dysfunction (e. g. due to a spinal cord injury, a stroke, Parkinson's disease, multiple sclerosis, spina bifida, or diabetic cystopathy)
- No bladder outlet obstruction (determined by urodynamic investigation)
- Men: no bacterial prostatitis for previous 6 months
- Absence of bladder, ureteral, or urethral calculi for previous 3 months
- No urethritis for previous 3 months
- Not having had a urethral dilation, cystometrogram, a bladder cystoscopy under full anesthesia, or a bladder biopsy in previous 3 months
- Never having had an augmentation cystoplasty, cystectomy, cystolysis, or neurectomy
- Not having a urethral stricture of less than 12 French

Control Group

The multipurpose nature of the ICDB, pending the formation of a wide range of research questions, posed a serious challenge related to the formation of a control group(s), especially because the choice of comparison groups depends precisely on which research question is under investigation. In the interest of being able to form various comparison subgroups, patients with IC-like symptoms, at various stages of symptom severity, are being recruited for the ICDB Study. Based on a subjective, patient-reported scale (ranging from 0 to 3) for each of three dimensions [frequency (F), urgency (U), and pain (P)], the patient's total FUP score (ranging from 0 to 9) is formed as a sum of the three individual scores. In order to capture a mild-symptom comparison group, eligibility requires a total FUP score of only 1 or greater. The recruitment net was widened even further by requiring patients to undergo a cystoscopy, hydrodistention, and biopsy under full anesthesia (CHB) only if clinically indicated. Patients whose symptoms do not warrant a CHB at baseline must be willing, however, to undergo these procedures when clinically indicated during the course of the study.

Sample Size Requirements

The ICDB Study was designed on the basis of the assumption that studying the associations between many possible variables is of primary interest. Therefore, with the assumption of a prevalence rate of 30% for one of the symptoms, sample size requirements were calculated so that statistical associations between any two binary variables, with an odds ratio of at least 1.5, could be detected with 80% power. The sample size calculations were performed for two-sided tests with a 0.05 significance level and adjusted for an assumed 6% annual attrition rate and for clustering of homogeneous patients within the nine hospitals. With these assumptions, the studywide sample size requirement was determined to be 1,365 patients. With the further assumption of equal recruitment among the five clinical centers, the accrual requirements were set at 273 subjects per center over the course of the study period.

THE ICDB STUDY PLAN

The ICDB Study comprises two distinct phases for each participating patient: the baseline screening phase and the longitudinal follow-up phase. The baseline screening phase is designed so that a patient's eligibility can be assessed and baseline data collected. Any candidate failing any of the eligibility criteria is treated according to usual clinical care, but is not eligible to participate in the follow-up phase. Patients passing all of the eligibility criteria move into the longitudinal follow-up phase.

Baseline Screening

The screening phase comprises from one to three clinic visits scheduled as closely together as possible. Extensive baseline data, consisting of approximately 1,025 data fields, are collected on each patient (Table 3). To ensure that each patient's baseline data are collected contemporaneously, each patient's screening phase must be completed within 13 weeks.

Longitudinal Follow-Up

Patients participating in the longitudinal follow-up phase are followed until the close of the ICDB Study, with four contacts annually, twice by telephone and twice by a physician's office visit. The phone calls take place during months 3 and 9 of every patient-year, and the clinic visit on months 6 and 12 of every patient-year (Table 3).

Recruitment and Retention

Both recruitment and retention provide a tremendous challenge to the clinical centers, as patients are charged in full for their care and are not provided additional remuneration for their study participation. Although secondary recruitment methods vary across clinical centers, the investigators' and their clinics' patient populations serve as the primary source of study participants for all centers. Television newscasts, articles in institutional research bulletins, and presentations at local Interstitial Cystitis Association (ICA) chapter meetings have also served as advertisement for the ICDB study and have helped to increase recruitment.

Investigators aim to achieve high patient retention on the ICDB Study by providing benefits to study participants that are not available to nonstudy patients. For example, each clinical center offers a dedicated study phone line, which allows patients direct and easy access to their Research Nurse Coordinator for daily support and care. Patients are also offered a free membership in the ICA for the duration of their study participation. Most patients are inspired solely by their desire to become actively involved in the research and care of their own debilitating disorder.

Data Quality

Because scientific results are only as valid as the quality of the data that produce them, the ICDB Study Group developed and implemented an extensive studywide Data Quality Assurance Program. Some of the main components of the Data Quality Assurance Program include (a) development and use of protocol adherence aids, such as

TABLE 3. *Data and specimen collection schedule*

	Study month[a]													
	B	1	3	6	9	12	15	18	21	24	27	30	33	36
Eligibility	x													
Demographics	x									x				
Patient medical history	x									x				
Family medical history	x													
Symptom history	x													
Prior diagnostic tests and treatments	x													
Pregnancy history[b]	x									x				
Voiding log	x	x	x	x	x	x	x	x	x	x	x	x	x	x
Dietary effects	x			x		x		x		x		x		x
Patient symptoms[c]	x	x	x	x	x	x	x	x	x	x	x	x	x	x
SF-36 quality of life	x			x		x		x		x		x		x
Pain and urgency scale	x	x	x	x	x	x	x	x	x	x	x	x	x	x
Concomitant medications	x	x	x	x	x	x	x	x	x	x	x	x	x	x
Treatments	x	x	x	x	x	x	x	x	x	x	x	x	x	x
Medical events	x	x	x	x	x	x	x	x	x	x	x	x	x	x
Physical exam[d]	x			x		x		x		x		x		x
Hematology	x													
Urinalysis	x			x		x		x		x		x		x
Urodynamic evaluation	x													
Cystoscopy and biopsy[e]	x													

[a]Months 3, 9, 15, 21, 27, 33 are telephone contacts. Months 6, 12, 18, 24, 30, and 36 are clinic visits. Baseline (B) visits are clinic visits; month 1 is a phone contact or clinic visit.
[b]Women only.
[c]Questionnaires for phone contacts are abbreviated from the questionnaires for clinic visits.
[d]Only if indicated for follow-up visits.
[e]When indicated at base-line or follow-up visits.

patient visit schedules and visit checklists; (b) a database management system that identifies gross data errors, such as incorrect patient IDs or invalid visit numbers; (c) a computerized data validation module that detects missing data points, out-of-range values, and illogical data; (d) computerized monitoring reports that identify protocol violations; (e) on-site data audits of each clinical center, during which data forms are compared to source documents for discrepancies; and (f) on-site audits of the datacoordinating center to ensure that sound data management procedures are practiced (11,12).

Functionally, the clinical centers and data coordinating center complement each other by providing a system of checks and balances within the Data Quality Assurance Program. The clinical centers are responsible for ensuring that high-quality data are collected by adhering to the standardized study protocol and data collection procedures, while the data coordinating center is responsible for monitoring the quality of the data collected and notifying clinical centers of data or procedural problems.

DATA COLLECTION AND CLINICAL PROCEDURES

Each patient enrolled in the ICDB Study contributes a wealth of information to the database by completing a variety of data forms and undergoing extensive clinical procedures (Table 3). At baseline alone, each patient contributes approximately 1,025 data fields. All data collected are transcribed onto ICDB data forms and mailed weekly from the clinical centers to the DCC for data processing. This section describes, in brief, some of the data collected on each patient.

Demographics and History

Standard demographic information is collected on each patient, including age, race, sex, state and country of birth, current zip code, religion, marital status, educational background, employment status, and household income. Patients provide extensive information on their medical history, including any intercurrent medical conditions such as gastrointestinal disorders, allergies, chronic fatigue syndrome, arthritis, and fibromyalgia. Patients who have intercurrent disorders indicate the timing of the disorder's onset relative to the onset of their urinary symptoms. Patients also provide information on frequency of previous bladder and respiratory infections as well as frequency of tobacco and alcohol use. Women provide additional information on their menstrual history, such as regularity of menses, tampon use, and previous abnormal pap smears.

In order to gain insight into the potential etiology of their urinary condition, each patient answers 19 questions on the history of their symptoms, such as age at onset and remission and flare history. Patients also report potential triggers of their symptoms, such as urinary tract infections, antibiotic use, sexually transmitted diseases, pelvic surgery, or illness. Patients indicate presence of 14 conditions in first-order blood relatives, including IC, Crohn's disease, irritable bowel syndrome, allergies, fibromyalgia, diabetes, and migraine headaches.

Female patients also provide information on their pregnancy history, such as number of live births, stillbirths, miscarriages, abortions, and ectopic pregnancies. Parous patients indicate the timing of their pregnancies relative to the onset of their urinary symptoms.

Symptoms and Quality of Life

Patients provide an assessment of their overall quality of life on the standard SF-36 questionnaire as well as report detailed information about their symptoms. Information is collected on frequency of specific symptoms, such as urgency, hesitancy, hematuria, involuntary loss of urine, pain relief on urination, and average daytime and nighttime frequencies. For each of six body parts, patients report the type, persistence, and intensity of pain. The body parts include urethra, lower back, lower abdomen, rectum, vagina (women), perineum (men), and an optional "other" body part. Possible choices for types of pain are dull, aching, bloating, pressure, stabbing, sharp, spasms, and burning. Persistence of pain is described as either intermittent or constant, and intensity as either mild, moderate, or severe.

Dietary Effects

For 35 different foods, patients indicate what effect they think the food has on their urinary symptoms. Foods include fruits and juices (e.g., cranberry, orange, pineapple), vegetables (e.g., avocados, corn, potatoes), dairy products (e.g., milk, sour cream, yogurt), beverages (e.g., beer, coffee, red wine), and others (e.g., chocolate, chilies, and aspartame).

Voiding Log

Each patient provides a 3-day voiding log at every study visit. Just before each visit, the patient records the date, time, and volume urinated every time she or he urinates for three consecutive days. The 3-day period includes only one of the two weekend days, so collection takes place on a Thursday, Friday, Saturday; or on a Sunday, Monday, Tuesday. At the end of each of the three days, the patient also indicates on linear analog scale the degree of her pain and urgency.

Urodynamic Evaluation

Each patient undergoes a cystometrogram with water, and some patients also undergo optional uroflowmetry. For patients undergoing uroflow, initial average uroflow rate, initial peak uroflow rate, and initial volume voided are recorded. For all patients, postvoid residual urine is recorded. Then, the investigator attempts to fill the bladder with water at a rate of 60 cc/min. During filling, the patient reports her first sensation to void and her maximal discomfort. The volumes at these two time points are recorded, as are any involuntary bladder contractions and the end filling pressure. At the time of micturition for all male patients and a subset of female patients, the opening pressure, average uroflow rate, peak uroflow rate, volume voided, peak flow, and maximum pressures are recorded.

Cystoscopy

A subset of patients, in whom it is clinically indicated, are cystoscoped under either local or general anesthesia. Data are collected on the presence of a variety of conditions, including urethral or prostatic calculi, urethral diverticulum, abnormal orfices, pseudomembranous trigonitis, bladder calculi, tumors, Hunner's patch, scars, and hyper- or hypovascularity. A smaller subset of patients are also clinically indicated for hydrodistention and biopsy under general anesthesia. For these patients, additional parameters are collected, including bladder capacity (at 80 to 100 cm H_2O), presence of bloody effluent, and type and severity of glomerulations. To standardize the determination of the presence of Hunner's patch and glomerulations, investigators refer to a set of photographs developed solely for the ICDB Study.

Concomitant Medications and Treatments

Because of the large number of treatment methods attempted for IC, extensive efforts are made to get an adequate treatment and medication profile on each patient. Therefore, at every clinic visit or telephone contact, patients report all treatment and concomitant medication use since their last study visit or contact. Drug or treatment name, start date, and stop date are collected.

BLADDER SPECIMEN BANK AND PANEL REVIEW

If these are clinically indicated, patients undergo a cystoscopy, hydrodistention, and biopsy under general anesthesia (CHB). Bladder tissue specimens are forwarded to, processed by, and banked at the anatomic pathology laboratory (APL) at the University of Pennsylvania Medical Center in Philadelphia. The Pathology Reading Group (PRG), an expert panel comprised of the Director of the APL (John Tomaszewski, M.D.), a pathologist and molecular biologist at the University of New Mexico (Thomas Williams, M.D.), and a cytopathologist at Scripps Institute (Valentina Russak, M.D.), evaluates each specimen for a broad panel of histopathologic features.

Biopsy Sampling Protocol

Three sets of tissue are sampled from each patient undergoing a CHB. A set comprises two samples of bladder tissue: the first is sampled superficially, and the second is sampled from deep bladder tissue (muscularis propria). The guidelines for sampling the bladder tissue are: (a) if the patient has a Hunner's patch, then two sets, not closer than 5 mm of each other, are sampled in the area of the patch; (b) if the patient does not have a Hunner's patch but has glomerulations, then two sets, not closer than 5 mm of each other, are sampled in the area of the glomerulations; (c) if the patient does not have a Hunner's patch or glomerulations, then two sets, not closer than 5 mm of each other, are randomly sampled from the posterior bladder wall. The third set of tissue is always sampled from the trigonal area.

Immediately following acquisition, the specimen set sampled from the most diseased area is forwarded to the clinical center's local pathology lab for clinical evaluation. Subsequently, the local pathology lab creates six to ten unstained microscope slides from the specimen set and forwards them to the APL for storage in the ICDB specimen bank. The other two specimen sets (one from a diseased area, one from the trigone) are forwarded immediately to the APL in paraformaldehyde-lysine, a weak cross-linking fixative. The vials are shipped in a polystyrene foam mailing box for express delivery to the APL within 24 hr. Specimens and slides shipped from the clinical centers to the APL are tracked to ensure safe delivery. To date, all shipments have been successful.

Specimen Processing and Banking

As soon as specimen sets arrive at the APL, a research technician processes the tissue and prepares an initial set of 56 serial 5-μm sections. Four (4) of the 56 sections are stained as follows: sections 1 and 56 are stained with hematoxylin and eosin (H&E) stain; section 20 is stained with trichrome stain, and section 25 with a long toluidine blue stain. Three of the 56 sections are used to perform the following immunohistochemical studies using an avidin–biotin complex technique: section 30 with LCA (CD45); section 31 with S-100; and section 32 with Factor VIII. If a section is technically inadequate, the next closest section is selected for staining. Slides are labeled by an identification number and then filed in a slide cabinet for later retrieval. To date, the APL has received 206 specimens and has prepared 23,062 slides.

The unsectioned tissue remaining in the paraffin blocks is logged and stored for future use. The vials containing the weak cross-linking fixative in which the specimens were transported are labeled by corresponding identification number and banked for future use. Pilot studies indicate that fixed proteins may be suitable for electrophoretic analysis.

Specimen Review by Pathology Reading Group

By way of a round-robin mailing, each member of the Pathology Reading Group independently evaluates each specimen set for various histopathologic features described in the next section. The first reviewer (Dr. Tomaszewski) evaluates the specimen set and completes the biopsy data form. He then forwards his completed data form to the DCC for immediate processing and data quality validation. Once the DCC confirms that there are no data quality problems, Dr. Tomaszewski forwards the specimen set to the second reviewer (Dr. Williams) for his review. Similarly, he reviews the slides, forwards his completed biopsy data form to the DCC for data quality confirmation, and then forwards the slides to the final reviewer (Dr. Russak) for similar handling. When the round-robin mailing is complete, the specimen set is placed back in storage at the APL bank, and the DCC is in possession of three independently completed biopsy data forms. The DCC runs a computerized algorithm to assess the level of agreement among the three reviewers for each specimen set. In cases of less than perfect agreement, statistically generated scores are created.

Biopsy Data

The PRG evaluates each specimen set on as many as 39 different histopathologic features (Table 4). The specimen set used by the clinical center's local pathology lab to prepare unstained slides is evaluated on 17 features, and the two specimen sets used by the APL to prepare stained slides are evaluated on 39 features. For most cases, the PRG evaluates the quantitative distribution of a feature using an asymmetric scoring system. For example, to perform a semiquantitative distribution of fibrosis of the detrusor muscle, the PRG must estimate whether fibrosis is represented in 0%, 1% to 10%, 11% to 40%, or more than 40% of the muscularis propria space.

In addition to the PRG review, slides stained with long toluidine blue and tryptase are also independently reviewed

TABLE 4. *Pathologic features evaluated by the pathology reading group*

Unstained and H&E-stained sections
- Status of urothelium: denuded? discontinuities? wedge-shaped ulcerations?
- Presence of granulation tissue lamina propria?
- Quantitative distribution of mucosa denuded of urothelium?
- Quantitative distribution of submucosal hemorrhage?
- Quantitative distribution of submucosal granulation tissue?
- Presence of hyperplastic muscularis mucosa?
- Presence of eosinophilia in urothelium, lamina propria or muscularis propria?
- Presence of mononuclear endothelitis?
- Presence of transmural mononuclear vasculitis?
- Presence of detrusor myopathy: vacuolar degeneration? nuclear pyknosis? nuclear karyorrhexsis?
- Presence of mucosal edema?
- Presence of urothelial metaplasia: squamous? mucinous? nephrogenic? glandular?
- Presence of reactive urothelial change?
- Presence of urothelial hyperplasia?

LCA-stained sections
- Quantitative distribution of urothelial, lamina propria, and muscularis propria hematopoietic cells?
- Qualitative distribution of lamina propria and muscularis propria infiltrate: diffuse? aggregated? diffuse and aggregated?

Trichrome-stained sections
- Dominant quality of the lamina propria collagen: dense? loose?
- Quantitative distribution of fibrosis of detrusor muscle?

S-100-stained sections
- Quantitative distribution of nerves in lamina propria and muscularis propria?
- Quantitative distribution of positive mononuclear cells in lamina propria?
- Presence of perineural inflammation?

F8-stained sections
- Quantitative distribution of vessels in muscularis propria and lamina propria?
- Qualitative distribution of vessels in muscularis propria and lamina propria: random? clustered?

by the research technician at the APL for mast cells. Quantitative counts of the number of mast cells/mm^2 in the detrusor muscle, urothelium, and lamina propria are made using an optical reticle.

STUDY TIMETABLE

Protocol and data forms development proceeded rapidly after the selection of the data coordinating center in the summer of 1992. The Steering Committee met frequently during the fall of 1992 in order to develop the protocol, data collection forms, and manual of operations. A brief pilot study to test data collection and processing procedures began in March 1993, immediately following a 2-day training program for the Research Coordinators in Hershey, PA. The final versions of the data forms were completed in time for the main study to begin on May 1, 1993, followed immediately by on-site training visits to each clinical center in May and June, 1993, by DCC staff. In October 1993, the Steering Committee decided to implement a major forms revision based on quality assurance issues identified during the early months of patient accrual. The second and final version of the data collection forms, representing a reduction from 2,315 baseline screening variables to approximately 1,025, was made operational on January 1, 1994. The ICDB Study finished accruing patients on Decedmber 31, 1996, and the NIDDK extended patient accrual and follow-up through November 30, 1997.

PRELIMINARY RESULTS: ACCRUAL AND BASELINE DEMOGRAPHICS

As of September 29, 1995, 377 patients have completed base-line screening and are therefore enrolled in the ICDB Study. Of the 377 patients, 193 (51.1%) have been followed for at least 1 year, and 24 (6.4%) have been followed for at least 2 years. Patients enrolled in the ICDB Study are predominantly female (343 or 91.0%), white (346 or 91.8%), and middle-aged (188 or 49.9% in the age group from 35 to 54 years). As these patients are followed further, and more are enrolled, this large, multicenter ICDB Study represents a unique, first-time opportunity to investigate the longitudinal course of patients with symptoms consistent with IC.

Acknowledgments

This work was supported entirely by NIH grant U01 DK45859.

REFERENCES

1. Hand JR. Interstitial cystitis: report on 223 cases (204 women and 19 men). *J Urol* 1949;61:291–310.
2. Messing EM, Stamey TA. Interstitial cystitis: early diagnosis, pathology, and treatment. *Urology* 1978;12:381–392.
3. Kastrup J, Hald T, Larsen S, Nielsen VG. Histamine content and mast cell count of detrusor muscle in patients with interstitial cystitis and other types of chronic cystitis. *Br J Urol* 1983;55:495–500.
4. Fall M, Johansson SL, Vahlne A. A clinicopathological and virological study of interstitial cystitis. *J Urol* 1985;133:771–773.
5. Fall M, Johansson SL, Aldenborg F. Chronic interstitial cystitis: a heterogeneous syndrome. *J Urol* 1987;137:35–38.
6. Holm-Bentzen M, Jacobsen F, Nerstrom B, et al. Painful bladder disease: clinical and pathoanatomical differences in 115 patients. *J Urol* 1987;138:500–502.
7. Hanno P, Levin RM, Monson FC, et al. Diagnosis of interstitial cystitis. *J Urol* 1990;143;278–281.
8. Hanno PM, Staskin DR, Krane RJ, Wein AJ, eds. *Interstitial Cystitis*. New York: Springer-Verlag, 1990.
9. Hanno PM, ed. *Interstitial Cystitis*. Philadelphia: WB Saunders, 1994.
10. Gillenwater JY, Wein AJ. Summary of the National Institute of Arthritis, Diabetes, Digestive and Kidney Diseases workshop on interstitial cystitis, National Institutes of Health, Bethesda, Maryland, August 28–29, 1987. *J Urol* 1988;140:203–206.
11. Meinert CL. Quality assurance. In: *Clinical Trials: Design, Conduct, and Analysis*. New York: Oxford University Press, 1986;166–176.
12. Gassman JJ, Owen WW, Kuntz TE, Martin JP, Amoroso WP. Data quality assurance, monitoring, and reporting. *Controlled Clin Trials* 1995; 16(Suppl):104–136.

Interstitial Cystitis, edited by Grannum R. Sant.
Lippincott–Raven Publishers, Philadelphia ©1997.

CHAPTER 4

Idiopathic Cystitis in Cats: An Animal Model of Interstitial Cystitis

C.A. Tony Buffington, Dennis J. Chew, Bruce E. Woodworth, and Stephen P. DiBartola

The features of lower urinary tract disease (LUTD) in cats that have come to be known as the feline urologic syndrome (FUS) have been recognized in the veterinary literature since at least 1925 (1). Despite many studies of FUS during the intervening 70 years, there still is no consensus among veterinary urologists regarding the cause, or even the definition, of this frustrating disorder. The term *feline urologic syndrome* was first used in 1970 by Osbaldiston and Taussig (2), who concluded that FUS may not be a single disease. More recently, the opinion has been expressed that FUS should be redefined as feline urologic *signs* to emphasize that it is not a specific lower urinary tract disease (3).

Cats with LUTD present with variable combinations of dysuria, hematuria, pollakiuria, and urination in inappropriate locations. These signs can result from urolithiasis, urinary tract infection, neoplasia, congenital anomalies, and idiopathic inflammation of the lower urinary tract. In 1985, Lawler (4) reported that the overall incidence of these signs was 0.85% in the United States cat population. During a similar time, Kruger et al. (5) found that of 141 cats presenting to the University of Minnesota Veterinary Hospital with signs of LUTD, approximately 23% had struvite urolithiasis, 2% had urinary tract infection, and none had neoplasia or a congenital anomaly. No diagnosis could be made in 58% of female and 79% of unobstructed male cats. Interestingly, although diet has long been thought to be associated with signs of LUTD in cats (6), it was not reported to be associated with disease in any of these animals. It recently has been shown that the primary influence of dietary ingredients on the urinary tract is largely limited to effects on urolith formation (7).

In 1990, Clasper (8) suggested that some cases of idiopathic LUTD (iLUTD) in cats may be similar to interstitial cystitis (IC) in humans. Cats with iLUTD meet all the criteria for diagnosis of IC established by the National Institutes of Arthritis, Diabetes, Digestive and Kidney Diseases to ensure that studies of IC include reasonably comparable groups of patients, including a number of exclusion criteria (9):

1. Bladder capacity of >350 cc on awake cystometry using either a gas or a liquid filling medium.
2. Absence of an intense urge to void with the bladder filled to 1,200 cc of gas or 150 cc of water during cystometry, using a fill rate of 30 to 100 cc/min.
3. The demonstration of phasic involuntary bladder contractions on cystometry using the fill rate described above.
4. Duration of symptoms less than 9 months.
5. Absence of nocturia.
6. Symptoms relieved by antimicrobials, urinary antiseptics, anticholinergics, or antispasmodics.
7. A frequency of urinations while awake of less than eight times per day.
8. A diagnosis of bacterial cystitis or prostatitis within a 3-month period.
9. Bladder or ureteral calculi.
10. Active genital herpes.
11. Uterine, cervical, vaginal, or urethral cancer.
12. Urethral diverticulum.
13. Cyclophosphamide or any type of chemical cystitis.
14. Tuberculous cystitis.
15. Radiation cystitis.
16. Benign or malignant bladder tumors.
17. Vaginitis.
18. Age less than 18 years.

C. A. T. Buffington, D. J. Chew, and S. P. DiBartola: Department of Veterinary Clinical Sciences, The Ohio State University, Columbus, Ohio 43210-1089.

B. E. Woodworth: Division of Urology, Department of Surgery, The Ohio State University, Columbus, Ohio 43214.

The above exclusion criteria were promulgated to assure that subjects in research studies of IC were reasonably comparable. In practice, criteria 4–6, 8, 9, 11, 12, 17, and 18 need not be ruled out to make the diagnosis (10). Cats with iLUTD meet all the criteria for diagnosis of IC that can be applied to animals. Although exclusion criteria 1 to 3 cannot be tested in awake cats, we have not observed involuntary contractions (at fill rates appropriate to cats) during urocystometric examination of 19 cats with iLUTD anesthetized with ketamine and xylazine *(unpublished observations).* Criterion 5 is hard to apply to cats because they are nondiurnal animals, so we have relied on client reports of increased frequency of urination. With the exception of criterion 18 (although the disease most commonly is seen in adult cats), the remaining criteria are met in cats with iLUTD. Unfortunately, as Hanno (10) recently concluded, "The diagnosis of interstitial cystitis is necessarily tightly linked to its definition, and until the latter is crystal clear, the former will continue to be murky." This conclusion surely also applies to the disease in cats.

The clinical presentation of iLUTD in cats and IC in human beings includes pain and increased urinary frequency and urgency. The increased licking of the caudal abdomen and genitalia by cats with iLUTD is consistent with reports of bladder pain experimentally induced in animals. For example, instillation of 30% xylene into the bladder of rats caused a significant increase in head turns toward the lower abdomen and licking of the lower abdomen or perineal region (11). In addition to these pain-like behaviors, cats with iLUTD usually resent handling and resist abdominal palpation, often vocalizing and attempting to bite during such examinations.

Although the frequency of efforts to urinate has not been quantitated in cats with iLUTD, owner reports and our clinical experience suggest that it is much greater than the normal frequency of two to three times per day. Urine volume produced during these episodes often is less than 2 ml. Urgency to urinate also may occur in cats with iLUTD, manifested by episodes of urination outside the litterbox. This behavior does not appear to be related to incontinence because only small volumes of urine usually are voided.

Results of urinalysis and urine culture in cats with iLUTD are similar to those in humans with IC. Microorganisms cannot reliably be cultured from the urine, and the urine is cytologically nondescript. Although iLUTD and IC are not thought to be infectious diseases, novel organisms reportedly have been cultured from some women with the disease (12). Whether these organisms are the cause or an effect of the disease remains to be determined. Moreover, some microorganisms might incite an inflammatory response that becomes self-sustaining but may no longer be present when the disease is recognized.

Hematuria is reported in patients of both species. Microscopic hematuria is reported more commonly in cats than it is in women, although it occurs in both species (5,13). This may be a result of etiologic differences between the two diseases, presentation at different stages of the disease, or the fact that veterinarians commonly collect urine by antepubic cystocentesis. For example, Kruger et al. (5) observed hematuria in 46% of urine samples collected from normal cats by cystocentesis. Macroscopic hematuria reportedly occurs in 11% to 35% of patients with IC (14). Similar data are not available for cats with iLUTD, but this range is in accord with our clinical experience.

Radiographic studies conducted in women to exclude other disorders are not helpful in diagnosing IC. Radiographic studies of cats for diagnosis of LUTD are much more common because of the limited availability of cystoscopy in veterinary medicine. Radiographic studies can be used to identify anatomic defects, neoplasia, and radiodense uroliths, which are not present in cats with iLUTD.

Although cystoscopy is required for diagnosis of IC in humans, the typical cystoscopic findings of prominent vascularity and submucosal petechial hemorrhages (glomerulations) following a second distention are shared with other bladder diseases (15). We and others (16) have observed lesions in cats with iLUTD that are indistinguishable from those found in humans. We have not observed them in the bladders of normal cats.

The diagnosis of iLUTD in cats thus rests on the same criteria as does the diagnosis of IC in humans: of "chronic irritative voiding symptoms, sterile and cytologically negative urine, and characteristic cystoscopic findings...along with failure to find a more objective cause for this clinical picture" (17).

Unfortunately, because the etiology of both diseases is unknown, similarities may be coincidental. To further examine the similarities and differences between iLUTD in cats and IC in human beings, we have evaluated cats with iLUTD for the presence of other abnormalities reported to occur in IC. To date, we have examined the histopathology, presence of substance-P-containing fibers in the bladder and substance P receptors in the bladder and spinal cord, urine glycosaminoglycan excretion, and bladder permeability of cats with iLUTD. We also have begun to study the differential effects of stress on normal cats and cats with iLUTD.

The histopathologic findings in patients with IC vary (18). The usual finding of a relatively normal epithelium and muscularis with submucosal edema and vasodilatation without remarkable inflammatory infiltrate is consistent with findings in many cats with iLUTD. These changes may result from release of substance P from sensory neurons in concentrations sufficient to produce vascular leakage, but not infiltration of granulocytes (19). Mast cells also have been found in bladder biopsy specimens of some (20) but not all women with IC (15) and in cats with iLUTD *(unpublished observations).* Problems with the study of mast cells include the presence of different subsets of mast cells that affect their detection by standard histologic techniques and the fact that their granules, to which commonly used stains bind, may be released by the distention that occurs before the biopsy specimen is obtained.

An increased density of nerve fibers containing substance P has been reported in some studies of the bladders of patients with IC (20–22), suggesting a role for neurogenic inflammation in the pathophysiology of IC. In contrast, others (23) have reported that the number of neurons positive for substance P immunoreactivity (SPIR) was not significantly greater in specimens from bladders of IC patients relative to bladders of patients with stress incontinence or vesicovaginal fistulas. Based on increased numbers of neurons positive for vasoactive intestinal polypeptide (VIP) and neuropeptide Y immunoreactivity, they concluded that the enhanced innervation of the bladder might represent an increase of sympathetic neurons. The absence of an increase in SPIR in specimens from the bladder of patients with IC was offered as evidence of the lack of effect of sensory nerve involvement in IC. Alternatively, reduced SPIR could have resulted from a disease-induced increase in neuropeptide release from sensory nerve fibers or from decreased storage of SP in these neurons (24,25). Moreover, Hohenfellner et al. (23) collected tissues from IC patients after hydrodistention, whereas control samples were collected from (presumably undistended) bladders during repair of stress incontinence. Bladder distention is known to stimulate release of substance P from sensory neurons (26), which would reduce SPIR.

To evaluate the role of substance P in the bladders of cats with iLUTD, we examined the presence and distribution of nerve fibers demonstrating SPIR by standard immunohistochemical methods in bladders from six normal cats and eight with LUTD presented to a local humane society for euthanasia. Presence of anatomic defects, neoplasia, urolithiasis, and urinary tract infection was ruled out in all animals. We found a modest increase in SPIR in the submucosa of bladders from cats with iLUTD relative to normal cats. We also examined bladder tissue of cats for the presence of SP receptors using ^{125}I-SP (27). Mammalian bladders usually express the NK_1 (high-affinity) or the NK_2 (low-affinity) SP receptor or both (28). In normal cat bladders, we identified the NK_2 receptor, but NK_1 receptors were at or below the threshold of detectability. In contrast, inflamed bladders had higher concentrations of NK_1 receptors, comparable to that of brain. These results suggest that increased expression of NK_1 SP binding sites is associated with inflammatory events in urinary bladders of cats. Whether they are a cause of, or are induced by, inflammation remains to be determined.

Further support for sensory neuron involvement in the pathogenesis of IC comes from studies of the effects of capsaicin, a pungent ingredient in hot peppers that stimulates a specific population of sensory neurons, on bladder function (29,30). Instillation of capsaicin into the bladders of five patients with hypersensitive bladders produced a concentration-dependent reduction in capacity and pressure threshold for micturition. Moreover, all patients reported disappearance or marked attenuation of their symptoms for a few days after capsaicin treatment, suggesting that capsaicin-sensitive sensory neurons are present in the human bladder (30). The urinary bladder of cats contains a similar population of neurons (31), which have been shown to respond to high intravesical pressure (80 cm water) and to intraluminal application of chemical irritants (32).

Stimulation of sensory neurons can induce local release of neurotransmitters even in the absence of a propagated action potential, a phenomenon referred to as the "axon reflex." This reflex appears to protect normal skin (33), stomach (34), and bladder (35) epithelium and also to play a role in neurogenic inflammatory processes in a variety of tissues, including skin (36), intestine (37), lung (38), joints (39), and bladder (26,40). Although neuropeptides are required for normal bladder function, neuropeptides released locally by sensory neurons after chemical or mechanical stimulation can dilate microvessels and increase vascular permeability, which may appear as glomerulations in the bladder wall (26). Neuropeptides also can degranulate mast cells (20,41), which may explain the finding of increased histamine concentrations in bladder effluent of IC patients after distention (42). Additionally, the depletion of neuropeptides shortly after distension may explain the reduction in pain reported by some IC patients after distension therapy.

Some patients with IC appear to have a functional defect of the urothelial glycosaminoglycan (GAG) layer (43). Such a defect might permit urine to penetrate the urothelium and induce inflammation. Studies in IC patients (44) have found urine GAG excretion to be lower than normal, which was attributed to increased binding of GAG to the damaged urothelium. Some qualitative differences in GAG composition between normal human beings and those with IC also have been reported (45). We also have found decreased GAG excretion in cats with iLUTD (46) (Fig. 1). Average urine GAG excretion was three times greater in 24-hr urine samples from normal cats than in urine from cats with iLUTD. In spot urine samples from normal cats, the GAG/Cr ratio was 2.4 times that found in symptomatic cats and twice that found in asymptomatic cats with iLUTD. Interestingly, although GAG excretion was less than normal in cats with iLUTD whether or not they were exhibiting signs of the disease at the time of urine collection, GAG excretion appeared to be further reduced by flares in signs of the disease. If this observation is confirmed by further study, it might suggest that some GAG-related abnormality predisposes patients to this disease.

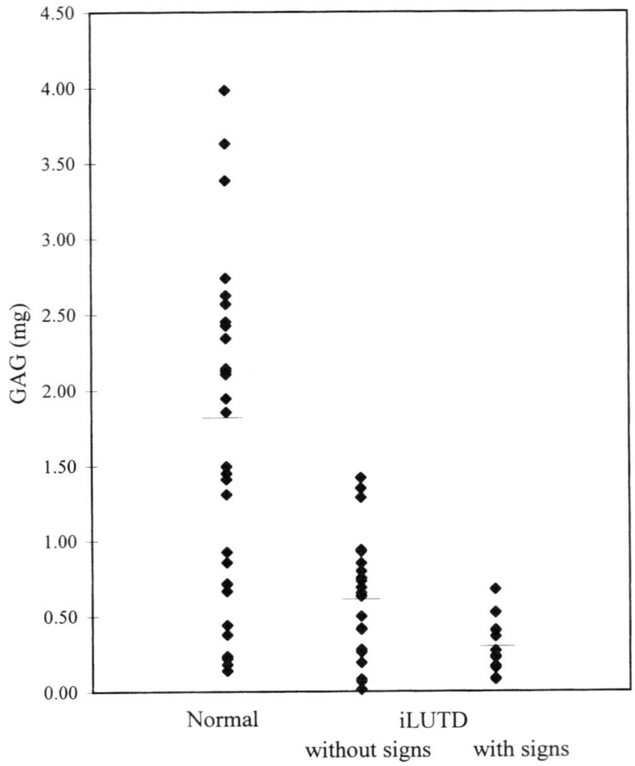

FIG. 1. Twenty-four-hour urine glycosaminoglycan (GAG) excretion in the urine of normal cats and cats with idiopathic lower urinary tract disease (iLUTD). Samples were collected from cats with iLUTD when they had signs of active disease as well as during periods of remission. (From Gao et al., ref. 51, with permission.)

As discussed above, one consequence of defects in the urothelial GAG layer is thought to be increased permeability (47,48). Parsons et al. (48) instilled urea into the bladders of normal subjects and patients with IC, drained the bladders after 45 min, and determined the amount of urea that could not be recovered. They found decreased urea recovery from the bladders of patients with IC, providing indirect evidence of differences in permeability. The smaller recovery of urea from IC patients than from normal controls may have resulted from the fact that patients, but not controls, underwent cystoscopy before the urea study. If greater bladder filling occurred in these patients, the permeability of their bladders might have been affected. In this regard, Tammela et al. (49) have shown that increasing intravesicular pressure of rabbit bladders *in vitro* to approximately 20 cm water can significantly increases bladder permeability.

Increased SP release from stimulated C-fibers also could influence bladder permeability; although SP probably plays a role in the maintenance of epithelial barrier function, it also can increase (pulmonary) epithelial permeability (50). These findings provide an additional possible mechanism for the increased bladder permeability found in patients with IC. To study bladder permeability more directly, we measured bladder epithelial permeability of healthy cats and cats with iLUTD using sodium salicylate (51) (Fig. 2). The apparent bladder absorption rate constant and the peak plasma concentration of sodium salicylate in cats with iLUTD were seven to eight times greater than those of healthy cats. These data indicate a significantly higher bladder permeability to salicylate in iLUTD.

The increased bladder permeability observed in cats with iLUTD and women with IC may result from local inflammation associated with increased activity of the disease or be part of some defect underlying the disease. Not all researchers have found increased permeability of bladders of patients with IC, however. When ^{99m}Tc-DTPA was used to assess bladder permeability for 30 min in women with IC, no statistically significant difference was found from women with normal urologic function (52). The average percentage absorption of the ten women with IC was 1.8 times that observed in the normal women, however, and a (two-tailed) p value of 0.075 was

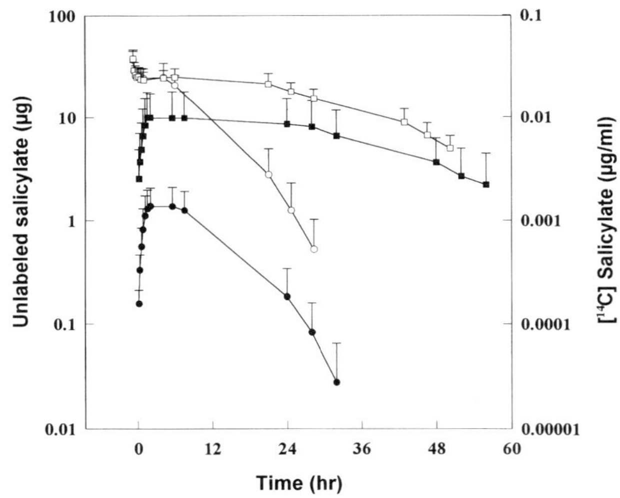

FIG. 2. Plasma concentration–time profiles of ^{14}C-salicylate and unlabeled salicylate after concomitant administration of intravenous and intravesical doses. Cats were given an intravesical dose of unlabeled sodium salicylate (25 mg/kg) via a urethral catheter and, 5 min later, an intravenous dose of ^{14}C-salicylic acid (6 mg/kg) via femoral vein. Data represent mean + 1 SD of five healthy cats *(circles)* and five iLUTD cats *(squares)*. ^{14}C-Salicylate concentrations are represented by *open symbols,* and unlabeled salicylate concentrations by *closed symbols.* Note that for two of the healthy cats, the salicylate concentrations were below the detection limit at 1920 min; these data were entered as 0 in the calculation of the mean concentration, which resulted in a mean concentration lower than the detection limit of 0.5 mg/ml.

reported. Because the absorption of the tracer from the bladder of patients was so much greater during the short period of study, the risk of a type II statistical error seems high. The molecular diameters of salicylate (~5 Å) and urea (~4 Å) are smaller than that of ^{99m}Tc-DTPA, the diameter of which is approximately 11 Å. Probe size has been suggested to be an important criterion for study of permeability of other epithelia (53,54) and may underlie differences in permeability studies of the bladder that have used molecules of differing sizes and geometries.

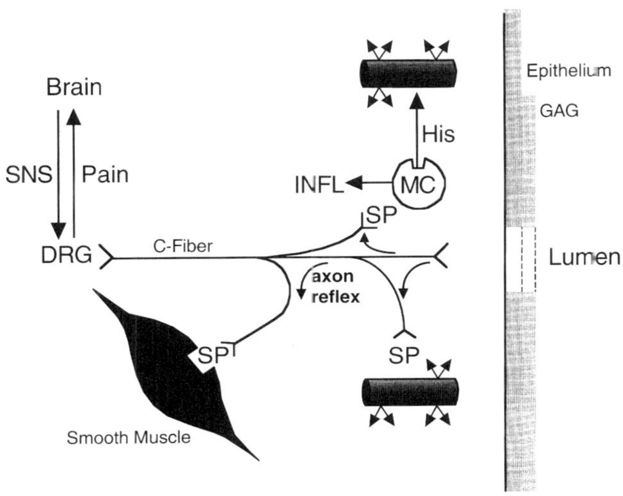

FIG. 3. Neurogenic inflammation as it affects the urinary bladder. Sensory neurons (C-fibers) seem to play a central role in transmission of action potentials via the dorsal root ganglia (DRG). These signals are perceived as painful by the brain. Sensory fibers also can propagate a local axon reflex without transmission of an action potential. The axon reflex results in release of peptide neurotransmitters such as substance P (SP) by the nerve endings. Interaction of SP with receptors on vessel walls results in vascular leakage that can be augmented by SP-induced release of histamine by mast cells. These actions may give rise to the submucosal petechial hemorrhages observed at cystoscopy. Receptors for SP also occur on smooth muscle and, when activated, stimulate muscle contraction. Also shown are the urothelium (epithelium) and the overlying glycosaminoglycan (GAG) layer adjacent to the bladder lumen. Damage or malfunction of either or both of these layers may permit constituents of the urine, such as protons, potassium ions, or hyperosmolar (>2,000 mOsm/liter) fluid to activate the sensory fibers. The effects of stress on sensory fibers may be related to descending efferent sympathetic (SNS) signals stimulating the DRG and inducing peripheral release of neuropeptides. Local release of neurotransmitters by bladder sympathetic fibers also could stimulate sensory fibers. Another factor probably involved in chronic bladder inflammation, but not shown, is local and systemic release of nerve growth factors, which may promote sensory fiber terminal sprouting to increase the size of sensory fiber receptive fields.

In both humans with IC and cats with iLUTD, symptoms of the disease tend to wax and wane. Whitmore (55) described IC as "...characterized by a flare and remission of irritative voiding symptoms..." and states that "remission occurs in 56.7% to 69% of patients (3 or more months without symptoms)..." and that "stress is likely the most significant flare factor for interstitial cystitis symptoms." Recurrence of clinical signs in association with aversive environmental stimuli also occurs in cats. For example, an increase in the number of cats presenting with signs of lower urinary tract disease was reported after the 1971 Sylmar–San Fernando earthquake in Southern California (56). Jones et al. (57) have reported that the two most common features of the history of cats presented for care of signs of LUTD are a move to a new home and a recent weather change. Many veterinarians have observed that increased numbers of cats present for care of signs of LUTD after major holidays and other disruptions in the cat's environment.

Based on the observed similarities in history, clinical signs, cystoscopy, bladder permeability, GAG excretion, sensory neuron changes, and exacerbation by stress, iLUTD in cats presents striking similarities to IC in humans. The occurrence of pain, submucosal petechial hemorrhages, and alterations in the innervation of the bladder of patients of both species suggests the participation of neurogenic inflammation (Fig. 3) in the pathophysiology of IC. If so, the bladder could be added to the list of other tissues, including the skin, lung, intestine, joint, and meninges, whose epithelia respond to some insults via this mechanism. It also may be relevant that patients with IC appear to be at increased risk for diseases of these other tissues (58). Moreover, all these diseases are exacerbated by stress in some humans and cats. This observation suggests that sensory nerve fibers may be activated by efferent sympathetic signals, either centrally or peripherally (23,59–61), and may partly explain the beneficial effects of antidepressant medications observed in both humans and cats (62). Finally, bladder pain is a well-recognized experimental example of visceral pain in cats (63). Visceral pain can sensitize both peripheral and central neurons, lowering the painful response threshold to subsequent noxious (hyperalgesia) and physiological (allodynia) stimulation. These and many other hypotheses concerning IC can be tested directly in subjects with the naturally occurring disease. The recognition that IC also may occur in cats may be exploited to study many of the chronic aspects of the disease in humans and possibly to test promising new therapies.

Acknowledgments

Research was supported by grants from the NIDDK (47538), the Interstitial Cystitis Association, and the Winn Foundation.

REFERENCES

1. DiBartola SP, Buffington CA. Feline urological syndrome. In: Slatter D, ed. *Textbook of Small Animal Surgery*, 2nd ed. Philadelphia: WB Saunders, 1993;1473–1487.
2. Osbaldiston GW, Taussig RA. Clinical report on 46 cases of feline urological syndrome. *Vet Med Small Anim Clin* 1970;65:461–468.
3. Osborne CA, Kruger JM, Lulich JP, Polzin DJ. Feline lower urinary tract diseases. In: Ettinger SJ, Feldman EC, eds. *Textbook of Veterinary Internal Medicine*, 4th ed. Philadelphia: WB Saunders, 1995; 1805–1832.
4. Lawler DF, Sjolin DW, Collins JE. Incidence rate of feline lower urinary tract disease in the United States. *Feline Pract* 1985;15:13–16.
5. Kruger JM, Osborne CA, Goyal SM. Clinical evaluation of cats with lower urinary tract disease. *J Am Vet Med Assoc* 1991;199:211–216.
6. Buffington CAT. Lower urinary disease in cats: new problems, new paradigms. *J Nutr* 1994;124:2643S–2651S.
7. Buffington CAT, Chew DJ, DiBartola SP. Lower urinary tract disease in cats: Is diet still a cause? *J Am Vet Med Assoc* 1994;205:1524–1527.
8. Clasper M. A case of interstitial cystitis and Hunner's ulcer in a domestic shorthaired cat. *N Z Vet J* 1990;38:158–160.
9. Gillenwater JY, Wein AJ. Summary of the National Institute of Arthritis, Diabetes, Digestive and Kidney Diseases workshop on interstitial cystitis. *J Urol* 1988;140:203–206.
10. Hanno PM. Diagnosis of interstitial cystitis. *Urol Clin North Am* 1994;21:63–66.
11. Abelli L, Conte B, Somma V, Maggi CA, Guiliani S, Meli A. A method for studying pain arising from the urinary bladder in conscious, freely-moving rat. *J Urol* 1989;141:148–151.
12. Domingue GJ, Ghoniem GM, Bost KL, Fermin C, Human LG. Dormant microbes in interstitial cystitis. *J Urol* 1995;153:1321–1326.
13. Holm-Bentzen M, Jacobsen F, Nerstrom B, et al. Painful bladder disease: clinical and pathoanatomical differences in 115 patients. *J Urol* 1987;138:500–502.
14. Koziol JA, Clark DC, Gittes RF, et al. The natural history of interstitial cystitis: A survey of 374 patients. *J Urol* 1993;149:465–469.
15. Pontari MA, Hanno PM. Interstitial cystitis. In: Walsh PC, Retik AB, Stamey TA, Vaughan ED, Wein AJ, eds. *Campbell's Urology*, update 14. Philadelphia: WB Saunders, 1995;1–19.
16. McCarthy TC, McDermaid SL. Cystoscopy. *Vet Clin North Am Small Anim Pract* 1990;20:1315–1339.
17. Messing EM. Interstitial cystitis and related syndromes. In: Walsh PC, Retik AB, Stamey TA, Darracott-Vaughan E Jr., eds. *Campbell's Urology, 3rd ed.* Philadelphia: WB Saunders, 1992;982–1005.
18. Johansson SL, Fall M. Pathology of interstitial cystitis. *Urol Clin North Am* 1994;21:55–62.
19. Walsh DT, Weg VB, Willams TJ, Nourshargh S. Substance P-induced inflammatory responses in guinea-pig skin: The effect of specific NK_1 receptor antagonists and the role of endogenous mediators. *Br J Pharmacol* 1995;114:1343–1350.
20. Pang X, Marchand J, Sant GR, Kream RM, Theoharides TC. Increased number of substance P positive nerve fibres in interstitial cystitis. *Br J Urol* 1995;75:744–750.
21. Hamid QA, Rode J, Flanagan AM, et al. Endocrine differentiation in inflamed urinary bladder epithelium with metaplastic changes. *Virchows Arch [A] Pathol Anat Histopathol* 1988;412:267–272.
22. Christmas, TJ, Rode, J, Chapple, CR, Milroy, EJG, Turner-Warwick, RT. Nerve fibre proliferation in interstitial cystitis. *Virchows Arch [A] Pathol Anat Histopathol* 1990;416:447–451.
23. Hohenfellner M, Nunes L, Schmidt RA, Lampel A, Thuroff JW, Tanagho EA. Interstitial cystitis: increased sympathetic innervation and related neuropeptide synthesis. *J Urol* 1992;147:587–591.
24. Mapp PI, Kidd BL, Gibson SJ, et al. Substance P–, calcitonin gene-related peptide-and C-flanking peptide of neuropeptide Y-immunoreactive fibres are present in normal synovium but depleted in patients with rheumatoid arthritis. *Neuroscience* 1990;37:143–153.
25. Donnerer J, Schuligoi R, Stein C. Increased content and transport of substance P and calcitonin gene-related peptide in sensory nerves innervating inflamed tissue: evidence for a regulatory function of nerve growth factor *in vivo*. *Neuroscience* 1992;49:693–698.
26. Maggi CA. The role of peptides in the regulation of the micturition reflex: an update. *Gen Pharmacol* 1991;22:1–24.
27. Wolfe SA, Sokolov AG, Buffington CAT: *Effects of interstitial cystitis on bladder and spinal cord tachykinin receptor concentrations in cats.* Paper presented at Society for Neuroscience meeting, San Diego, CA, 1995.
28. Maggi CA, ed. *Nervous Control of the Urogenital System.* Chur: Harwood Academic Publishers, 1993.
29. Maggi CA, Lecci A, Abelli L, Guiliani S. The role of capsaicin-sensitive afferents in the genesis of visceral pain and inflammation. In: Vecchiet L, Albe-Fessard D, Lindblom V, Gamberardino MA, eds. *New Trends in Referred Pain and Hyperalgesia.* New York: Elsevier Science, 1993;161–175.
30. deGroat WC, Fowler CJ, Jewkes D, McDonald WI, Lynn B. Intravesical capsaicin for neurogenic bladder dysfunction. *Lancet* 1992;339: 1239.
31. deGroat WC, Kawatani M, Houston MB, Rutigliano M, Erdman S. Identification of neuropeptides in afferent pathways to the pelvic viscera of the cat. In: Ciriello J, Calaresu F, Renaud L, Polosa C, eds. *Organization of the Autonomic Nervous System: Central and Peripheral Mechanisms, Neurology and Neurobiology.* New York: Alan R Liss, 1987;81–90.
32. Habler HJ, Janig W, Koltzenburg M. Activation of unmyelinated afferent fibres by mechanical stimuli and inflammation of the urinary bladder in the cat. *J Physiol* 1990;425:545–562.
33. Maggi CA, Borsini F, Santicioli P, et al. Cutaneous lesions in capsaicin-pretreated rats—a trophic role of capsaicin-sensitive afferents? *Naunyn Schmiedebergs Arch Pharmacol* 1987;336:538–545.
34. Holzer P, Livingston EH, Saria A, Guth PH. Sensory neurons mediate protective vasodilatation in rat gastric mucosa. *Am J Physiol* 1991;260: G363–G370.
35. Maggi CA, Meli A. The sensory–efferent function of capsaicin-sensitive nerves. *Gen Pharmacol* 1988;19:1–43.
36. Breneman DL, Cardone JS, Blumsack RF, Lather RM, Searle EA, Pollack VE. Topical capsaicin for treatment of hemodialysis-related pruritus. *J Am Acad Dermatol* 1992;26:91–94.
37. Eysselein VE, Reinshagen M, Patel A, Davis W, Nast C, Sternini C. Calcitonin gene-related peptide in inflammatory bowel disease and experimentally induced colitis. *Ann NY Acad Sci* 1992;657:319–327.
38. Barnes PJ. Neuropeptides and asthma. *Am Rev Respir Dis* 1991;143: S28–S32.
39. Larsson J, Ekblom A, Henriksson K, Lundberg T, Theodorsson E. Concentration of substance P, neurokinin A, CGRP, NPY, and VIP in synovial fluid from knee joints in patients suffering from rheumatoid arthritis. *Scand J Rheum* 1991;20:326–335.
40. Maggi CA. Capsaicin and primary afferent neurons, from basic science to human therapy. *J Auton Nerv Syst* 1991;33:1–14.
41. Dray A. Neuropharmacological mechanisms of capsaicin and related substances. *Biochem Pharmacol* 1992;44:611–615.
42. Yun SA, Laub DJ, Weese DL, Lad PM, Leach GE, Zimmern PE. Stimulated release of urine histamine in interstitial cystitis patients. *J Urol* 1992;148:1145–1148.
43. Parsons CL. A model for the function of glycosaminoglycans in the urinary tract. *World J Urol* 1994;12:38–42.
44. Hurst RE, Parsons CL, Roy JB, Young JL. Urinary glycosaminoglycan excretion as a laboratory marker in the diagnosis of interstitial cystitis. *J Urol* 1993;149:31–35.
45. Holm-Bentzen M, Ammitzboll T, Hald T. Glycosaminoglycans on the surface of the human urothelium: a preliminary report. *Neurourol Urodyn* 1986;5:519–523.
46. Buffington CAT, Blaisdell JL, Binns SP, Woodworth BE. Decreased urine glycosaminoglycan excretion in cats with inflammatory bladder syndrome. *J Urol* 1996;155:1801–1804.
47. Lilly JD, Parsons CL. Bladder surface glycosaminoglycans: A human epithelial permeability barrier. *Surg Gynecol Obstet* 1990;171:493–496.
48. Parsons CL, Lilly JD, Stein P. Epithelial dysfunction in nonbacterial cystitis. *J Urol* 1991;145:732–735.
49. Tammela T, Wein AJ, Monson FC, Levin RM. Urothielial permeability of the isolated whole bladder. *Neurourol Urodyn* 1993;12:39–47.
50. Petersson G, Svensjo E. Nasal mucosal permeability after methacholine, substance P, and capsaicin challenge in the rat. *Int J Microcirc Clin Exp* 1992;9:205–212.
51. Gao X, Buffington CAT, Au JLS. Effect of interstitial cystitis on drug absorption from urinary bladder. *J Pharmacol Exp Ther* 1994;271: 818–823.

52. Chelsky MJ, Rosen SI, Knight LC, Maurer AH, Hanno PM, Ruggieri MR. Bladder permeability in interstitial cystitis is similar to that of normal volunteers: direct measurement by transvesical absorption of ^{99m}technetium-diethylenetriaminepentaacetic acid. *J Urol* 1994;151: 346–349.
53. Hollander D. The intestinal permeability barrier. A hypothesis as to its regulation and involvement in Crohn's disease. *Scand J Gastroenterol* 1992;27:721–726.
54. Malik A, Lynch J, Cooper J. Endothelial barrier function. *J Invest Dermatol* 1989;93:62S–67S.
55. Whitmore K. Self-care regimens for patients with interstitial cystitis. *Urol Clin North Am* 1994;21:121–130.
56. Caston HT. Stress and the feline urological syndrome. *Feline Pract* 1973;4(6):14–22.
57. Jones BR, Sanson RL, Morris RS. *Elucidating the risk factors of feline urologic syndrome.* Paper presented at WSAVA, Durban South Africa, 1994.
58. Koziol JA. Epidemiology of interstitial cystitis. *Urol Clin North Am* 1994;21:7–20.
59. Weihe E. Neurochemical anatomy of the mammalian spinal cord: functional implications *Ann Anat* 1992;174:89–118.
60. Jänig W, McLachlan EM. The role of modifications in noradrenergic peripheral pathways after nerve lesions in the generation of pain. In: Fields HL, Liebeskind JC, eds. *Progress in Pain Research and Management, Vol 1. Pharmacological Approaches to the Treatment of Chronic Pain: New Concepts and Critical Issues*. Seattle: IASP Press, 1994;163–192.
61. Perl ER. A reevaluation of mechanisms leading to sympathetically related pain. In: Fields HL, Liebeskind JC, eds. *Progress in Pain Research and Management, Vol 1. Pharmacological Approaches to the Treatment of Chronic Pain: New Concepts and Critical Issues*. Seattle: IASP Press, 1994;163–192.
62. Huangfu D, Goodwin WB, Guyenet PG. Sympatholytic effect of tricyclic antidepressants: site and mechanism of action in anesthetized rats. *Am J Physiol* 1995;268:R1429–R1441.
63. Koltzenburg M, McMahon SB. Mechanically insensitive primary afferents innervating the urinary bladder. In: Gebhart GF, ed. *Progress in Pain Research and Management, Vol 5. Visceral Pain*. Seattle: IASP Press, 1995;163–192.

Interstitial Cystitis, edited by Grannum R. Sant.
Lippincott–Raven Publishers, Philadelphia ©1997.

CHAPTER 5

Experimental Autoimmune Cystitis: An Autoimmune Model for Interstitial Cystitis

Carl G. Klutke, Arnold D. Bullock, and Timothy D. Ratliff

Interstitial cystitis (IC) is a condition of unknown etiology that has several features of an autoimmune disease. Equivocal evidence and lack of a suitable animal model to study this pathogenetic hypothesis have hampered investigation. Recently, several animal models have been introduced that may provide insight into the role of the immune response in interstitial cystitis. In this chapter we review some general concepts of autoimmunity, look at what evidence does exist for and against IC as a disease of inappropriate immunologic responsiveness, and finally review the autoimmune mouse model: experimental autoimmune cystitis .

GENERAL CONCEPTS OF AUTOIMMUNITY

Immunologic reactivity to self antigens is well described for a number of diseases. Of these various autoimmune diseases, the common pathologic flaw is that circulating antibodies react with normal body constituents. Patients frequently have increased immunoglobulins in the serum, and these antibodies may appear in each of the main immunoglobulin classes. There is a greater incidence of autoimmune diseases in women. The disease process is not always progressive: exacerbations and remissions, sometimes complete, are frequently seen. Autoantibody tests are of diagnostic value (1).

On the basis of clinical, serologic, and genetic criteria, the immunologic response is customarily divided into organ-specific (thyrogastric) and non-organ-specific (lupus) groups (2). The organ-specific group of autoimmune diseases is notable for antibodies that are organ-specific and have a familial tendency. In this group of autoimmune diseases, although the affected organ is removed or the disease destroys the tissue antigens, the antibodies nevertheless remain constant or decrease slowly in the course of years. Therapy for the disease is usually aimed at replacing specific hormones. Examples of organ-specific autoimmune disease include myasthenia gravis, Graves' disease, insulin-resistant diabetes, and diabetes mellitus. In the latter disease, a cell-mediated response to islet cells destroys the insulin-producing capacity of the individual. In the remaining autoimmune disorders, antibody to the acetylcholine receptor, thyroid-stimulating hormone receptor, or insulin receptor, respectively, induces the disease.

By comparison, the non-organ-specific immune diseases are characterized by the presence of serum antibodies to intracellular components. Examples include rheumatoid arthritis and systemic lupus erythematosis (SLE). Rheumatoid arthritis is characterized by the presence of autoantibodies to the Fc region of IgG (rheumatoid factor). Although this antibody is characteristic of the disease, it may not be the cause of the disorder. Trentham and associates have observed T-cell reactivity to type II or III collagen in 75% of patients tested to date, suggesting a cellular cause (3). In SLE, high serologic titers of antinuclear antibodies are characteristic of the disease; however the specific inducing agent is unknown.

The type of immune response can also be classified as to the effector arm responsible for the immune reaction. These can be humoral, cellular, or both. The humoral response involves antibody production from B lymphocytes, whereas a primarily cell-mediated response involves the actions of T cells. The T cells responsible for cell-mediated response are further divided into two main regulatory lymphocyte phenotypes, the helper and suppressor/cytotoxic T cells. The various T-lymphocyte phe-

C. G. Klutke: Department of Surgery/Division of Urology, Washington University Medical Center, St. Louis, Missouri, 63110.

A. D. Bullock: Department of Surgery/Division of Urology, Washington University School of Medicine, St. Louis, Missouri 63110.

T. L. Ratliff: Department of Urology, University of Iowa, Iowa City, Iowa, 52242.

notypes can be differentiated by monoclonal antibodies against cell markers. The helper/inducer T cells are predominantly CD4-positive (cluster designation nomenclature) and are detected by antibodies specific for that marker (4). Similarly, suppressor/cytotoxic T cells are predominantly CD8-positive (5). Although much attention has been given to a possible antibody-related mechanism in interstitial cystitis, few studies have addressed the role of cell-mediated immunity.

INTERSTITIAL CYSTITIS

What is interstitial cystitis? Probably the clearest answer at present is that interstitial cystitis is one of the most disabling nonmalignant disorders seen by the urologist. It is an uncommon disease whose hallmarks are a triad of irritative voiding symptoms, sterile cytologically negative urine, and characteristic cystoscopic appearance. The fact that the diagnosis of interstitial cystitis is first and foremost made by exclusion results from the lack of a distinctive marker of the disease. Variable signs of chronic inflammation within the bladder are frequently seen with IC, and although the mast cell seems to play a role in some cases, it is conspicuously absent in others. Although numerous theories of pathogenesis have been proposed, the etiology of this disorder remains unknown, and, therefore, interstitial cystitis at present represents little more than a symptom complex. The hypothesized causes of interstitial cystitis include infectious, lymphovascular obstructive, neurogenic, endocrinologic, psychoneurotic, inflammatory, and autoimmune pathologies.

One well-known aspect of this enigmatic disease is that it can be classified into two rather distinct groups—classic and early—based on cystoscopic findings, histology, and, to a certain extent, clinical behavior (6). Classic or ulcer-type interstitial cystitis is identified by the presence of a single or multiple ulcerations within the bladder seen on cystoscopy. This so-called Hunner's ulcer is described as an area of reddened mucosa with central scar that ruptures with increasing bladder distention. Histologically, classic interstitial cystitis is associated with marked infiltration with chronic inflammatory cells including mast cells (7). In contrast, early or nonulcer-type interstitial cystitis exhibits only petechial mucosal bleeding (glomerulations) on distention cystoscopically and, when biopsied, shows no or mild inflammatory changes such as edema and vascular dilation. The fact that the same symptom complex can be divided into groups on clinical and histologic grounds has led many researchers to believe that multiple disease processes may possibly be involved. More than one pathogenesis may very well be responsible for the symptoms and signs of interstitial cystitis, with an autoimmune mechanism being one of them.

Interstitial Cystitis as an Autoimmune Disease

Much clinical evidence has accumulated to support the hypothesis that IC is an immunologically mediated disease. From a clinical perspective, IC fits well with the typical picture of an autoimmune process. Up to 90% of patients are middle-aged or elderly women, and in many there is a high incidence of other autoimmune diseases such as rheumatoid arthritis, polyarteritis nodosa, and Hashimoto's thyroiditis (8). A history of drug hypersensitivity can be found in up to 70% of patients (9), and other atopic reactions are also more common (10). The disease process tends to wax and wane, and spontaneous remissions are not unusual (8,11,12). In some cases treatment with corticosteroids has been associated with amelioration of symptoms (13).

As with other autoimmune diseases, interstitial cystitis is associated with an accumulation of lymphocytes, plasma cells, and mast cells within the bladder (14,15). In this respect, there appear to be significant differences between the early and classic types of the disease. In a study by Harrington and associates, the nonulcer group had rare mucosal ruptures but no ulcers, slightly increased lymphoid cells, occasional T-cell aggregates, no B-cell nodules, and rare plasma cells. No statistically significant difference between control and nonulcerative interstitial cystitis patients was identified histologically. In contrast, the classic interstitial cystitis group had ulcers, intense inflammation with focal sheets of plasma cells, aggregates of T cells, B-cell nodules including germinal centers, a decreased or normal helper-to-suppressor cell ratio, and suppressor cytotoxic cells in germinal centers (16). Observations of increased mast cell density in biopsies of IC patients suggest that these cells may be important in pathogenesis (17,18). Here again, however, there appears to be a dichotomy between early and classic forms of the disease. In studies involving patients divided into classic versus early forms of interstitial cystitis, only those with the classic disease have elevated mast cells in the bladder (6,19). In peripheral blood, interstitial cystitis patients appear to exhibit essentially normal numbers of lymphocyte subsets (20).

Interstitial Cystitis as an Organ-Specific Autoimmune Disorder

Bladder-specific antibodies have been reported in IC, implying an antibody-mediated organ-specific autoimmune mechanism. Using indirect immunofluorescence, Silk and associates found circulating humoral antibodies reactive with allogeneic bladder in nine of 20 patients with interstitial cystitis (11). Similarly, Gordon and associates found deposits of immunoglobulin, particularly IgG and IgM, in the connective tissue of the lamina propria and most strikingly in some cases in sarcolemma or subsarcolemmal sites in the bladder muscle of patients with interstitial cystitis, further suggesting a specific response to bladder antigens (21). These findings stand in contrast, however, to reports by Jokinen et al., who found no organ-specific antibodies in their patients. Although tissue antibodies were found in serum samples with an incidence exceeding those in the control groups, they were only against non-organ-specific antigens (22).

Serum antibodies to Tamm–Horsfall protein, a glycoprotein produced in the ascending thick limb of the loop of Henle and released in substantial amounts into the urine, have been noted in patients following pyelonephritis (23). Antibodies to Tamm–Horsfall protein have also been found in a small subset of patients with severe interstitial cystitis in the absence of pyelonephritis, raising the possibility that interstitial cystitis involves the immune system reacting to this self protein and the bladder serving as a nonspecific target organ (24). These findings stand in contrast to those of Stone et al., however, who compared bladder biopsies from 14 interstitial cystitis patients to those from 11 normal controls and found neither a high incidence of Tamm–Horsfall protein in the mucosa of IC patients nor a significant difference in the incidence compared to control patients (25).

Interstitial Cystitis as a Non-Organ-Specific Autoimmune Process

Antinuclear antibodies, typical of SLE, have been identified in IC patients: Oravisto and associates noted antinuclear antibodies in 85% of patients tested (10). Further reports from this same group inferred that the increased antibodies suggest that IC belongs to that group of autoimmune diseases in which the disease is restricted to one organ, whereas the autoantibodies are non-organ-specific (26). This finding, however, remains controversial. In a study by Anderson et al., although IC patients demonstrated a nonspecific increase in antibody formation, this was not significantly different from a similar group of other urologic patients without IC. This lack of specificity implied that the immunologic response was more likely to be a secondary phenomenon associated with inflammatory damage to the bladder rather than the primary cause of the disease (27).

The deposition of immunoglobulins within the bladder vasculature was first reported by Helin et al. Immunofluoresence examination of biopsy specimens from IC patients and controls identified vascular deposition of immunoglobulin and complement, suggesting an immunologically mediated vascular injury (28). Subsequently, Gillespie and associates used immunofluorescent staining to identify immunoglobulins in biopsy specimens taken from patients with the diagnosis of interstitial cystitis compared to specimens taken from normal volunteers. The immunofluorescent staining patterns observed fell into four distinct categories: group 1, IgA and fibrinogen; group 2, IgM and fibrinogen; group 3, IgA, IgM, and fibrinogen; group 4, fibrinogen only, no control bladder biopsies exhibited immunoglobulin, complement, or fibrinogen (29).

Cell-Mediated Immunity in Interstitial Cystitis

A role for cell-mediated immune mechanisms in interstitial cystitis, at least in the classic form, can be inferred from the histopathology of the disease. Work by Harrington, Fall, and Johansson has shown intense inflammation with focal sheets of plasma cells, aggregates of T cells, B-cell nodules including germinal centers, a decreased or normal helper-to-suppressor cell ratio, and suppressor cytotoxic cells in germinal centers (16). Christmas et al. found infiltration of $CD4^+$, $CD8^+$ T cells and, unlike in normal control and bacterial cystitis bladders, $TCR\text{-}1^+$ (a type of $CD3^+/CD4^-/CD8^-$ T cell) T cells present (30).

Periperal blood examined in the study by Harrington et al. with flow cytometry revealed increased numbers of Ig-positive B cells and activated lymphocytes compared to controls. Looking only at early-type IC patients, another group has demonstrated normal lymphocyte populations in the peripheral blood, which is not supportive of an autoimmune mechanism in the disease (20). This same group has reported on the absence of increased T-cell proliferation or cytokine production in response to mitogen. In this study by Miller et al. comparing the *in vitro* function of peripheral blood lymphocytes from patients with early-type IC to those from healthy female controls, there was no difference in the rate of proliferation of the various lymphocyte phenotypes between the two groups in any of the culture media. Similarly, there was no difference between the two groups in the degree of lymphocytic activation after incubation. The authors thus concluded that there is no primary immunologic disorder evident in patients with interstitial cystitis and that the urine does not act as an immune stimulant (31). Unfortunately, this study does not look at classic-type IC, which appears to have a different histologic appearance.

Thus, the literature supporting immunologic mechanisms in interstitial cystitis is at best tenuous and often contradictory. Studies so far, however, have involved evaluating patients with IC, and the ability to identify fundamental biological mechanisms using clinical specimens has inherent limitations. Clinical specimens often extrapolate poorly to biological mechanisms. The introduction of artifact by nonphysiological conditions is an unavoidable condition when one deals with human subjects. Furthermore, when one is looking for something as subtle as immunologic evidence, human patients make difficult study subjects. These difficulties all emphasize the need for a laboratory animal model of IC.

EXPERIMENTAL AUTOIMMUNE INFLAMMATION

The murine experimental autoimmune cystitis model has its origins 100 years earlier in the field of neuroimmunology, when it was noted that sometimes fatal paralytic accidents occurred following immunization with the Pasteur rabies vaccine. The Pasteur rabies vaccine was prepared in rabbit CNS tissue, and subsequent experimental trials using either rabbit CNS tissue alone or killed virus in rabbit CNS yielded paralysis, indicating that the causative factor was related to the CNS tissue itself. This postrabies immunization encephalomyelitis eventually became known as experimental autoimmune neuritis and has proven to be the precursor of a vast field of research on delayed-hypersensitivity-type reactions, particularly to myelin antigens(32).

Experimental autoimmune neuritis (EAN) is an organ-specific, delayed-hypersensitivity-type disease inducible in a number of species by inoculation with a basic protein from myelin. It was formally described in 1955 by Waksman and Adams, who produced a fulminant inflammatory demyelinating condition in the rabbit with inoculum containing peripheral nerve (33). This model received relatively little attention until the late 1960s, when Ballin and Thomas and also Lampert, while characterizing the spontaneous demyelination and remyelination in the disease, noted selective removal of myelin by macrophages and relative preservation of axons (34,35). It is widely believed that multiple sclerosis, a disease associated with inflammatory demyelination, is the delayed clinical expression of an unknown acquired childhood infection and that the disease course, which is more typically chronic progressive or chronic relapsing, commonly spans three or more decades. In view of the existence of chronic, relapsing idiopathic polyneuritis in man, these animal diseases provided useful models.

Experimental allergic neuritis and, more importantly, the later developed experimental autoimmune encephalomyelitis (EAE) epitomize the cross-fertilization of neurology and immunology and have become the major applied models in multiple sclerosis research. The models involve induction of an active autoimmunogenic demyelination by the inoculation of animals with an encephalitogenic emulsion. The emulsion can contain whole white matter, spinal cord, or purified myelin and is organ-specific. In EAE, unequivocal roles for T and B cells are well documented (36). Firm parallels between EAE and multiple sclerosis cannot be drawn at this time, although points of similarity clearly exist between EAE and acute multiple sclerosis.

Attempts to manipulate the course of EAE and EAN in terms of both acceleration and suppression of the disease have been documented. The suppression of antibody responses by surgical destruction of the posterior hypothalamus in EAN-sensitized animals, a technique that is claimed to leave T-cell-mediated responses unimpaired, causes earlier, more severe onset of EAN (37). Modulation and suppression of acute EAE has been achieved with a wide variety of compounds including myelin basic protein, immunosuppressive drugs, and synthetic peptides (38–40). Although the evidence for specific immunologic changes in the human demyelinating diseases is still largely indirect, against the background of experimental autoimmune demyelination, the disease mechanism can be studied, and tools for manipulation can be tested.

AN EXPERIMENTAL AUTOIMMUNE CYSTITIS MODEL

With experimental autoimmune encephalomyelitis as a guide, we attempted to create experimental autoimmune cystitis in the mouse as a model for interstitial cystitis. An animal model for this disorder has not been developed in the past, for it was impossible to establish criteria for this poorly defined clinical entity. However, several histologic and immunologic features have been described in numerous studies using human tissue (19). Our goal was the development of a murine experimental autoimmune cystitis model with an immune-mediated inflammatory reaction within the bladder in response to antigen stimulation that correlated with the histologic features observed in interstitial cystitis and was associated with the functional and behavioral changes of IC (41).

Our specific objectives for the immunologically induced murine model were:

1. Develop a model with the typical histologic features of IC.
2. Identify susceptible strains of mice.
3. Determine time and dose curves for the appearance of the histologic changes.
4. Isolate the factor in the inoculum capable of inducing the cystitis.
5. Evaluate the immunologic basis for the histologic changes by defining the humoral and cell-mediated factors involved.
6. Perform adoptive transfer.

INDUCTION OF EXPERIMENTAL AUTOIMMUNE CYSTITIS

Mice

Young female mice from 8 to 10 weeks of age are used as syngeneic donors and recipients. In the initial study, several different inbred strains of mice were studied for their susceptibility to induction of immunologically induced cystitis (41). Mice of strains Balb/cANN, C57BL/6J, and C3H/HEN are obtained from the animal facility of Barnes-

Jewish Hospital of St. Louis, and Balb/cBYJ are obtained from the Jackson Laboratory, Bar Harbor, Maine. All animals were maintained in an environment with controlled temperature and light and with food and water available *ad libitum*.

Immunization

Syngeneic mouse bladder homogenate is prepared using tissue from inbred strains. The pooled fresh bladders are minced thoroughly using sterile technique over ice. This material is homogenized at 1,000 rpm in distilled water with 0.5% Triton X-100. After centrifugation at 1,000 rpm for 10 min, a microprotein assay is performed on the supernatant (Bio Rad, Richmond, CA), and aliquots can be stored at −70°C.

For immunization, the bladder homogenate is diluted in phosphate-buffered saline (PBS), 0.1 M, pH 7.2 for a final concentration of antigen of 0.5 mg in 50 μl. Immediately before immunization, the homogenate is emulsified with an equal volume of complete Freund's adjuvant (CFA, Difco Laboratories, Detroit, Michigan). The 0.1 ml of the emulsion is injected in divided dose into the hind footpads (intradermal) and the base of the tail (subcutaneous).

Control animals include normal mice, mice with bacterial cystitis *(Escherichia coli)*, and mice immunized with 0.1 ml of (1:1) PBS emulsified in CFA. Experimental *E. coli* cystitis is produced in BALB/c mice by subjecting them to urethral catheterization and instillation of approximately 10,000 colony-forming units of *E. coli* three times a week. Bacterial urinary tract infection was confirmed by urine culture postcatheterization.

Rabbits, guinea pigs, and mice have been used unsuccessfully in the past in efforts to develop immunologically induced animal models for interstitial cystitis (11). Similar to our model, Silk et al. subcutaneously injected syngeneic bladder extracts in rabbits, but their attempts failed to induce a reproducible cystitis. We used strains of mice that had been previously used to induce an experimental interstitial nephritis (42) and autoimmune orchitis (43).

Passive Sensitization (Adoptive Transfer)

The adoptive transfer of experimental autoimmune cystitis was performed according to a procedure described by Mahi-Brown et al. (43). Spleens and draining lymph nodes (popliteal, inguinal, and paraaortic) from mice of a reactive BALB/cANN group were isolated under sterile conditions 7 days after a booster immunization (0.5 mg homogenate in CFA, 1:1). Spleens and lymph nodes from animals immunized with CFA only were used as controls. The tissues were placed in PBS with 5% fetal calf serum (FCS), ground, and filtered through nylon gauze to produce single-cell suspensions of lymph nodes (LNC) and spleen cells (SpC). Erythrocytes in the SpC suspension were lysed with ACK, and both SpC and LNC were washed three times with PBS-FCS. The cells were suspended at 1.5×10^6 cells/ml in complete RPMI 1640 medium and cultured in 75-cm^2 plastic culture flasks with 25 ml of cells at 37°C, 5% CO_2 in air. To each flask concanavalin A at 3 μg/ml was added (Calbiochem, LaJolla, CA). After 2 days of culture, dead cells were removed by centrifugation on Hypaque 1083 (Sigma Chemical, St. Louis, MO). Viable cells were washed three times in PBS-FCS. Syngeneic recipients were injected intraperitoneally with 2.5×10^7 cells in 0.5 ml of PBS. The recipients were sacrificed 10 days to 1 month after cell transfer, and histologic quantitation was performed.

CLINICAL PARAMETERS OF EXPERIMENTAL AUTOIMMUNE CYSTITIS

In the initial study comparing various strains of mice, animals were injected at 2-week intervals for a maximum of three immunizations. We have subsequently observed that a comparable degree of cystitis can be induced with only a single injection. In the initial study, mice were sacrificed at 2 weeks, 4 weeks, 2 months, 4 months, and 6 months. Similar to the natural history of interstitial cystitis, experimental autoimmune cystitis was observed at 2 weeks and reaches a maximum at 4 weeks. This induced cystitis persists without progression for at least 6 months, and there is no spontaneous remission.

Grossly, the immunologically induced cystitis exhibits features found in interstitial cystitis including a contracted bladder capacity, fibrous thickening, increased vascularity and glomerulations after hydrodistention (Fig. 1). Measurements of bladder capacity in anesthetized control and antigen-immunized mice objectively

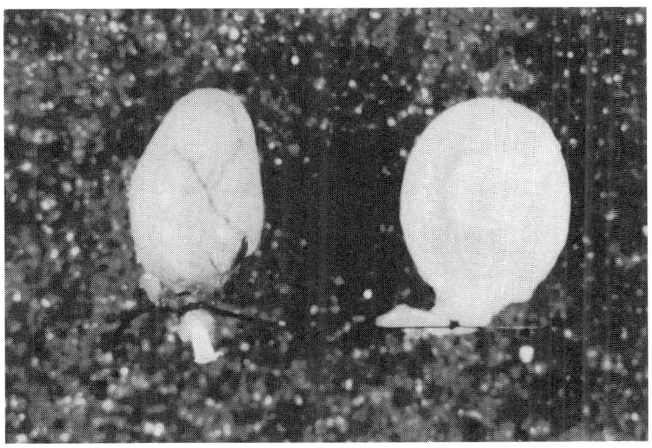

FIG. 1. The experimental autoimmune cystitis (EAC) bladder **(left)** is fibrotic and contracted with increased vascularity compared to the thin-walled normal bladder. See color plate 1.

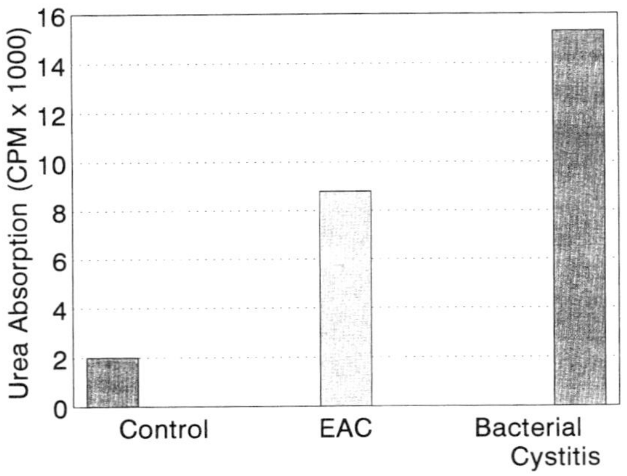

FIG. 2. Carbon 14-Urea Absorption. ^{14}C-Urea absorption studies show that the increased epithelial absorption in EAC bladders is not as extensive as in bacterial cystitis (which has greater epithelial destruction).

demonstrated the diminished bladder capacity that resulted from fibrosis and edema.

Two weeks after immunization with antigen or complete Freund's adjuvant only (control animals), mice were studied for bladder capacity. After the animal had been anesthetized with sodium pentobarbitol, the urethra was catheterized with a 24-gauge angiocatheter, and residual urine was withdrawn. A 1-ml syringe and PBS under approximately 40 cm of pressure were used to measure bladder capacity. There was a significant difference in bladder capacity between the immunized mice (mean volume 358 ± 29 µl), and the CFA-only controls (mean volume 462 ± 24 µl, $p < 0.02$).

Glomerulations after hydrodistention are a pathognomonic feature of interstitial cystitis. To aid in the demonstration of this characteristic of our EAC model, carbon black was injected intravenously in the antigen-immunized mice before bladder distention under anesthesia.

The studies by C. L. Parsons et al. that demonstrated increased permeability of the interstitial cystitis bladder are frequently referenced (43a–c). Similarly, we have demonstrated an increased permeability of the EAC bladders using ^{14}C-urea transport testing. ^{14}C-Urea (0.05 µCi in 100 µl) was placed intravesically into normal control mice, control mice with bacterial cystitis, and BALB/cANN mice with EAC. After 90 min, the kidneys and bladders were recovered. After rinsing of the tissues with PBS and tissue degradation in Scintigest (Fisher Scientific, St. Louis, MO), urea content was measured with a liquid scintillation counter. The absorption of ^{14}C-urea was significantly increased in mice immunized with syngeneic bladder extracts but not in the adjuvant-only control animals (Fig. 2).

HISTOPATHOLOGY

Cystectomy specimens from mice were fixed in 10% phosphate-buffered formalin for 24 to 36 hr before paraffin embedding. The fixed tissues were processed through xylene, embedded in paraffin, and sectioned at 6 µm for hematoxylin and eosin staining, and 7 µm for Mallory's trichrome staining.

For each specimen examined, at least two appropriately stained slides were prepared from different sampling areas of the bladder. Bladders were graded using an additive histologic scoring system. The histologic features are graded on a scoring system form 0 to +3, where 0 represents absence or nonpathologic involvement. The features are equally weighted and include:

1. Mucosal ulceration.
2. Acute inflammation (polymorphonuclear neutrophils).
3. Chronic inflammation (mononuclear inflammatory cells).
4. Volume density of mast cells, fractionated into:
   a. Detrusor mast cells.
   b. Submucosal and subserosal (extradetrusor) mast cells.
5. Superficial vascular ectasia.
6. Plasma cell density.
7. Edema.
8. Sub-basal-lamina (sub-basement-membrane) fibrosis.
9. Nerve fiber hypertrophy (in detrusor).

Marked variability was observed in the three mouse strains tested, and presently only the BALB/c mice are used, for only this strain reproducibly demonstrated histologic features similar to those observed in interstitial cystitis (19). In the initial studies, all specimens were

TABLE 1. *Comparative features of experimental autoimmune cystitis and interstitial and bacterial cystitis*

Features	Experimental autoimmune cystitis	Interstitial cystitis	Bacterial cystitis
Mucosal ulceration	Mild; urothelium remains intact	Variable	Severe; urothelial destruction
Submucosal fibrosis	Marked	Prominent	Minimal
Vascular ectasia	Prominent	Prominent	Minimal
Inflammatory infiltrate	Submucosal mononuclear cells; perivascular	Submucosal mononuclear cells; perivascular	Polymorphoneutrophils in all layers
Submucosal deposition	Collagen	Collagen	Fibrin
Detrusor mast cells	Numerous	Numerous	Rare
Glomerulations	Present	Present	Absent
Bladder capacity	Decreased	Decreased	Decreased

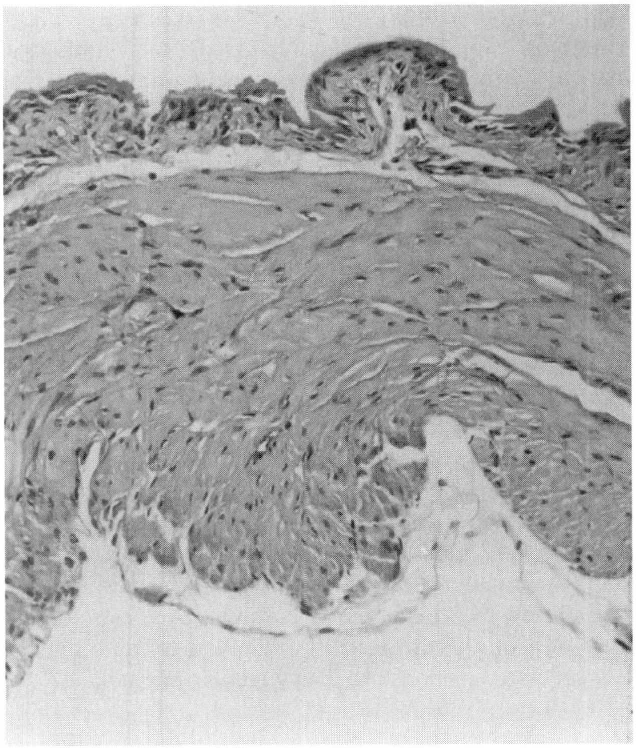

A

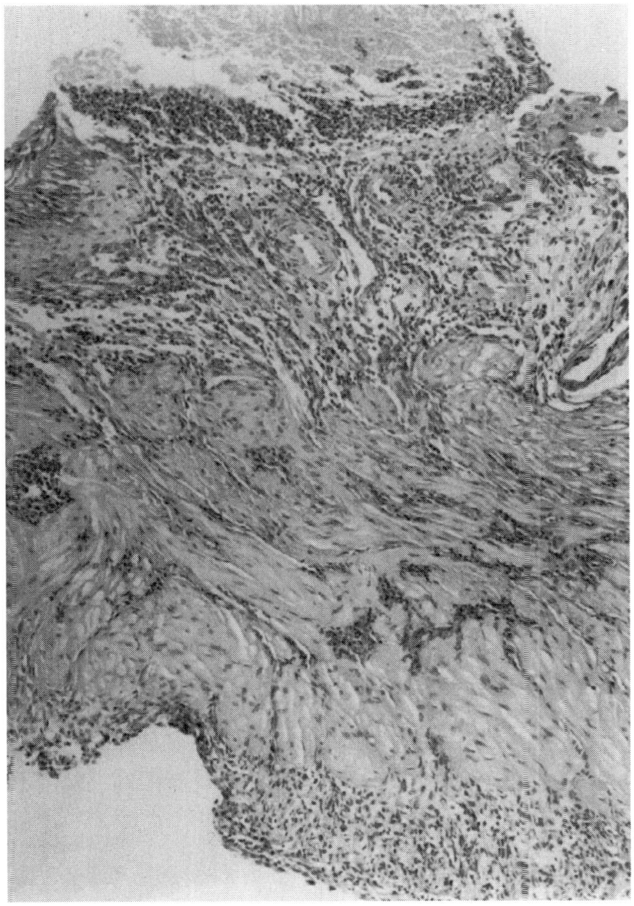

B

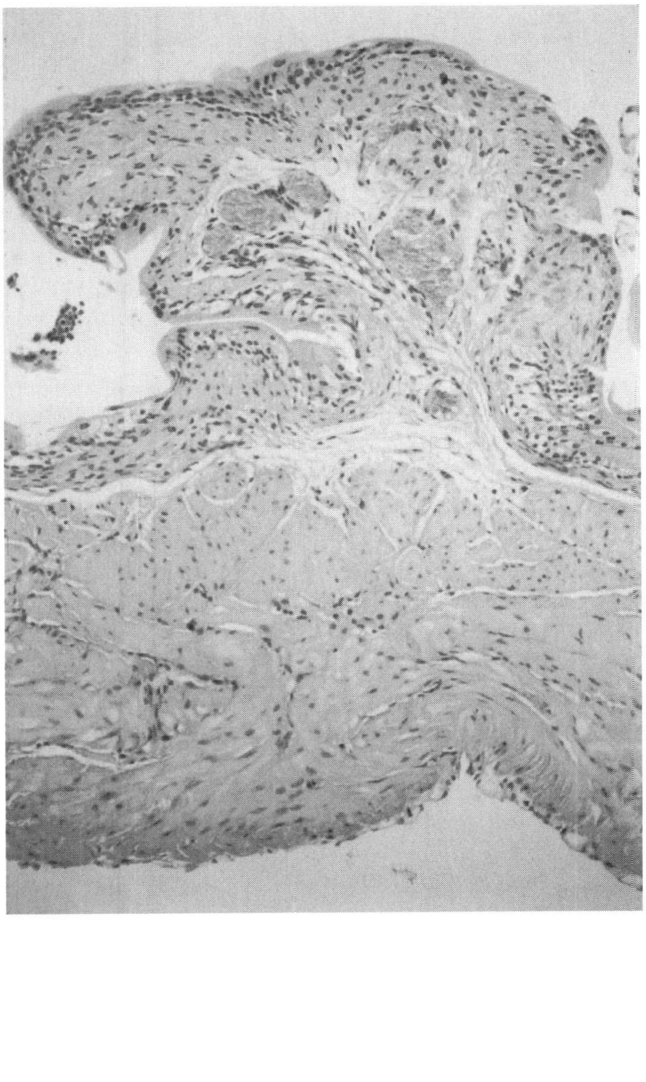

C

FIG. 3. (A) Normal bladder with small mucosal folds without edema or fibrosis. **(B)** Chronic bacterial cystitis shows extensive mucosal destruction and frank ulceration. **(C)** Bladder with EAC displays prominent, large mucosal folds with edema, fibrosis, and increased vascularity.

reviewed in a blinded fashion by a single pathologist (Michael J. Becich, M.D.).

Classic (ulcerative) interstitial cystitis does not have a single diagnostic histologic characteristic, but mastocytosis is a prominent feature. In multifactorial pathologic reviews of ulcerative IC, a constellation of pathologic features in all layers of the bladder wall have been defined that together provide the histologic identification of this unique form of cystitis (15,19,44,45). In blinded studies, the classic interstitial cystitis bladders could be identified histologically from the nonulcer IC and control bladders.

Histologically, the experimental autoimmune cystitis bladder correlates with the features seen in ulcerative interstitial cystitis, and these features are quite distinct from a bacterial cystitis control model (Table 1). The reactive EAC bladders demonstrate inflammation that is localized to the submucosa with detachment of an intact urothelium from the lamina propria (Fig. 3). The inflammatory infiltrate in EAC is primarily mononuclear cells in perivascular areas confined to the submucosa (Fig. 4). In the bacterial cystitis model, there is mainly polymorphonuclear inflammatory reaction diffusely involving all bladder layers with diffuse destruction of the urothelium. The EAC bladder has redundant mucosal folds with marked submucosal fibrosis, whereas minimal fibrosis is found in the bacterial cystitis model. In EAC, the interstitial response involves collagen deposition, and in bacterial interstitial cystitis, the interstitial changes are primarily fibrin deposition (Fig. 5). Vascular ectasia in the submucosa with evidence of submucosal hemorrhage is seen only in the EAC model (Fig. 6). The most pathognomonic feature of our model is mastocytosis. Mast cells were prominent in the detrusor muscle layer, which is different from the usual small number of mast cells in the submucosa and serosa in bacterial cystitis and normal controls (Fig. 7).

Experimental autoimmune cystitis can be transferred to naive, syngeneic Balb/cANN mice using spleen cells and lymphocytes from antigen-immunized mice. This transfer is tissue- and strain-specific, and the cystitis induced by adoptive transfer is indistinct from the primary disease. The ability to transfer EAC passively suggests that the induction of this disorder is based on an autoimmune, cell-mediated response to the syngeneic antigen.

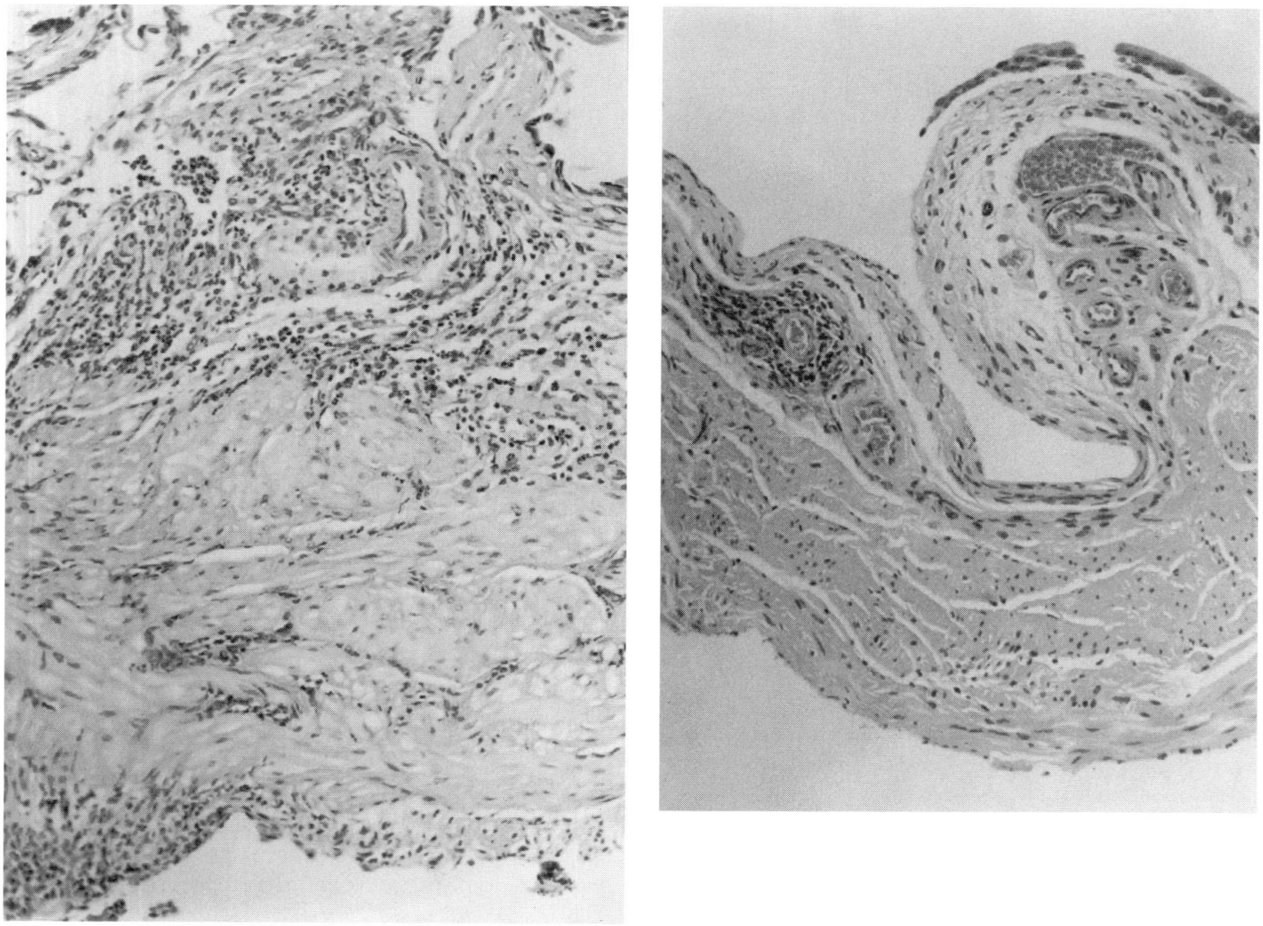

A B

FIG. 4. (A) Bladder with bacterial cystitis has a diffuse polymorphonuclear infiltrate involving all layers. **(B)** Bladder with EAC shows perivascular inflammation of mononuclear cells confined to the submucosa.

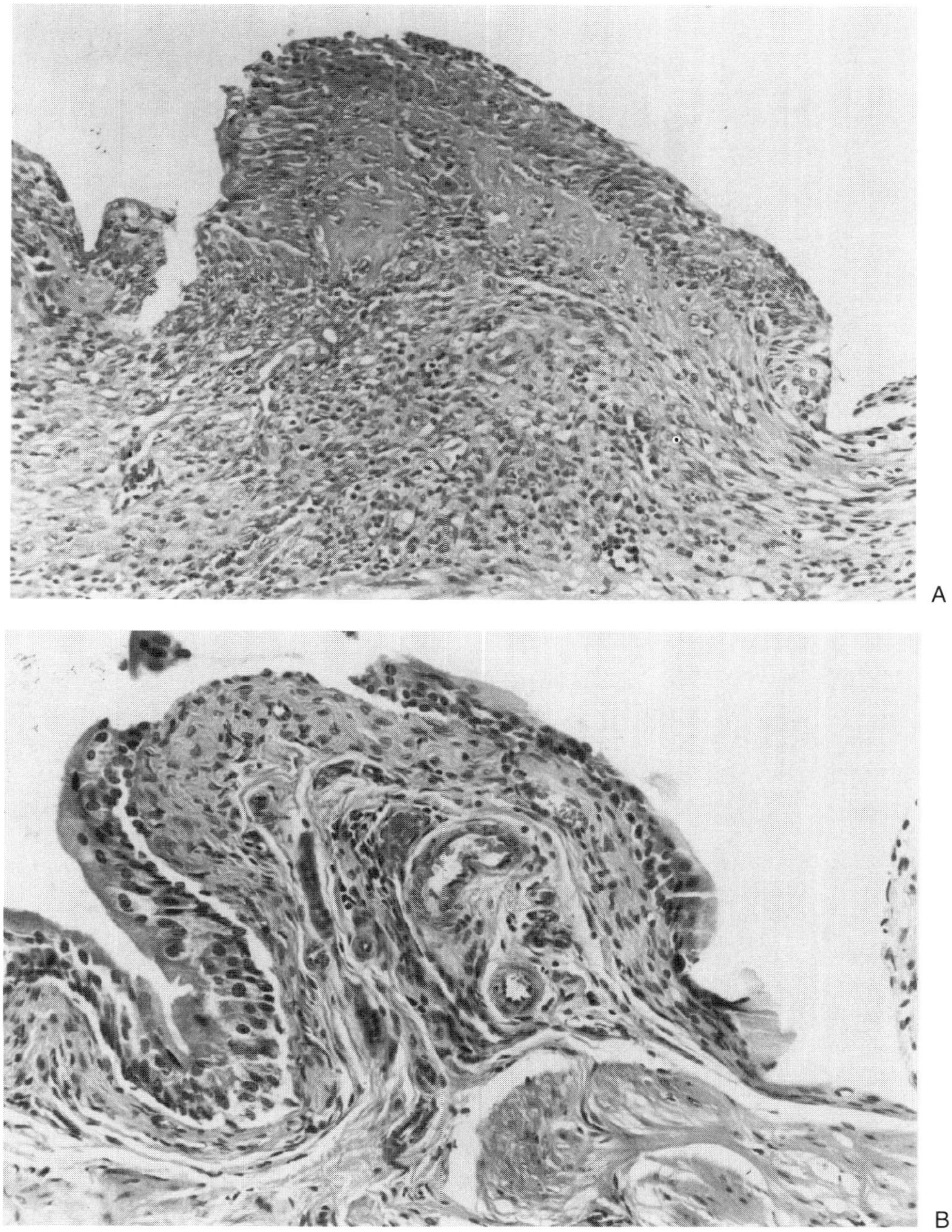

FIG. 5. (A) The submucosal deposits seen in bacterial cystitis are composed mainly of fibrin. **(B)** The submucosal fibrosis in EAC is predominantly collagen.

In the initial report, adoptive transfer studies suggested that EAC was induced by activated T lymphocytes (42). We performed additional studies to assess the T-lymphocyte subset responsible for the induction of EAC. Before immunization, mice were treated with specific monoclonal antibodies to deplete either all T cells (30H12), helper T cells (GK 1.5), or cytotoxic T cells (2.43) (46). After depletion, mice were immunized as described above with the bladder extract. At day 28, mice were sacrificed, and bladders were subjected to histologic analysis. The data showed that depletion of either all T lymphocytes or helper T lymphocytes significantly reduced the presence of inflammation and mast cell numbers in the detrusor muscle. In contrast, depletion of cytotoxic T cells or administration of an isotype control antibody had no significant effect on inflammation. These data confirm the requirement of T lymphocytes for induction of EAC and suggest that helper T lymphocytes are necessary for induction of the disease.

We observed a strong correlation between the development of bladder inflammation and the accumulation of mast cells in the bladder wall. This observation, which

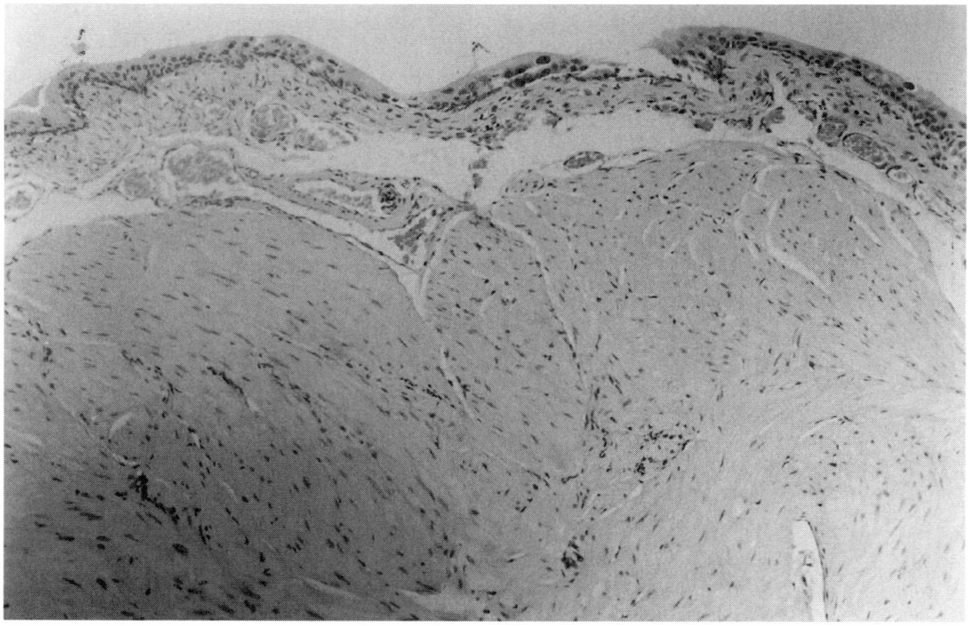

A

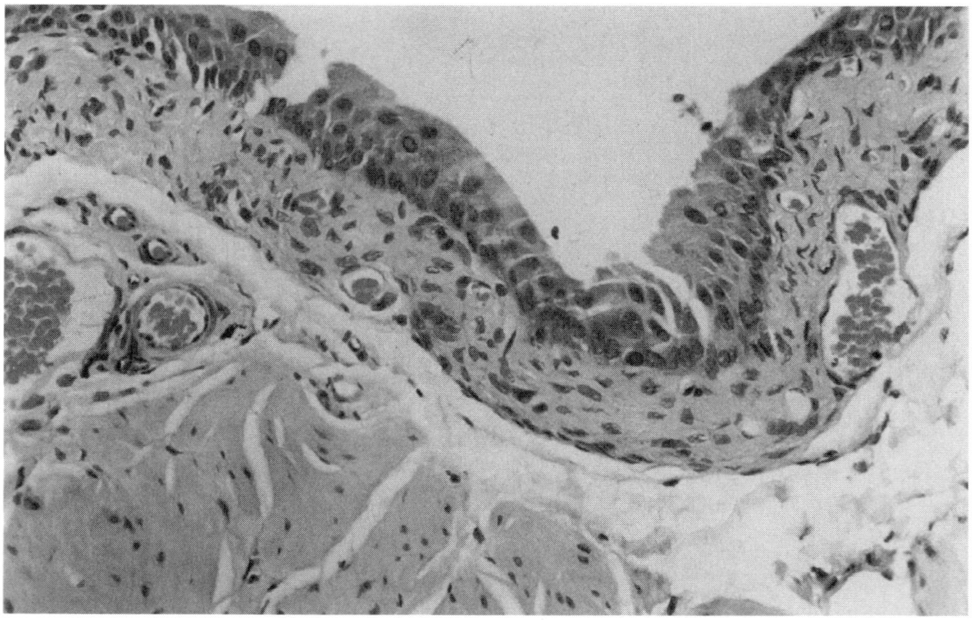

B

FIG. 6. The EAC bladders have prominent vascular ectasia with numerous dilated submucosal venules.

also has been reported by others, catalyzed studies to characterize bladder mast cells in IC patients and EAC (47). Specimens from IC patients and from mice with EAC were evaluated by electron microscopy. Mast cells in IC patients contained a heterogeneous mixture of cytoplasmic granules including homogeneous, scroll, particle, and dense-core types. No crystalline-type granules, which are commonly seen in human skin mast cells, were noted. Large cytoplasmic lipid bodies, which rarely exist in mast cells, were frequently identified in the mast cells of IC and EAC specimens. We observed that subpopulations of mast cells located in the detrusor muscle showed reduced numbers of granules, alveolar profiles in cytoplasm, and severe degranulation. These changes suggest that mast cells in IC patients and mice with EAC may undergo chronic degranulation, leading to the secondary histologic changes observed in IC and EAC (mucosal injury, detrusor muscle fragmentation/fibrosis, vasodilatation, and increased numbers of inflammatory cells). Interestingly, the mast cells in the detrusor were frequently observed in close proximity to nonmyelinated nerve fibers, many of which showed evidence of cellular

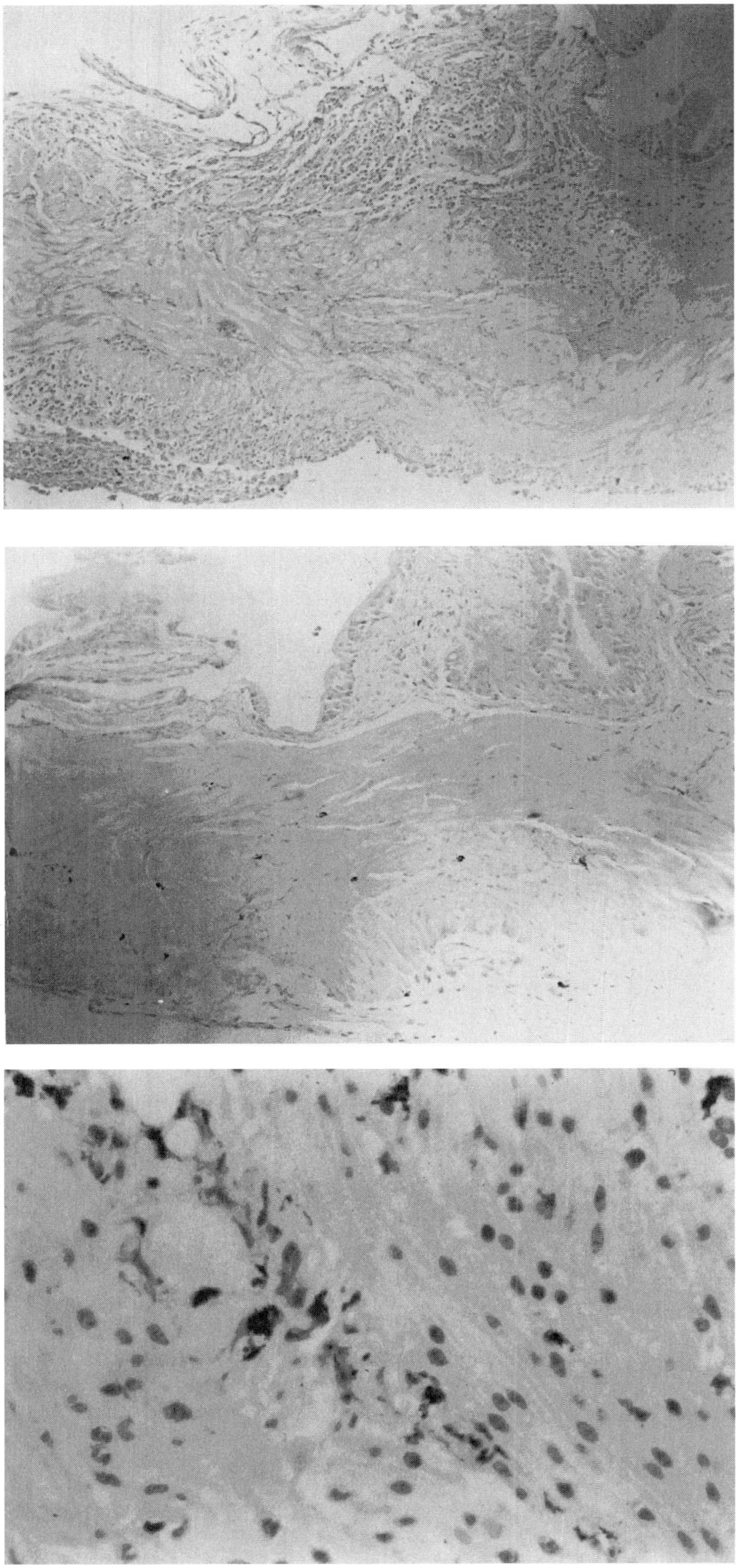

FIG. 7. (A) Bladder with bacterial cystitis displays small numbers of connective tissue mast cells with few in the detrusor muscle. **(B)** Bladder with EAC shows numerous mast cells concentrated in the detrusor muscle layer. **(C)** The mast cells in EAC are often degranulated. See color plate 2.

injury. Taken together, these data suggest that helper T cells of the Th2 subtype activate an immediate hypersensitivity response to autologous antigens that results in mast cell accumulation and their degranulation. The comparative features of EAC, IC, and bacterial cystitis are listed in Table 1.

PERSPECTIVE

After numerous successful runs, the experimental autoimmune cystitis model has become difficult to reproduce in our laboratory. Whether this is a problem of murine strain specificity, of antigen processing, or of another procedural variable is presently unclear. Efforts are ongoing to return the experimental autoimmune cystitis model to operation. Luber-Narod et al., using a similar immunization protocol in Lewis rats, have found comparable behavioral effects and pathology to that of patients with the early (nonulcer) form of interstitial cystitis (48). In their hands, bladders from experimental inflammatory cystitis exhibited vascular congestion and edema but not the perivascular cuffing or chronic inflammatory cell infiltrate as evidenced in the Bullock model. Urinary frequency in experimental inflammatory cystitis as measured by urine spots on filter paper per unit time was significantly increased compared to sham-operated animals. Furthermore, splenocytes cultured from animals with EAC transferred to naive recipients were capable of transferring the urinary frequency and histologic changes, indicative of a cell-mediated immune response.

Although premature, ultimate goals for this new immune cystitis model are easy to foresee. Following the establishment of the murine autoimmune cystitis model in a reproducible manner, the antigen responsible remains to be characterized. Once this is achieved, the disease may be more carefully scrutinized for clues to the lymphocytic function and interactions. By then, attempts to modulate the immune response—both suppression and acceleration—should be possible. The most important and certainly most difficult step will be to extrapolate findings in the animal model to human interstitial cystitis.

One of the main problems in interstitial cystitis vis-à-vis understanding its pathogenesis resides in the fact that interstitial cystitis is essentially a diagnosis of exclusion and nonuniform criteria are used to diagnose the disease. Unfortunately, at present there are no objective markers other than clinical signs and symptoms to label the disease. Thus, without a clear handle on the disease process, the pathophysiology remains debatable. Indeed, most researchers presently feel there may not be a single underlying mechanism for all interstitial cystitis sufferers rather a number of causes with similar symptomatic effects. There are already established types of interstitial cystitis (classic versus early). Should an autoimmune mechanism be proven as one of the causes of interstitial cystitis, its curtailment will likely be first achieved in the experimental autoimmune cystitis model.

REFERENCES

1. Roitt IM, Doniach D, eds. *Textbook of Immunopathology, Vol II: Gastric Autoimmunity.* New York: Grune & Stratton, 1969.
2. Donach D, Roitt IM. Auto-immunity in Hashimoto's disease and its implications. *J Clin Endocrinol* 1957;17:1293–1304.
3. Trentham D. Adverse reactions to bovine collagen implants: Additional evidence for immune response gene control of collagen reactivity in humans. *Arch Dermatol* 1986;122:643–644.
4. Reinherz EL, Kung PC, Goldstein G, Schlossman SF. Separation of functional subsets of human T cells by a monoclonal antibody. *Proc Natl Acad Sci USA* 1979;76:4061–4065.
5. Reinherz EL, Hussey RE, Fitzgerald K, Snow P, Terhorst C, Schlossman SF. Antibody directed at a surface structure inhibits cytolytic but not suppresser function of human T lymphocytes. *Nature* 1981; 294:168–170.
6. Fall M, Johansson SL, Aldenborg F. Chronic interstitial cystitis: A heterogeneous syndrome. *J Urol* 1987;137:35–38.
7. Johansson SL, Fall M. Pathology of interstitial cystitis. *Urol Clin North Am* 1994;21(1):55–62.
8. Shipton EA. Hunner's ulcer (chronic interstitial cystitis). A manifestation of collagen disease. *Br J Urol* 1965;37:443–449.
9. Rosin RD, Griffiths T, Sofras F, et al. Interstitial cystitis. *Br J Urol* 1979;51:524–527.
10. Oravisto KJ, Alfthan OS, Jokinen EJ. Interstitial cystitis. Clinical and immunological findings. *Scand J Urol Nephrol* 1970;4:37–42.
11. Silk MR. Bladder antibodies in interstitial cystitis. *J Urol* 1970;103: 307–309.
12. Fister GM. similarity of interstitial cystitis (Hunner ulcer) to lupus erythematosis. *J Urol* 1938;40:37–51.
13. Kerr WS Jr. Interstitial cystitis: treatment by transurethral resection. *J Urol* 1971;105:664–666.
14. Larsen S, Thompson SA, Hald T, et al. Mast cells in interstitial cystitis. *Br J Urol* 1982;54:283–286.
15. Fall M, Johansson SL, Aldenborg F. Chronic interstitial cystitis: a heterogeneous syndrome. *J Urol* 1987;137:35–38.
16. Harrington DS, Fall M, Johansson SL. Interstitial cystitis: bladder mucosa lymphocyte immunophenotyping and peripheral blood flow cytometry analysis. *J Urol* 1990;144:868–871.
17. Lynes WL, Flynn SD, Shortliffe LD, Lemmers M, Zipser R, Roberts LJ, Stamey TA. Mast cell involvement in interstitial cystitis. *J Urol* 1987; 138:746–752.
18. Aldenborg F, Fall M, Enerback L. Proliferation and trans epithelial migration of mucosal mast cells in interstitial cystitis. *Immunology* 1986;58:411–415.
19. Johansson SL, Fall M. Clinical features and spectrum of light microscopic changes in interstitial cystitis. *J Urol* 1990;143:1118–1124.
20. Macdermott JP, Miller CH, Levy N, Stone AR. Cellular immunity in interstitial cystitis. *J Urol* 1991;145:274–278.
21. Gordon HL, et al. Immunologic aspects of interstitial cystitis. *J Urol* 1973;109:228–233.
22. Jokinen EJ, Oravisto KJ, Alfthan OS. The effect of cystectomy on antitissue antibodies in interstitial cystitis. *Clin Exp Immunol* 1973;15: 457–460.
23. Fasth A, Hanson LA, Jodal U, Peterson H. Autoantibodies to Tamm–Horsfall protein associated with urinary tract infections in girls. *J Pediatr* 1979;95:54–60.
24. Neal DE, Dilworth JP, Kaack MB. Tamm–Horsfall autoantibodies in interstitial cystitis. *J Urol* 1991;145:37–39.
25. Stone AR, Vogelsang P, Miller CH, Macdermott JP. Tamm–Horsfall protein as a marker in interstitial cystitis. *J Urol* 1992;148:1406–1408.
26. Jokinen EJ, Alfthan OS, Oravisto KJ. Antitissue antibodies in interstitial cystitis. *Clin Exp Immunol* 1972;11:333–339.
27. Anderson JB, Parivar F, Lee G, Wallington TB, Maciver AG, Bradbrook RA, Gingell JC. The enigma of interstitial cystitis—an autoimmune disease? *Br J Urol* 1989;63:58–63.

28. Helin H, Mattila J, Rantala I, Vaalast T. *In vivo* binding of immunoglobulin and complement to elastic structures in urinary bladder vascular walls in interstitial cystitis: demonstration by immunoelectron microscopy. *Clin Immunol Immunopathol* 1987;43:88–96.
29. Gillespie L, Said J, Sostrin S, Kleiwer K. Immunofluoresent and histochemical staining confirm the identification of the many diseases called interstitial cystitis. *Br J Urol* 1990;66:265–273.
30. Christmas TJ, Rode J, Bottazo GF, Milroy E, Turner-Warwick RT. Cellular infiltration in interstitial cystitis; a study of T-cell subpopulation and mast cells. *J Urol* 1990;143(4):373A.
31. Miller CH, Macdermott JP. Lymphocyte function in patients with interstitial cystitis. *J Urol* 1992;147:592–595.
32. Raine CS. Experimental allergic encephalomyelitis and experimental allergic neuritis. In: Koetsier JC, ed. *Handbook of Clinical Neurology,* Vol 3(47). Amsterdam: Elsevier, 1985; 429–466.
33. Waksman BH, Adams RD. Allergic neuritis—experimental disease of rabbits induced by the injection of peripheral nervous tissue and adjuvants. *J Exp Med* 1955;102:213–230.
34. Ballin RHM, Thomas PK. Electron microscope observations on demyelination and remyelination in experimental allergic neuritis. II. Remyelination. *J Neurol Sci* 1969;8:225–237.
35. Lampert PW. Mechanisms of demyelination in experimental allergic neuritis—electron microscopic studies. *Lab Invest* 1969;20: 127–138.
36. Traugott U, Raine CS. Further lymphocyte characterization in the central nervous system in multiple sclerosis. *Ann NY Acad Sci* 1984;436: 163–180.
37. Konovalov GV, Korneva EA, Khai LM. Effect of destruction of the posterior hypothalamus on the experimental allergic polyneuritis. *Brain Res* 1971;29:383–397.
38. Driscoll BF, Kies MW, Alvord EC. Successful treatment of experimental allergic encephalomyelitis (EAE) in guinea-pigs with homologous myelin basic protein. *J Immunol* 1974;112:392–397.
39. Raine CS, Snyder DH, Stone SH, Bornstein MB. Suppression of acute and chronic experimental allergic encephalomyelitis in strain 13 guinea-pigs. *J Neurol Sci* 1977;31:355–367.
40. Arnon R. Experimental allergic encephalomyelitis—susceptibility and suppression. *Immunol Rev* 1981;55:5–30.
41. Bullock AD, Becich MJ, Klutke CG, Ratliff TL. Experimental autoimmune cystitis: A potential murine model for ulcerative interstitial cystitis. *J Urol* 1992;148:1951–1956.
42. Ueda S, Wakashin M, Wakashin Y, et al. Autoimmune interstitial nephritis induced in inbred mice. *Am J Pathol* 1988;132:304–318.
43. Mahi-Brown C, Yule T, Tung K. Adoptive transfer of murine autoimmune orchititis to naive recipients with immune lymphocytes. *Cell Immunol* 1987;106:408–419.
43a. Parsons CL, Stein PC, Lilly JD. Epithelial dysfunction in nonbacterial cystitis (interstitial cystitis). *J Urol* 1990;143:690–693.
43b. Parsons CL, Boychuck D, Jones S, Hurst R, Callahan H. Bladder surface glycosaminoglycans: An epithelial permeability barrier. *J Urol* 1990;143:139–142.
43c. Stein PC, Pham H, Ito T, Parsons CL. Bladder injury model induced in rats by exposure to protamine sulfate followed by bacterial endotoxin. *J Urol* 1996; 155:1133–1138.
44. Messing EM, Stamey TA. Interstitial cystitis: Early diagnosis, pathology and treatment. *Urology* 1978;12:381–392.
45. Smith BH, Dehner LP. Chronic ulcerating interstitial cystitis (Hunner's ulcer). *Arch Pathol* 1972;93:76–81.
46. Ratliff TL, Ritchey JK, Yuan JJJ, Andriole GL, Catalona WJ. T-cell subsets required for intravesical BCG imunotherapy for bladder cancer. *J Urol* 1993;150:1018–1023.
47. Sant GR, Theoharides TC. The role of the mast cell in interstitial cystitis. *Urol Clin North Am* 1994;21:41–53.
48. Luber-Narod J, Austin-Ritchie T, Banner B, et al. Experimental inflammatory cystitis; an animal model for IC. NIDDK/ICA Interstitial Cystitis Scientific Workshop, San Diego;1995;45(abst).

Interstitial Cystitis, edited by Grannum R. Sant.
Lippincott–Raven Publishers, Philadelphia ©1997.

CHAPTER 6

Autoimmunity and Interstitial Cystitis

Robert L. Ochs and Eng M. Tan

Interstitial cystitis (IC) is a chronic inflammatory disease of the bladder characterized by symptoms of pain, urgency, and frequent urination (1–4). A clinical diagnosis is supported by cystoscopic findings of focal glomerulations or ulcers (Hunner's ulcer) in the bladder wall. Interstitial cystitis is primarily found in women (90%) who are 30 to 45 years old at first onset of symptoms. Although the cause of IC is currently unknown, previously mentioned etiologic agents/causes include bacteria (4), viruses (4), toxic substances in the urine (4), direct physical trauma to the bladder wall (5), and bladder-specific autoimmune disease (6,7). Pathologically and histologically, the IC bladder has been variously reported to have a defective glycosaminoglycan layer, widening of the interstitium, increased numbers of mast cells, inflammatory mononuclear cell infiltration, endothelial cell injury with immune deposits, and widespread fibrosis in end-stage disease (8–12).

A number of reports document the existence of autoantibodies in some patients with IC (6,13–15), but the identity of these autoantibodies has been largely undetermined. Because infection, viruses, and toxic insult have not proven to be causative agents in the pathophysiology of IC, and because the disease presents many of the clinical and pathologic features of autoimmune conditions such as episodic/remissive chronic inflammation, infiltration with inflammatory mononuclear cells (lymphocytes, monocytes, plasma cells), and the presence of antinuclear antibodies (ANAs), it is reasonable to suspect that IC may be a bladder-specific autoimmune disease or a chronic inflammatory condition of the bladder involving an autoimmune response. In view of a potentially complex etiology with multiple causes, autoimmune phenomena could account for a number of the common clinical and pathologic features observed in the IC patient population (4,16).

R. L. Ochs and E. M. Tan: W. M. Keck Autoimmune Disease Center, Department of Molecular and Experimental Medicine, The Scripps Research Institute, La Jolla, California 92037.

AUTOANTIBODIES IN IC

In our previous studies, we identified and partially characterized autoantibodies from the sera of patients with interstitial cystitis. Of the 96 IC patients enrolled in our initial study (17), 38 (39%) had detectable levels of autoantibodies by immunofluorescence on HEp-2 cells (ANA slides) or Western blotting on whole-cell extracts of T24 bladder cells. None of the patients had detectable bladder-tissue-specific autoantibodies. Most of the autoantibodies were against nuclear or nucleolar antigens, but in addition there were three autoantibodies detected against mitochondria and three autoantibodies against unknown cytoplasmic antigens. The incidence of ANAs was somewhat higher than the value of 25% previously reported by Oravisto (6). We attributed this to the combination of ANA testing on HEp-2 and Western blotting on cultured T24 bladder cells, with the added ability to detect nucleolar or cytoplasmic antigens. All but four of the 35 ANA-positive sera were exclusively of the IgG class, and we were unable to detect any low-titer IgM autoantibodies to intermediate filaments as previously reported (11).

Similar to systemic autoimmune diseases such as lupus and scleroderma (18,19), the autoantibody profile among IC patients consisted mainly of antinuclear antibodies of defined types, either nuclear speckles or nucleolar. These results were strikingly similar to those of Jokinen et al. (14), who reported that seven of 33 (21%) IC patients had ANAs of titer 1:160 or greater, with fine-speckled nuclear staining being the most common pattern. Another interesting feature was the relatively high percentage of nucleolar ANAs that occurred in IC patients (20% of IC ANAs were nucleolar). Nucleolar ANA staining patterns are rare in lupus but occur quite commonly in scleroderma (18,19). Whether this observation means that the pathophysiology of IC is in some way related to that of scleroderma is not yet clear, but further characterization of these antibodies may prove informative. At the present time, however, the molecular identity of IC autoantigens is unknown, but as determined by unique ANA staining patterns and by specificities on Western blots, IC autoantibodies appeared to recognize novel autoantigens not previously described in patients with systemic autoimmune diseases such as lupus, scleroderma, and Sjögren's syndrome (18,19).

AUTOANTIBODIES OF IgG, IgM, AND IgA ISOTYPE IN THE SERA OF IC PATIENTS

As discussed in the previous section, we initially characterized autoantibodies in the sera of IC patients by immunofluorescence (ANAs) and Western blotting (17). We now add to that initial characterization by describing further refinements in technique that enhance detection of low-titer autoantibodies or autoantibodies to minor proteins as well as detecting antibodies of different isotypes. Previous Western blotting studies were done with ^{125}I-protein A as the detecting reagent for antibody binding, but important minor autoantibodies could have been missed by not using a more sensitive technique. Therefore, we repeated our Western blotting experiments with the more sensitive and specific enhanced chemiluminescence technique for antibody detection. And unlike ^{125}I-protein A, which detects only IgGs, chemiluminescence used in conjunction with different peroxidase-conjugated secondary antibodies also has the capability of detecting antibodies of different isotypes.

Figure 1 is a direct comparison of the sera from 33 previously characterized ANA-positive IC patients (see ref. 17) by Western blotting using ^{125}I-protein A (A) and chemiluminescence for the detection of IgG (B), IgM (C), or IgA (D). Arrowheads in Fig. 1B indicate protein bands from patients 8, 22, and 29 that were not detected by ^{125}I-protein A (A). Patients 21, 23, and 30 in Fig. 1C had demonstrable IgM autoantibodies (arrowheads) by chemiluminescence Western blotting, and patients 20, 23, and 25 had IgA autoantibodies (arrowheads in Fig. 1D). In addition to these major bands, approximately ten of the 33 IC patients had IgA autoantibodies that recognized a band of 40 kDa (double arrowheads in Fig. 1D).

Although the significance of finding autoantibodies of different isotypes in select patients is not apparent at this time, it is perhaps worthwhile to hypothesize that patients with IgM autoantibodies may be early in the disease process, and those with secretory IgA autoantibodies may be more likely to represent individuals with potentially pathogenic autoantibodies localized in the bladder or urine. Longitudinal studies focusing on autoantibody isotypes during the development of IC could prove to be very informative.

ANALYSIS OF PAIRED LONGITUDINAL SAMPLES

Analysis of paired longitudinal samples from eight IC patients showed that some autoantibodies remained con-

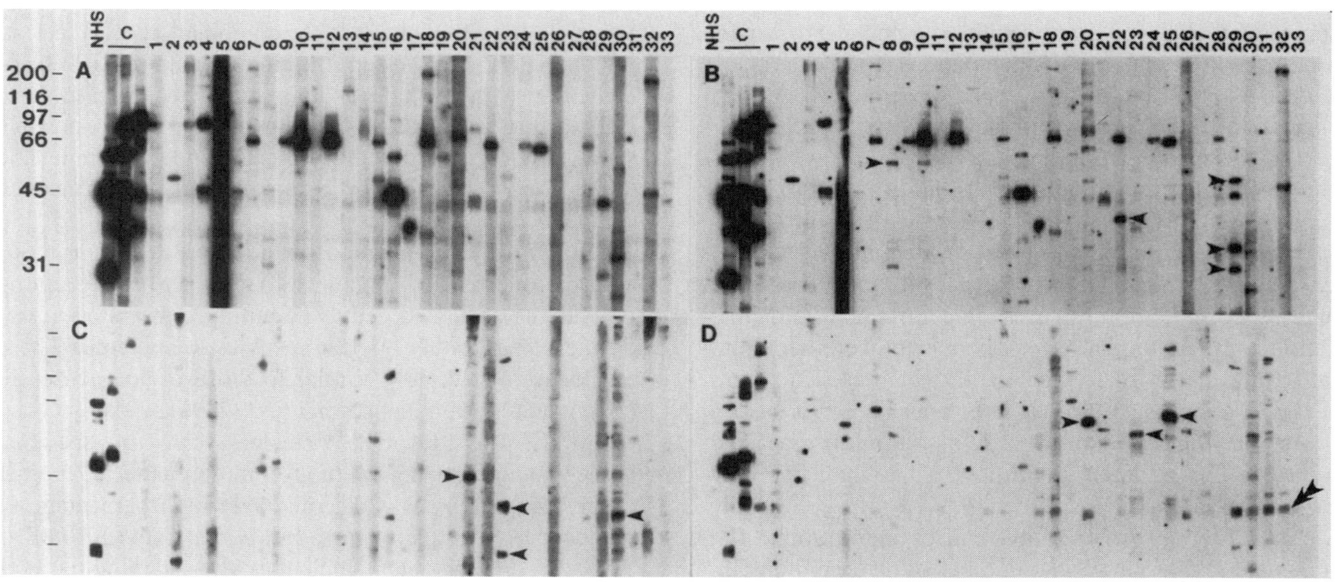

FIG. 1. Direct comparison of the sera from 33 previously characterized ANA-positive IC patients (see ref. 17) by Western blotting using ^{125}I-protein A **(A)** or chemiluminescence **(B–D)** for the detection of IgG **(A,B)**, IgM **(C)**, or IgA **(D)** autoantibodies. *Arrowheads* ***(B)*** indicate protein bands from patients 8, 22, and 29 that were not detected by ^{125}I-protein A **(A)**. Patients 21, 23, and 30 **(C)** had demonstrable IgM autoantibodies *(arrowheads)* by chemiluminescence Western blotting. Patients 20, 23, and 25 **(D)** had IgA autoantibodies *(arrowheads)* in addition to a number of patients who also recognized a 40-kDa antigen (*double arrowheads* in **D**). NHS, normal human serum; C, positive control antibodies.

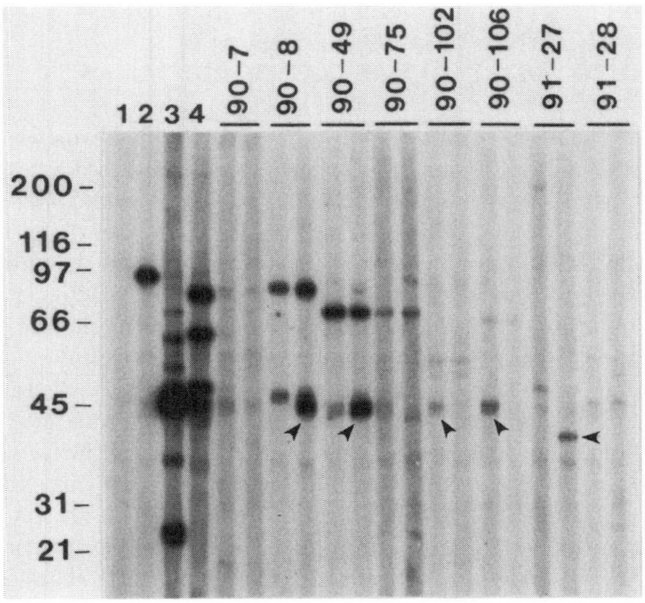

FIG. 2. Western blotting of longitudinal serum samples from eight IC patients. Of each pair of samples, the one on the **left** was the original, and the one on the **right** was obtained 3 to 4 years later. Some autoantibody profiles remained relatively unchanged with time (patients 90-7, 90-75, and 91-28). In others, certain protein bands became stronger (*arrowhead* in 90-49), new bands appeared (*arrowheads* in 90-8 and 91-27), and some bands disappeared (*arrowheads* in 90-102 and 90-106). **Lane 1,** normal human serum; **lanes 2 to 4,** positive control antibodies.

stant with time, some increased or decreased in amount, some disappeared, and other autoantibodies appeared *de novo.*

Figure 2 shows ^{125}I-protein A Western blotting analysis of longitudinal serum samples from eight IC patients. In each pair of samples, the one on the left was the original serum sample, and the one on the right was obtained 3 to 4 years later. Some autoantibody profiles remained relatively unchanged with time (patients 90-7, 90-75, and 91-28). In others, certain protein bands became stronger (arrowhead in 90-49), new bands appeared (arrowheads in 90-8 and 91-27), and some bands disappeared (arrowheads in 90-102 and 90-106). Although the significance of these results is presently unknown, it is tempting to speculate that individual changes in autoantibody expression could be a reflection of an ongoing disease process and may relate to disease symptoms and severity.

AUTOANTIBODIES AS CORRELATES OF DISEASE ACTIVITY: A POTENTIAL ROLE FOR AUTOANTIBODIES IN IC DIAGNOSIS AND TREATMENT

Even if autoimmunity is not the direct cause of interstitial cystitis, there may still be a role for serum autoantibodies in IC diagnosis and treatment. For example, those patients with autoantibodies may represent a separate subpopulation of the IC patient group with a different set of symptoms and perhaps a need for different treatment modalities. The presence or absence of a particular autoantibody may indicate a better or worse prognosis. As described in the systemic autoimmune diseases (18,19), sets or profiles of specific disease-related autoantibodies may also be important in classifying different groups of IC patients. For instance, in scleroderma, autoantibodies to centromere proteins are associated with the CREST form of the disease, whereas autoantibodies to DNA topoisomerase I (so-called Scl-70) are associated with diffuse scleroderma. This degree of specificity is difficult to explain unless the pathophysiology of each of these forms of scleroderma is unique, resulting in an "antigen-driven" (18) autoimmune response to different cellular components. Thus, the different autoantibody responses may reflect subtly different forms or categories of the same disease. Likewise, in IC, patients with nuclear autoantibodies, as distinct from those with nucleolar autoantibodies, may distinguish different forms of the disease. We have identified several potential candidate autoantibody–autoantigen systems that seem to occur in more than one patient. If further work indicates that these occur in a significant number of patients, and if they demonstrate specificity for IC, then they could prove to be useful in diagnosis. Objective laboratory findings such as these would augment what is currently a symptomatic diagnosis (1,3).

Among the IC patient population with autoantibodies, it is still not known when antibodies first appear in the course of the disease—whether they precede, coincide with, or occur after the onset of symptoms. This information could be informative because their occurrence before symptom onset might indicate a causal and direct role in disease, whereas coincident appearance could mean they play a contributory role, and appearance at a time significantly after symptom onset could indicate their appearance as a direct result of disease (so-called epiphenomenon).

Fundamental questions are still unanswered. For example, once it is detectable, is the autoantibody profile constant, or does it change with time? Does the autoantibody disappear or get weaker (lower titer) in remission and then reappear or become stronger during exacerbation of symptoms? From our results illustrated in Fig. 2, it is quite likely that autoantibodies do indeed reflect an ongoing disease process and could be used to monitor disease progression, and perhaps treatment as well.

THE ROLE OF AUTOIMMUNITY IN INTERSTITIAL CYSTITIS

Although the role of autoimmunity in interstitial cystitis is controversial and may be indirect in nature, it is obvious that patients with serum autoantibodies are manifesting components of an autoimmune response that may be contributing directly or indirectly to disease progression and symptomology. At least three different possibilities exist:

- Interstitial cystitis is caused by a *direct* autoimmune attack on the bladder.
- Some of the autoimmune symptoms and pathology of IC arise *indirectly* as a result of tissue destruction and inflammation from other, as yet unknown, causes.
- Autoimmune phenomena in IC patients are coincident and unrelated to the disease.

In the first scenario, an autoimmune response would be mounted against the bladder, and autoantibodies would be pathogenic, causing *direct* cell death and tissue destruction. Because there is no compelling evidence for bladder-specific autoantibodies, and only a portion of IC patients have autoantibodies (17), this is unlikely to be the universal explanation for IC. More complicated might be a case of immunologic attack on a bladder infected by viruses or bacteria. Similar to tuberculosis, the infectious agent is the actual cause of disease, but the pathology and major symptoms arise as a result of the ensuing immunologic response to what may now be altered or diseased tissue. More complicated still is the case of "molecular mimicry," where circulating antibodies against a past or present foreign organism can cross-react with "self" antigens (in this case a bladder antigen), causing inflammation and cell and tissue destruction. In the absence of strong proof for bladder-specific autoantibodies, molecular mimicry as a mechanism for immune attack on the bladder is not likely.

In the second scenario, the autoimmune response in IC is *indirect*, and autoantibodies arise as a result of cell and tissue destruction caused by chronic inflammation. In this case, autoantibodies could be targeted to the bladder in an attempt to "clean up" cellular debris, and their presence would be considered an "epiphenomenon" as a result of the massive tissue destruction. In the presence of antibody and complement, and other cytokines and chemoattractants, even more cell and tissue destruction could occur, "adding insult to injury." In this case, not every IC patient would necessarily have serum autoantibodies, depending on the individual immune response and the amount of tissue damage involved. In fact, the titers or presence of autoantibody could be a reflection of disease severity and may fluctuate during the disease course.

Finally, the presence of autoantibodies in some IC patients may have nothing to do with the disease, and their presence is *coincident*, being the result of another coexisting condition or disease process. This possibility seems unlikely because the incidence of autoantibodies in the IC patient population can be relatively high, and the types of autoantibodies observed are unlike those found in well-defined autoimmune diseases (17).

INTERSTITIAL CYSTITIS AS A BLADDER-SPECIFIC AUTOIMMUNE DISEASE: AUTOANTIBODIES AS PATHOGENIC AGENTS

Interstitial cystitis demonstrates some of the characteristics of an autoimmune disease, such as autoantibodies in association with chronic inflammation, episodic waxing and waning of the disease, and in some cases its resolution by antiinflammatory agents and steroid therapy (4,6,15). And because IC is confined to the bladder, it could possibly be considered a bladder-specific autoimmune disease. Compared to other organ-specific autoimmune diseases such as thyroiditis and diabetes, however, IC lacks evidence for a directed autoimmune attack on the bladder that would then result in disease. In fact, no bladder-specific autoantibodies were detected in our prior studies (17), but anecdotal reports have surfaced from time to time indicating that they could be present (10,13), and a recent paper by Golan et al. (20) suggests that some autoantibodies can enter live cells *in vitro* and *in vivo.* Even if this were the case, we would still be required to explain bladder-specific effects.

Autoantibodies could arise secondarily in IC as a result of tissue and cell destruction from chronic inflammation caused by some as yet unknown primary insult or injury (15). Consequently, they may function to "clear" cellular debris, and if this is the case, their specificities may reflect a unique and ongoing disease process for each individual patient. Autoantibodies would contribute indirectly to the pathophysiology of IC by perpetuating an already ongoing inflammatory process (10,12). In this scenario, a primary insult or injury to the bladder elicits a chemotactic response by mast cells, neutrophils, macrophages, and lymphocytes, with an initial local release of cytokines and inflammatory mediators followed by a secondary autoimmune response to self antigens that are derived from the injured bladder cells but are not necessarily bladder-specific. This local autoimmune response would involve components of the complement system, resulting in even more inflammation and tissue destruction. Finally, the end-product of this chronic inflammatory process is a widespread fibrosis.

It is interesting to note that mononuclear cell infiltration, mastocytosis, immune complex deposition, and fibrosis have all been reported at times, although not consistently, in biopsies of IC bladders (4,8–12), perhaps reflecting the complexity and diversity of this disease syndrome. Therefore, much as occurs in other chronic inflammatory diseases such as chronic active hepatitis (21), inflammatory bowel disease (16), and rheumatoid arthritis, diseases in which non-organ-specific autoantibodies have been identified, IC might belong to the group of autoimmune diseases in which the disease is confined to a single organ but the autoantibodies are not organ-specific (6,14).

ANIMAL STUDIES

The most compelling evidence for an autoimmune causation of interstitial cystitis was provided in animal studies by Bullock et al. (22,23), who immunized mice with autologous bladder antigens and then observed histologic evidence of IC-like disease. Further proof of autoimmune causation was provided by adoptive transfer of disease following the injection of lymphocytes from immunized animals into naive mice. However, no evidence was provided for the presence or absence of any autoantibodies. Animal studies such as these may provide the ultimate test for hypotheses involving autoimmune causation for the development of human IC.

INFECTION, AUTOIMMUNITY, AND INTERSTITIAL CYSTITIS

As detailed in a recent report by Warren (24), a unifying theory to explain the etiology, symptoms, and progression of IC could involve a role for infectious organisms that act as initiating and/or persistent agents for bladder inflammation. It has already been pointed out (24) that patients with IC are twice as likely to have a history of urinary tract infection as control subjects and 10 to 12 times as likely to have a history of childhood urinary tract disorders. In addition, the predominance of women with the syndrome, the acute onset of symptoms, the inflammatory histologic evidence, and the presence of IgA deposits in the bladder epithelium all suggest that IC may be caused by an infectious microorganism. The concept of IC as an infectious disease is further supported by recent data from Keay et al. (25) indicating that IC patients as a group have more bacteria in their urine than do controls, and data from Domingue et al. (26), who report the presence of unculturable dormant microbes in IC bladders as detected by polymerase chain reaction (PCR) for bacterial 16S rRNA genes and by direct visualization using electron microscopy. There could also be a primary defect in the bladder cell wall that would allow bacteria to enter from the urine of these patients. Such a defect could be caused by physical damage to the bladder surface or by a defect in the glycosaminoglycan (GAG)-containing mucosal outer layer that provides a protective barrier to entry of bacteria (5). Once bacteria are resident in the bladder, a self-perpetuating chronic inflammatory process could be initiated with autoantibodies produced to “altered” bladder antigens or produced as a result of cell and tissue destruction, as already discussed (24).

Another set of observations compatible with a role for infection in the etiology of IC is the finding of specific IgA autoantibodies in the sera (shown in Fig. 1) and IgA antibody deposits (27) and IgA plasma cells (28) in bladders of some IC patients. The IgA antibodies are often of a local secretory type that provide an immunologic barrier in epithelial tissues to entry of bacteria, viruses, and other foreign invaders (29), but elevated serum levels of IgA can also be indicative of a mucosal infection such as might occur in the bladder wall. It has also been shown recently that IgA relies on the cytokine IL-6 for its synthesis (30), and elevated IL-6 levels were detected in the urine of IC patients and were correlated positively with pain scores and disease severity (31). On the basis of *in situ* hybridization studies for the detection of IL-6 mRNA, it was concluded that the source of urinary IL-6 was immune-activated cells in the bladder urothelium. Therefore, elevated levels of IgA and IL-6 could be a result of bacterial infection in the bladder wall whether or not organisms can be isolated or cultured from the urine.

SUMMARY

In summary, a body of evidence exists to indicate that interstitial cystitis is a bladder-specific autoimmune disease or that the autoimmune response that is present contributes to the symptomology and progression of the disease. The evidence for autoimmune involvement can be summarized as follows:

- Presence of autoantibodies whose titer may be correlated with disease severity (11–15,17,32).
- Histologically, plasma cells and antibody deposits are found in the bladder (8,9,28).
- Clinically, some of the symptoms resemble those observed in the systemic autoimmune diseases lupus and scleroderma, and remissions have been reported with cortisone treatment (15).
- Abnormal HLA-DR expression and immunotyping of cells in the bladder indicate immune activation (16,33, 34).
- Immunization of a mouse with autologous bladder antigens results in IC-like bladder changes that can be adoptively transferred (22,35).
- Interstitial cystitis has been reported in association with other autoimmune diseases such as Sjögren’s (36), rheumatoid arthritis (37), lupus (37), and Hashimoto’s thyroiditis (13).
- Other organ-specific autoimmune conditions exist, such as primary biliary cirrhosis, chronic inflammatory bowel disease, thyroiditis, and diabetes (15).

Conversely, a number of studies have examined the issue of autoimmunity and IC and have concluded that there is no autoimmune component to this disease. These findings are summarized as follows:

- No elevation in the urinary immune cytokine marker IL-1β (38).
- Lymphocytes from the bladder and blood of IC patients being of normal type and not capable of being stimulated (39,40).

In conclusion, the exact role of autoimmunity in interstitial cystitis is controversial and is likely to remain so until bona fide animal models are developed for this disease. For our part, we have provided evidence and argued for a role for autoantibodies in diagnosis, treatment, and classifiction of the IC patient population.

Acknowledgments

This work was supported by grant DK49413 from the NIDDK, NIH. The authors wish to acknowledge Thomas W. Stein, Jr. for excellent technical assistance. The Interstitial Cystitis Association aided in the recruitment of patients for our studies.

REFERENCES

1. Messing EM, Stamey TA. Interstitial cystitis: early diagnosis, pathology, and treatment. *Urology* 1978;12:381–392.
2. Gillenwater JY, Wein AJ. Summary of the National Institutes of Arthritis, Diabetes, Digestive and Kidney Diseases Workshop on Interstitial Cystitis. National Institutes of Health, Bethesda, Maryland, August 28–29, 1987. *J Urol* 1988;140:203–206.
3. Hanno P, Levin RM, Monson FC, Teuscher C, Zhou ZZ, Ruggieri M, Whitmore K, Wein AJ. Diagnosis of interstitial cystitis. *J Urol* 1990; 143:278–281.
4. Sant GR. Interstitial cystitis. In: Stamey TA, ed. *Monographs in Urology,* Vol 12. Montverde, FL: Medical Direction Publishing, 1991;37–63.
5. Parsons CL, Lilly JD, Stein P. Epithelial dysfunction in nonbacterial cystitis (interstitial cystitis). *J Urol* 1991;145:732–735.
6. Oravisto KJ. Interstitial cystitis as an autoimmune disease: a review. *Eur Urol* 1980;6:10–13.
7. Stone AR, Quattrocchi KB, Miller CH, MacDermott JP. Role of the immune system in interstitial cystitis. *Semin Urol* 1991;9:108–114.
8. Johansson SL, Fall M. Clinical features and spectrum of light microscopic changes in interstitial cystitis. *J Urol* 1990;143:1118–1124.
9. Lynes WL, Flynn SD, Shortliffe LD, Stamey TA. The histology of interstitial cystitis. *Am J Surg Pathol* 1990;14:969–976.
10. Gordon HL, Rossen RD, Hersh EM, Yium JJ. Immunologic aspects of interstitial cystitis. *J Urol* 1973;109:228–233.
11. Mattila J, Linder E. Immunoglobulin deposits in bladder epithelium and vessels in interstitial cystitis: possible relationship to circulating anti-intermediate filament autoantibodies. *Clin Immunol Immunopathol* 1984;32:81–89.
12. Helin H, Mattila J, Rantala I, Vaalasti T. *In vivo* binding of immunoglobulin and complement to elastic structures in urinary bladder vascular walls in interstitial cystitis: demonstration by immunoelectron microscopy. *Clin Immunol Immunopathol* 1987;43:88–96.
13. Silk MR. Bladder antibodies in interstitial cystitis. *J Urol* 1970;103: 307–309.
14. Jokinen EJ, Alfthan OS, Oravisto KJ. Antitissue antibodies in interstitial cystitis. *Clin Exp Immunol* 1972;11:333–339.
15. Anderson JB, Parivar F, Lee G, Wallington TB, MacIver AG, Bradbrook RA, Gingell JC. The enigma of interstitial cystitis—an autoimmune disease? *Br J Urol* 1989;63:58–63.
16. Harrington DS, Fall M, Johansson SL. Interstitial cystitis: bladder mucosa lymphocyte immunophenotyping and peripheral blood flow cytometry analysis. *J Urol* 1990;144:868–871.
17. Ochs RL, Stein TW Jr, Peebles CL, Gittes RF, Tan EM. Autoantibodies in interstitial cystitis. *J Urol* 1994;151:587–592.
18. Tan EM. Antinuclear antibodies: diagnostic markers for autoimmune diseases and probes for cell biology. *Adv Immunol* 1989;44:93–151.
19. vonMühlen CA, Tan EM. Autoantibodies in the diagnosis of systemic rheumatic diseases. *Semin Arthritis Rheum* 1995;24:323–358.
20. Golan TD, Gharavi AE, Elkon KB. Penetration of autoantibodies into living epithelial cells. *J Invest Dermatol* 1993;100:316–322.
21. Imai H, Ochs RL, Kiyosawa K, Furuta S, Nakamura RM, Tan EM. Nucleolar antigens and autoantibodies in hepatocellular carcinoma and other malignancies. *Am J Pathol* 1992;140:859–870.
22. Bullock AD, Becich MJ, Klutke CG, Ratliff TL. Experimental autoimmune cystitis: a potential murine model for ulcerative interstitial cystitis. *J Urol* 1992;148:1951–1956.
23. Ratliff TL, Klutke CG, McDougall EM. The etiology of interstitial cystitis. *Urol Clin North Am* 1994;21:21–30.
24. Warren JW. Interstitial cystitis as an infectious disease. *Urol Clin North Am* 1994;21:31–39.
25. Keay S, Schwalbe RS, Trifillis AL, Lovchik JC, Jacobs S, Warren JW. A prospective study of microorganisms in urine and bladder biopsies from interstitial cystitis patients and controls. *Urology* 1995;45:223–229.
26. Domingue GJ, Ghoniem GM, Bost KL, Fermin C, Human LG. Dormant microbes in interstitial cystitis. *J Urol* 1995;153:1321–1326.
27. Said JW, Van de Velde R, Gillespie L. Immunopathology of interstitial cystitis. *Mod Pathol* 1989;2:593–602.
28. Christmas TJ. Lymphocyte sub-populations in the bladder wall in normal bladder, bacterial cystitis and interstitial cystitis. *Br J Urol* 1994; 73:508–515.
29. Mazanec MB, Nedrud JG, Kaetzel CS, Lamm ME. A three-tiered view of the role of IgA in mucosal defense. *Immunol Today* 1993;14:430–435.
30. Ramsay AJ, Husband AJ, Ramshaw IA, Bao S, Matthaei KI, Koehler G, Kopf M. The role of interleukin-6 in mucosal IgA antibody responses *in vivo. Science* 1994;264:561–563.
31. Lotz M, Villiger P, Hugli T, Koziol J, Zuraw BL. Interleukin-6 and interstitial cystitis. *J Urol* 1994;152:869–873.
32. Neal DE Jr, Dilworth JP, Kaack MB. Tamm–Horsfall autoantibodies in interstitial cystitis. *J Urol* 1991;145:37–39.
33. Christmas TJ, Bottazzo GF. Abnormal urothelial HLA-DR expression in interstitial cystitis. *Clin Exp Immunol* 1992;87:450–454.
34. Liebert M, Wedemeyer G, Stein JA, Washington R Jr, Faerber G, Flint A, Grossman HB. Evidence for urothelial cell activation in interstitial cystitis. *J Urol* 1993;149:470–475.
35. Ratliff TL, Klutke CG, Hofmeister M, He F, Russell JH, Becich MJ. Role of the immune response in interstitial cystitis. *Clin Immunol Immunopathol* 1995;74:209–216.
36. Van de Merwe J, Kamerling R, Arendsen E, Mulder D, Hooijkaas H. Sjögren's syndrome in patients with interstitial cystitis. *J Rheumatol* 1993;20:962–966.
37. Golstein MA, Manto M, Noel JC, Appleboom T. Chronic interstitial cystitis occurring during the shift between rheumatoid arthritis and lupus. *Clin Rheumatol* 1994;13:119–122.
38. Martins SM, Darlin DJ, Lad PM, Zimmern PE. Interleukin-1B: A clinically relevant urinary marker. *J Urol* 1994;151:1198–1201.
39. MacDermott JP, Miller CH, Levy N, Stone AR. Cellular immunity in interstitial cystitis. *J Urol* 1991;145:274–278.
40. Miller C, MacDermott J, Quattrocchi K, Broderick GA, Stone AR. Lymphocyte function in patients with interstitial cystitis. *J Urol* 1992; 147:592–595.

Interstitial Cystitis, edited by Grannum R. Sant.
Lippincott–Raven Publishers, Philadelphia ©1997.

CHAPTER 7

Neuropeptide–Mast Cell Interaction in Interstitial Cystitis

Ricardo Saban, Ingegerd M. Keith, and Dale E. Bjorling

Mast cells are strategically localized in the urinary bladder close to blood vessels, lymphatics, nerves, and detrusor smooth muscle. Mast cell response to alterations in bladder microenvironment (e.g., by urinary or blood-borne substances) normally leads to short-term inflammation contributing to resolution or consequent removal of inciting irritants. mast cell responses can be modified by local sensory peptides; if this occurs in a disproportionate manner, chronic bladder changes such as persistent inflammation and increased detrusor reactivity may result. Fundamental work regarding the participation of sensory nerves and mast cells in interstitial cystitis (IC) has provided evidence of mast cell activation and degranulation (1,2), increased nerve density (3,4), increased mast cell–nerve proximity in biopsy material from IC patients (5), and a selective role of mast cells in the inflammatory process of IC (6).

In this chapter, we review current information and present new data on the participation of mast cells and sensory nerves in IC with special emphasis on mast cell–nerve interaction, its modulation by peptidergic and trophic factors, and its pathophysiological consequences. It is clear that future investigations will focus on how this interaction is regulated during acute and chronic disease at the tissue, cellular, and molecular levels.

R. Saban and D.E. Bjorling: The Smooth Muscle Laboratory, Department of Surgical Sciences, School of Veterinary Medicine, University of Wisconsin-Madison, Madison, Wisconsin 53706.

I.M. Keith: Laboratory for Neuroendocrine Physiology and Neurochemistry, Department of Comparative Biosciences, School of Veterinary Medicine, University of Wisconsin-Madison, Madison, Wisconsin 53706.

NEUROANATOMIC BASIS FOR NERVE–MAST CELL INTERACTION: PEPTIDERGIC INNERVATION OF THE URINARY BLADDER

The urinary bladder is innervated by sensory, noradrenergic, and cholinergic systems. Neuropeptides found in nerve fibers supplying the bladder include substance P (SP), neurokinin A (NKA), calcitonin gene-related peptide (CGRP), vasoactive intestinal peptide (VIP), neuropeptide Y (NPY), somatostatin (SOM), and enkephalin (7–15).

Both SP- and NKA- but not neurokinin B (NKB)-immunoreactive nerves and fibers are reported in all layers of the bladder wall and form a suburothelial plexus that branches into the urothelium and occasionally reaches the bladder lumen; nerve fibers displaying CGRP-like and VIP-like immunoreactivity (LI) follow a similar distribution pattern (4,14,16–18). Although sensory fibers (e.g., those containing SP, NKA, CGRP, VIP, SOM, or NPY) primarily innervate the mucosal and submucosal layers, these and other peptidergic nerves may also originate from peripheral autonomic ganglia (8) and are therefore found in fibers innervating vessels and detrusor smooth muscle. The presence of the enzymes tyrosine hydroxylase (TH) and dopamine β-hydroxylase (DBH) confirms a noradrenergic motor fiber contribution, probably from the pelvic ganglia (11). Nerve fibers displaying immunoreactivity to SP, NKA, CGRP, and SOM antisera also innervate perikarya of intramural autonomic (parasympathetic) ganglia (8,12). The CGRP-LI in these perikarya (19) suggests that neurons of the intramural ganglia exert CGRP-mediated relaxing effects on both vascular and detrusor smooth muscle in addition to the cholinergic role of these ganglia. Finally, the potent vasoconstrictor and mitogen endothelin-1 (ET-1) is synthesized in bladder epithelia such as vascular endothelium, urothelial cells, and serosal mesothelium in addition to vascular and detrusor smooth muscle (20).

Endothelin-1 has also been described as a putative sensory neuropeptide with high content in the intact peripheral nervous system of guinea pigs (21).

MAST CELL INNERVATION BY SENSORY NERVES

Anatomic Evidence

Biopsies from IC patients have revealed increased nerve density within the bladder wall, specifically increased numbers of sympathetic nerves and fibers containing SP (2–5,7,22). In one study, the number of nerve fibers correlated positively with the number of mast cells and amount of histamine in suburothelial connective tissue and detrusor smooth muscle (5). Furthermore, Ratliffe and co-workers reported that nerve fibers classified as peptide-containing because of the presence of dense-core vesicles were more frequently in close apposition to degranulating mast cells in the urinary bladders of IC patients (23). They argued for a role of autoimmunity in IC and its expression being mediated by mast cells. In an experimental model of noninfectious bladder inflammation [ovalbumin sensitization followed by repeated challenge (24)], guinea pigs developed pathophysiological changes similar to those of IC patients and also had increased numbers of bladder mast cells in close contact with nerve fibers displaying CGRP-LI than did controls (Fig. 1). Moreover, in sensitized animals, these fibers were thicker and had frequent immunoreactive dilations, suggesting storage of CGRP in nerve varicosities.

A close spatial relationship between mast cells and nerve fibers has been described in normal and diseased tissues of various organ systems (25–28). For example, increased mucosal/epithelial innervation and nerve–mast cell associations have been reported in patients with ulcerative colitis and Crohn's disease (29,30), beneath psoriasis lesions of the skin (31), in arthritic rat synovium (32), and in the intestines of animals infected with *Nippostrongylus brasiliensis* and *Trichinella spiralis* (both potent allergens that elicit strong immune responses) (33–35).

In normal guinea pig urinary bladder, nerve fibers containing the sensory peptides CGRP, SP, and VIP contact mast cells identified histochemically with toluidine blue and alcian blue (SP and CGRP) and with serotonin immunohistochemistry (VIP) (19). Also in these bladders, presumed sensory nerve fibers were observed ultrastructurally deep inside mast cells (Fig. 2), with evidence suggesting paracrine, bidirectional (mutual) exchange (19). This finding is supported by the observation that mast cells may affect neuronal transmission in a bidirectional system (36). Although true synapses have not been found between nerve fibers and mast cells (19,37–39), paracrine transmission by peptides and neurotransmitters is possible. Despite numerous studies demonstrating the effects of SP on mast cells, a tachykinin receptor has not been found on the surface of mast cells. The interaction of SP with mast cells may represent an adaptive response to environmental changes not restricted by a requirement for synaptic junctions or membrane-bound receptors. This enigma has led to suggestions that SP (and other cationic amphiphilic neuropeptides) may directly activate G proteins present in the cell membrane (40). As conventional characteristics of innervation (e.g., synapses) do not appear to exist here, this uniquely intimate paracrine form of innervation could be classified as a new concept, endonervation, which refers to the internal localization of neurites within the mast cells enabling paracrine bidirectional exchange.

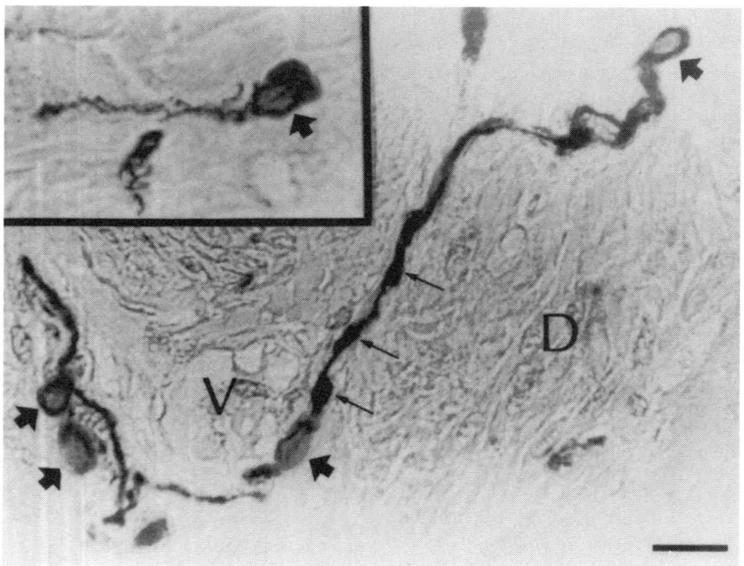

FIG. 1. Nerve fiber in guinea pig detrusor muscle (D) displaying immunoreactivity to rabbit antiserum for CGRP (1:1,000, Incstar Corporation, Stillwater MN) here seen trailing past, and in close apposition to, numerous mast cells *(fat arrows)* in ovalbumin-sensitized/challenged bladder. In nonsensitized control bladders, few nerve–mast cell contacts were seen **(inset).** Note that the nerve fiber in sensitized/challenged bladder is thicker and has numerous immunoreactive swellings *(thin arrows),* probably representing stored CGRP. Immunoreactivity was detected with the peroxidase–antiperoxidase method *(dark reaction product);* preabsorption of diluted antiserum with 50 μg of CGRP abolished immunoreactivity. Mast cells were detected with toluidine blue (1% toluidine blue in 0.5 M HCl, pH 0.5), Bouin's fixation, 5-μm-thick paraffin sections. Scale bar, 100 μm.

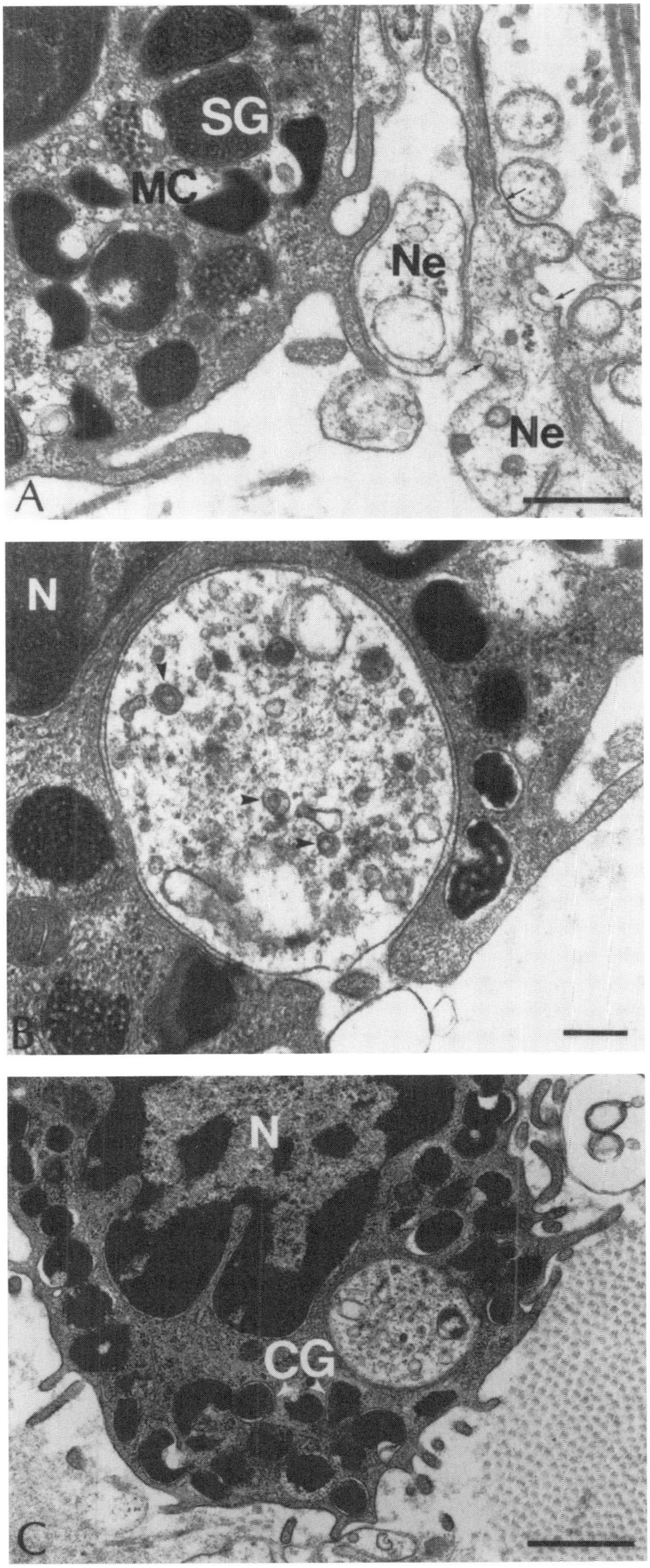

FIG. 2. (A) Electron micrographs from normal guinea pig bladder showing mast cell (MC) processes contacting neuritic process (Ne). Note neurite branching and vesicles fused with neural plasmalemma suggesting transmitter release or pinocytosis *(thin arrows)*. SG, simple granule. Examination of another mast cell **(B,C)** shows a different stage in nerve–mast cell interaction. The mast cell has almost completely enveloped a neural process that contains dense-core *(arrowheads)* and clear vesicles that may contain neuropeptide and neurotransmitter, respectively **(B)**; this is also seen in additional serial section completely embracing the fiber **(C)**, supporting the novel innervation mode, endonervation. Note the close proximity of neuritic process to nucleus. Compound granules (CG) are present. Scale bars, 0.5 μm **(A),** 0.25 μm **(B),** 1.0 μm **(C).** (Altered from Keith et al., ref. 19, with permission.)

The close nerve–mast cell proximity in normal urinary bladder suggests a purposeful and significant role in maintenance of local tissue homeostasis as proposed for the normal rat intestine and respiratory tract (33). In addition to interactions with peripheral nerves, mast cells have been reported in close association with intramural autonomic bladder ganglia (19). Histaminergic excitation of ganglionic neurons has been shown in the nodose and superior cervical ganglia, further supporting the concept of neuronal interaction with ganglionic mast cells in the urinary bladder (36,41).

Functional Evidence

A functional consequence of nerve–mast cell interaction is the peptide-induced mast cell release of inflammatory mediators known to occur in many tissues (42,43). In the urinary bladder, SP, NKA, and VIP induce histamine release in a time-dependent fashion (Fig. 3). Conversely, products of mast cell degranulation such as histamine, prostaglandin D_2, and leukotriene C_4 are able to stimulate sensory neurons and induce SP release (Fig. 4) (44), thus creating a self-perpetuating cycle (Fig. 5). Although the concentrations of SP used to elicit *in vitro* mast cell histamine release exceed normal tissue concentrations, the capacity of endogenous neuropeptide, primarily SP, to induce histamine release was confirmed by exposure of guinea pig bladder to a concentration of capsaicin known to stimulate sensory nerves and cause release of endogenous SP (D. E. Bjorling and R. Saban, *unpublished data*). Also, because of the close proximity between mast cells and sensory nerves in the urinary bladder (endonervation) (Fig. 3), directed and precise paracrine release of endogenous SP could achieve mast cell activation at significantly lower concentrations. This is further supported by the fact that mast cells can be primed to degranulate by picomolar concentrations of SP (45) and by observations within bladders of IC patients that suggest "intragranular activation" of mast cells frequently associated with neuronal processes (2).

In addition, it has been shown that mast cells are present in the guinea pig lung within parasympathetic ganglia and that antigenic challenge of actively sensitized lungs causes mast cell-mediated excitation of vagal neurons innervating the airways (46). In the gut, mast cell activation by antigen challenge alters ion transport and epithelial permeability (47). Moreover, indirect evidence for functional nerve–mast cell interaction is provided by the observation of acetylcholine-induced histamine release

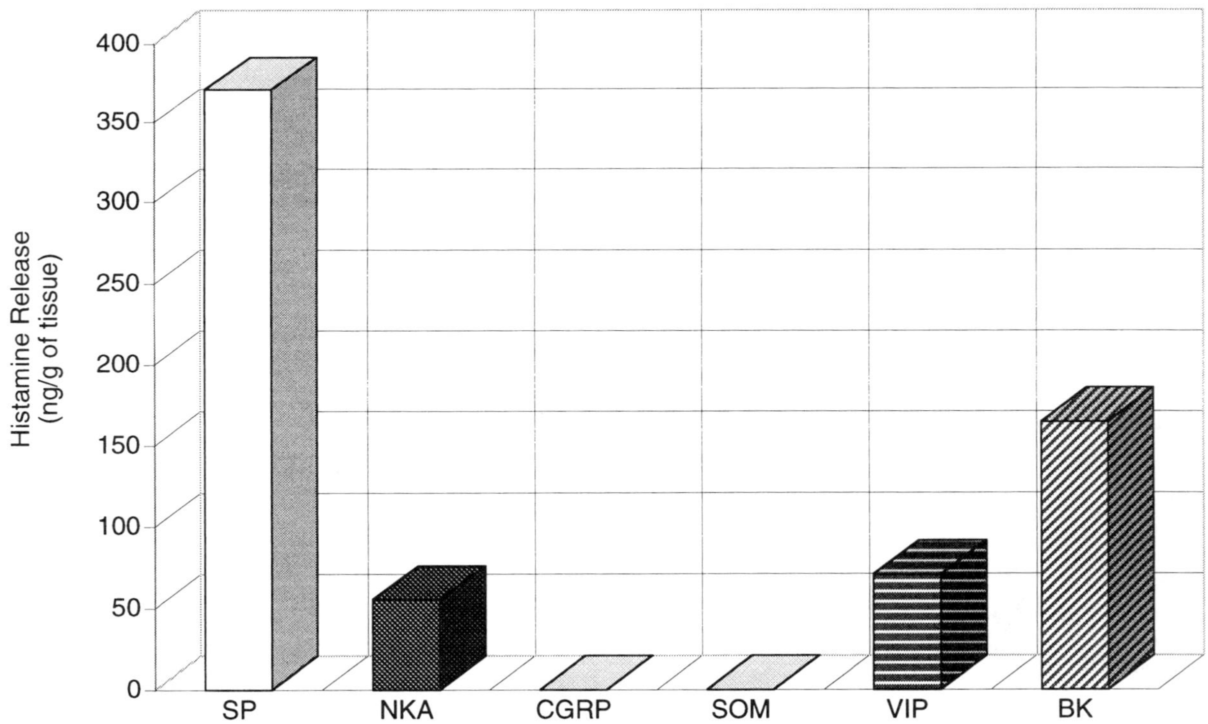

FIG. 3. Release of histamine from isolated guinea pig bladder in response to neuropeptides. Strips of normal guinea pig bladder were incubated in tissue baths with 1 μM concentrations of substance P (SP), neurokinin A (NKA), calcitonin gene-related peptide (CGRP), somatostatin (SOM; octreotide, a long-acting analog of somatostatin), vasoactive intestinal peptide (VIP), or bradykinin (BK) for 30 min, and histamine release (ng/g tissue) was determined by ELISA (Miles Inc., West Haven, CT); $n = 6$ animals.

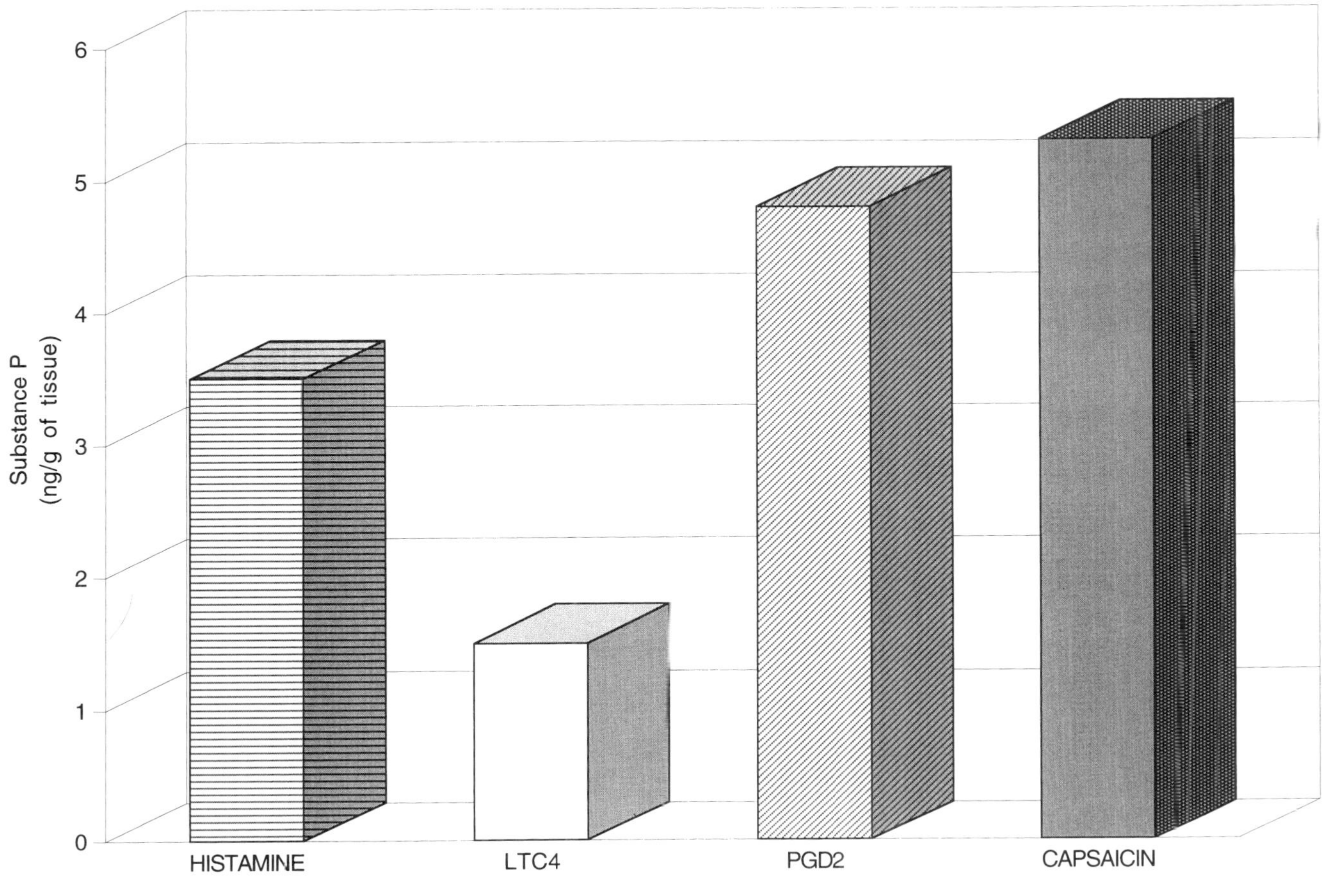

FIG. 4. Release of substance P from isolated guinea pig bladder in response to inflammatory mediators and capsaicin. Strips of normal guinea pig bladder were incubated in tissue baths with histamine (1 μM), leukotriene C_4 (LTC_4; 1 μM), prostaglandin D_2 (PGD_2; 1 μM), or capsaicin (3 μM) for 30 min, and substance P release (ng/g tissue) was determined by radioimmunoassay; $n = 8$ animals. (Altered from Bjorling et al., ref. 39, with permission.)

from intestinal mast cells (48) and mast cell degranulation by antidromic cutaneous nerve stimulation (49).

MAST CELLS AND THE AXON REFLEX

Localization of SP-, CGRP-, and VIP-immunoreactive nerves in the bladder mucosa, their contact with mast cells and vasculature, and the close mast cell proximity to bladder vessels support the concept of mast cell participation in axon-reflex-mediated vasodilation (49,50) on exposure to noxious stimuli in urine or blood. Such interaction was recently proposed (33,51). Participation of mast cells in the axon reflex is supported by the observation that intradermal SP injection in rats causes mast cell histamine release, mimicking injection of histamine or compound 48/80 (a mast cell secretagogue) (52), and that its effect is attenuated in guinea pigs by the SP-cleaving enzyme, neutral endopeptidase (53). Moreover, antidromic stimulation of afferent sensory nerves of the guinea pig bladder causes increased vascular permeability attributed to release of neuropeptides (54), which act directly on the vasculature and indirectly through histamine release from juxtavascular mast cells. The role of neuronal SP in this response has been well documented. However, other tachykinins, and CGRP, generally do not induce mast cell histamine release, although plasma extravasation in response to SP is augmented by CGRP (55–58). Axon-reflex-mediated vasodilation can be significantly inhibited by pretreatment with antihistamine (also suggesting mast cell involvement) or capsaicin (which depletes sensory nerves of SP and CGRP) (49,59).

Functional results of interaction between ET-1 and mast cells further support a role for mast cells in axon-reflex-mediated vasodilation and plasma extravasation. For example, a major component of flare induced by ET-1 results from mast cell activation that is secondary to direct ET-1 stimulation of sensory nerves (60). Although ET-1 had minimal effect on spontaneous neuropeptide release, pretreatment of cultured rat sensory neurons with 500 nM ET-1 resulted in a 50% augmentation of SP and CGRP release in response to 50 nM capsaicin (61). These findings suggest that ET-1 may act as a paracrine sub-

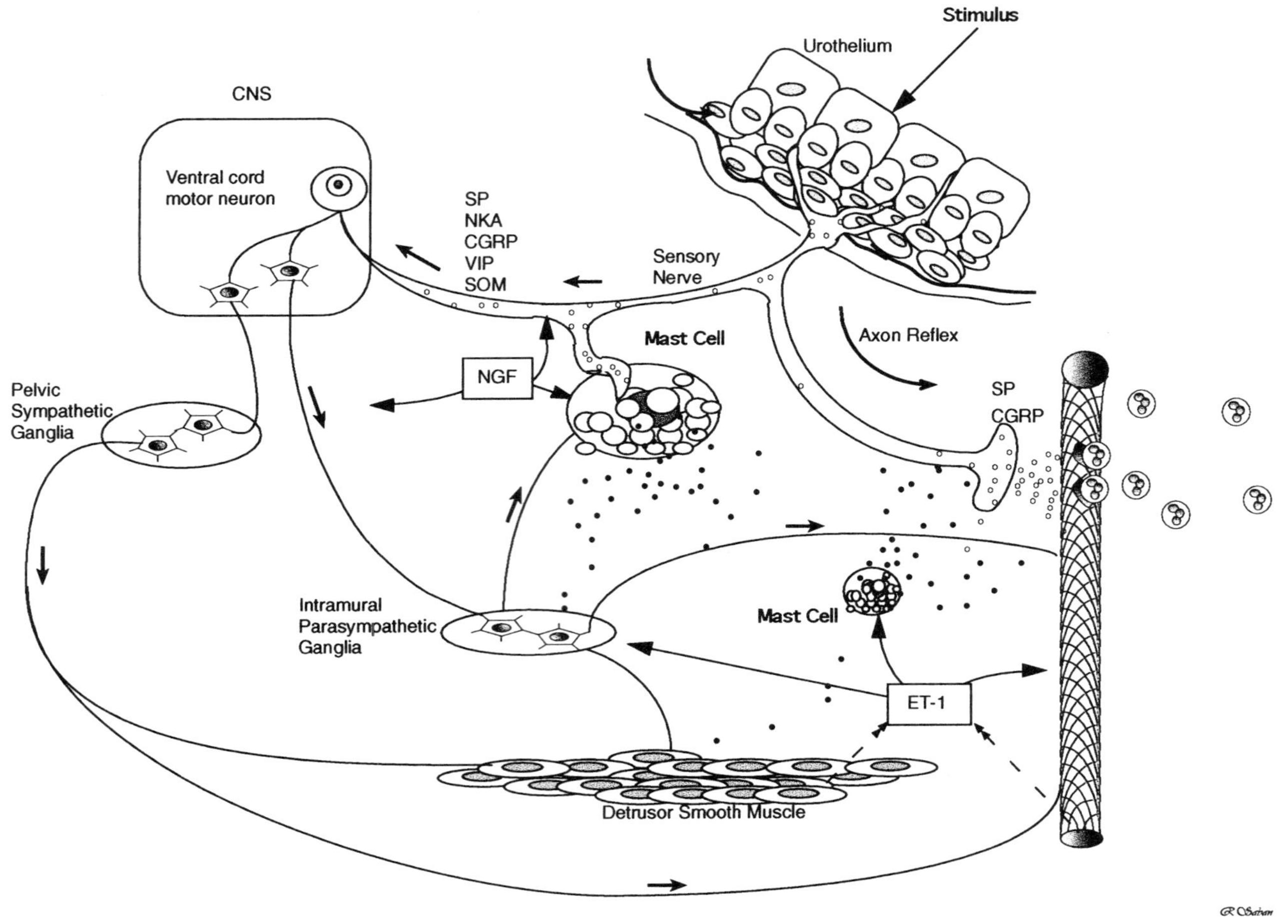

FIG. 5. Schematic illustration of the neural circuitry and its interaction with mast cells in the bladder. An irritant stimulus to the urothelium is perceived by the sensory nerve and transmitted to the central nervous system, initiating a reflex arc that involves motor efferents from the spinal cord to pelvic ganglia and bladder ganglia, resulting in vascular and detrusor smooth muscle effects. In addition, urothelial stimulation may directly affect these tissues via an axon reflex, resulting in release of neuropeptides *(open circles)* that induce mast cell release of other vasoactive agents, peptidases, and inflammatory mediators *(filled circles)* adjacent to vessels, nerves, and detrusor. Inflammatory mediators and neuropeptides cause increased vascular permeability and ingress of leukocytes or may stimulate further neural release of neuropeptides (particularly substance P). This axon-reflex-mediated event may become a self-perpetuating cycle leading to chronic changes. Endothelin-1 (ET-1) released from the detrusor or endothelium causes vasoconstriction, activation of mast cells (via stimulation of sensory nerves), and stimulation of intramural ganglia, amplifying the response. Nerve growth factor (NGF), produced by the nerves or mast cells, stimulates mast cell hyperplasia and synthesis of neuropeptides and likely contributes to neuronal proliferation. The interrelationship of these processes with neural control of the bladder contributes to detrusor hyperreactivity associated with IC and other inflammatory processes of the bladder.

stance, neurotransmitter, or neuromodulator by augmenting axon-reflex-mediated histamine release. In fact, ET-1 is one of the most potent stimulants of histamine release from mouse peritoneal mast cells discovered to date (62). In the urinary bladder, axon reflexes can also cause noninfectious, neurogenic inflammation (54), and the influx of inflammatory cells from the blood vasculature via diapedesis could be enhanced by mast cell involvement (Fig. 5). Neurogenic inflammation is extensively reviewed in Chapter 8.

MAST CELLS AND NEURONAL PLASTICITY IN THE URINARY BLADDER

The bidirectional interaction between mast cells and nerves can be modulated by various mechanisms. For example, mast cell-induced neuronal growth could amplify functional nerve–mast cell interactions. The potential for neural plasticity within the urinary bladder is evidenced by increased innervation in bladders of patients with chronic IC (2). Specifically, increased numbers of fibers containing VIP and NPY were reported in submucosa and detrusor muscle of IC patients (7), at the same anatomic location where contact between nerve fibers with VIP-LI and mast cells have been reported (19). This increased nerve density suggests enhanced sympathetic outflow to the bladder (3). Moreover, time-lapse studies of murine sympathetic neurons cocultured *in vitro* with murine leukemia (RBL-2H3) cells (homologs of mucosal mast cells) showed 60% to 100% neurite–mast cell contact within 17 hr (63). That study proposed a neurotrophic effect of mast cells, also suggested by ultrastructural evidence in the guinea pig urinary bladder (17). Endothelin-1 may modulate the process of neuritic outgrowth (64), and bone-marrow-derived mast cells have been identified as a source of ET-1 (62).

The recent observation that peritoneal mast cells synthesize and store nerve growth factor (NGF) (65) and the findings that NGF stimulates synthesis of sensory peptides (66) and induces mast cell hyperplasia (67) indicate significant participation of NGF in mast cell interaction with local primary sensory afferent nerves. Nerve growth factor is a neurotrophic protein essential for the development, functional maintenance, and regeneration of the peripheral sympathetic nervous system (68–71) and the central nervous system (72). It also promotes survival and integrity of a large percentage of sensory neurons, including small-fiber pain-transmitting neurons often prominently affected in diabetic neuropathy (73). Recent observations in our laboratory of increased NGF content in mast cells contacting nerves and intramural ganglia in urinary bladders after sensitization to the bacterial product hemolysin (Fig. 6) suggests that mast cell-mediated neuronal plasticity can occur in the urinary bladder on mast cell activation by antigen. Not only may peripheral

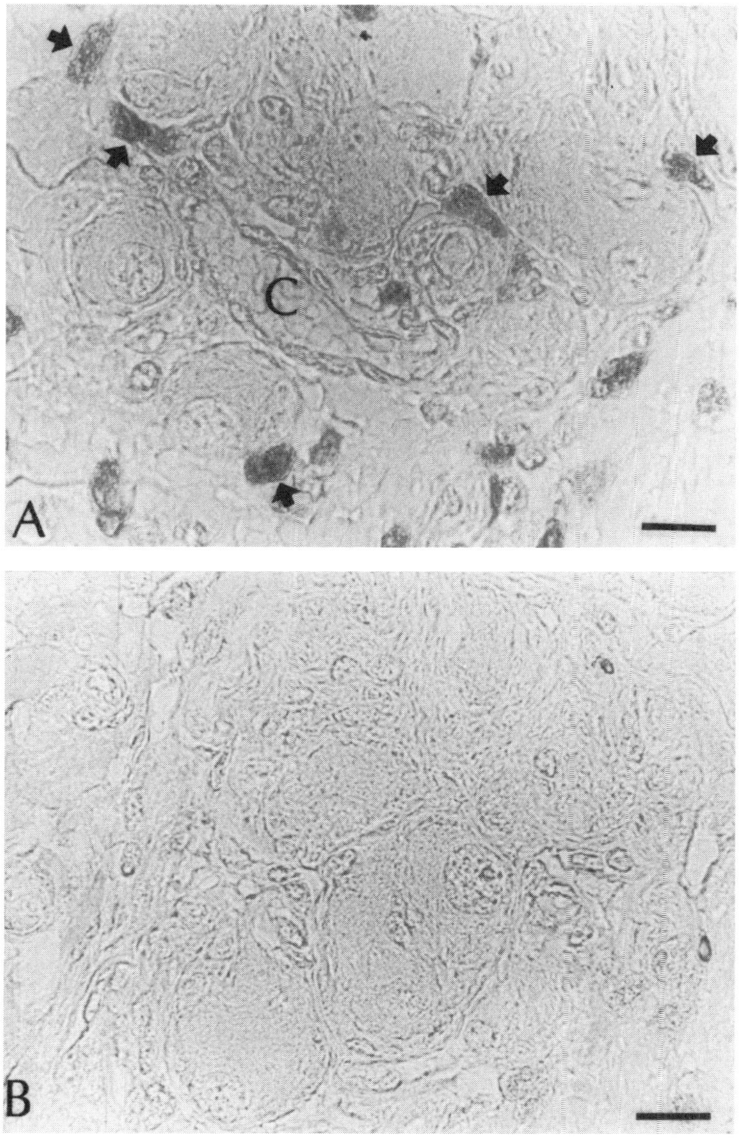

FIG. 6. (A) Intramural parasympathetic ganglion in urinary bladder of hemolysin-sensitized guinea pig immunoreacted with monoclonal antibodies raised against human nerve growth factor (NGF) (500 ng/ml, Promega Corporation, Fitchburg, WI, followed by the ZYMED histostain kit). Note numerous immunopositive mast cells around and within the ganglion, many in close apposition to perikarya *(fat arrows).* **(B)** Mast cells in bladders of control, nonsensitized guinea pigs were fewer and did not display NGF-like immunoreactivity. Omission of the specific primary antibody completely abolished any immunoreactivity. C, capillary. Bouin's fixation, 5-μm-thick paraffin sections. Scale bar, 100 μm.

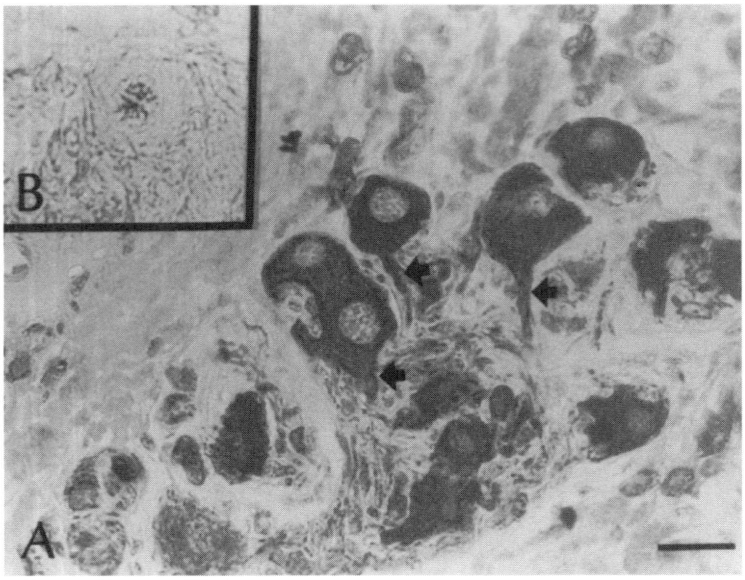

FIG. 7. Intramural parasympathetic ganglion in urinary bladder of ovalbumin-sensitized/challenged guinea pig immunoreacted with rabbit antiserum against the neuronal marker, neurofibrillary protein (NFP, 1:50, Accurate Chemical & Scientific Corp., Westburg, NY). Perikarya, axons *(arrows),* and other nerve fibers appear dark. Note a perikaryon with two nuclei sharing the same cytoplasm, suggestive of incomplete mitotic division or increased synthetic activity. Double nuclei were frequently observed in perikarya of these antigen-sensitized/challenged guinea pigs, and visible chromosomes in these nerve cell bodies **(inset)** were immunochemically enhanced using monoclonal antibodies to the endogenous cyclin D_3 expressed during mitosis (5 µg/ml, Transduction Laboratories, Lexington, KY). Bouin's fixation, 5-µm-thick paraffin sections and peroxidase–antiperoxidase method. Scale bar, 80 µm.

nerve fibers become more numerous and branched, but frequent small intramural autonomic ganglia were noted in bladders from ovalbumin-sensitized/challenged guinea pigs, some having perikarya with two nuclei sharing the same cytoplasm (Figs. 7 and 8), suggestive of ganglionic recruitment of new perikarya by mitosis or increased neuronal synthetic activity. Visible chromosomes in some nuclei of these perikarya, emphasized by immunoreactivity with antibodies against chromosomal cyclin D_3 (which occurs naturally only during cell division) (Fig. 7) further support mitotic activity in these ganglionic neuronal cell bodies. This was not observed in control bladders not sensitized to ovalbumin.

The stimulating effect of mast cells on neuronal growth is substantiated by the observation of mast cell-induced neuronal growth of neurofibromas (74) and neuromas (75). Moreover, NGF is critically involved in mast cell-associated peripheral thermal, but not mechanical, hyperalgesia (76). Profound behavioral hyperalgesia by excess NGF administration (77) addresses the possibility of mast cell/NGF involvement in the suprapubic bladder pain typical of IC and provides further evidence of an effect of NGF on sensory nerves. Temporary relief of symptoms in five patients with hypersensitivity disorders of the lower urinary tract was observed after intravesical capsaicin, confirming the participation of sensory nerve fibers in bladder pain (78). Mast cell-mediated increased sensory innervation could be associated with increased pain sensation. These data argue strongly for mast cell-mediated neuronal plasticity in the urinary bladder, and

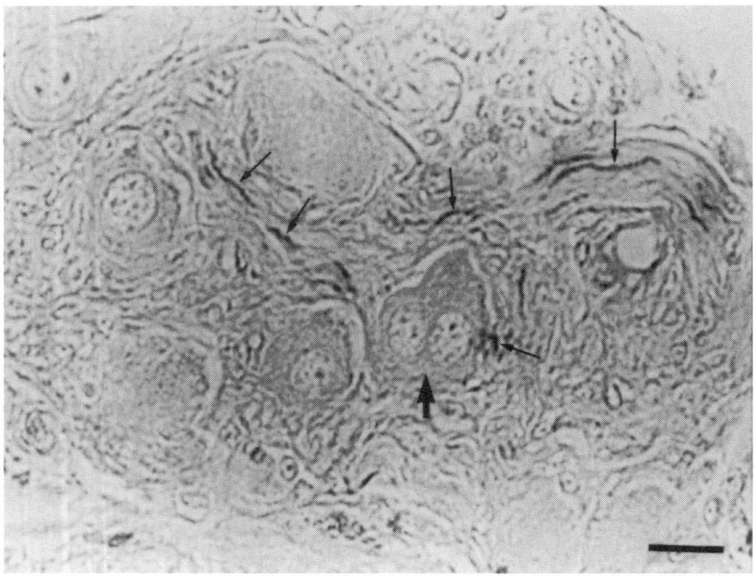

FIG. 8. Intramural parasympathetic ganglion in urinary bladder of ovalbumin-sensitized/challenged guinea pig displaying nitric oxide syntase-like immunoreactivity (1:500, rabbit b-NOS antiserum, Transduction Laboratories, Lexington, KY) in nerve fibers of a proximal nerve and in individual nerve fibers in close proximity to perikarya *(arrows).* Note one perikaryon has two nuclei *(fat arrow).* Bouin's fixation, 5-µm-thick paraffin sections and peroxidase–antiperoxidase method. Scale bar, 100 µm.

this has pathophysiological consequences in IC and other chronic inflammatory disorders.

DYSFUNCTIONAL NERVE–MAST CELL INTERACTION: A PUTATIVE BASIS FOR BLADDER DISEASE

The role of mast cells in IC is discussed in detail in Chapter 12. The intimate mast cell innervation (endonervation) described in the urinary bladder wall in conjunction with excessive neuronal proliferation and mast cell activation by peptidergic, antigenic, and bacterial stimulation suggest that disproportionate interactions between these structures may be pathogenic or may contribute to local chronic disease involving the mucosa and detrusor smooth muscle. It is likely that mast cell degranulation contributes significantly to the pathogenesis of cystitis, but this is obviously not the sole pathogenic process in bladder disorders such as IC. In most studies, SP stimulates histamine release from mast cells isolated from a variety of tissues and species, but NKA and CGRP generally fail to stimulate mast cell histamine release (56,57). Although SP was described as a histamine-releasing agent at least 18 years ago, the mechanism of its action on mast cells is not fully understood. Mast cells from IC bladders were more responsive than mast cells from normal bladder to calcium ionophore A23187 and anti-IgE, as measured by histamine release (79). Mast cell activation in IC is also indicated by a fourfold increase in urinary methylhistamine (the major metabolite of histamine) and tryptase and by ultrastructural evidence of profound degranulation in bladders of IC patients (1).

Histamine can cause vasodilation and plasma extravasation (edema) as a result of increased vascular permeability, modulate neurotransmitter release, and act as a spasmogen on nonvascular smooth muscle (Fig. 5) (42,50,59,80,81). Imbalance in the mutual exchange and feedback system between nerves and mast cells could thus result in vasodilation or constriction, edema, ulceration, increased detrusor reactivity (resulting in increased voiding frequency), inflammation, and pain, all symptoms of IC.

Mucosal Ulceration

Sensory innervation protects the bladder mucosa against noxious stimuli. Findings in intestinal tract biopsies from patients with ulcerative colitis and Crohn's disease, as well as cutaneous biopsies of psoriasis lesions, suggest that abnormal nerve–mast cell interactions may cause mucosal and epidermal ulceration (29–31). Capsaicin-sensitive nerves have been observed in the bladders of various species (78,82). The recent discovery of specific capsaicin-sensitive receptors (vanilloid receptors, 260 kDa) on primary afferent neurons in the urinary bladder (83) suggests that repeated activation of these receptors, perhaps by ET-1 (61), could lead to abnormal mast cell stimulation and bladder disease Ulcerative lesions in the bladder mucosa [Hunner's ulcer (84)] occur in about 10% of IC cases (85) and may be caused by the same dysfunction proposed in the intestine and skin. However, acute release of sensory peptides protects the mucosa against damage. Calcitonin gene-related peptide (exogenously applied or released by topical capsaicin treatment) is known to mediate protection against gastric mucosal ulceration by increasing gastric blood flow and SOM secretion (86–88). Removal of sensory nerve influence by capsaicin treatment leads to loss of the protective action, presumably by depletion of protective neuropeptides (89), suggesting that CGRP is essential for mucosal protection. The CGRP may act directly or may facilitate acetylcholine-induced vasodilation, probably by activation of K^+ (90). In the bladder, SP-evoked mast cell release of proteolytic enzymes, as described in the skin (91), may accelerate CGRP degradation, thus facilitating mucosal ulceration.

Experimentally, the acute protective effect of capsaicin seems to depend in part on the release of nitric oxide (NO), because blockade of nitric oxide synthase (NOS) reduces the protective effect of acute capsaicin but not prostaglandin E_2 (92). Nitric oxide has also been shown to inhibit leukocyte adhesion in postcapillary venules *in vivo,* similar to the effect of superoxide dismutase (93), thereby preventing diapedesis and inflammation. This has been attributed in part to NO scavenging of the proadhesive mast cell activator molecule, superoxide. Moreover, inhibition of NO synthesis with either L-NMMA or L-NAME increased leukocyte adhesion fourfold, mimicking the effect of the mast cell activator 48/80. The response was abolished by the mast cell stabilizer ketitofen (94). These data indicate that NO has a functional relationship with mast cells. Immunohistochemistry using antiserum to the neural form of NOS revealed localization of NOS-LI in nerve fibers of vessels and intramural parasympathetic ganglia (Fig. 8), where presumptive motor CGRP fibers are also found, suggesting additional sources of NO within the urinary bladder. Effective NO–mast cell interaction could thus be facilitated by the close neural contact with mast cells. Nitric oxide may also contribute to mucosal protection by its vasodilatory effect on mucosal vessels. In fact, NO regulates gastric mucosal blood flow during both the resting and the secretory phase (95). Although NO donors have been shown to protect against ulceration, unregulated release of high levels of NO can lead to mucosal injury (95).

The neuropeptide SOM has also been shown to prevent experimental injury of the gastric mucosa *in vivo,* probably through inhibition of mast cell activation (96–98) and interaction with other mucosal sensory peptides, e.g., CGRP release and inhibition of SP (99). The use of a

SOM antagonist confirms the specific role of SOM by inhibition of its protective effect (99). Moreover, SOM selectively antagonizes SP, a neutrophil chemoattractant, thus modulating SP-induced inflammatory cell influx (100), and can also inhibit VIP release (101). Both SP and VIP have been shown to stimulate histamine secretion from rat peritoneal mast cells (102). Mast cell participation in gastric mucosal injury is indicated by observations of a high inverse correlation ($r = -0.85$) between degree of hemorrhagic mucosal ulceration and number of mast cells present; i.e., mast cell depletion was correlated with decreased mucosal injury (97). On the other hand, at higher doses (10^{-7} mol/rat, i.p.), SOM can exacerbate ethanol-induced gastric injury; both SOM-14 and SOM-28 were shown to induce mast cell degranulation at a rate that corresponded with severity of lesions (96). This dose-dependent effect was also observed in peritoneal mast cells (102,103). However, the effects of SOM on mast cells may be tissue-specific, because mast cells from intestine and many other human tissues did not respond to SOM (104). Preliminary studies suggest that SOM, administered subcutaneously to OVA-sensitized guinea pigs, reduced mast cell ingress to the urinary bladder on OVA challenge, and pretreatment of mice with a SOM analog (octreotide acetate; 50 μg subcutaneously) caused a significant decrease in Evans blue dye extravasation and ingress of MCs into the bladder wall in response to subsequent intravesical capsaicin (D. E. Bjorling and R. Saban, *unpublished data*). It appears that endogenous SOM may act to limit the severity of neurogenic inflammation.

Endothelin-1 is known to exert long-lasting vasoconstriction. Synthesis and secretion of this peptide have been reported in bone-marrow-derived mast cells that also express ET_A receptors having high affinity for ET-1 (62). Thus, mast cells may be a source of ET-1 in addition to that produced by bladder epithelia and smooth muscle. Local ET-1 availability can be increased by extracellular cleavage of the precursor big ET into ET-1 by mast cell-derived chymase, as demonstrated in a perfused rat lung preparation (105). Endothelin-1 is known to induce mast cell histamine secretion, block orthodromic action potentials in colonic parasympathetic ganglia (106), modulate peptide release from primary sensory afferent neurons (61), and directly vasoconstrict mucosal vessels, potentially contributing to ulcerative lesions. In fact, ET-1 induces mucosal injury following local administration (95).

Investigations utilizing bladder biopsies from IC patients and experimental models of IC provide further evidence for mast cell involvement in mucosal lesions. For example, mast cell numbers specifically beneath the mucosal lesions increased by 90% (107) and conformational changes were described in detrusor mast cells in biopsies from IC patients (108,109). Mast cell degranulation and increased mast cell size in the detrusor were also reported in the ovalbumin-sensitized/challenged guinea pig model of increased detrusor contractility and chronic bladder inflammation (24).

Increased Detrusor Contractility

Increased mast cell–nerve association can lead to a decrease in the threshold of stimuli necessary to trigger bladder contraction. Increased bladder contraction, increased frequency of micturition, and decreased voiding volumes were observed when sensitized animals were challenged intravesically with antigen (110). Bladder contractility was found to be enhanced in sensitized guinea pigs on antigen challenge *in vitro* (24). Edema and increased detrusor contractility (instability) typically occur in IC. This is also supported by the findings that activation of bladder sensory C-fibers initiates reflex micturition (78,111,112), mediates pain sensation (54), and causes local release of SP and NKA (77). Cystometric evidence in humans specifically reveals that capsaicin-sensitive nerves may modulate the afferent branch of micturition (78). Both histamine and tachykinins have been shown to induce contraction of urinary bladder smooth muscle (12,24,113), and CGRP has been proposed as a regulator of bladder smooth muscle tone (114). Furthermore, mast cells have been implicated in refractory idiopathic detrusor instability (115) and in detrusor changes associated with IC (116–118).

Increased bladder contractility could also be caused by changes in availability of and response to ET-1. This potent constrictor peptide was demonstrated to induce concentration-dependent contraction of isolated human detrusor strips (119). Endothelin-1 may also act through enhancement of sensory peptide release induced by stimulation of capsaicin-sensitive receptors (61) or by modulation of adrenergic neurotransmission at the neuroeffector junction (120). Enhancement of smooth muscle tone by these peptides may be direct or through the release of histamines or prostaglandins (primarily PGD_2) from local mast cells, mediating long-lasting changes in the microenvironment.

CONCLUDING REMARKS

As described in this chapter and illustrated in Fig. 5, neuropeptide–mast cell interaction may affect bladder inflammation by various mechanisms. There appears to be an intimate anatomic relationship between afferent sensory nerve fibers and mast cells, and trophic factors produced by mast cells or trophic effects of neuropeptides themselves may induce neuronal proliferation and infiltration of the bladder wall during IC. It must be assumed that, under normal circumstances, homeostatic mechanisms limit the proinflammatory effects of neuropeptides and substances produced by mast cells, and failure of these mechanisms contributes to chronic inflammatory disorders. The processes that result in failure of homeostasis are unclear but may be related in part to alterations in peptide degradation or desensitization. Peptidases, in particular neutral endopeptidase (EC 3.4.24.11) located primarily in the mucosa, degrade neuropeptides, terminating their biological effects (121,122). Removal or damage of the mucosa or inhibition of these peptidases significantly prolongs or amplifies the effects of neuropeptides (12). Exposure of tissues to neuropeptides commonly results in desensitization of the tissues to subsequent exposure to the same compounds, and this phenomenon has been attributed to occupation of receptors or alteration of receptor numbers, geometry, or binding capacity (123). Recently, it has been observed that when SP binds to neurokinin-1 (NK-1) receptors, the receptor complex is internalized into early endosomes, and SP is degraded (124). Tissues remain desensitized to SP until receptors are restored to the surface. Alterations in peptide degradation or receptor number and function may profoundly affect the ability of the bladder to limit the inflammatory response to various irritants.

We have presented anatomic evidence for bidirectional exchange of substances between afferent sensory nerves and mast cells (19), and a reciprocal relationship appears to exist between SP and inflammatory mediators released by mast cells (44). Failure of mechanisms that inactivate neuropeptides may amplify this phenomenon. Neuropeptides also indirectly facilitate mast cell activation by priming mast cells to the effects of other stimuli (125), thereby enhancing mast cell responsiveness. The net result appears to be activation of processes that lead to histologic alterations commonly found in bladder biopsies from IC patients: edema, areas of increased leukocytic infiltration, mastocytosis, and increased numbers of nerve fibers. Therapy specifically targeted at preventing or halting abnormal or undesirable neuropeptide–mast cell interaction has the potential of being an effective component of IC treatment. This requires a more complete understanding of the processes that regulate this interaction during health and disease.

Acknowledgments

We wish to thank Jie Jin and Marcia Saban for excellent technical assistance. Supported by the University of Wisconsin School of Veterinary Medicine and NIH grant DK 42897.

REFERENCES

1. Theoharides TC, Sant GR, El-Mansoury M, Letourneau R, Ucci AA Jr, Meares ER Jr. Activation of bladder mast cells in interstitial cystitis: a light and electron microscopic study. *J Urol* 1995;153:629–636.
2. Letourneau R, Pang X, Sant GR, Theoharides TC. Intragranular activation of bladder mast cells and their association with nerve processes in interstitial cystitis. *Br J Urol* 1996;77:41–54.
3. Christmas TJ, Rode J, Chapple CR, Milroy EJ, Turner-Warwick RT. Nerve fibre proliferation in interstitial cystitis. *Virchows Arch [A] Pathol Anat* 1990;416:447–451.
4. Pang X, Marchand J, Sant GR, Theoharides TC. Increased number of substance P positive fibres in interstitial cystitis. *Br J Urol* 1995;75: 744–750.
5. Lundeberg T, Liedberg H, Norling L, Theodorsson E, Owzarski A, Ekman P. Interstitial cystitis: correlation with nerve fibres, mast cells and histamine. *Br J Urol* 1993;71:427–429.
6. Lynes WL, Flynn SD, Shortliffe LD, Lemmers M, Zipser R, Roberts LJ II, Stamey TA. Mast cell involvement in interstitial cystitis. *J Urol* 1987;138:746–752.
7. Hohenfeller M, Nunes L, Schmidt RA, Lampel A, Thuroff JW, Tanagho EA. Interstitial cystitis: increased sympathetic innervation and related neuropeptide synthesis. *J Urol* 1992;147:587–591.
8. Hökfelt T, Schultzberg M, Elde R, et al. Peptide neurons in peripheral tissues including the urinary tract: immunohistochemical studies. *Acta Pharmacol Toxicol* 1978;43(Suppl)2:79–89.
9. Jen PY, Dixon JS, Gosling JA. Immunohistochemical localization of neuromarkers and neuropeptides in human fetal and neonatal urinary bladder. *Br J Urol* 1995;75:230–235.
10. Maggi CA, Gepetti P, Santicioli P, et al. Tachykinin-like immunoreactivity in the mammalian bladder: correlation with the functions of the capsaicin-sensitive sensory nerves. *Neuroscience* 1988;27:233–242.
11. Mattiasson A, Ekblad E, Sundler F, Uvelius B. Origin and distribution of neuropeptide Y-, vasoactive polypeptide- and substance P-containing nerve fibers in the urinary bladder of the rat. *Cell Tissue Res* 1985; 239:141–146.
12. Saban R, Keith IM, Nielsen K, Christensen M, Rhodes P, Bruskewitz R. *In vitro* effects of bladder mucosa and an enkephalinase inhibitor on tachykinin induced contractility of the dog bladder. *J Urol* 1992;147: 750–755.
13. Sharkey KA, Williams RG, Schultzberg M, Dockray GJ. Sensory substance P innervation of the urinary bladder: possible site of action in causing urine retention in rats. *Neuroscience* 1983;10:861–868.
14. Su HC, Wharton J, Polak JM, et al. Calcitonin gene-related peptide immunoreactivity in afferent neurons supplying the urinary tract: Combined retrograde tracing and immunohistochemistry. *Neuroscience* 1986;18:727–747.
15. Yokokawa K, Sakanaka M, Shiosaka S, Tohyama M, Shiotani Y, Aonoda T. Three-dimensional distribution of substance P-like immunoreactivity in the urinary bladder of the rat. *J Neural Transm* 1985;63: 209–222.
16. de Groat WC, Kawatani M, Hisamitsu T, et al. The role of neuropeptides in the sacral autonomic reflex pathways of the cat. *J Auton Nerv Syst* 1983;7:339–350.
17. Keast JR, De Groat WC. Segmental distribution and peptide content of primary afferent neurons innervating the urogenital organs and colon of male rats. *J Comp Neurol* 1992;319:615–623.
18. Lasanen LT, Tammela TLJ, Liesi P, Waris T, Polak JM. The effect of acute distension on vasoactive intestinal polypeptide (VIP), Neuropeptide Y (NPY) and substance P (SP) immunoreactive nerves in the female rat urinary bladder. *Urol Res* 1992;20:259–263.
19. Keith IM, Jin J, Saban R. Nerve–mast cell interaction in guinea pig urinary bladder. *J Comp Neurol* 1995;363:28–36.
20. Saenz de Tejada I, Mueller JD, de Las Morenas A, Machado M, Moreland RB, Krane RJ, Wolfe HJ, Traish AM. Endothelin in the urinary bladder. I. Synthesis of endothelin-1 by epithelia, muscle and fibroblasts suggests autocrine and paracrine cellular regulation. *J Urol* 1992; 148:1290–1298.
21. Franco-Cereda A, Rydh M, Lou YP, Dalsgaard CJ, Lundberg JM. Endothelin as a putative sensory neuropeptide in the guinea pig. *Regul Pept* 1991;32:253–265.
22. Pang X, Boucher W, Triadafilopoulos G, Sant GR, Theoharides TC. Mast cell and substance P-positive nerve involvement in a patient with both irritable bowel syndrome and interstitial cystitis. *Urology* 1996; 47:436–438.
23. Ratliff TLl, Klutke CG, Hofmeister M,He F, Russell JH, Becich MJ. Short analytical review: Role of the immune response in interstitial cystitis. *Clin Immunol Immunopathol* 1995;74:209–216.
24. Saban R, Christensen M, Keith M, et al. Experimental model for the study of bladder mast cell degranulation and smooth muscle contraction. *Semin Urol* 1991;9:88–101.
25. Kruger L, Silverman JD, Mantyh PW, Sternini C, Brecha NC. Peripheral patterns of calcitonin gene-related peptide general somatic sensory innervation: cutaneous and deep terminations. *J Comp Neurol* 1989;280:291–302.

26. Arizono N, Matsuda S, Hattori T, Kojima Y, Maeda T, Galli S. Anatomical variation in mast cell nerve associations in the rat small intestine, heart, lung, and skin. *Lab Invest* 1990;62:626–634.
27. Stead RH, Perdue MH, Blennerhassett MG, Kakuta Y, Sestini P, Bienenstock J. The innervation of mast cells. In: Freir S, ed. *The Neuroendocrine–Immune Network.* Boca Raton: CRC Press, 1990;19–37.
28. McKay DM, Bienenstock J. The interaction between mast cells and nerves in the gastrointestinal tract. *Immunol Today* 1994;15(11): 533–538.
29. Dvorak AM, McLeod RS, Onderdonk AB, et al. Human gut mucosal mast cells: ultrastructural observations and anatomic variation in mast cell–nerve associations. *Int Arch Allergy Immunol* 1992;98:158–168.
30. Yonei Y. Autonomic nervous alterations and mast cell degranulation in the exacerbation of ulcerative colitis. *Jpn J Gastroenterol* 1987;84: 1045–1056.
31. Naukkarinen A, Harvima IT, Aalto ML, Harvima RJ, Horsmanheimo M. Quantitative analysis of contact sites between mast cells and sensory nerves in cutaneous psoriasis and lichen planus based on a double staining technique. *Arch Dermatol Res* 1991;283:433–437.
32. Hukkanen M, Grönblad M, Rees R, et al. Regional distribution of mast cells and peptide containing nerves in normal and adjuvant arthritic rat synovium. *J Rheumatol* 1991;18:177–183.
33. Bienenstock J, MacQueen G, Sestini P, Marshall JS, Stead RH, Perdue MH. Mast cell/nerve interactions *in vitro* and *in vivo. Am Rev Respir Dis* 1991;143:S55–S58.
34. Stead RH, Tomioka M, Quinonez G, Simon GT, Felten SY, Bienestock J. Intestinal mucosal mast cells in normal and nematode-infected rat intestines are in intimate contact with peptidergic nerves. *Proc Natl Acad Sci (USA)* 1987;84:2975–2979.
35. Stead RH, Tomioka M, Riddell RH, Bienenstock J. Substance P and/or calcitonin gene-related peptide are present in subepithelial enteric nerves apposed to intestinal mucosal mast cells. In: MacDermott RP, ed. *Inflammatory Bowel Disease: Current Status and Future Approach.* Amsterdam: Elsevier, 1988;43–48.
36. Christian EP, Undem BJ, Weinreich D. Endogenous histamine excites neurones in the guinea pig superior cervical ganglion. *J Physiol (Lond)* 1989;409:297–312.
37. Newson B, Dahlström A, Enerbäck L, Ahlman H. Suggestive evidence for a direct innervation of mucosal mast cells. *Neuroscience* 1983;10: 565–570.
38. Skofitsch G, Savitt JM, Jacobowitz DM. Suggestive evidence for a functional unit between mast cells and substance P fibers in the rat diaphragm and mesentery. *Histochemistry* 1985;82:5–8.
39. Wiesner-Menzel L, Schultz B, Vakildazeh F, Czarnetzki BM. Electron microscopical evidence for a direct contact between nerve fibres and mast cells. *Acta Dermatovener (Stockh)* 1981;61:465–469.
40. Mousli M, Bueb JL, Bronner C, Rouot B, Landry Y. G protein activation: A receptor-independent mode of action for cationic amphiphilic neuropeptides and venom peptides. *Trends Pharmacol Sci* 1990;11: 358–362.
41. Undem BJ, Weinreich D. Electrophysiological properties and chemosensitivity of guinea pig nodose ganglion neurons *in vitro. J Auton Nerv Syst* 1993;44:17–34.
42. Johnson D, Krenger W. Interactions of mast cells with the nervous system—recent advances. *Neurochem Res* 1992;17:939–951.
43. Shanahan F, Denburg J, Fox J, Bienenstock J, Befus AD. Mast cell heterogeneity: Effects of neuroenteric peptides on histamine release. *J Immunol* 1985;135:1331–1337.
44. Bjorling DE, Saban MR, Saban R. Neurogenic inflammation of guinea pig bladder. *Mediators Inflam* 1994;3:189–197.
45. Janiszewski J, Bienenstock J, Blennerhassett MG. Activation of rat peritoneal mast cells in coculture with sympathetic neurons alters neuronal physiology. *Brain Behav Immun* 1990;2:139–150.
46. Undem B, Weinreich D, Ellis J, Meyers A. Neuronal consequences of the allergic response in the airways. In: Holgate FT, Austin KF, Lichtenstein LM, Kay AB, eds. *Asthma: Physiology, Immunopharmacology, and Treatment. Fourth International Symposium.* London: Academic Press, 1993;275–286.
47. Crowe SE, Perdue MH. Functional abnormalities in the intestine associated with mucosal mast cell activation. *Reg Immunol* 1992;4: 113–117.
48. Yonei Y, Oda M, Nakamura M, et al. Evidence for direct interaction between the cholinergic nerve and mast cells in rat colonic mucosa. An electron microscope cytochemical and autoradiographic study. *J Clin Electr Microsc* 1985;18:560–561.
49. Lembeck F, Holzer P. Substance P as neurogenic mediator of antidromic vasodilation and neurogenic plasma extravasation. *Naunyn-Schmiedebergs Arch Pharmacol* 1979;310:175–183.
50. Kiernan JA. A pharmacological and histological investigation of the involvement of mast cells in cutaneous axon reflex vasodilation. *Q J Exp Physiol* 1975;60:123–130.
51. Marshall JS, Waserman S. Mast cells and the nerves—potential interactions in the context of chronic disease. *Clin Exp Allergy* 1995;25: 102–110.
52. Hagermark O, Hökfelt T, Pernow B. Flare and itch induced by substance P in human skin. *J Invest Dermatol* 1978;71:233–235.
53. Rubenstein I, Iwamoto I, Ueki IF, Borson B, Nadel JA. Recombinant neutral endopeptidase attenuates substance P-induced plasma extravasation in the guinea pig skin. *Int Arch Allergy Appl Immunol* 1990;91: 232–238.
54. Lundberg JM, Brodin E, Hua X, Saria A. Vascular permeability changes and smooth muscle contractions in relation to capsaicin-sensitive substance P afferents in the guinea pig. *Acta Physiol Scand* 1984;120:217–227.
55. Brain SD, Williams TJ. Inflammatory oedema induced by synergism between calcitonin gene-related peptide (CGRP) and mediators of vascular permeability. *Br J Pharmacol* 1985;86:855–860.
56. Foreman JC, Jordan CC, Oehme P, Renner H. Structure–activity relationships for some substance P-related peptides that cause wheal and flare reactions in human skin. *J Physiol* 1983;335:449–465.
57. Foreman JC. Peptides and neurogenic inflammation. *Brain Res Bull* 1987;43:386–398.
58. Gamse R, Saria A. Potentiation of tachykinin-induced plasma protein extravasation by calcitonin gene-related peptide. *Eur J Pharmacol* 1985;114:61–66.
59. Kiernan JA. The involvement of mast cells in vasodilatation due to axon reflexes in injured skin. *Q J Exp Physiol* 1972;53:311–317.
60. Brain SD, Thomas G, Crossman DC, Fuller R, Church MK. Endothelin-1 induces a histamine-dependent flare *in vivo,* but does not activate human skin mast cells *in vitro. Br J Clin Pharmacol* 1992;33: 117–120.
61. Dymshitz J, Vasko MR. Endothelin-1 enhances capsaicin-induced peptide release and cGMP accumulation in cultures of rat sensory neurons. *Neurosci Lett* 1994;167:128–132.
62. Yamamura H, Nabe T, Kohno S, Ohata K. Endothelin-1, one of the most potent histamine releasers in mouse peritoneal mast cells. *Eur J Pharmacol* 1994;265:9–15.
63. Blennerhasset MG, Tomioka M, Bienenstock J. Formation of contacts between mast cells and sympathetic neurons *in vitro. Cell Tissue Res* 1991;265:121–128.
64. Hsu L, Savage P, Jeng AY. Dual effects of endothelin-1 (ET-1) on neurite outgrowth induced by 12-O-tetradecanoylphorbol-13-acetate. *Neurosci Lett* 1992;136:219–222.
65. Leon A, Buriani A, Dal Toso R, Fabris M, Romanello S, Aloe L, Levi Montalcini R. Mast cells synthesize, store, and release nerve growth factor. *Proc Natl Acad Sci (USA)* 1994;91:3739–3743.
66. Vedder H, Affolter HU, Otten U. Nerve growth factor (NGF) regulates tachykinin gene expression and biosynthesis in rat sensory neurons during early postnatal development. *Neuropeptides* 1993;24:351–357.
67. Marshall JS, Stead RH, McSharry C, Nielsen L, Bienenstock J. The role of mast cell degranulation products in mast cell hyperplasia. I. Mechanism of action of nerve growth factor. *J Immunol* 1990;144:1886–1892.
68. Chalazonitis A, Kalberg J, Twardzik DR, Morrison RS, Kessler JA. Transforming growth factor beta has neurotrophic actions on sensory neurons *in vitro* and is synergistic with nerve growth factor. *Dev Biol* 1992;152:121–132.
69. Levi-Montalcini R, Callissano P. Nerve growth factor as a paradigm of other polypeptide growth factors. *Trends Neurosci* 1986;9(10): 275–286.
70. Levi-Montalcini R. The nerve growth factor. Thirty five years later. *EMBO J* 1987;6:1145–1154.
71. Vantini G. The pharmacological potential of neurotrophins: A perspective. *Psychoneuroendocrinology* 1992;17:401–410.
72. Yoshida K, Kakihana M, Chen LS, Ong M, Baird A, Gage FH. Cytokine regulation of nerve growth factor-mediated cholinergic neurotrophic activity synthesized by astrocytes and fibroblasts. *J Neurochem* 1992;59:919–931.
73. Lindner MD, Gordon DD, Miller JM, et al. Increased levels of truncated nerve growth factor receptor in urine of mildly demented patients with Alzheimer's disease. *Arch Neurol* 1993;50:1054–1058.

74. Kawamura K, Jono M, Katsuragi M, Baba S, Shida K. A case of neurofibromatosis with occlusion of multiple cerebral artery, moyamoya phenomenon and scoliosis. *No To Shinkei* 1994;46:1163–1168.
75. Zochodne DW, Nguyen C, Sharkey KA. Accumulation and degranulation of mast cells in experimental neuromas. *Neurosci Lett* 1994; 182:3–6.
76. Lewin GR, Rueff A, Mendell LN. Peripheral and central mechanisms of NGF-induced hyperalgesia. *Eur J Neurosci* 1994;6:1903–1912.
77. Ritter AM, Lewin GR, Mendell LM. Regulation of myelinated nociceptor function by nerve growth factor in neonatal and adult rats. *Brain Res Bull* 1993;30:245–249.
78. Maggi CA, Barbanti G, Santicioli P, et al. Cystometric evidence that capsaicin-sensitive nerves modulate the afferent branch of micturition reflex in humans. *J Urol* 1989;142:150–154.
79. Frenz AM, Christmas TJ, Pearce FL. Does the mast cell have an intrinsic role in the pathogenesis of interstitial cystitis? *Agents Actions* 1994;41(Spec No):C14–C15.
80. Dzeliak DJ, Thureson-Klein A, Klein RL. Local modulation of neurotransmitter release in bovine splenic vein. *Blood Vess* 1983;20:122–134.
81. Kiernan JA. Interaction between mast cells and nerves—neurogenic inflammation. *Trends Pharmacol Sci* 1990;11:316.
82. Maggi CA, Santicioli P, Giuliani Furio S, Meli A. The capsaicin-sensitive innervation of the rat urinary bladder. Further studies on mechanisms regulating micturition treshold. *J Pharmacol Exp Ther* 1986; 136:696–700.
83. Szallasi A, Conte B, Goso C, Blumberg PM, Manzini S. Vanilloid receptors in the urinary bladder: regional distribution, localization on sensory nerves, and species-related differences. *Naunyn Schmiedebergs Arch Pharmacol* 1993;347:624–629.
84. Hunner GL. A rare type of bladder ulcer in women; report of cases. *Boston Med Surg J* 1915;172:660–664.
85. Sant GR, Theoharides TC. The role of the mast cell in interstitial cystitis. *Urol Clin North Am* 1994;21:41–53.
86. Brzozowsky T, Konturek SJ, Pytko-Polonczyk J, Warzecha Z. Gastric adaptation to stress: role of sensory nerves, salivary glands, and adrenal glands. *Scand J Gastroenterol* 1995;30:6–16.
87. Gray JL, Bunnett NW, Orloff SL, Mulvihill SJ, Debas HT. A role for calcitonin gene-related peptide in protection against gastric ulceration. *Ann Surg* 1994;219:58–64.
88. Kinoshita Y, Inui T, Chiba T. Calcitonin gene-related peptide: a neurotransmitter involved in capsaicin-sensitive afferent nerve-mediated gastric mucosal protection. *J Clin Gastroenterol* 1993;17(Suppl)1: S27–S32.
89. Goso C, Evangelista S, Tramontana M, Manzini S, Blumberg PM, Szallasi A. Topical capsaicin administration protects against sulfonic acid-induced colitis in the rat. *Eur J Pharmacol* 1993;249:185–190.
90. Scott MA, Fone KC. Modulation of calcitonin gene-related peptide release from dorsal thoraco-lumbar spinal cord slices by 5-HT_3 receptors. *Neurosci Lett* 1994;175:5–8.
91. Wallengren J, Wang ZY. Interaction between tachykinins and CGRP in human skin. *Acta Derm Venereol* 1993;73:259–261.
92. Konturek SJ, Brzozovsky T, Stachura J, Majka J. Role of neutrophils and mucosal blood flow in gastric adaptation to aspirin. *Eur J Pharmacol* 1994;253:107–114.
93. Kubes P, Suzuki M, Granger DN. Nitric oxide: an endogenous modulator of leukocyte adhesion. *Proc Natl Acad Sci (USA)* 1991;88: 4651–4655.
94. Kubes P, Kanwar S, Niu S-X-F, Gaboury JP. Nitric oxide inhibition induces leukocyte adhesion via superoxide and mast cells. *FASEB J* 1993;7:1293–1299.
95. Whittle BJ, Lopez-Belmonte J. Actions and interactions of endothelins, prostacyclin and nitric oxide in the gastric mucosa. *J Physiol Pharmacol* 1993;44:91–107.
96. Diehl F, Borch H, Hosenfeld S. Effects of somatostatin on ethanol-induced gastric erosions in the rat: role of mast cells. *Agents Actions* 1986;18:273–275.
97. Diehl F, Szabo S. Dose-dependent effects of linear and cyclic somatostatin on ethanol-induced gastric erosions: the role of mast cells and increased vascular permeability in the rat. *Regul Pept* 1986;13:235–243.
98. Laszlo F, Pavo I, Penke B, Balint GA. Protective effect of an orally administered, highly potent somatostatin analog (RC-121) against absolute ethanol-induced hemorrhagic erosions of the rat gastric mucosa. *Life Sci* 1989;44:1573–1578.
99. Karmeli F, Eliakim R, Okon E, Rachmilewitz D. Somatostatin effectively prevents ethanol- and NSAID-induced gastric mucosal damage in rats. *Dig Dis Sci* 1994;39:617–625.
100. Kolasinski SL, Haines KA, Siegel EL, Cronstein BN Abramson SB. Neuropeptides and inflammation. A somatostatin analog as a selective antagonist of neutrophil activation by substance P. *Arthritis Rheum* 1992;35:369–375.
101. Grosman I, Simon D. Potential gastrointestinal uses of somatostatin and its synthetic analogue octreotide. *Am Gastroenterol* 1990;85: 1061–1072.
102. Piotrowski W, Foreman JF. On the actions of substance P, somatostatin, and vasoactive intestinal polypeptide on rat peritoneal mast cells and in human skin. *Naunyn Schmiedebergs Arch Pharmacol* 1985;331: 364–368.
103. Theoharides TC, Douglas WW. Somatostatin induces histamine secretion from rat peritoneal mast cells. *Endocrinology* 1992;102: 1637–1640.
104. Church MK, Lowman MA, Robinson C, Holgate ST, Benyon CR. Interactions of neuropeptides with human mast cells. *Int Arch Allergy Appl Immunol* 1989;88:70–78.
105. Wypij DM, Nichols JS, Novak PJ, Stacy DL, Berman J, Wiseman JS. Role of mast cell chymase in the extracellular processing of big-endothelin-1 to endothelin-1 in the perfused rat lung. *Biochem Pharmacol* 1992;43:845–853.
106. Nishimura T, Krier J, Akas T. Endothelin causes prolonged inhibition of nicotinic trancmission in feline colonic parasympathetic ganglia. *Am J Physiol* 1991;261:G628–G633.
107. Aldenborg F, Fall M, Enerbäck L. Proliferation and transepithelial migration of mucosal mast cells in interstitial cystitis. *Immunology* 1986;58:411–416.
108. Christmas TJ, Rode J. Characteristics of mast cells in normal bladder, bacterial cystitis and interstitial cystitis. *Br J Urol* 1991;68:473–478.
109. Larsen S, Thompson SA, Hald T, et al. Mast cells in interstitial cystitis. *Br J Urol* 1982;54:283–286.
110. Kim YS, Longhurst PA, Wein AJ, Levin RM. Effects of sensitization on female guinea pig urinary bladder function: *In vivo* and *in vitro* studies. *J Urol* 1991;146:454.
111. Holzer-Petsche U, Lembeck F. Systemic capsaicin treatment impairs the micturition reflex in the rat. *Br J Pharmacol* 1984;83:935–941.
112. Maggi CA, Meli A. The role of neuropeptides in the regulation of the micturition reflex. *J Auton Pharmacol* 1986;6:133–162.
113. Christensen M, Keith I, Rhodes P, et al. A guinea pig model for study of mast cell function: histamine release and smooth muscle contraction. *J Urol* 1990;144:1293–1300.
114. Stief CG, Bernard F, Bosch RJLH, Aboseif SR, Lue RF, Tanagho EA. A possible role for calcitonin gene-related peptide in the regulation of smooth muscle tone of the bladder and penis. *J Urol* 1990;143: 392–397.
115. Moore KH, Nickson P, Richmond DH, Sutherst JR, Manasse PR, Helliwell TR. Detrusor mast cells in refractory idiopathic instability. *Br J Urol* 1992;70:17–21.
116. Feltis JT, Perez-Marrero R, Emerson LE. Increased mast cells of the bladder in suspected cases of interstitial cystitis: a possible disease marker. *J Urol* 1987;138:42–43.
117. Kastrup J, Hald T, Nielsen VG. Histamine content and mast cell count of detrusor muscle in patients with interstitial cystitis and other types of chronic cystitis. *Br J Urol* 1983;55:495–500.
118. Letourneau R, Sant GR, El-Mansory M, Theoharides TC. Activation of bladder mast cells in interstitial cystitis. *Int J Tissue React* 1992;14: 307–312.
119. Maggi CA, Giuliani S, Patacchini R, et al. Heterogeneity of tachykinin NK-2 receptors and human smooth muscles. *Neuropeptides* 1992;23:181–186.
120. Bull HA, Dowd PM. Endothelin-1 in human skin. *Dermatology* 1993; 187:1–5.
121. Devillier P, Advenier C, Drapeau G, et al. Comparison of the effects of epithelium removal and of an enkephalinase inhibitor on the neurokinin-induced contractions of guinea pig isolated trachea. *Br J Pharmacol* 1988;94:675–684.
122. Maggi CA, Astolfi M, Santicioli P, et al. Effect of thiorphan on the response of guinea-pig isolated urinary bladder to exogenous and endogenous tachykinins. *J Urol* 1990;144:1546–1549.
123. Rang HP, Dale MM, Ritter JM, Gardner P. *Pharmacology*. New York: Churchill Livingstone, 1995;19–20.
124. Garland AM, Grady EF, Payan DG, Vigna SR, Burnett NW. Agonist-induced internalization of the substance P (NK1) receptor expressed in epithelial cells. *Biochem J* 1994;303:177–186.
125. Hökfelt T. Neuropeptides in perspective: the last ten years. *Neuron* 1991;7:867–879.

Interstitial Cystitis, edited by Grannum R. Sant.
Lippincott–Raven Publishers, Philadelphia ©1997.

CHAPTER 8

Neurogenic Inflammation and Nerve Growth Factor: Possible Roles in Interstitial Cystitis

William D. Steers and Jeremy B. Tuttle

Neurogenic inflammation is the process whereby stimulation of peripheral nerves elicits vasodilation, plasma extravasation, and other inflammatory changes in the skin or viscera (1). Neurogenic inflammation can be evoked in the bladder by antidromic stimulation of visceral afferents in the pelvic nerve (1,2). Although bladder afferents relay information to the central nervous system, they also act in the periphery to alter mucosal permeability, smooth muscle contractility, and local blood flow and to influence cellular mediators of the immune system (Fig. 1). These effects of afferent stimulation result from the release of substances from peripheral terminals. Peripheral nociceptive (pain) nerves and their central connections are subject to alterations in function following any insult, including that caused by the mediators of neurogenic inflammation. Therefore, an initial inflammatory event may be reinforced by neurogenic mechanisms. The resulting changes in neural processing affect the pain pathways in particular, and perturbations in the function of peripheral and central elements of the nociceptive system can be durable, outlasting the initial inflammation.

Neurogenic inflammation may participate in the pathophysiology of interstitial cystitis (IC). The histologic features of neurogenic inflammation bear a striking resemblance to the cystoscopic and pathologic findings reported in IC. Hyperemia, inflammatory infiltrate, and disrupted mucosa develop in bladders with that condition (3). Interstitial cystitis has been associated with an increase in the number of nerves in the submucosa and muscle of the bladder (4–6). Furthermore, immunoreactivity for substance P and other tachykinins found in afferent terminals is increased in bladders from patients with IC (6). The location of these nerves and their increased tachykinin content suggest that patients with interstitial cystitis possess altered afferent innervation. Last, therapies for interstitial cystitis often rely on anesthetizing or sectioning nerves to the bladder. On the basis of animal models, acute inflammatory stimuli in the bladder can lead to short- and long-term alterations in sensory nerves. This review focuses on those potential mechanisms whereby acute neurogenic inflammation may lead to chronic changes in innervation, resulting in a persistent pain syndrome.

BLADDER AFFERENTS

Neuroanatomy

The urinary bladder receives input from parasympathetic and sympathetic nerves (7). The parasympathetic preganglionics responsible for micturition originate in the sacral spinal cord (S_2 to S_4). The pelvic nerve conveys these cholinergic preganglionic axons as well as peptidergic afferents and some sympathetic postganglionic neurons from the chain ganglia. Sympathetic input to the bladder arises from the thoracic and lumbar spinal cord (T_{10} to L_2). These preganglionics are relayed by lumbar splanchnics, which proceed anterior to the aorta and coalesce to form the hypogastric nerves. The hypogastric nerve carries sympathetic preganglionic input to pelvic ganglia and afferent input from the bladder to the thoracolumbar spinal cord. Neurons in the pelvic plexus as well as bladder wall contain a mixture of cholinergic and adrenergic neurons that provide motor input to the bladder. Afferents travel in close proximity to pre- and postganglionic axons.

Structurally, bladder afferents are either lightly myelinated (Aδ fibers) or unmyelinated (C fibers) (8). The prop-

W. D. Steers: Department of Urology, University of Virginia Health Sciences Center, Charlottesville, Virginia 22908.
J. B. Tuttle: Departments of Urology and Neuroscience, University of Virginia Health Sciences Center, Charlottesville, Virginia 22908.

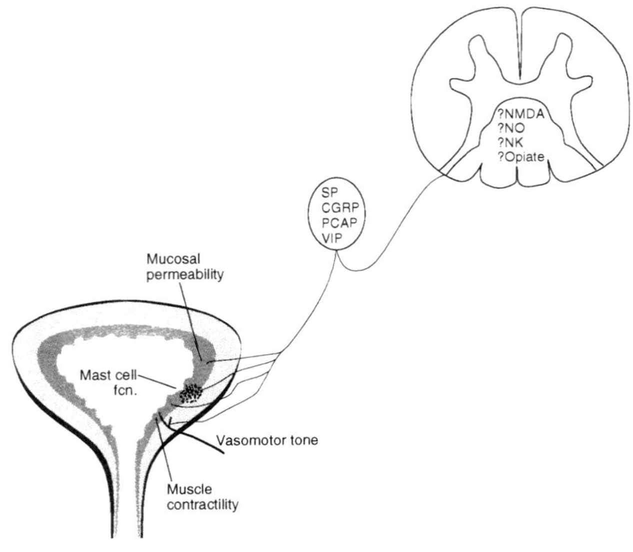

FIG. 1. Neurogenic inflammation and central hyperalgesia. Sacral dorsal root ganglia (DRG) contain substance P (SP), calcitonin gene-related peptide (CGRP), dynorphin (DYN), and vasoactive intestinal polypeptide (VIP), which are transported to afferent terminals via the pelvic nerve to the bladder. Release of these substances in the bladder increases mucosal permeability, degranulates mast cells, alters contractility, and produces vasodilation. Release of these substances from afferent terminals in the spinal cord acts on second-order neurons that act through glutamate (NMDA), nitric oxide (NO), neurokinin (NK), or opiate nociceptive (pain) pathways.

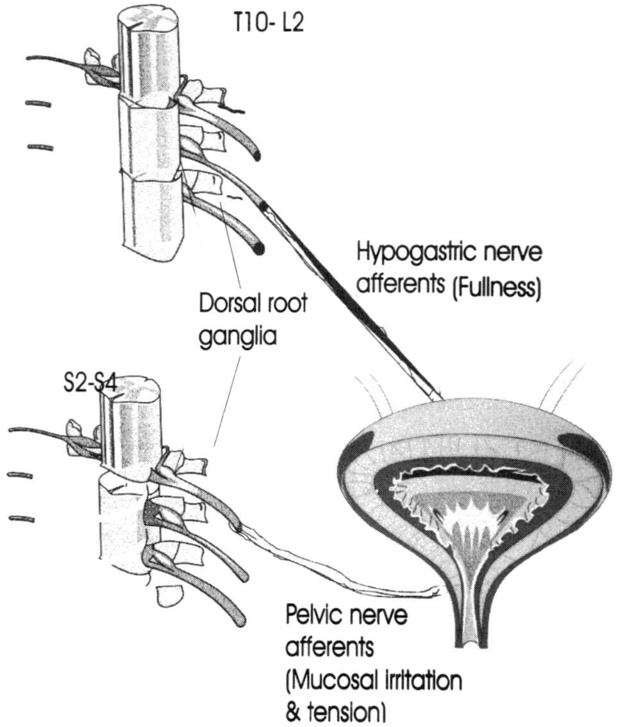

FIG. 2. Neural substrates for bladder sensation. Afferents in the pelvic nerve projecting to the sacral (S_2 to S_4) spinal cord transmit sensations of mucosal irritation and tension, triggering voiding. Afferents in the hypogastric nerve convey sensations of bladder overdistention or fullness to the thoracolumbar (T_{10} to L_2) spinal cord.

erties of these two types of axons differ. Myelinated fibers conduct action potentials more rapidly than unmyelinated axons, and both relay distinct information. Voiding relies on activation of mechanoreceptive Aδ fibers in the pelvic nerve, which trigger a supraspinal micturition reflex (9,10). Following spinal cord injury, C-fiber afferents trigger a spinal reflex responsible for bladder contraction (11). In addition, Aδ- and C-fiber afferents in the pelvic and hypogastric nerves can transmit nociceptive input to the spinal cord (12–14).

On the basis of lesioning studies, Learmonth proposed in 1931 that the sensations of suprapubic pain from overdistention of the bladder are transmitted by sensory fibers in the hypogastric nerves (Fig. 2) (15). This is consistent with the pattern of referred pain for the bladder, which corresponds to the T_{10} to T_{12} dermatomes (16,17). In contrast, the sensations signaling mucosal irritation or inflammation are relayed by afferents in the pelvic nerve. This neuroanatomic distribution explains referred pain to the vagina, rectum, and perineum with bladder irritation.

Bladder afferents project to characteristic regions of the dorsal horn of the thoracolumbar and sacral spinal cord segments (18,19). Nociceptive (i.e., pain) processing is subserved by Lissauer's tract and laminae I and II (Fig. 3). Other axonal projections terminate in autonomic nuclei and the dorsal gray commissure. Sensations of bladder pain and fullness are transmitted by the lateral spinothalamic tract to the brain (16). Spinothalamic tracts terminate in the thalamus and periaqueductal gray of the pons, which are associated with pain processing (16) (Fig. 4). Thus, anterolateral cordotomies for control of chronic lower extremity pain also abolished bladder and pelvic sensation (20). The afferent fibers serving the bladder, and viscera in general, are fewer and are organized somewhat differently than those serving cutaneous fields of similar size. Bladder afferent input to the spinal cord is more overlapped in different laminae and has wider rostral–caudal and medial–lateral extent than the precise somatotopic organization of similar cutaneous fibers (21).

Afferent Neurotransmitter Mechanisms

Bladder afferents express pituitary adenylate cyclase activating peptide (PCAP) substance P, neurokinin A, neurokinin B, calcitonin gene-related peptide (CGRP), vasoactive intestinal polypeptide (VIP), dynorphins, nitric oxide synthase (Table 1) (21–25). In the human,

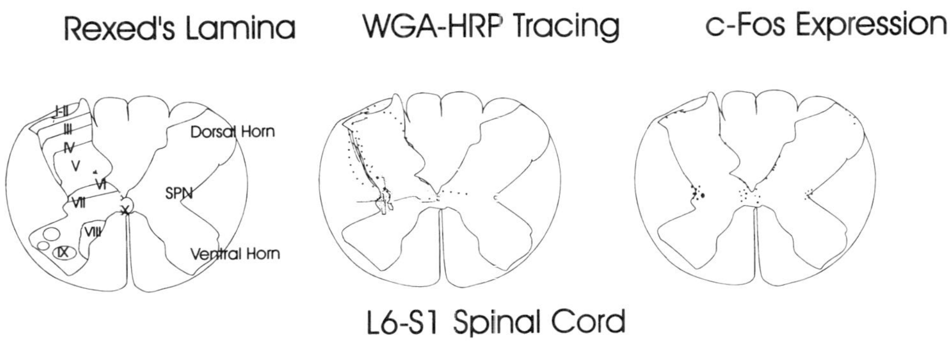

FIG. 3. Summary of retrograde axonal tracing experiments in lumbosacral spinal cord of the rat. Wheat germ agglutinin–horseradish peroxidase (WGA–HRP) tracers injected into the bladder appear in afferent projections conveyed by pelvic nerve to the spinal cord from L_6 to S_1. Reaction product is found in laminae I, II, V, and X. Neurons in the same regions express immediate early gene (IE6) products such as c-fos, c-jun, and Krox-24 within 2 hr of introduction of chemical irritants in the urinary bladder. IE6 activation could play a role in long-term alterations in receptor expression by neurons in pain pathways.

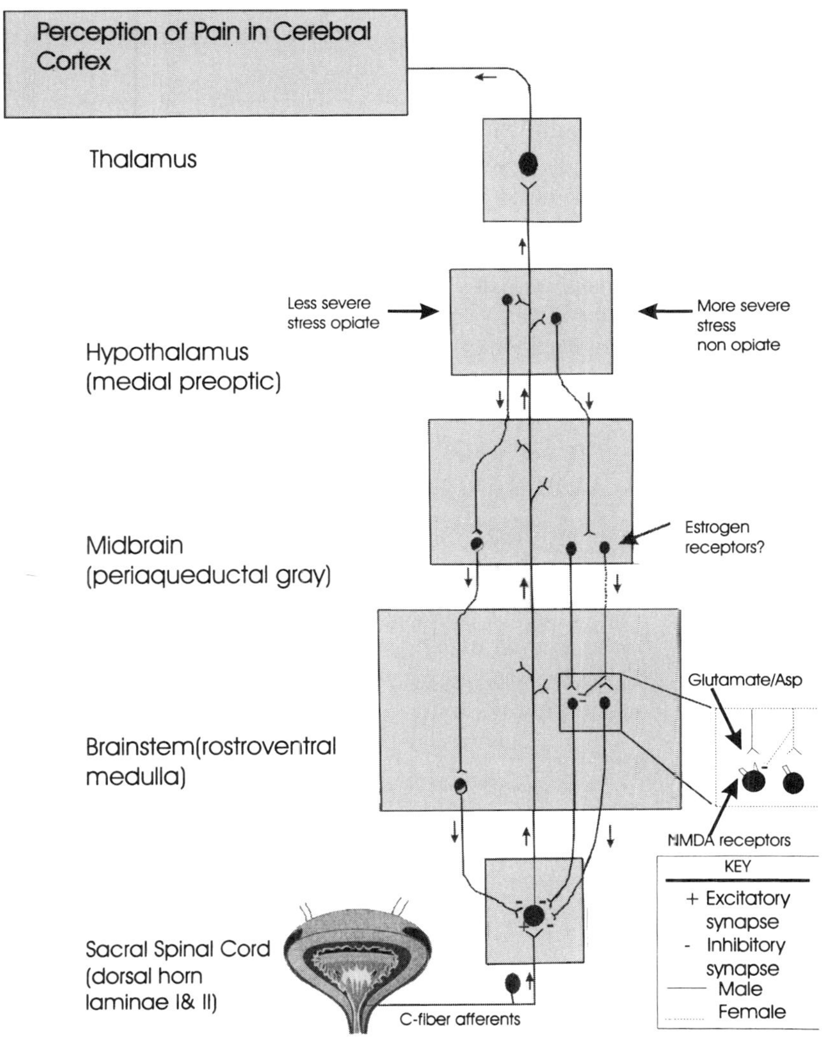

FIG. 4. Postulated networks involved in pain transmission and inhibition and role of sex hormones. Noxious stimuli from the bladder enter the sacral spinal cord and terminate in laminae I and II of the dorsal horn. Second-order neurons project via spinothalamic tracts to the thalamus as well as cortical sensory and limbic areas of the brain, where pain perception occurs. Environmental and emotional stressors activate neurons in the hypothalamus and other regions that activate descending nociceptive inhibitory circuits that inhibit ascending spinothalamic neurons. Opiate systems in the dorsal horn also inhibit spinothalamic neurons. Men possess more powerful opiate inhibition than women. The male system *(solid line)* also invokes glutamate inhibition, whereas the female system uses a yet-undefined system *(dashed line).* Estrogen may activate receptors in midbrain that inhibit male systems. In absence of estrogen, the female nonglutamate system is inactive. (Modified from a scheme proposed by Steinberg et al., ref. 86, with permission.)

TABLE 1. *Neurotransmitters in bladder afferents*

Substance P
Neurokinins A and B
Calcitonin gene-related peptide
Vasoactive intestinal polypeptide
Enkephalin
Dynorphin
Somatostatin
Galanin
Bombesin
Neuromedin U
Cholecystokinin
Nitric oxide synthase (NOS)
Pituitary adenylate cyclase activating peptide (PCAP)

substance-P-immunoreactive nerves ramify beneath the urothelium and course through the bladder wall (26). Nerves containing VIP, found throughout the human bladder, are more prevalent than those with substance P or CGRP (27). Vasoactive intestinal polypeptide is also synthesized by cholinergic postganglionic neurons (28). Investigators have attempted to assign different functions to nerves corresponding to this chemical encoding (29). For example, pain associated with irritation might be conveyed by substance P nerves, whereas thermal hypersensitivity is relayed by VIP axons. However, a unifying scheme for chemical encoding in sensory nerves has not been delineated.

Chemical, mechanical, or electric stimulation of afferent axons releases substance P and other tachykinins and neuropeptides from terminals in the target organ (2, 30–32). In addition to mediating the aforementioned characteristics of neurogenic inflammation, substance P and tachykinins contract smooth muscle (33). Tachykinins produce detrusor contraction in the human bladder by activating NK-2 receptors (33). In the dorsal horn of the spinal cord, substance P and tachykinins primarily activate NK-1 receptors (34). Combined blockade of NK-2 and NK-1 receptors fails to abolish micturition (34). However, intrathecal NK-1 and NK-2 antagonists inhibit hyperreflexia induced by chemical irritation (35). Therefore, although substance P may influence voiding, tachykinin-containing afferents do not convey the mechanoreceptive input that triggers a voiding reflex. Spinal neurokinin receptors appear to be involved in hyperactivity associated with chemical cystitis (35,36).

Capsaicin-Sensitive Afferents

Understanding the function of peptide-containing afferents has been hampered by lack of potent and specific antagonists. One pharmacologic probe used to study afferent function has been capsaicin and the related, more potent compound resiniferotoxin (30). Capsaicin is the active ingredient of many hot peppers. Capsaicin binds to specific vanilloid receptors on small-diameter unmyelinated or lightly myelinated afferents. Capsaicin initially releases afferent neurotransmitters and induces pain. This effect is followed by period of anesthesia as a result of desensitization.

The properties of capsaicin suggest that this compound can be used to treat pain. Indeed, a topical preparation of capsaicin is approved for the treatment of pain from herpes zoster (37). Likewise, intravesical administration of capsaicin can eradicate bladder pain or sensations of urgency for weeks or months (38). This latter effect confirms that the human bladder contains capsaicin-sensitive afferents that are involved in pain. Detrusor hyperreflexia, especially after spinal cord injury, has also been treated with intravesical capsaicin (39). This additional finding suggests that capsaicin-sensitive afferents, most likely C fibers, are involved in hyperreflexia and, as in animals, initiate the spinal reflex responsible for voiding in paraplegics (9–11,40). However, capsaicin must be dissolved in ethanol before instillation. This solubility vehicle alone may itself contribute to the clinical efficacy of capsaicin.

Another link between capsaicin-sensitive afferents and interstitial cystitis is the action of substance P on mast cells. Some patients with interstitial cystitis demonstrate increased numbers or function of mast cells (41–43). Substance P or capsaicin administration causes degranulation of mast cells and histamine release (43). One can envision a vicious cycle in which substance P causes mast cell release, which in turn evokes further activation of bladder afferents.

BLADDER INFLAMMATION

Models

A number of models have been used to create bladder inflammation in order to study its effect on nerves (Table 2). Intravesical instillation of chemical irritants (mustard oil, turpentine, xylene, acetic acid, formalin, and cyclo-

TABLE 2. *Animal models of bladder inflammation and pain*

Animal Model
Mustard oil
Xylene
Acetic acid
Turpentine
Formalin
Cyclophosphamide
Lipopolysaccharide
Suture
Feline cystitis
Ovalbumin

phosphamide), immune sensitizers (ovalbumin), suture, and infectious toxins [endotoxin or lipopolysaccharide (LPS)] have been used to induce bladder inflammation (35,36,46–52). Histologic examination of the bladders following intravesical irritants reveals changes that resemble interstitial cystitis, including a profuse inflammatory infiltrate, submucosal edema, and mucosal erosion (49). Behavioral responses in animals following intravesical irritants include hypertension and tachycardia as well as licking of the suprapubic and perineal regions (36,49).

Consistent with the release of substance P and related tachykinins from bladder afferents, intravesical irritants increase mucosal permeability as measured by extravasation of Evans blue dye (2). Prior administration of capsaicin abolishes extravasation of Evans blue dye, confirming that densitization of afferents has a modulating effect on the increase in mucosal permeability.

However, these models are not identical to interstitial cystitis, as they do not always induce chronic urinary frequency, a hallmark of interstitial cystitis (50,51). Similarly, intravesical formalin instillation, a foreign body, or LPS, although producing inflammation, fails to alter cystometry performed weeks later (50,51). Histologic examination weeks after intravesical instillation of irritants failed to increase bladder innervation (51). In fact, staining for catecholamine-fluorescent fibers decreases. Furthermore, acute inflammation does not increase responses of bladder smooth muscle to contractile agents such as acetylcholine, norepinephrine, or potassium. Thus, although bladder inflammation in models does not represent interstitial cystitis, it provides valuable information on the nerve response to inflammation.

Inflammation and Neural Hypertrophy

Although inflammation fails to alter bladder contractility or nerve content, neuronal plasticity occurs within dorsal root ganglia (DRG) and sensory receiving areas of the spinal cord (Table 3). Bladder afferent cell bodies in thoracolumbar and sacral dorsal root ganglia hypertrophy in response to intravesical irritants (50,51). Similar enlargement has been reported in other hyperactive bladder states such as obstruction, partial denervation, spinal cord injury, or in spontaneously hypertensive rats with urinary frequency (19,53–56).

The mechanism whereby DRG cells enlarge in animal models could provide insight into potential sensory remodeling that occurs with chronic pain in humans. Nerve growth factor (NGF) is a trophic signaling protein responsible for the growth and normal function of sensory and noradrenergic nerves, and NGF is manufactured by bladder smooth muscle (57,58). Nearly 80% of DRG cells labeled from the bladder express the NGF receptor known as *trkA* (59). After obstruction or denervation of the bladder, hypertrophy of afferents corresponds to a rise in NGF within the bladder. Blockade of NGF prevents hypertrophy of DRG cells and expression of growth-associated protein (GAP-43) within the sacral spinal cord (60). Following inflammation, levels of NGF in the bladder rise and then fall (51–54). Inflammatory mediators may contribute to this rise in NGF. Exposure of cultured bladder smooth muscle to interleukin-1 increases NGF in the medium (61). Furthermore, inflammation increases expression of the NGF receptor in the bladder (62). Although a rise in NGF has not yet been demonstrated in a purely neuropathic pain model, the association between NGF and alterations in nociceptive signaling rests on firm experimental grounds (63–66). Nerve growth factor has been shown to alter nociceptive signaling at peripheral sites and to affect central processing of afferent signals. Mast cells contain and respond to NGF with degranulation, releasing, among other substances, serotonin, which causes a potent and long-lasting lowering of nociceptive afferent thresholds (43). Through this mechanism, a single systemic injection of NGF alters nociceptive thresholds for several days (63–66). The effect is reduced by treatments that deplete mast cells, block 5-HT receptors, or inhibit NGF.

A central site of action for NGF is indicated by NGF-induced cutaneous hyperalgesia that can be modulated by spinal blockade of NMDA-type glutamate receptors and by hyperalgesia resistant to NMDA receptor antagonists (67,68). Thus, in addition to the effects of NGF on peripheral afferents, this signaling factor triggers long-lasting alterations in the central circuitry serving pain sensation. It does so by at least two pharmacologically distinct mechanisms (63–66).

What evidence is there that bladder afferents can change their function in the adult? Patch-clamp electrophysiological analysis of sacral DRG cells labeled from the bladder show that these neurons are small, quiescent, and possess high thresholds for firing (69). Such cells are

TABLE 3. *Potential mechanisms of afferent signaling plasticity*

	Description and site	Timing
Afferent sensitization	Decreased threshold to stimuli; peripheral	Rapid
Afferent “reassignment”	Respond to novel stimuli; peripheral/central	Slow
Afferent transfer function	Novel impact of activity; central	Slow
Sympathetic maintained pain (SMP, RSD)	Sympathetic/afferent loop; peripheral/central	Slow
Central nociceptive sensitization	Supraspinal, brain processing; central	Rapid circuit; slow plasticity

believed to be the source of "silent C fibers" (12–14). Many of these afferents express sodium channels resistant to tetrodotoxin. Following inflammation, spontaneous activity develops with expression of tetrodotoxin-sensitive sodium channels. Thus, changes in afferent function occur in response to changes in the bladder (55). Unfortunately, no mechanism for the deactivation of such cells, once they have been activated, has yet been described.

These structural and functional alterations in afferent pathways rely on changes in gene expression. Chemical cystitis increases immediate early gene expression in the sacral spinal cord (45,46,49) (Fig. 3). Increases in c-fos, Krox-24, and c-jun proteins localize to lamina I, sacral parasympathetic nucleus, and dorsal gray commissure regions of the spinal cord, which receive bladder afferent input (Fig. 4). The degree and localization of gene expression are related to the severity and duration of bladder inflammation (49). In contrast to mucosal irritation, overdistention of the bladder increases c-fos in the thoracolumbar rather than sacral spinal cord (46). These data are consistent with the concept of differential functional encoding by hypogastric versus pelvic nerve afferents, described by Learmonth (15).

Receptor Plasticity

Immediate early gene activation could play a role in long-term alterations in receptor expression, neurotransmitter synthesis, or mechanisms governing transmitter release. For example, tissue damage and/or inflammation up-regulates tachykinin receptors (NK-2) located on axons in the bladder (35). Similar stimuli evoke changes in NK-1 receptors in the sacral spinal cord (35). Likewise, chronic NGF administration enhances the function of NK-1 receptors in the spinal cord (70). These perturbations in tachykinin receptors may promote increased susceptibility to substance P released from bladder afferents, causing pain and urinary urgency.

Nitric oxide synthase (NOS) is also expressed by some bladder afferents. However, the role of these nerves is unclear. In the normal bladder, NO donors or activators of NO pathways do not affect smooth muscle contractility or cystometry (71). However, following inflammation or injury to the bladder or its innervation, activators of NO inhibit bladder hyperactivity (23,72). This observation suggests that NO may play a role in inflammation-induced bladder hyperactivity.

Glutamate is an excitatory amino acid that functions as a neurotransmitter in the brain and spinal cord. Glutamate acts on NMDA, AMPA, and kainate receptors. There are substantial data indicating that events mediated by the NMDA receptor contribute to spinal hyperalgesia associated with pain and inflammation. The NMDA receptor antagonists AP-5 and MK-801 prevent bladder hyperreflexia associated with chemical cystitis (67,68); MK-801 also prevents immediate early gene expression in the spinal cord following chemical cystitis (68).

Humoral Modulation of Pain Signaling

The incidence of interstitial cystitis is much higher in women than in men. Furthermore, changes in bladder sensation have been reported in different stages of the menstrual cycle and with varying emotional or stress states. What evidence exists for hormonal modulation of nociception, and can this be linked to inflammatory modulation of nociception? It is well known that estrogen and progesterone can affect adrenergic receptors in the bladder (74,75). Dorsal root ganglion cells also express the mRNA for the estrogen receptor (76). These female hormones affect neurotransmitter receptors and central processing of pain afferent signals (77–79). Estrogen amplifies glutamate responses and produces increased sensorimotor activation. The effects are mediated via NMDA-type receptors. This effect is sufficient to increase responsiveness of CNS neurons to the stimulation of peripheral afferents 15 min after a single estradiol injection (78). One theory holds that inhibition of pain processing is greater in women than men because of the effect of estrogen on NMDA and non-NMDA receptors (Fig. 4). This causes less noxious stimuli to seem more painful. In contrast, the progestins, in particular one metabolite of progesterone, have anesthetic actions at $GABA_A$ receptors (78) and also reduce glutamate responses. However, the effects of these steroid sex hormones are influenced by previous history and the hormonal milieu present. Thus, the effects of one steroid can be prevented by prior administration of other hormones. It is provocative that these sex steroids influence the same receptor systems that are involved in the central sensitization to pain associated with inflammation. It certainly seems likely that individual differences in susceptibility to interstitial cystitis may reflect individual variation in the strength and impact of such modulatory processes.

The profuse sensory innervation of the lower urinary tract with its potential exposure to the constituents of urine, including pH, ions, dietary substances, and infectious agents, may explain the common occurrence of irritative disorders such as interstitial cystitis, prostatitis, and urethritis. In addition, interactions between the autonomic centers in the brain, such as the hypothalamus and amygdala, that control emotions and micturition provide an anatomic link between daily variations in voiding symptoms and effects of stress or emotions on urination and pain.

FUTURE DIRECTIONS

If one accepts the notion that inflammatory painful stimuli, especially if repeated, can chronically alter innervation, central pain-processing mechanisms, and tissue responses, then therapy must be targeted beyond the level of the bladder. Indeed, although therapies for interstitial cystitis often rely on their ability to block bladder sensation, the effects are uniformly transient. Intravesical DMSO and lidocaine, which act as local anesthetics, hydrodistension, which destroys sensory terminals in the bladder wall, and intravesical capsaicin, intended to silence nociceptive afferents, produce only temporary relief (38,39,80,81). More disturbing is the fact that in many experimental situations, injury (redistension) and inflammation can result from the treatments used to initiate processes that result in sensory remodeling. Thus, over the long term, many of the current therapies may actually exacerbate the symptoms much the same way that repeated reading reinforces memory through neural plasticity in the occipital and hippocampal regions of the brain. Even the most radical of neurolytic procedures, such as sacral rhizotomy or radical cystectomy, fail to abolish bladder pain in 30% to 50% of patients (82). This can be taken as very suggestive evidence that nociceptive processing in the spinal cord or brain contributes to the persistent sensations of bladder discomfort, and these events cannot be permanently silenced by targeting only the bladder for treatment. A useful analogy is that of the phantom limb, in which a patient may experience the presence of many sensations, including pain, localized to an amputated limb. In this case, the central nervous system circuitry that maintains an internal, neural representation of the limb was not removed by the amputation. For interstitial cystitis patients, treatment of only the peripheral structures serving bladder pain leaves the central circuitry unaffected. Therapies targeted at multiple levels of the neuraxis and at probable participants in nociceptive processing offer the best hope for treatment of chronic visceral pain syndromes such as interstitial cystitis.

In this regard, Table 4 lists potential neural therapeutic targets. Likely candidates are the neurotransmitters and neuromodulators responsible for signaling in nociceptive afferents and their central circuits. These networks have recently been shown to have significant plasticity in the adult in that synaptic strength or connections can be affected by levels of activity. Mechanisms of change similar to those hypothesized to serve memory in the central nervous system are thought to modulate sensitivity to and transmission of pain information.

Nerve growth factor has emerged as a key player capable of linking inflammation or intensely painful events to altered pain signaling. The processes that govern NGF synthesis, its release, and its effect are therefore intriguing targets for therapeutic intervention. An interesting tactic might be to affect many of these processes simultaneously. For example, neurons rely on a rise in intracellular calcium to release neurotransmitters, to regulate NGF synthesis, and for the processes serving activity-dependent synaptic plasticity. Experimental evidence shows that calcium channel blockers lower NGF in the bladder (83). Thus, it is of interest that long-term treatment with calcium channel blockers has been associated with isolated successes in eliminating the symptoms of interstitial cystitis (84).

TABLE 4. *Neural therapeutic targets in IC*

Target	Peripheral	CNS
Anesthetics/neural blockade: Intravesical		
Lidocaine	++	--
DMSO	++	--
Capsaicin	++	--
Substance P and other tachykinins		
Production	++	++
Release	++	++
Receptors	++	++
GABA	--	++
Opiates/enkephalins/endorphins		
Receptors	?	++
NOS/NO	++	++
Serotonin		
Receptors	++	++
Excitatory amino acids		
Synthesis	--	++
Degradation	--	++
Receptors (NMDA)	--	++
Histamine		
Receptors	++	++
Release	++	?
Nerve growth factor		
Synthesis	++	?
trkA	++	?
Other?	?	?
Ca^{2+} channels	++	?
Inducible cyclooxygenase (COX-2)	?	++

Another approach would be to prevent growth factor access by neurons or its effects responsible for the upregulated function. Antagonists to *trkA* receptors or NGF offer intriguing experimental approaches. On the basis of anecdotal reports, it seems possible that protein kinase inhibition is relatively benign and may be a useful therapeutic target. An interesting but much more speculative target may be the inducible cyclooxygenase (COX-2) involved in the signaling for prostaglandin synthesis in the spinal cord. The prostaglandins have been shown experimentally to influence bladder contractility and mucosal permeability as well as to regulate NGF synthesis (52). Prostaglandins may also be involved in the upregulation of central pain pathways that serve neurogenic pain mechanisms. Last, a physiological basis for behavioral and electric stimulation exist. Transdermal elecric neural stimulation (TENS) units can diminish the increase in c-fos expression in the spinal cord following peripheral inflammation (85). It may be that the best therapies target multiple potential sites of action in the peripheral and central nervous systems.

Intuitively, it seems that pharmacologic or behavioral therapies are optimally suited to treat the chronic visceral pain syndromes such as interstitial cystitis. Formulation of uniformly successful medical therapy has been hampered by a lack of understanding of the basic biology of chronic pain. Moreover, our understanding of the fundamental neurophysiology of pain and altered pain processing has advanced rapidly. This understanding has offered multiple possibilities for basic mechanisms operative in interstitial cystitis. The next phase of investigation should focus on revealing which of these possibilities can best be exploited to provide effective medical therapy.

REFERENCES

1. Pinter E, Szolcanyi J. Plasma extravasation in the skin and pelvic organs evoked by antidromic stimulation of the lumbosacral dorsal roots in the rat. *Neuroscience* 1995;68:603–614.
2. Koltzenburg M, McMahon SB. Plasma extravasation in the rat urinary bladder following mechanical, electrical, and chemical stimuli: evidence for a new population of chemosensitive primary sensory neurons. *Neurosci Lett* 1986;72:352–356.
3. Johansson SL, Fall M. Clinical features and spectrum of light microscopic changes in interstitial cystitis. *J Urol* 1990;143:1118–1124.
4. Christmas TL, Rode J, Chapple CR, Milroy EJ, Turner-Warwick RT. Nerve fiber proliferation in interstitial cystitis. *Virchows Arch [A] Pathol Anat* 1990;416:447–451.
5. Lundeberg T, Liedberg H, Nordling L, Theodorsson E, Owzarski A, Ekman P. Interstitial cystitis: correlation with nerve fibers, mast cells and histamine content. *Br J Urol* 1993;71:427–429.
6. Hohenfellner M, Nunues L, Schmidt RA, Lampel A, Thuroff JW, Tanagho EA. Interstitial cystitis: increased sympathetic innervation and related neuropeptide synthesis. *J Urol* 1992;147:587–591.
7. Steers WD. Physiology of the urinary bladder. In: Walsh PC, Retik AB, Stamey TA, Vaughan ED, eds. *Campbell's Urology.* Philadelphia: WB Saunders, 1992;142–176.
8. Gosling JA, Dixon JS. Sensory nerves in the mammalian urinary tract. An evaluation using light and electron microscopy. *J Anat* 1974;117: 133–144.
9. de Groat WC. Nervous control of the urinary bladder of the cat. *Brain Res* 1975;87:201–211.
10. Mallory B, Steers WD, de Groat WC. Electrophysiological study of micturition reflexes in the rat. *Am J Physiol* 1989;257:R410–R421.
11. de Groat WC, Kawatani M, Hisamitsu T, Cheng CL, Ma CP, Thor K, Steers WD, Roppolo JR. Mechanisms underlying the recovery of urinary bladder function following spinal cord injury. *J Auton Nerv Syst* 1990;30:S71–S78.
12. Habler HJ, Janig W, Koltzenburg M. Receptive properties of myelinated primary afferents innervating the inflamed urinary bladder of the cat. *J Neurophysiol* 1993;69:395–405.
13. Habler HJ, Janig W, Koltzenburg M. Activation of unmyelinated afferent fibers by mechanical stimuli and inflammation of the urinary bladder in the cat. *J Physiol (Lond)* 1990;425:545–567.
14. Janig W, Koltzenburg M. Pain arising from the urogenital tract. In: Maggi CA, ed. *The Autonomic Nervous System: Nervous Control of the Urogenital System.* London: Harwook Academic Publisher, 1992; 525–570.
15. Learmonth JR. A contribution to the neurophysiology of the urinary bladder in man. *Brain* 1931;54:147–178.
16. Bors E, Comarr AE. *Neurological Urology.* Baltimore: University Park Press, 1971.
17. Milne RJ, Foreman RD, Giesler GJ, Willis WD. Convergence of cutaneous and pelvic visceral nociceptive inputs onto primate spinothalamic neurons. *Pain* 1981;11:163–183.
18. Morgan C, Nadelhaft I, de Groat WC. The distribution of visceral primary afferents from the pelvic nerve within Lissauer's tract and the spinal gray matter and its relationship to sacral parasympathetic nucleus. *J Comp Neurol* 1981;201:415–421.
19. Steers WD, Ciambotti J, Etzel B, Erdman S, de Groat WC. Alterations in afferent pathways from the urinary bladder in response to partial urethral obstruction. *J Comp Neurol* 1991;310:401–410.
20. Nathan PW, Smith MC. The centrifugal pathway for micturition within the spinal cord. *J Neurol Neurosurg Psychiatry* 1958;21:177–180.
21. de Groat WC. Neuropeptides in pelvic afferent pathways. *Experientia* 1987;43:801–813.
22. Keast JR, deGroat WC. Segmental distribution and peptide content of primary afferent neurons innervating the urogenital organs and colon of male rats. *J Comp Neurol* 1992;319:615–623.
23. Vizzard MA, Erdman S, de Groat WC. Increased expression of neuronal nitric oxide synthase (NOS) in visceral neurons after nerve injury. *J Neurosci* 1995;15:4033–4045.
24. McNeill DL, Harris CH, Holzbeierlein JM, Shew RL, Traugh NE, Papka RE. CGRP-immunoreactive primary afferent nerve fibers in the rat urinary bladder: effects of dorsal rhizotomy and MK-801. *Exp Neurol* 1992;118:317–323.
25. Gibson SJ, Polak JM, Anand P, Blank MA, Yiangou Y, Su HC. A VIP/PHI containing pathway links urinary bladder and sacral spinal cord. *Peptides* 1986;7:205–219.
26. Wakabayashi Y, Tomoyoshi T, Fujimiya M, Arai R, Maeda T. Substance P-containing axon terminals in the mucosa of the human urinary bladder: pre-embedding immunohistochemistry using cryostat sections for electron microscopy. *Histochem J* 1993;100:401–407.
27. Gu J, Blank MA, Huang WM, Islam KN, McGregor GP, Christofides N, Allen JM, Bloom SR, Polak JM. Peptide containing nerves in the human urinary bladder. *Urology* 1984;24:353–357.
28. Keast J, de Groat WC. Immunocytochemical characterization of pelvic neurons which project to the bladder, colon, and penis in rats. *J Comp Neurol* 1989;288:387.
29. Costa M, Furness JB, Gibbins IL. Chemical encoding of enteric neurons. *Prog Brain Res* 1986;68:217–239.
30. Maggi C, Abelli L, Giuliani S, Geppetti P. Capsaicin-sensitive afferents and pain arising from the urinary bladder. *Adv Pain Res Ther* 1992;20: 71–80.
31. Maggi C, Santicioli P, Patacchini R, et al. Contractile response of the human isolated urinary bladder to neurokinins: involvement of NK-2 receptors. *Eur J Pharmacol* 1988;145:335–340.
32. Maggi C, Meli A. The sensory-efferent function of capsaicin-sensitive sensory neurons. *Gen Pharmax* 1988;19(1):1–43.
33. Maggi CA, Parlani M, Astolfi M, Santicioli P, Rovero P. Neurokinin receptors in the rat lower urinary tract. *J Pharmacol Exp Ther* 1988;246: 308–315.
34. Ishizuka O, Igawa Y, Lecci A, Maggi CA, Mattiasson A, Andersson KE. Role of intrathecal tachykinins for micturition in unanesthetized rats with and without outlet obstruction. *Br J Pharmacol* 1994;113:111–117.
35. Lecci A, Guiliani S, Santicioli P, Maggi CA. Involvement of spinal tachykinin NK1 and NK2 receptors in detrusor hyperreflexia during chemical cystitis in anesthetized rats. *Eur J Pharmacol* 1994;259: 129–135.
36. Abelli L, Conte B, Somma V, et al. The contribution of capsaicin-sensitive sensory nerves to xylene-induced visceral pain in conscious, freely moving rats. *Arch Pharmacol* 1988;337:545–551.
37. Maggi C. Therapeutic potential of capsaicin-like molecules: studies in animals and humans. *Life Sci* 1992;51:1777–1781.
38. Fowler CJ, Jewkes D, McDonald WI. Intravesical capsaicin for neurogenic bladder dysfunction. *Lancet* 1992;339:1239–1240.
39. Fowler C, Beck RO, Gerrard S, Betts CD, Fowler CG. Intravesical capsaicin for treatment of detrusor hyperreflexia. *J Neurol Neurosurg Psychiatry* 1994;57:169–173.
40. Chen C, Ma C, de Groat WC. Effects of capsaicin on micturition and associated reflexes in rats. *Am J Physiol* 1993;265:R132–R138.
41. Larsen S, Thompson SA, Hald T, et al. Mast cells in interstitial cystitis. *Br J Urol* 1982;54:283–286.
42. Kastrup J, Hald T, Larsen S, Nielsen VG. Histamine content and mast cell count of detrusor muscle in patients with interstitial cystitis and other types of chronic cystitis. *Br J Urol* 1983;55:495–500.
43. Purcell WM, Atterwill CK. Mast cells in neuroimmune function: neurotoxicological and neuropharmacological perspectives. *Neurochem Res* 1995;20:521–532.
44. Cruz F, Avelino A, Lima D, Coimbra A. Activation of c-fos proto-oncogene in the spinal cord following noxious stimulation of the urinary bladder. *Somatosens Mot Res* 1994;11:319–325.
45. Birder LA, de Groat WC. Increased c-fos expression in spinal neurons after chemical irritation of the lower urinary tract of the rat. *J Neurosci* 1992;12:4878–4889.
46. Birder LA, de Groat WC. The effect of glutamate antagonists on c-fos expression induced in spinal neurons by irritation of the lower urinary tract. *Brain Res* 1992;580:115–120.
47. Maggi CA, Lecci A, Santicioli P, Del Bianco E, Giuliani S. Cyclophosphamide cystitis in rats: involvement of capsaicin-sensitive primary afferents. *J Auton Nerv Syst* 1992;38:201–208.

48. McMahon SB. Neuronal and behavioral consequences of chemical inflammation of rat urinary bladder. *Agents Actions* 1988;25:231–233.
49. Lanteri-Minet M, Bon K, de Pommery J, Michiels JF, Menetrey D. Cyclophosphamide cystitis as a model of visceral pain in rats: model elaboration and spinal structures involved as revealed by the expression of c-Fos and Krox-24 proteins. *Exp Brain Res* 1995;105;220–232.
50. Dupont MC, Steers WC, Tuttle JB. Inflammation induced neural plasticity in autonomic pathways supplying the bladder may depend on NGF. *Soc Neurosci Abstr* 1994;20:53.1.
51. Dupont M, Steers WD, McCarty R, Tuttle JB. Neural plasticity and alterations in nerve growth factor and norepinephrine in response to bladder inflammation. *J Urol* 1994;151:284.
52. Saban R, Undem BJ, Keith I, et al. Differential release of prostaglandins and leukotrienes by sensitized guinea pig urinary bladder layers upon antigen challenge. *J Urol* 1994;152:544–549.
53. Tuttle JB, Steers WD, Albo M, Nataluk E. Neural input regulates tissue NGF and growth of the adult rat urinary bladder. *J Autonom Nerv Syst* 1994;49:147–158.
54. Dupont M, Persson K, Spitsbergen J, Tuttle JB, Steers WD. The neuronal response to bladder outlet obstruction. A role for NGF. *Adv Exper Med Bio* 1995;385:41–44.
55. Yoshimura N, Yoshida O, de Groat WC. Regional differences in plasticity of membrane properties of rat urinary bladder afferent neurons following spinal cord injury. *J Urol* 1995;153:262a.
56. Spitsbergen JM, McCarty RC, Steers WD, Tuttle JB. Nerve growth factor, sympathetic innervation and voiding frequency in spontaneously hypertensive rats. *Soc Neurosci Abstr* 1995;21:761.
57. Steers WD, Kolbeck S, Creedon D, Tuttle JB. Nerve growth factor in the urinary bladder of the adult regulates neuronal form and function. *J Clin Invest* 1991;88:1709–1715.
58. Persson K, Sando J, Tuttle JB, Steers WD. Protein kinase C in cyclic stretch-induced nerve growth factor production by urinary tract smooth muscle cells. *Am J Physiol* 269:C1018–C1024.
59. McMahon SB, Armanimi MP, Ling LH, Phillips HS. Expression and coexpression of *trk* receptors in subpopulations of adult primary sensory neurons projecting to identified peripheral targets. *Neuron* 1994; 12:1161–1171.
60. Steers WD, Creedon D, Tuttle JB. Immunity to NGF prevents afferent plasticity following hypertrophy of the urinary bladder. *J Urol* 1996;155:379–386.
61. Persson K, Herrell D, Tuttle JB, Steers WD. Regulation of NGF secretion by urinary tract smooth muscle cells. *J Urol* in press, 1997.
62. Andreev NY, Bennett D, Priestly J, Rattray M, McMahon SB. NGF mRNA is increased by experimental inflammation of adult rat urinary bladder. *Abstr Soc Neurosci* 1993;19:248.
63. Lewin GR, Mendell LM. Nerve growth factor and nocioception. *Trends Neurosci* 1993;16:353–359.
64. Lewin GR, Rueff A, Mendell LM. Peripheral and central mechanisms of NGF induced hyperalgesia. *Eur J Neurosci* 1994;6:1903–1912.
65. Lewin GR, Ritter AM, Mendell LM. Nerve growth factor induced hyperalgesia in the neonatal and adult rat. *J Neurosci* 1993;13:2136–2148.
66. Lewin GR, Ritter AM, Mendell LM. On the role of nerve growth factor in the development of myelinated nociceptors. *J Neurosci* 1992;12: 1896–1905.
67. Rice AS, McMahon SB. Pre-emptive intrathecal administration of an NMDA receptor antagonist AP-5 prevents hyper-reflexia in a model of persistent visceral pain. *Pain* 1994;57:335–340.
68. Kakizaki H, Yoshiyama M, de Groat WC. c-Fos expression in spinal neurons after irritation of the lower urinary tract depends on synergistic interactions between NMDA and AMPA glutamatergic transmission. *Soc Neurosci Abstr* 1995;21:1872.
69. Yoshimura N, deGroat WC. Patch clamp analysis of afferent and efferent neurons that innervate the urinary bladder of the rat. *Soc Neurosci Abstr* 1992;18:127.
70. Thompson SWN, Dray A, McCarson KE, Krause JE, Urban L. Nerve growth factor induces mechanical allodynia associated with novel A fibre-evoked spinal reflex activity and enhanced neurokinin-1 receptor activation in the rat. *Pain* 1995;62:219–231.
71. Andersson KE, Persson K. Nitric oxide synthase and nitric oxide-mediated effects in lower urinary tract smooth muscles. *World J Urol* 1994; 12:274–280.
72. Kahizaki H, de Groat WC. Possible involvement of nitric oxide in the facilitation of the micturition reflex by bladder irritation. *J Urol* 1995; 153:459A.
73. Tang LH, Erdman S, de Groat WC, Vizzard M. Increased expression of nitric oxide synthase and growth associated protein (GAP-43) in visceral neurons after nerve injury. *Soc Neurosci Abstr* 1994;20:617.
74. Levin R, Jacobowitz D, Wein A. Autonomic innervation of rabbit urinary bladder following estrogen administration. *Invest Urol* 1981;XVIII(5): 449–453.
75. Ekstrom J, Iosif CS, Malmberg L. Effects of long-term treatment with estrogen and progesterone on *in vivo* muscle responses of the female rabbit urinary bladder and urethra to autonomic drugs and nerve stimulation. *J Urol* 1993;150:1284–1288.
76. Sohrabji F, Miranda RC, Toran-Allerand CD. Estrogen differentially regulates estrogen and nerve growth factor receptor mRNAs in adult sensory neurons. *J Neurosci* 1994;14:459–471.
77. Frye CA, Bock BC, Kanarek RB. Hormonal milieu affects tailflick latency in female rats and may be attenuated by access to sucrose. *Physiol Behav* 1992;52:699–706.
78. Smith SS. Female sex steroid hormones: from receptors to networks to performance-actions on the somatosensory system. *Prog Neurobiol* 1994;44:55–86.
79. Martinez-Gomez M, Cruz Y, Salas M, Hudson R, Pacheco P. Assessing pain threshold in the rat: changes with estrus and time of day. *Physiol Behav* 1994;55:651–657.
80. Stewart BH, Branson AC, Hewitt CB, Kiser WS, Straffon RA. The treatment of patients with interstitial cystitis with special reference to intravesical DMSO. *J Urol* 1972;107:377–380.
81. Asklin B, Cassuto J. Intravesical lidocaine in severe interstitial cystitis. *Scand J Urol Nephrol* 1989;23:311–312.
82. Baskin LS, Tanagho EA. Pelvic pain without pelvic organs. *J Urol* 1992;147:683–686.
83. Steers WD, Tuttle JB, Albo M. Calcium channel antagonists prevent urinary bladder growth and neuroplasticity following mechanical stress. *Am J Physiol* 1994;266:R20–R26.
84. Fleischmann JD, Huntley HN, Shingleton WB, Wentworth DB. Clinical and immunological response to nifedipine for the treatment of interstitial cystitis. *J Urol* 1991;146:1235–1239.
85. Wei F, Zhao ZQ. Effect of TENS-like stimulation on C afferent induced c-fos expression in the rat spinal cord. *Neuroreport* 1995;6:1659–1663.
86. Steinberg W, Mogil J, Liebeskind UCLA. Estrogen and pain. *J NIH Res* 1993;5:55–56.

Interstitial Cystitis, edited by Grannum R. Sant.
Lippincott–Raven Publishers, Philadelphia ©1997.

CHAPTER 9

Occult Infection in Interstitial Cystitis

Gerald J. Domingue, Sr., and Gamal M. Ghoniem

It was Darwin's concept that life forms are infinitely diverse in nature and that those suited to a particular environment are most likely to persist; any change in the environment tends to change the character of the selection. This dynamic has been further extended by the observation that living biological forms continually alter their morphology and metabolism. Therefore, in the context of clinical pathology, both bacteria and host are interacting in a kaleidoscopic, qualitative relationship.

The defenses of the host against invasion and injury by bacteria include the degradation of their cell wall by such metabolites as lysozyme and complement. In addition, antibody absorption and/or various drugs and antimicrobial agents can cause such injury that phagocytosis and intralysosomal digestion occur. If such functions fail to operate optimally, variant bacterial forms with morphologically altered cell walls can be sequestered within the tissues of the host; such forms cause minimal host inflammatory reaction and, because of their aberrant appearance, are not recognized by conventional laboratory techniques.

Over the life of every host, disturbances of immunity occur so that variant forms episodically develop and accumulate. The most resistant variants are benign seedlike elementary bodies whose tiny packets of DNA, no larger than some viruses, can persist as long as their cellular locus does. Only mechanisms compromising the cell's function activate the elementary variant's metamorphosis toward a free-living form. The nature, location, and number of activated organisms determine clinical sequelae, producing, at worst, serious foci or systemic pathology; at best, an endogenous microboost of immunity against kindred organisms. Many autoimmune illnesses are probably the consequence of such activation.

G. J. Domingue, Sr.: Departments of Urology and Microbiology and Immunology, Tulane University School of Medicine, New Orleans, Louisiana 70112-2699.

G. M. Ghoniem: Department of Urology, Tulane University School of Medicine, New Orleans, Louisiana 70112-2699.

Some aberrant bacteria can be recognized, even identified, by increasingly sophisticated biological techniques, the most recent of which is nucleic acid analysis. However, many forms can not be classified by any technique. It is probable that DNA analysis will finally reveal the overwhelming load of microbes we all carry about and make clear that the products of host and parasitic DNA can sometimes neutralize and sometimes generate pathologic sequelae, echoing the unpredictable behavior of the population of our planet.

There are numerous diseases of humans exhibiting symptomatology suggestive of a bacterial etiology in which routine bacteriologic methods fail to demonstrate causative organisms in culture. These diagnostic failures often lead to frustrating clinical diagnoses and to difficulty in management of the patient's illness. It is our working hypothesis that interstitial cystitis (IC) fits this category of disease.

THE DISEASE, HISTORY OF INFECTION, AND ETIOLOGIC THEORIES

The etiology of interstitial cystitis is unknown. Disease states predominate in women and have varying degrees of morbidity. In the most severe cases, the disease is debilitating and characterized by small bladder capacity, ulcers, severe frequency, nocturia, dysuria, and pain. Quality of life scores in these patients have been measured to be lower than in chronic renal disease patients. Treatment for the disease is varied and includes bladder distension, intravesical instillation therapy, and sometimes cystectomy. The limitations of current therapies result in part from the unknown cause of the disease. The primary focus of this chapter is (a) to consider IC as an infectious disease; (b) to present microbiological cultural and molecular evidence for the association of microorganisms with diseased tissue; and (c) to propose mechanisms by which a host–pathogen interaction could result in IC.

Hunner, in 1915, was the first to suspect that a bacterial infection was the cause of interstitial cystitis. He attempted to implicate infection from the teeth and tonsils as a cause of the elusive ulcer (1,2). Approximately four decades later, Smith reported two incidences of IC in which the exacerbation of bladder symptoms followed the extraction of infected teeth (3). He also reported on the treatment of IC with multiple antibacterial agents without achieving favorable results. Early microbiological studies that have searched for bacteria, fungi, and viruses have failed to identify a microbial cause for IC (4–6). However, these studies were performed before established clinical criteria were available for defining the disease. It is possible that many of the patients in the early microbiological studies had a urinary tract infection only and not IC.

Recognition of urethral syndrome as an early stage of interstitial cystitis was postulated by Wilkins et al. in 1989 (7). In their study seven of ten patients with IC were shown to have fastidious bacterial growth, mainly *Gardnerella vaginalis*. Also, one of six patients with urethral syndrome showed the presence of fastidious organisms. The presence of fastidious bacteria was demonstrated in both urine and bladder biopsy cultures. Fastidious bacteria were absent in four patients with bacterial cystitis. These authors postulated that urethral syndrome is an early stage of IC.

Unfortunately, microorganisms as possible etiologic agents in IC have received little attention in comparison with other leading theories: (a) bladder mastocytosis and mast cell activation (8), (b) a glycosaminoglycan deficiency (a mucopolysaccharide complex lining normal urinary bladders) (9), and (c) autoimmunity (10). Proponents of the glycosaminoglycan (GAG) deficiency theory argue that bacteria are not likely to be involved as causative agents because the GAG deficiency would also lead to diminished bacterial adherence, preventing colonization. It is possible that the GAG deficiency could be brought about by repeated bacteriuric episodes or persistent, intracellular, mucosal epithelial cell infections with dormant bacteria secreting enzymes and toxins that destroy the GAG. Studies by Ruggieri et al. (11) have shown that bacteria inoculated into normal and GAG-deficient rabbit bladders were 100 times more adherent to the GAG-deficient bladders than to the normal bladders. Possibly all proposed theories may be operative in IC if infectious agents or their antigens or metabolic products cause the initial insult to the uroepithelium. It is logical to assume that a number of cascading pathologic events could occur as a result of infection and lead to chronic bladder inflammation.

Although there are no accurate data to determine whether all patients correctly diagnosed with IC had a history of urinary tract infections, many have a history of bacteriuria. It has been reported by Held et al. (12) that urinary infection is twice as common among IC patients as among controls. It is also likely that those who deny a history of bacteriuria may have had asymptomatic disease.

PROBLEMS ASSOCIATED WITH ROUTINE MICROBIOLOGY AND MICROSCOPY

It has been suggested that the inability to culture "significant" numbers of bacteria routinely from urine specimens of IC patients indicates that bacteria are not involved in the etiology or morbidity associated with the disease. However, the clinical and pathologic findings in IC could be compatible with an infectious etiology: the Hunner's ulcer and the petechial hemorrhages called glomerulations. When a patient is first diagnosed with IC, the symptoms are highly suggestive of a urinary tract infection—pain and irritated voiding. The epidemiology is similar to bacteriuria in that 90% of IC patients are women, who also have a higher incidence of bacteriuria and are at a higher risk of developing a urinary tract infection because the short female urethra is easily colonized by organisms from vaginal and perineal sites.

Often, positive microbiological culture results in IC are interpreted as representing normal urethral microbiota contaminating the urine specimen. In our opinion, it is unwise to dismiss the pathogenic potentialities of any microbe in a patient with a mysterious disease. Normal microbiota is a statistical concept that derives from the immune competence of most of the human population. Repeated isolation of identical organisms in small numbers could increase the confidence level. Inability to culture microorganisms routinely from IC urines does not negate the role of difficult- or impossible-to-culture microorganisms. The standard quantitative and qualitative criteria for defining bacteriuria may not be applicable to infectious agents with a tropism for urinary bladder tissue. If microorganisms are intracellular or cell-associated or adhere rigidly to the bladder mucosa, urine may not adequately reflect the microbial content of the tissue. The pathology that can be produced by dormant bacteria cannot be appreciated unless clinical laboratories provide the methodology for their detection. Bacteria with aberrant cell wall morphology can be so dysmorphic as to resemble debris when viewed by bright light microscopy.

Oil-immersion phase microscopy of a wet preparation of the urine sediment often allows their recognition. Such a specimen stained with the fluorescent dye acridine orange and viewed with ultraviolet light microscopy will reveal the content of nucleic acids. Urine sediment, heat fixed on a slide and Gram stained, is a routine technique for visualizing bacteria; fragile wall-defective bacteria are totally disrupted by this method. Fastidious microorganisms, such as rickettsia, spirochetes, mycoplasmas, and chlamydia, would not be detected on a Gram stain. These microorganisms cannot be visualized by light microscopy at ×400 magnification on an unstained wet mount of sedimented or unsedimented urine, as is the usual practice in most clinics. Many dormant bacteria are cell-associated and may require rapid lysis of host cells to demonstrate their presence. These host cell lysates require immediate culture on enriched media and under conditions suitable for growth of osmotically fragile or nutritionally deficient microbial forms. Most laboratories do not employ these practices. That something of microbiological importance may have been overlooked in IC seems plausible.

A critique and review of the literature on microbial studies in IC was published in 1994 (13). This chapter focuses primarily on newly published papers, abstracts, and presentations at scientific meetings. Additionally, emphasis is on the use of specialized culture methods and molecular technology that may be of value in searching for buried bacterial genomes in urinary bladder tissue of patients with IC. To date, none of the routine microbiological studies that have been published implicate a single organism or a group of microorganisms in the etiology of IC. Therefore, the relationship of microbes to the disease has not been proved or disproved. Nevertheless, isolation of low concentrations of bacteria has been shown in some studies to be greater in the urine of IC patients than of control subjects (14). These findings have generated hypotheses that these microorganisms and/or their antigens and products could be involved in the pathogenesis of IC.

RECENT RESEARCH POSTULATING A ROLE FOR BACTERIA IN INTERSTITIAL CYSTITIS

The first report of molecular evidence demonstrating the presence of bacterial DNA in urinary bladder tissue of IC patients was presented at a meeting in 1993 (15) and in a published paper in 1995 (16). These data are presented later in the section on molecular bacteriology of IC. Subsequent scientific reports suggest that microorganisms may have a role in the etiology of IC. Provocative observations have been reported by Abrahams et al. (17) concerning activation of mast cells by type 1 fimbriated *Escherichia coli.* They examined the effect *in vitro* of adding type 1 fimbriated *E. coli* to a murine mast cell line, CFTL-12, and observed a strong proliferative response in the mast cells.

> It is of interest that when an isogenic mutant strain deficient in the fimbrial adhesive subunit FimH was employed, no mast cell proliferation was observed. Thus, direct binding of bacteria to the mast cell was required for mast cell activation, and the bacterial determinant for mast cell activation is FimH. Since mast cells are known to spontaneously proliferate as a result of the secretion of IL-3, by the activated mast cells, they reasoned that there was a possibility that type 1 fimbriated bacteria were inducing IL-3 production in CFTL-12 cells. Total RNA purified from bacteria-activated mast cells was subjected to reverse transcription-PCR using specific primers for mouse IL-3 mRNA transcripts in mast cells after 1 hr exposure to type 1 fimbriated bacteria but not in mast cells exposed to FimH-bacteria.

Taken together, their data suggest that type 1 fimbriated *E. coli* triggered bladder mast cell proliferation, possibly by inducing mast cell release of IL-3. Fimbrial antigens, particularly the P fimbriae, have received much attention as determinants of virulence in the pathogenesis of pyelonephritis. The above findings with type 1 fimbriae warrant extensive studies to determine whether repeated infections with fimbriated organisms could lead to the pathologic findings associated with IC.

Keay et al. (18) described a putative urinary antiproliferative factor of low molecular weight (<10 kDa) that is trypsin-sensitive and stable to 70°C for 2 hr. These authors have hypothesized that IC is caused by a low-molecular-weight stable protein in urine that caused decreased bladder epithelial cell proliferation. Their theory is that injury to the bladder epithelium such as occurs during bacteriuria might result in a chronically damaged epithelium that cannot adequately regenerate. It would be important to determine whether this protein is derived from host cells or tissues or microorganisms as well as to search for this protein in the urine of patients with other types of inflammatory diseases.

Elgavish et al. (19) propose that chronic inflammation results as an aftermath of recurrent infections. They hypothesize a mechanism by which bacteria cause injury that persists after they are no longer in the urine. Along those lines, they have been investigating the role of lipoteichoic acids (LT) from gram-positive bacteria and lipopolysaccharides (LPS) from gram-negative bacteria in basal urothelial cell proliferation, differentiation, and adhesion properties. Briefly, their proposed model centers on exposure of the basal urothelial cells to LT and/or LPS, with cytokine and nitric oxide synthase induction, activation of apoptosis, and incomplete healing of earlier foci of infection that possibly results in ulcers. They further speculate that more differentiated basal urothelial cells with low adhesive ability in the basal layer may cause focal detachments in distended IC bladders and provide a putative pathway for induction of an autoimmune response. This model is attractive because it is possible that the low concentrations of bacteria that are more often found in IC urine than controls could serve as a continual source of LT and LPS in the basal urothelial cells. It would therefore be important to determine whether LT and LPS persist in urinary bladder tissue of IC patients at different stages of the disease, using molecular and immunologic techniques.

Our focus at Tulane University School of Medicine is on buried bacterial genomes as a possible cause of occult infection that may have been missed or overlooked in the pathogenesis of IC. Specialized culture methods using enriched media and a polymerase chain reaction designed to detect a gene common to most bacteria of medical significance have provided new information on the microbiology of IC (16).

ANALOGS OF BACTERIAL PERSISTENCE IN DISEASES OF THE URINARY TRACT

We demonstrated in 1974 (20) the phenomena of bacterial persistence and reversion with cell-wall-deficient bacteria in a human embryonic kidney tissue culture system. Intracytoplasmic bodies derived from relatively cell-wall-deficient enterococci were demonstrated as persisters in a tissue culture infected with a wall-deficient *Enterococcus faecalis*. These intracytoplasmic bodies (0.05 to 0.15 μm) were nonculturable; however, there was continual persistence of these small bodies in the tissue culture cells despite disintegration of the cell-wall-deficient enterococci. Twenty-five days after initial infection, there was conversion of the tiny bodies to the parent, wall-containing enterococcus from which the wall-deficient forms had been derived. An indirect immunofluorescent technique with specific immune serum to the wall-deficient form proved that the persisting bodies were of bacterial origin and not host-cell organelles. Although persistence of the small bodies appeared to render no visible pathology, reversion to the wall-containing enterococci resulted in death of the tissue culture cells. Unlike the relatively stable wall-deficient form, a stable, nonreverting, wall-deficient enterococcal strain could be cultured 73 days after initial infection of the tissue culture, indicating that the organisms had survived and multiplied *in vivo*. At no time during the course of the study did the stable wall-deficient forms revert to their parent wall-containing bacterial forms. Throughout all of the cell infection experiments, the stable form grew out more readily on specialized media and in greater numbers than did the reverting wall-deficient enterococcal strain. These findings documented for the first time that intracytoplasmic dense bodies derived from cell-wall-deficient bacteria are a mechanism for bacterial persistence. It is further suggested that cell-wall-defective bacteria may be involved in latent and chronic infection and that these organisms may retain their pathogenicity. Persisting small electron-dense bacterial elementary bodies may have cellular and tissue tropisms that correlate with a variety of chronic human diseases, notably dormant and persistent infections of the urinary tract. Furthermore, these dense bodies bear a remarkable resemblance to the membrane-bonded core particles of unknown origin demonstrated at the infrastructural level in various tissues.

We extended our experimental studies on bacterial persistence to include investigations of patients with diseases of the urinary tract whose etiologies were enigmatic. Our aim was to determine whether cryptic bacterial persistence could be demonstrated in patients suspected of having a bacterial infection of the urinary tract although routine cultures were negative. Over a period of several years, we have demonstrated the presence of dormant bacteria in the urine of patients with idiopathic hematuria (21), in patients with nephrotic syndrome (22), and in urinary casts in a patient with renal Fanconi syndrome (23). Often the clinical course in these conditions is highly suspicious of urinary tract infection. However, negative urine cultures and the absence of ordinary bacteria and white blood cells in the urine sediment as well as failure of therapeutic approaches should lead to extensive urologic, nephrologic, and microbiological laboratory investigation. Many idiopathic collagen disorders and a disease such as IC could have a related pathogenesis. Confirmation of this dynamic is possible only if occult infection is considered in the differential diagnosis and clinical laboratories are prepared to recognize it. Many examples exist of persistent infections that produce only episodic illness. A possible mechanism for activation of an occult bacterial infection is transient immune dysfunction (possibly undetected by available laboratory tests) that can be brought about by severe physical or emotional stress, not unlike that seen in patients suffering with interstitial cystitis. In addition, the introduction of a coinfecting symbiotic organism could adversely alter the relationship of host and microbe. Our findings of dormant bacteria in idiopathic hematuria and nephrotic syndrome supported our earlier work on the persistence of intracytoplasmic bodies in kidney fibroblasts infected with cell-wall-deficient enterococci (20).

The above clinical examples are presented because they and other studies in numerous patients with idiopathic urinary infections by cryptic bacteria illustrate the need to search exhaustively for dormant bacteria in IC patients. It has been clearly established that morphologically aberrant bacteria can be induced within a suitable host; they can survive and persist in a latent state within the host; and they can induce pathologic responses compatible with disease (24). Unfortunately, the process of cryptic parasitization is an important bacteriologic phenomenon too often overlooked in clinical medicine. These dormant forms could account for chronicity of an inflammatory disease such as IC. It is possible that certain morphologically altered bacteria have a tropism for uroepithelial cells, resulting in an epitheliosis. This may be unrecognized because the persisting microbial forms could mimic host-cell organelles in morphologic appearance. Therefore, there is a need to search for microbial DNA and/or antigens that may persist in diseased urinary bladder tissue of IC patients.

MOLECULAR BACTERIOLOGY OF INTERSTITIAL CYSTITIS

One of the most sensitive methods for amplifying gene sequences is the polymerase chain reaction (PCR) (25). We hypothesized that a possible bacterial etiology for IC may have been overlooked because the methods of detection for pathogens may not have been adequate (16). We proposed to use PCR to detect the presence of bacterial DNA sequences in urinary bladder biopsies of patients with IC along with a group of control subjects, mainly those seeking medical attention for stress incontinence. If DNA sequences were present, we reasoned that the sensitivity of this method should allow us to detect its presence, and positive PCR results would strongly suggest a bacterial association with this disease.

Perhaps the most important consideration in the design of an optimal PCR strategy for amplifying a particular DNA segment is the selection of appropriate sequences to serve as primers. Because the amount of biopsy material available (1 to 5 mg) from patients with IC is limited, we selected pairs of primers that had the potential to amplify a large number of different bacterial genera. This required selection of a DNA sequence that was relatively conserved among bacterial genera, and we chose the DNA encoding 16S rRNA because this gene fulfilled that criterion. For example, searching gene bank version 65 homology of a segment of DNA encoding *E. coli* 16S rRNA demonstrated substantial homology with many other bacterial genera, including *Proteus, Pseudomonas, Klebsiella, Neisseria, Lactobacillus, Chlamydia, Streptococcus, Staphylococcus,* and *Bacterioides,* among others. Thus, it should have been possible to design PCR primers that have the ability to amplify DNA from a wide variety of bacterial genera. Thirty nucleotide segments of *Escherichia coli* DNA encoding 16S rRNA were screened for homology with (a) all known bacterial sequences and (b) all known primate sequences using MacVector version 3.5 sequence analysis software (IBI, New York, NY) and the Genbank version 65 data base. From these data-base searches, several pairs of oligonucleotide primers were selected that had high melting temperatures, no significant self-complementarity, and would result in the amplification of DNA segments of approximately 400 to 600 base pairs. In theory, these primer pairs should be optimal for these purposes, and the ultimate test was that they did function as expected.

Patients were diagnosed with IC according to the criteria set forth by the National Institutes of Arthritis, Diabetes, Digestive and Kidney Diseases as reported by Gillenwater et al. in 1988 (26). Three separate cold-cup biopsies (approximately 1 to 5 mg) were surgically removed from inflamed sites in the bladder wall of IC patients or from the normal bladder wall of control subjects using sterile techniques. One biopsy sample was homogenized immediately and was exhaustively evaluated for the presence of bacteria by routine and specialized methodology for demonstrating the presence of morphologically aberrant bacteria (24). The second biopsy specimen was stored as a coded sample at –70°C until total DNA was extracted. The third biopsy was evaluated histopathologically. The molecular methodology that we used was recently published (16). Briefly, we extracted DNA from cold-cup biopsies of bladder tissue of IC and control subjects and performed PCR using nested primers for the amplification of bacterial 16S rRNA genes. The amplified bacterial gene encoding 16S rRNA was detected by electrophoresis on agarose/ethidium bromide gels. Southern blot analyses were done to demonstrate hybridization of the amplified DNA fragments with oligonucleotide specific for bacterial 16S rRNA genes. To identify the type(s) of bacteria present in bladder biopsies that had 16S rRNA genes amplified, these gene fragments were cloned and sequenced. The sequences were compared with known bacterial sequences from the Ribosomal RNA database, University of Illinois, and the BLAST (National Center for Biotechnology Information, NCBI), Bethesda, MD. Extreme precautions were used to assure that no cross-contamination occurred. Optimization of the PCR and methods to detect amplified products gave a high probability of being able to amplify small amounts of bacterial DNA should it be present in biopsy samples. Because of the sensitivity of this assay, it was necessary that precautions be taken to eliminate any potential for contaminating experimental samples with DNA from cultured bacteria. This was easily and effectively accomplished because of the availability of two laboratories to carry out this work. Separate laboratory work areas were used to separate pre-PCR experimentation from post-PCR. Also, dedicated pipettes and specially equipped filter pipette tips were used in all experiments to prevent cross-contamination.

Of 49 patient IC biopsies extracted for bacterial DNA and subjected to primary and nested PCR, 18 IC patients showed presence of bacterial DNA (37%). The primary PCR was negative, but further amplification of the primary reaction with nested primers produced amplifiable gene fragments. All reactions with no input DNA (negative controls) were negative by both primary and nested PCR, and all positive bacterial DNA controls were positive by PCR. Tissue from two of 44 control subjects gave a positive PCR for bacterial DNA (4.5%). It was shown that the amplified fragments from IC patients represented gram-negative bacteria: *Pseudomonas* and *Escherichia* species, with *Pseudomonas* species predominating.

It is likely that the number of IC patients determined to be positive for the presence of bacterial 16S rRNA genes by this methodology is a minimal estimate. This likelihood is based on several technical considerations, which include (a) the limited amount of biopsy tissue available for study, (b) the limitation of using a single biopsy as representative of bacterial DNA in the entire bladder, (c) the need for bacterial DNA in the tissues to be sufficiently intact so that PCR amplification can occur, (d) the necessity in treating *Taq* DNA polymerase preparations with DNAase to eliminate *Thermas aquatius* DNA contamination before use in PCR, which reduced the sensitivity of the assay, and (e) the possibility that the primers selected may not be suitable for PCR amplification of all possible bacterial species that might be present. For example, we have found that *Mycoplasma genitalium* cannot be amplified with these primers.

It is unlikely that contamination by exogenous bacterial DNA could account for these results because great care was taken to eliminate this possibility. If contamination were a factor, one would expect that the multiple samples with no input DNA (negative control) would have also shown amplified DNA, but they did not. One might also argue that damaged urothelium such as is found in IC would be less resistant to the adherence of bacteria and that the bacterial DNA found is uninvolved in the IC process. We employed sensitive methodology to demonstrate the presence of ordinary bacteria by culture, and these routine cultures on the tissues processed for PCR were negative according to the usual criteria for interpreting routine culture findings in a clinical microbiology laboratory. All tissue samples were incubated in culture medium for prolonged periods of time (several months in broth culture). Final analyses on these cultures are presently in progress. It is also possible that the amplified nucleic acid represents DNA from nonviable bacteria remaining in the tissues from previous colonization or infection of the damaged tissue. It is impossible to completely rule out persistent DNA from a previous infection. However, a control subject had a *Proteus* infection 2.5 months before the biopsy; yet *Proteus* were not amplified from the biopsy tissue specimen, suggesting that bacterial DNA did not persist for prolonged periods after the infection had been cleared. This example would tend to argue against "leftover" DNA from a previous infection accounting for the positive PCR findings in patients. Nevertheless, deposition of microbial antigens, toxins, and metabolic products from a previously cleared infection should not be overlooked as factors in the pathogenesis of IC.

It is clear that the use of routine culture techniques to detect the presence of bacteria in the urine or bladder biopsies of patients with IC does not accurately reflect a possible bacterial presence in the tissue. There are at least two possible explanations for the molecular evidence of bacterial DNA in these patients. The presence of bacterial DNA could indicate that bacteria present in the bladder are viable but not culturable on media even using exhaustive culture methods. Alternatively, the inability to grow bacteria from the bladders of patients positive for gram-negative DNA by PCR may indicate that these organisms are not viable, perhaps because they have been destroyed by the resulting immune response. Either of these two possibilities could account not only for the lack of culturable bacteria but also for the presence of an inflammatory response in urinary bladder tissue.

ROUTINE MICROBIOLOGY CULTURES

Routine cultures on biopsy bladder tissue and urine from the above IC patients and control subjects revealed the following data. Four of 53 IC patients and one of 47 control subjects had positive bacteriologic findings (>100 colonies) and were not included in the PCR analysis of data. The organisms isolated from the IC patients were *Serratia marscescens, Staphylococcus haemolyticus, Escherichia coli,* and *Enterococcus faecalis*. The control subject specimen grew *Staphyloccocus epidermidis* and *Candida albicans.* Nine of the 53 IC patients and three of 47 control subjects had <100 colony-forming units per milliliter of urine. The organisms isolated in small numbers were identified as *Escherichia coli, Enterococcus faecalis, Staphylococcus haemolyticus, Acinetobacter* species, *Corynebacterium* species, *Bacteroides fragilis,* and *Fusobacterium falcifarium* from the IC patients and *Staphylococcus haemolyticus, Staphylococcus epidermidis,* and *Candida albicans* from the control subjects. Regardless of the type of specimen and numbers of bacteria isolated from the specimens, 34% of the IC patients had specimens from which bacteria were grown as compared with 15% for the controls. It is also possible that the organisms isolated in small numbers (<100 colonies) may represent urethral contamination of the specimens in both IC and control subjects. Except for *Escherichia coli* from biopsy tissue (negative routine cultures), none of the organisms isolated on routine culture were detected by PCR on biopsy tissue. Anaerobes and *Mycoplasma* species were not grown from the biopsy tissue. *Chlamydia* tests on urine sediments utilizing a fluorescent monoclonal antibody were all negative from both IC and control subjects. There may be some significance to the findings that the prevalence of bacteria in the urine and biopsy tissue of IC patients is greater than that of controls. These data would require confirmation with larger populations of diseased and control subjects. Clearly, some IC patients do develop urinary infections, and attention should be directed to whether these infections (demonstrable on routine culture or at times cryptic) represent an infectious etiology for IC or a result of IC.

FILTERABLE FORMS IN SPECIMENS FROM IC PATIENTS

We have demonstrated novel 0.22-µm filterable forms in modified PPLO medium inoculated with serum from the majority of IC patients and rarely from control subjects (16). Similar morphologic structures were also demonstrated in biopsy tissue and urine of IC patients. These forms resemble cell-wall-deficient bacteria in gross colony morphology on solid media and in liquid culture. The forms contain DNA as detected by fluorescent nucleic acid stains and are not osmotically fragile (unlike known cell-wall-deficient bacteria). They can be demonstrated in nonosmotically stabilized media (approximately 300 mOsm/kg H_2O). These forms have an absolute requirement of serum for growth. This growth requirement is not fulfilled by substituting cholesterol for serum in the medium, suggesting that they are not mycoplasmas. They are difficult to propogate in subculture. They do not Gram stain but are stained by malachite green. The preliminary ultrastructural studies suggest a heretofore unclassified form consisting of myelin-like swirls forming a central core-like structure and a tail. However, contrary to true myelin double-membrane spacing, spacing of the form's membrane-like sheets is tighter. No molecular relationship between myelin structure and these cultured filterable forms is implied. It is only mentioned as a guide for spacing between lamellae. Nevertheless, it would be of interest to determine whether these cultured forms have a tropism for nervous tissue.

At this time, it is not possible to fully determine the significance of these findings because we have demonstrated a similar morphologic form in commercially available pooled horse and human sera. Their presence in horse serum complicate interpretation of the findings from biopsy tissue and urine because 25% horse serum was incorporated in the medium. Heating the serum at 60°C for 2 hr is 90% effective in eliminating growth of the forms in culture. It is unclear whether heated horse serum can substitute for unheated serum in culture media in attempts to grow these forms from human specimens. To eliminate the problem of interpreting whether the forms arose from human or animal serum, it is preferable to employ high concentrations (25% or more) of the patient's own unheated serum in the culture medium. Preliminary immunologic studies suggest that the human and horse forms are antigenically different because antibodies generated to the human and horse forms do not cross-react. Additionally, the relationship (if any) of the amplified gram-negative bacterial DNA to the unidentified 0.22-μm filterable form remains to be determined. The extent of the presence of unusual filterable forms in the serum of healthy and diseased humans should be fully explored. Although specialized culture methods demonstrated their presence in specimens, we have not been successful in consistently amplifying DNA encoding for the 16S rRNA gene from extracts of these structures. This might indicate that the 16S rRNA gene may not be present in these forms, or, if it were present, the experimental conditions used for amplification may have to be modified. It remains to be determined whether these bizarre structures are symbionts found in a variety of hosts.

ANTIBIOTICS IN THE TREATMENT OF IC

In our studies, a strong microbial association with IC has been demonstrated. At least 37% of IC patients showed the presence of bacterial 16S rRNA genes in bladder biopsies, and PCR and subsequent cloning and sequencing of these gene fragments indicated that they were derived from gram-negative bacteria.

To assess the possible antimicrobial treatment of interstitial cystitis, six patients (four women and two men) with interstitial cystitis were enrolled. Their mean age was 54 years, with a mean duration of symptoms of 8 years and mean follow-up of 15 months. Their chief complaints were suprapubic pain with a visual analog score (VAS) of 90%. Frequency averaged 14 per day, and nocturia averaged three per night. Urinalysis and urine cultures were all negative. Four of the six patients demonstrated the presence of 16S rRNA genes in their bladder biopsies.

All patients received 1 month of oral ciprofloxacin (500 mg twice a day). Rifampin (600 mg/day) was given starting the second week of the ciprofloxacin treatment and continued for 3 weeks. This combination was chosen because rifampin is the most potent inhibitor of DNA-dependent RNA polymerase in bacteria; it is selectively toxic for bacterial but not for human cells. Ciprofloxacin interferes with the enzyme DNA gyrase, which is needed for the synthesis of bacterial DNA.

During the clinical course of treatment, all patients demonstrated increased irritative symptoms on the first week, ranging from mild to severe, with hemorrhagic cystitis in one patient. All patients demonstrated improvement of their symptoms gradually from the second to the fourth week. Overall results showed improvement of the suprapubic pain with a VAS score of 25%, improved frequency with a mean of seven per day, and nocturia with a mean of one. Relapse of symptoms was noticed in two patients after temporary improvement of 1 to 2 months. Partial improvement in one patient, with decreased need for intravesical DMSO instillation and a significant improvement of the suprapubic pain. Three patients demonstrated durable cure (more than 1 year) and required no treatment of their IC symptoms. Such a prolonged response strongly supports that it is not secondary to a placebo effect. Complications consisted of irritative bladder symptoms (four patients), vaginal yeast infection (two patients), and intolerance to rifampin administration because of mild skin itching in two patients.

Rifampin is a semisynthetic broad-spectrum bactericidal antibiotic. It inhibits bacterial but not human RNA synthesis. This is achieved by binding strongly with the β subunit of DNA-dependent RNA polymerase, preventing attachment of the enzyme to DNA and thus blocking initiation of RNA transcription. Eighty percent of rifampin is protein bound in the serum. Most of the unbound fraction is not ionized and therefore diffuses freely into tissues. It is particularly active against rapidly growing extracellular organisms but also has an intracellular bactericidal activity against susceptible organisms. It achieves a high contraction in macrophages. Unfortunately, resistance to rifampin has been demonstrated. This is because bacterial resistance occurs as a single step mutation of DNA-dependent RNA polymerase.

Ciprofloxacin has a wide spectrum of activity against gram-negative and gram-positive organisms. Its bactericidal action results from interference with the enzyme DNA gyrase, which is needed for synthesis of bacterial DNA.

The combination of ciprofloxacin and rifampin prevents the emergence of resistant bacteria not only to rifampin but also to ciprofloxacin. This is an important feature, especially with the new reports of emergence of bacteria resistant to ciprofloxacin. Ciprofloxacin and rifampin are ideal for long-term therapy of serious infections such as bacterial endocarditis. They are bactericidal, have good oral bioavailability, and are well tolerated over prolonged courses.

From this study, it seems that there is a role for antimicrobial treatment of interstitial cystitis. However, the most appropriate antimicrobial agents and the duration of the treatment need further study.

HYPOTHESES FOR THE ROLE OF BACTERIA AS INFECTIOUS AGENTS IN INTERSTITIAL CYSTITIS

We are proposing four mechanisms that may be operative if interstitial cystitis is an infectious disease.

1. Are difficult- or impossible-to-culture viable bacteria (cell-wall-defective or nutritionally deficient) the cause of IC? The bacteria may be dormant in the tissues. They may have been overlooked by light and electron microscopic methods because bacteria with aberrant cell-wall morphology often resemble host cell organelles. They are very difficult to culture and sometimes cannot be grown. It is possible that antimicrobial therapy could effect a cure.

2. Is IC a disease of "dysregulation" of the immune system? Is this disease brought about by a parallel set of antiidiotypic reactions induced by a self and a foreign bacterial antigen(s)? This theory would be analogous to that proposed by Kantor (27) and Dwyer et al. (28). Briefly, an antibody in one set may recognize the idiotype of an antibody in the other set. The two antibodies interact, thereby allowing one set of reactions to influence the other. If one of the interacting antibodies is directed against the self-antigen, the other could stimulate B cells bearing the autoantibody. The resulting response against the self-antigen would thus be based on a series of antiidiotypic reactions that begin with otherwise unrelated foreign antigen(s): whole, partially degraded, or completely degraded bacteria. These could include immunogenic bacterial intracellular or extracellular metabolic products, toxins, and antigens and bacterial DNA. Parallel-sets phenomenon has been demonstrated in other systems.

> Clinically, what causes anti-acetylcholine-receptor autoantibody production, the immunopathologic hallmark of myasthenia gravis, is unknown. A study by Dwyer et al. (28) found an antiidiotypic connection between separate immune responses—one against alpha 1,3 dextran (an antigen present on *Enterobacter* and *Serratia* species) and one against the acetylcholine receptor. Particularly interesting were findings with a monoclonal antibody designated SR11, obtained from a patient with myasthenia gravis and selected because of its specificity for a murine antiacetylcholine monoclonal antibody. SR11 was found to bind to dextran as well and to agglutinate both *Enterobacter* and *Serratia* species. In competitive binding assays, a murine antidextran monoclonal antibody inhibited SR11's binding to dextran, but acetylcholine receptor did not, which suggested that different parts of the SR11 idiotype recognized dextran and anti-acetylcholine-receptor. The clinical relevance was demonstrated in 60 myasthenic patients and 40 controls tested for antidextran antibodies. Ten of the patients were seropositive, compared with none of the controls. The implication was that a bacterial infection could indirectly initiate myasthenia gravis by stimulating production of antiidiotypes that also happen to be autoantibodies (27).

Because of the microbiological findings in IC, it would be worthwhile to search for antibodies to bacterial antigens that cross-react with urinary bladder tissue antigens. Such cross-reactions might result in a parallel set phenomenon in IC. By this mechanism, presence of bacterial antigen(s) that are immunogenic would participate in immunologic events, resulting in an autoimmune phenomenon in which bacteria (viable or nonviable) are involved. Deposition of bacterial antigen(s) in the urinary bladder or circulation via repeated bacteriuric episodes (symptomatic or asymptomatic) might be the only prerequisite for initiating this type of immunopathology.

3. Does IC occur as a result of an allergic and/or inflammatory reaction to bacterial antigen(s)? This hypothesis is based on the elegant representation of the effect of cell adhesion on mast cell and basophil function as proposed by Hamawy (29). Abbreviated to illustrate how this might be applicable to IC, tissue injury could be caused by bacteria, their extracellular or intracellular metabolic products, antigens, or toxins, or possibly by the persistence of their DNA (even in the absence of viable bacteria). Inflammatory mediators and cytokines secreted by mast cells and basophils could invade the site of injury. This may be followed by adherence of mast cells and basophils to other cells via surface adhesion receptors that mediate binding to other cells and to extracellular matrix. Modulation of the function of basophils and mast cells may follow, including adhesiveness, migration, secretion, and proliferation. These effects may be important in *in vivo* distribution, localization, function, and survival of these cells in tissue. Factors released at the site of injury could result in an increase in the number of different types of cells including mast cells and basophils. Enhanced secretion could lead to elimination of tissue injury or a chronic inflammatory response. Therefore, if the source of bacterial antigen is eliminated, and mast cell and basophil adhesion are manipulated, one might control the outcome of these cascading reactions that lead to allergic and/or inflammatory responses. Interstitial cystitis may be an analog of this type of inflammatory reaction (5). Invoking this mechanism would not require the presence of living organisms as long as bacterial antigens have been deposited in the tissues. Therefore, an infection (viable organisms) could have been cleared, yet bacterial antigens persist to cause tissue injury.

4. Is neurogenic detrusor inflammation triggered and escalated by infection? Neurogenic inflammation and local immune responses can be medicated by the release of sub-

stance P contained in afferent neurons and urothelial cells of the bladder. The neuropeptide substance P has excitatory effects on neurons and pain perception (nociception). In addition, substance P mediates muscle contraction, vasodilation, plasma extravasation, and local immune and inflammatory responses in nonneuronal tissues.

CONCLUSIONS

The presence of gram-negative bacterial DNA in urinary bladder tissue does not prove that they are the cause of IC. However, it would be difficult to imagine that such a microbial presence in the bladder has no effect on the disease and its resulting morbidity. By identifying patients having microbes in the bladder, it should be possible to determine if antimicrobials aid in the treatment of the disease. It is logical to suggest that even if organisms are not causative agents, their presence may lead to immune and host-cell responses that could initiate or exacerbate an inflammatory state. Thus, it would be predicted that appropriate treatments to minimize microbial presence in the tissue may significantly improve the morbidity associated with IC.

FUTURE RESEARCH

Future research should be directed at continuing to utilize molecular techniques to search for the presence of microorganisms and/or their metabolic products and antigens directly in urinary bladder tissue, particularly intracellular or cell-associated organisms. It might also be meaningful to search carefully for microorganisms in the blood of patients. It would be of value to determine whether bacterial antigens present in IC patient tissues can be linked with any immunopathologic event(s) in these patients. Studies should be undertaken at the light and ultrastructural microscopic level utilizing appropriate labeled antibodies to bacterial antigens in an effort to identify cryptic bacteria in tissue. It is possible that morphologically aberrant dormant bacteria may have been overlooked in earlier studies because of the morphologic resemblance of these forms to host-cell structures.

Definitive qualitative and quantitative data linking microorganisms with diseased urinary bladder tissue might lead to a better understanding of the pathogenesis of IC as well as its prevention. Molecular modifications of Koch's postulates may have to be invoked in IC if aberrant bacterial forms are the causative agents because of difficulty in repeatedly culturing these unusual bacteria from diseased tissues and body fluids. It would be important to explore the host and its reaction to dormant bacteria: immune system, phagocytosis, chemotaxis, complement, macrophage activation, adaptive immune responses, cell-mediated responses, and consequences of a compromised host. Factors that favor bacterial persistence in IC would need investigation, particularly into how dormant aberrant bacteria protect their selective advantage when establishing tissue tropisms.

Acknowledgments

We are grateful to Liset G. Human, M.P.H., and Kucting Wu for expert technical assistance. We thank Kenneth Johnston, Ph.D., Kenneth L. Bost, Ph.D., Cesar D. Fermin, Ph.D., Yoshihiro Mizuma, M.D., and Shinichi Makinose, M.D., for their collaboration. This work was supported by grants from the NIH: NIDDK RO1 DK44812-04, and the Interstitial Cystitis Association and a donation from Mr. and Mrs. W. Russell Harp.

REFERENCES

1. Hunner G. A rare type of bladder ulcer in women: Report of cases. *Boston Med Soc J* 1915;172:660–664.
2. Hunner G. Elusive ulcer of the bladder. *Am J Obstet* 1918;78:374–395.
3. Smith GG. Interstitial cystitis. *J Urol* 1952;67:903–915.
4. Hanash KA, Pool TL. Interstitial and hemorrhagic cystitis: Viral, bacterial and fungal studies. *J Urol* 1970;104:705–706.
5. Hedelin HH, Mardh P-A, Brorson J-E, et al. *Mycoplasma hominis* and interstitial cystitis. *Sex Transm* 1983;10:327–330.
6. Fall M, Johansson SL, Vahlne A. A clinicopathological and virological study of interstitial cystitis. *J Urol* 1985;133:771–773.
7. Wilkins E, Payne S, Pead P, et al. Interstitial cystitis and the urethral syndrome: A possible answer. *Br J Urol* 1989;64:39–44.
8. Sant GR, Theoharides TC. The role of the mast cell in interstitial cystitis. *Urol Clin North Am* 1994;21:41–53.
9. Parsons CL, Stouffer JD, Schmidt JD. Bladder surface glycosamimoglycans: An efficient mechanism of environmental adaptation. *Science* 1980;208:605–607.
10. Ratliff TL, Klutke CG, McDougall EM. The etiology of interstitial cystitis. *Urol Clin North Am* 1994;21:21–30.
11. Ruggieri MR, Balagani RK, Rajter JJ, et al. Characterization of bovine bladder mucin fraction that inhibits *Escherichia coli* adherence to the mucin deficient rabbit bladder. *J Urol* 1992;148:173–178.
12. Held PJ, Hanno PM, Weirr AJ, et al. Epidemiology of interstitial cystitis: 2. In: Hanno PM, Staskin DR, Krane RJ, et al., eds. *Interstitial Cystitis*. London, Spinger-Verlag, 1990.
13. Warren, JW. Intersititial cysitis as an infectious disease. *Urol Clin North Am* 1994;21:31–39.
14. Keay S, Schwalbe RS, Triffilis AL, et al. A prospective study of microorganisms in urine and bladder biopsies from interstitial cystitis patients and controls. *Urology* 1995;45:223–229.
15. Domingue GJ et al. NIH-NIDDK/ICA Interstitial Cystitis Scientific Workshop, Orlando, 1993;27 (abst).
16. Domingue GJ, Ghoniem GM, Bost KL, et al. Dormant microbes in interstitial cystitis. *J Urol* 1995;153:1321–1326.
17. Abraham SN, Shah A, Malaviya R. Mast cell-Bacteria in IC: Mastocytosis induced by type 1 fimbriated *E. coli*. NIH-NIDDK/ICA Interstitial Cystitis Scientific Workshop, San Diego, 1995;12 (abst).
18. Keay S et al. Evidence for a low molecular weight, heat stable antiproliferative protein in urine from IC patients. NIH-NIDDK/ICA Interstitial Cystitis Scientific Workshop, San Diego, 1995;14 (abst).
19. Elgavish A et al. A model for the etiology of interstitial cystitis (IC). NIH-NIDDK/ICA Interstitial Cystitis Scientific Workshop, San Diego, 1995;26 (abst).
20. Green MT, Heidger PM Jr., Domingue GJ. Demonstration of the phenomena of microbial persistence and reversion with bacterial L-forms in human embryonic kidney cells. *Infect Immun* 1974;10:889–914.
21. Domingue GJ, Thomas R, Walters F, et al. Cell wall-deficient bacteria as a cause of idiopathic hematuria. *J Urol* 1993;150:483–485.

22. Woody HB, Walker PD, Domingue GJ. Genesis of the urinary oval fat body by intracellular lipid absorbing cell wall-deficient bacteria. In: Domingue GJ, ed. *Cell Wall-Deficient Bacteria: Basic Prinicples and Clinical Significance*. Reading, MA: Addison-Wesley, 1982; 219–230.
23. Domingue GJ, Woody HB, Farris KB, et al. Bacterial variants in urinary casts and renal epithelial cells. *Arch Intern Med* 1979;139:1355–1360.
24. Domingue GJ. Filterable cell-associated cell wall-deficient bacteria in renal diseases. In: Domingue GJ, ed. *Cell Wall-Deficient Bacteria: Basic Principles and Clinical Significance*. Reading, MA: Addison-Wesley, 1982;121–148.
25. Mullis K, Faloona F, Scharf S, et al. Specific enzymatic amplification of DNA *in vitro:* The polymerase chain reaction. *Cold Spring Harbor Symp Quant Biol* 1986;51:263–273.
26. Gillenwater JY, Wein AJ. Summary of the national institute of arthritis, diabetes, digestive and kidney disease workshop on interstitial cystitis. *J Urol* 1988;140:203–206.
27. Kantor FS. Autoimmunities: Diseases of "dysregulation." *Hosp Pract* 1988;23:75–84.
28. Dwyer DS, Vakil M, Kearney JF. Idiopathic network connectivity and a possible cause of myasthenia gravis. *J Exp Med* 1986;164:1310–1318.
29. Hamawy MM, Mergenhagen SE, Siraganian RP. Adhesion molecules as regulators of mast cell and basophil function. *Immunol Today* 1994;15:62–66.

Interstitial Cystitis, edited by Grannum R. Sant.
Lippincott–Raven Publishers, Philadelphia ©1997.

CHAPTER 10

Disintegrity of the Vesical Blood–Urine Barrier in Interstitial Cystitis: A Vicious Circle

Gero Hohlbrugger

The urothelium separates urine from the bladder wall. Potassium (K^+, with a concentration as much as 10 times higher than in blood plasma) and organic nitrogen metabolites tend to have remarkable transurothelial concentration gradients from urine toward blood. Facilitated by the respective concentration gradients during urine storage in the bladder, any permanent and significant recirculation of substances already excreted by the kidneys would hardly be conducive to life. The primary function of the vesical blood–urine barrier is therefore to hold recirculation. Since the urothelium, under totally tension-free *in vitro* conditions, proved to be only slightly more permeable than skin, it was concluded that this structure alone represents the blood–urine barrier (1). For the same reason, the common view of bladder function excludes any involvement of urine composition in urge development; rather, it considers tension and pressure perception (= mechanoception or proprioception within the detrusor) for normalcy and detrusor hyperactivity or pathologically increased sensitivity for increased urge, as is the case with interstitial cystitis (IC) (2,3).

Relative impermeability of the urothelium is not only provided by its "tight junctions," but also by its delimiting heparin-containing glycosaminoglycans(GAG)-layer (4). The increased presence of mast cells in the submucosa of the bladder of patients with IC and their topographical closeness to sensory nerve endings, as well as their obvious cytoplasmic discharge, led to the consideration of pathophysiological relevance in referral to urge and pain symptoms (5). On the other hand, mast cells contain tremendous amounts of heparin. Therefore, it is quite possible that the heparin supply, which comes with cytoplasmic discharge, can also be seen as an attempt to compensate for insufficient GAG-expression of the urothelium (6). Since reduced vesical blood flow could easily compensate for leakiness of the primary barrier, increased urothelial permeability need not necessarily correspond with an increased transurothelial net flow. This means that vesical blood flow, as well as the urothelium, defines the efficiency of the blood–urine barrier. Therefore, unchanged urine-to-blood, or vice versa, tracer flows should not be interpreted as unchanged transurothelial permeability (7). This chapter deals with the normal, as well as pathophysiological, interdependency of urothelial permeability and vesical blood flow, and focuses on its importance for normal urge control and its loss.

G. Hohlbrugger: Department of Urology, University of Innsbruck, A-6020 Innsbruck, Austria.

NORMAL BLOOD–URINE BARRIER AND URGE CONTROL

In vivo experiments in normal rat bladders have shown that urothelial permeability increases with the filling volume (8). A decrease of the transurothelial electrical resistance in normal human bladders with increasing filling volume leads to the assumption of similar permeability dynamics for humans (9). Moreover, individuals with healthy bladders are able to notice that the voided volumes with increased urine coloring (= increase in urine concentration) are lower. On the other hand, forced diuresis after excessive beer consumption, for example, leads to significantly higher volumes (8,10). This fact can be proven quite easily through cystometry in the normal rat bladder. If 0.15 M KCl (30 times higher K^+ concentration than in blood plasma) is introduced, and if the resulting pressure curve is then compared with water cystometry (0.15 M NaCl = normal saline), one can see that the course of the curve differs from the very beginning, and that onset of voiding contractions occurs at significantly lower filling volumes (Fig. 1) (8). This can be considered

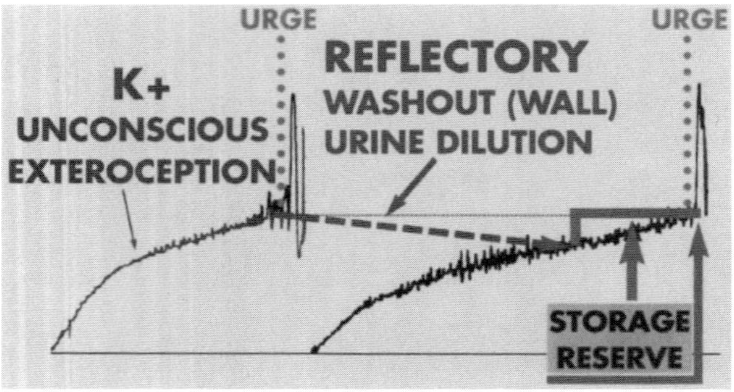

FIG. 1. Comparative cystometry in the normal rat bladder; the difference in compliance is obvious from the onset (6).

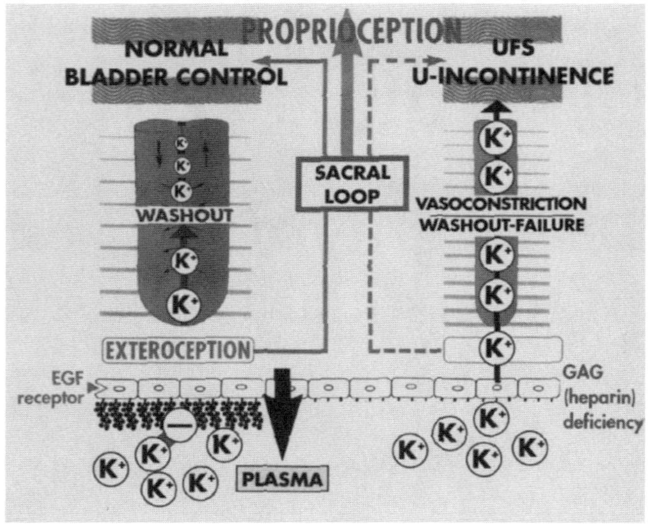

FIG. 2. The new concept of normal bladder control: urinary potassium only affects mucosal exteroceptors. Any impulses from there unconsciously trigger parasympathetic inflow to the detrusor in order to induce urge (conscious pressure reception) at a lower filling volume. Increased urothelial permeability and relative vesical ischemia in UFS and IC allow direct access of urinary K^+ to the detrusor.

as clear evidence that even the normal urothelium can never be absolutely tight, and that the change of the pressure curve has nothing to do with tension or pressure perception. Since direct contact of urine (high K^+ and hyperosmolarity) with the detrusor would result in its excitation, with concomitant severe urge and so-called unstable contractions which could not be inhibited by any endogenous neurotransmitter, this suggests that intravesical K^+ could not directly induce this change. Neurotransmitted detrusor inhibition or urge control can only function in the presence of a normal extracellular electrolyte and osmolarity environment within the smooth muscle syncytium of the detrusor (11,12).

In order to answer the question of why urge, despite increasing urothelial permeability and the influence of urine composition on the development of urge, can usually be controlled over a longer period of time, the dynamics of normal vesical blood flow had to be investigated. By applying an endorectal probe attached to a color Doppler unit (Acuson 128 XP 10), we have found that vesical blood flow increases and accelerates with filling (normal saline), and that this is amplified by intravesical K^+ (0.2 M KCl) (13). It is highly probable that the increase in blood flow with filling is caused mechanically by stretching the vessels, which in flaccid conditions are arranged in spirals (14,15,16). Since slight increases in perivascular K^+ concentration cause vasodilation, it can be assumed that no further vasomotor reflex is necessary for the increase in blood flow secondary to high intravesical K^+ (17). However, the dynamics of normal blood flow should be sufficient to wash out increasingly reabsorbed K^+, in order to keep the intramural extracellular environment as the prerequisite for normal urge control in balance. On the other hand, the opposing findings that have also been reported for the normal canine bladder must be taken into account (18). Since rapid filling reduces blood flow (19), one can assume that this experimental design might have been the reason for those controversial results. If our results are correct, it still remains to be explained how urinary K^+ contributes to the development of urge. Since direct contact of urinary K^+ with the detrusor does not come into question, urinary K^+ must have challenged exteroceptive nerve endings which are located in and below the urothelium (Fig. 2). Therefore, any impulses derived from there trigger the parasympathetic inflow to the detrusor with consequent urgency (conscious intramural pressure reception) at a lower filling volume. Since the concentration and the amount of urine stored in the bladder is not known, and since, at least in the rat bladder, "comparative" cystometry revealed differing pressures from the very beginning, it can, with great certainty, be stated that this primary exteroceptive reflex avoids the cortical micturition center (Fig. 3). According to W.E. Bradley and F.B. Scott, impulses derived from exteroceptors do not reach the cerebral cortex (20). Urge control, however, most likely is not only of a neuromuscular (hypogastric nerve) nature because: (a) hyperosmolar urine creates an osmotic gradient toward the bladder lumen, (b) there is a hydrostatic (filtration) pressure in the same direction, and, (c) vesical blood flow increases additionally after electrical stimulation of the hypogastric nerve, due to the conveyance of vasoactive intestinal peptide (21). Therefore, one may assume that neuromuscular urge suppression and transurothelial plasma filtration take place synchronously. Subsequent urine dilution could represent the key mechanism that keeps the bladder under control for a while. Only during forced diuresis (diluted urine), is it probable that only mechanic stretching, in conjunction with pressure, cause urgency. With already low osmolar

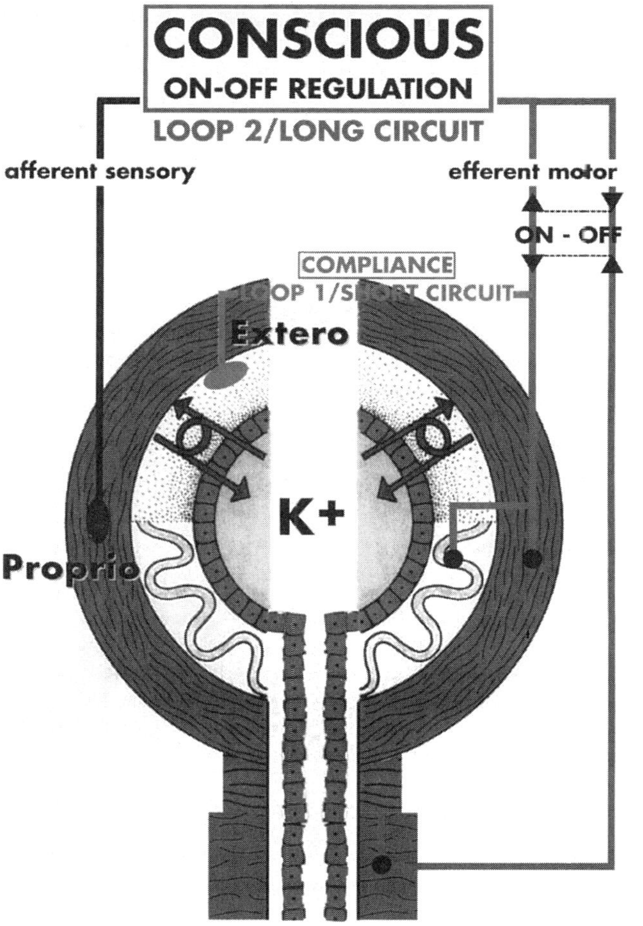

FIG. 3. Diagrammatic representation of conscious pressure and tension reception (proprio) and unconscious exteroception (extero) in relation to the relevant pathways of the micturition reflex (6).

urine, however, there is nothing more left to be diluted or to be washed out from the bladder wall. Hence, under these circumstances, pain quickly arises from urge.

IMPAIRED BLOOD–URINE BARRIER AND LOSS OF URGE CONTROL

In most patients with urgency/frequency syndrome (UFS) and IC, urothelial permeability is pathophysiologically increased (22,23); at the same time, the increase of the blood flow during filling, as well as through intravesical K^+, is missing (16,24). Following increased permeability, perivascular K^+ concentration increases far more extensively than normal with consequent vasoconstriction (25), and this again leads to a washout failure of reabsorbed K^+. Thus, increased urothelial permeability and relative vesical ischemia allow direct access of urine to the detrusor and its proprioception, with consequent excitation of both (see Fig. 2). The preceding safety mechanisms are undermined, and urge gets out of control, even at low filling volumes. This also helps to explain why so many patients with urgency do not satisfactorily respond to anticholinergics. Even if, through conventional water cystometry, neuromuscular drugs have proven to be beneficial, it is doubtful that these measured facts really correspond to any change toward a physiologic state (normalized urothelial permeability and vesical blood flow). On the other hand, micturition amplifies urgency, which will stop abruptly, however, with the onset of urine flow and during the highest intravesical pressures. One can consider this a significant indication that excitation (K^+ = urge) and contraction (calcium) have to be strictly separated. Ambulatory monitoring has quite clearly shown that unstable contractions occur, even in normal bladders (26,27). As a result of very efficient urethral opening, women frequently void at low to very low pressures, solely with the aid of isovolumetric (isotonic) contractions (28). Furthermore, according to micromotion investigations, local contractions can occur without an increase in tension or pressure, because other parts are in antiphase (29). Considering these circumstances, and taking into account that in UFS and IC, contrary to the neuropathic reflex bladder, urgency, not pressure (= harm to the kidneys, absence of urge), has to be treated; one can be certain that the present differentiation between sensory and motor urgency does not make sense. Besides neuromuscular drugs, estrogen substitution is also recommended in the treatment of UFS and IC in postmenopausal women. Estrogens not only promote the normalization of the urethral mucous membrane (30), but also bladder circulation (31). Since electrostimulation of the hypogastric nerve accelerates vesical blood flow (21,32), one might conclude that the success of temporary transdermal electrotherapy (33), as well as of permanent neuromodulation (34), is mainly caused by this and not only by interference with sensory afferents or by support of inhibitory impulses. Pelvic floor training seems to show similar effects (35). Impaired perfusion of the bladder affects the urothelium far more than the detrusor (36). Since Ca antagonists not only block detrusor contractions, but also widen spastic vessels, and since topical therapy of IC with these substances is also successful (37), it is highly probable that improved blood flow can help reestablish a damaged urothelium. Detrusor and vessels react to K^+ channel openers such as Ca antagonists (38). Topical installations of heparin (39), elmiron (40), hyaluronic acid (41), D-glucosamin (42) or DMSO-cocktails (43) primarily target the urothelial barrier. At present, whether normal blood flow and normal urothelial permeability can be reestablished in advanced stages of IC is doubtful. Capsaicin (44), overdistension procedures (45), and surgical or chemical denervation (46) solely interfere with sensory afferents. Therefore, these therapeutic regimens should be used only when irreversibility of a damaged blood–urine barrier is ascertained.

DIAGNOSIS OF IMPAIRED BLOOD–URINE BARRIER

Urothelial permeability of the bladder has so far been evaluated through measuring the concentration differences of instilled solutions, bladder-to-blood tracer studies, both in a relation to time and volume (= surface), as well as through measuring transurothelial electrical resistance (4,8,9,23,47). Examination of the penetration depth of color substances was also considered as a criterion for the changes of permeability (48). These different techniques, however, have hardly contributed to a better understanding of the pathophysiology of the urge bladder. For UFS, as well as IC patients, only the question of the extent to which urinary K^+ is responsible for urge and pain symptoms should be of clinical interest. In order to answer this question, C. L. Parsons instilled 50 ml water, and 50 ml 0.4 M KCl thereafter, into the bladders of healthy probands and of IC patients for ten minutes(22). Since only IC patients were able to state the difference of urge and pain symptoms clearly, it became obvious that their urothelial permeability for K^+ was increased. Following this examination, we have introduced "comparative" cystometry (50 ml/min, normal saline versus 0.2 M KCl) in our urodynamic laboratory. With regard to maximum capacity, normal volunteers showed minimal differences (0% to 14%) while UFS patients showed 44% (19% to 75%) lower volumes when filled with KCl (49). In order to prove an increased transurothelial permeability with "comparative" cystometry, we have decided temporarily to fix the difference of maximum capacity at > 20% for the urgency bladder. Based on ongoing urodynamic investigations (presently about 150), we have to admit that the K^+ provocation decreases with increasing denervation (residual urine), and remains fully absent after complete denervation. To the same degree that afferent denervation can hide urothelial disintegrity during "comparative" cystometry, cystoscopically visible alterations such as angiogenesis, for example, do not often correlate with the symptom score. However, in addition to "comparative" cystometry, cystoscopy is highly recommended for diagnosis of UFS and IC patients, because carcinoma *in situ* can be excluded, and the eye of the examiner learns to judge the difference between normal and affected bladders more sensitively.

PATHOPHYSIOLOGICAL INTERDEPENDENCE OF UROTHELIAL PERMEABILITY AND VESICAL BLOOD FLOW: A VICIOUS CIRCLE

Since intravesical neutralization of GAG–heparin with protamin sulfate induces urgency, which will abate after heparin-substitution, it is probable that there is a GAG deficiency in most cases of UFS and IC (50). This GAG deficiency can originate either from the urothelium itself, or can appear due to relative ischemia (36). Increased permeability seems, however, to induce deficient circulation (24). Therefore, UFS and IC can be caused by many basically different pathogens (51). According to transurothelial dialysis experiments in rats and in patients with normal vesical blood flow but with a "leaky" urothelium, a high percentage of renal waste may be recirculated within 2 to 3 hours (8). This means that increased urothelial permeability, in conjunction with relative vesical ischemia, make urge control impossible, while relative vesical ischemia and frequency protect against recirculation of renal waste. The pathophysiological interdependence of urothelial disintegrity and vesical ischemia, as a principle of survival in terms of nonrecirculation, therefore may do nothing, but in the sense of a vicious circle, permanently worsen urge and pain symptoms of IC (Fig. 4). Those assumptions were strongly confirmed by a preliminary cohort of our UFS patients, in which both vesical blood flow and "comparative" cystometry became normal, in addition to remission of symptoms, 8 weeks after topical heparin therapy (5,000 IU per day) (39).

Years of suffering with steadily increasing symptoms of IC sometimes require cystectomy. Intestinal augmentation has not proven to sufficiently rescue patients from urgency; patients either get a continent pouch or an ileal-neobladder, and forever spend their lives as bladder cripples, with or without intermittent catheterization (52). One must pose the question, if, in view of a nononcologic and a facultatively nonneuropathic disease, this is the only scenario? Does not each case of IC start with a sim-

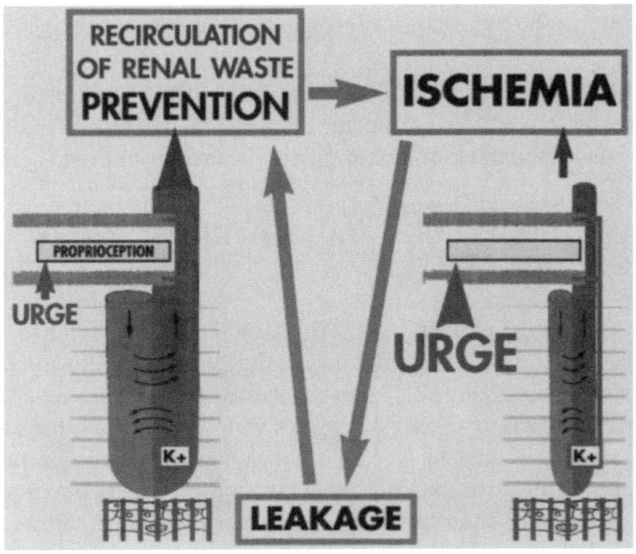

FIG. 4. The vicious circle in IC: recirculation of renal waste secondary to urothelial leakage is avoided by relative ischemia. On the other hand, ischemia can induce leakage and amplifies urge (48).

ple urgency bladder (53)? Is IC indeed a special disease, or is it simply the often irreversible final stage of an urgency bladder? After an impaired blood–urine barrier has been diagnosed, shouldn't earlier treatment be directed to the GAG-layer and vesical blood flow, instead of, or at least as a supplement to, different neuromuscular or even psychiatric therapy concepts, to break up that vicious circle for simple urgency bladders and therefore prevent irreversible final stages? Wouldn't it be better, in this sense, to leave the present inclusion criteria of IC (54) in order to establish reliable criteria for an irreversible IC? Only irreversibility allows invasive and irreversible therapy.

REFERENCES

1. Lewis SA. A reinvestigation of the function of the mammalian urinary bladder. *Am J Physiol* 1977;232:F187–F195.
2. Steers WD. Physiology of the urinary bladder. In: Walsh PC, Retic AB, Stamey TA, Vaughan ED Jr, eds. *Campbell's Urology.* Philadelphia: WB Saunders Company, 1992;142–169.
3. Hohenfellner M, Nunes L, Schmidt RA, Lampel A, Thüroff JW, Tanagho EA. Interstitial cystitis: increased sympathetic innervation and related neuropeptide synthesis. *J Urol* 1992;147:587–58.
4. Parsons CL, Boychuk D, Jones S, Hurst R, Callahan H. Bladder surface glycosaminoglycans: an epithelial permeability barrier. *J Urol* 1990; 143:139–142.
5. Theoharides TC, Sant GR, El-Mansoury M, Letournau R, Ucci AA Jr, Meares EM. Activation of bladder mast cells in interstitial cystitis: a light and electron microscopic study. *J Urol* 1995;153:629–636.
6. Moskowitz MO, Byrne DS, Callahan HJ, Parsons CL, Valderrama E, Moldwin RM. Decreased expression of a glycoprotein component of bladder surface mucin (GP1) in interstitial cystitis. *J Urol* 1994; 151:343–345.
7. Hohlbrugger G. Bladder permeability in interstitial cystitis is similar to that of normal volunteers: Direct measurement by transvesical absorption of 99m technetiumdiethylenetriaminepentaacetic acid (letter). *J Urol* 1994;152:2105–2106.
8. Hohlbrugger G. The vesical blood–urine barrier: a relevant and dynamic interface between renal function and nervous bladder control. *J Urol* 1995;154:6–15.
9. Birch BR, Brindley GS, Miller RA: The electrical resistance of the vesical epithelium. *J Urol* 1990;143:369A.
10. Kayada K, Yamaguchi O, Yoshimura Y. Effect of diuresis on frequency-volume chart in normal volunteers and patients with hyperactive detrusor. *Neurourol Urodyn* 1996;15:429–431.
11. Angelico P, Guaneri L, Fredella B, Testa R. In vivo effects of different antispasmodic drugs on the rat bladder contractions by topically applied KCl. *J Pharmacol* Toxicol 1992;27:33–39.
12. Uvelius B. Effect of variations in extracellular osmolality on spontaneous contractile activity and response to nerve stimualtion in rat detrusor muscle in vitro. *Urol Int* 1985;40:196–200.
13. Hohlbrugger G, Frauscher F, Strasser H, Colleselli K, Corvin S, Bartsch G. Vesical blood flow is modified by distension and intravesical potassium. *J Urol* 1997;(Suppl) 157:664 (abst).
14. Mehrotra RLM. An experimental study of the vesical circulation during distension and in cystitis. *J Pathol* 1953;66:79–89.
15. Andersson PO, Bloom SR, Mattiasson A, Uvelius B. Changes in vascular resistance in the feline urinary bladder in response to bladder filling. *J Urol* 1985;134:1041–1046.
16. Irwin P, Galloway NTM. Impaired bladder perfusion in interstitial cystitis: a study of blood supply using laser doppler flowmetry. *J Urol* 1993;149:890–892.
17. McCarron JG, Halpern W. Potassium dilates rat cerebral arteries by two different mechanisms. *Am J Physiol* 1990;259(part 2) :H902–H908.
18. Azadzoi KM, Pontari M, Vlachiotis J, Shiroky MB. Canine bladder blood flow and oxygenation: changes induced by filling, contraction and outlet obstruction. *J Urol* 1996;155:1459–1465.
19. Greenland JE, Brading AF. Urinary bladder blood flow changes during the micturition cycle in a conscious pig model. *J Urol* 1996;156: 1858–1861.
20. Bradley WE, Scott FB. Physiology of the urinary bladder. In: Harrison JH, Gittes RF, Perlmutter AD, Stamey TA, Walsh PC, eds. *Campbell's Urology.* Philadelphia: WB Saunders Company, 1978;87–124.
21. Andersson PO, Sjögren C, Uvnäs B, Uvnäs-Moberg K. Urinary bladder and urethral responses to pelvic and hypogastric nerve stimulation and their relation to vasoactive intestinal polypeptide in the anaesthetized dog. *Acta Physiol Scand* 1990;138:409–416.
22. Parsons CL, Stein PC, Bidair M, Lebow D. Abnormal sensitivity to intravesical potassium in interstitial cystitis and radiation cystitis. *Neurourol Urodyn* 1994;13:515–520.
23. Völter D, Weisswange V, Ziegler H, Schubert GE. Die Xenon-Exhalationsmessung im Rahmen der Diagnostik von Harnblasenerkrankungen. *Urologe A* 1975;14:38–40.
24. Hohlbrugger G, Frauscher F, Strasser H, Corvin S, Bartsch G. Nicht neuromuskuläre Dysregulation sondern erhöhtes extrazelluläres Kalium in der Blasenwand verursacht idiopathische Reizblase und Dranginkontinenz. *J Urol Urogynäkol Sonderheft* 1997;4:41.
25. Trautwein W, Gauer OH, Koepchen HP. Herz und Kreislauf. In: Gauer OH, Kramer K, Jung R, eds. *Physiologie des Menschen.* München-Berlin-Wien: Urban & Schwarzenberg, 1972;3:1–418.
26. Robertson AS, Griffiths CJ, Ramsden PD, Neal DE. Bladder function in healthy volunteers: ambulatory monitoring and conventional urodynamic studies. *Br J Urol* 1994;73:242–249.
27. van Waalwijk van Doorn ESC, Remmers A, Janknegt RA. Conventional and extramural ambulatory testing of the lower urinary tract in female volunteers. *J Urol* 1992;147:1319–1326.
28. McGuire EJ, Cespedes RD, O'Connel HE. Leak point pressures. *Urol Clin North Am* 1996;23:253–262.
29. Coolsaet BLRA, Van Duyl WA, Van Os-Bossagh P, De Bakker HV. New concepts in relation to urge and detrusor activity. *Neurourol Urodyn* 1993;12:463–471.
30. Cardozo L. Role of estrogens in the treatment of female urinary incontinence. *J Am Geriatr Soc* 1990;38:326–328.
31. Batra S, Bjellin L, Sjögren C, Iosif S, Widmark E. Increases in blood flow of the female rabbit urethra following low dose estrogens. *J Urol* 1986;136:1360–1362.
32. Hofmann R, Gomez R, Schmidt R, Tanagho EA. Effects of nerve stimulation on blood flow in the urinary bladder, urethra and pelvic floor in the dog. *J Urol* 1993;150:1945–1949.
33. Primus G, Kramer G. Maximal external electrical stimulation for treatment of neurogenic or nonneurogenic urgency and/or urge incontinence. *Neurourol Urodyn* 1996;15:187–194.
34. Hasan ST, Robson WA, Pridie AK, Neal DE. Transcutaneous electrical nerve stimulation and temporary S3 neuromodulation in idiopathic detrusor instability. *J Urol* 1996;155: 2005–2011.
35. Nygaard IE, Kreder KJ, Lepic MM, Fountain KA, Rhomberg AT. Efficacy of pelvic floor muscle exercises in women with stress, urge, and mixed urinary incontinence. *Am J Obstet Gynecol* 1996;174:120–125.
36. Levin RM, Hypolite JA, Haugaard N, Wein AJ. Comparative response of rabbit bladder smooth muscle and mucosa to anoxia. *Neurourol Urodyn* 1996;15:79–84.
37. Fleischmann JD, Huntley HN, Shingleton WB, Wentworth DB. Clinical and immunological response to nifedipine for the treatment of interstitial cystitis. *J Urol* 1991;146:1235–1239.
38. Edwards G, Henshaw M, Miller M, Weston AH. Comparison of the effects of several potassium-channel openers on rat bladder and portal vein in vitro. *Br J Pharmacol* 1991;102:679–686.
39. Parsons CL, Housley T, Schmidt JD, Lebow D. Treatment of interstitial cystitis with intravesical heparin. *Br J Urol* 1994;73:504–507.
40. Bade JJ, Laseur M, Nieuwenburg A, van der Weele LT, Mensink HJA. A placebo-controlled study of intravesical pentosanpolysulfate for the treatment of interstitial cystitis. *Br J Urol* 1997;79:168–171.
41. Morales A, Emerson L, Nickel JC, Lundie M. Intravesical hyaluronic acid in treatment of refractory interstitial cystitis. *J Urol* 1996; 156:45–48.
42. Bichler K-H, Strohmaier WL, Nelde HJ, Korn S, Keil R. Glykosaminoglykane. Sub-stanzen mit urothelprotektiver Wirkung. *TW Urologie Nephrologie* 1991;6:350–362.
43. Gillespie L, Said J, Cain W, VanDerVeld R. Antibiotic-induced interstitial cystitis: a model for cell membrane instability. *J Urol* 1985;133: 177A.

44. Cruz F, Guimaraes M, Silva C, Rio MA, Coimbra A, Reis M. Desensitization of bladder sensory fibers by intravesical capsaicin has long lasting clinical and urodynamic effects in patients with hyperactive or hypersensitive bladder dysfunction. *J Urol* 1997;157:585–589.
45. Lloyd SN, Lloyd SM, Rogers K, Deane RF, Kirk D, Kyle KF. Is there still a place for prolonged bladder distension? *Br J Urol* 1992;70:382–386.
46. Sant GR. Interstitial cystitis. *Monogr Urol* 1991;12:37–63.
47. Chelsky MJ, Rosen SI, Knight LC, Maurer AH, Hanno PM, Ruggieri MR. Bladder permeability in interstitial is similar to that of normal volunteers: Direct measurement by transvesical absorption of 99m technetiumdiethylenetriaminepentaacetic acid. *J Urol* 1993;151:346–349.
48. Monson FC, Wein AJ, McKenna BAW, Whithmore K, Levin RM. Indigocarmine as a quantitative indicator of urothelial integrity. *J Urol* 1991;145:842–845.
49. Hohlbrugger G, Strasser H, Colleselli K, Höltl L, Bartsch G. Comparative (normal saline vs. 0.2 M potassium chloride) cystometry in the normal bladder and in females with idiopathic urgency/frequency syndrome. *J Urol* 1997;(Suppl)157: 725(abst).
50. Lilly JD, Parsons CL. Bladder surface glycosaminoglycans: a human epithelial permeability barrier. *Surg Gynecol Obstet* 1990;171:493–497.
51. Hohlbrugger G. Leaky urothelium and/or vesical ischemia enable urinary potassium to cause idiopathic urgency/frequency syndrome and urge incontinence. *Int Urogyn J* 1996;7:242–255.
52. Christmas TJ, Holmes SAV, Hendry WF. Bladder replacement by ileocystoplasty: the final treatment for interstitial cystitis. *Br J Urol* 1996;78:69–73.
53. Frazer MI, Haylen BT, Sissons M. Do women with idiopathic sensory urgency have early interstitial cystitis? *Br J Urol* 1990;66:274–278.
54. Gillenwater JY, Wein AJ. Summary of the NIADDK diseases workshop on interstitial cystitis. *J Urol* 1988;140:203–205.

Interstitial Cystitis, edited by Grannum R. Sant.
Lippincott–Raven Publishers, Philadelphia ©1997.

CHAPTER 11

The Role of Glycosaminoglycans in Normal Bladder Physiology and the Pathophysiology of Interstitial Cystitis

Robert E. Hurst, Johnny B. Roy, and C. Lowell Parsons

The bladder is a specialized organ, well suited to its function of storing and then rapidly expelling urine. The bladder epithelium performs the essential functions of preventing the resorption of solutes from the urine and inhibiting attachment of bacteria or microcrystals (1,2). In the urinary tract, the epithelia are progressively more impermeable, starting with the extremely permeable kidney glomerular membrane and proceeding to the transitional epithelium, which normally is virtually impermeable to all solutes but is permeable to water. In the glomerular membrane, loss of the membrane proteoglycans results in a large increase in permeability (3). The urinary epithelium is specialized, with tight junctions, specialized cell-surface proteins, and ion pumps plus proteoglycans and glycoproteins, all of which function together to maintain the impermeability of the membrane (2,4–8). These same molecules also present an active defense against bacterial colonization.

The bladder lumen is coated with a thick layer of proteoglycan and glycoprotein (glycosaminoglycans, GAGs), and the evidence is strong that this layer plays an important role in antibacterial defenses and bladder impermeability. Because the bladders of interstitial cystitis patients seem to be more permeable than normal (9–11), and because such patients often seem to respond to therapy with exogenous sulfated polysaccharides such as heparin or Elmiron (SP-54) (12–15), the GAG-layer model has emerged. This theory states that the bladder surface proteoglycans play a physiological role in maintaining the impermeability of the bladder epithelium and that a functional deficiency of such proteoglycans is related to the etiology of as many as 60% to 70% of interstitial cystitis cases (11). However, recent physiological studies demonstrating that the membrane itself is highly impermeable to small ions suggests an interactive and interdependent system involving the proteoglycan layer, the lipid bilayer, and the tight junctions and ion pumps.

In this chapter we examine what is known about bladder glycosaminoglycans in the normal and interstitial cystitis bladder, the use of GAGs as therapeutic agents, and the role of GAGs and proteoglycans in bladder physiology.

R. E. Hurst and J. B. Roy: Department of Urology, University of Oklahoma Health Sciences Center, Oklahoma City, Oklahoma 73190.

C. L. Parsons: Division of Urology, Department of Surgery, University of California, San Diego, San Diego, California 92103.

STRUCTURE OF PROTEOGLYCANS AND GLYCOSAMINOGLYCANS

Glycosaminoglycans are linear copolymers formed from alternating hexosaminyl and uronyl residues or, in the case of keratan sulfate, hexosaminyl and galactosyl residues. Glycosaminoglycans are usually found as constituents of proteoglycans rather than as free chains. Proteoglycans are proteins containing one or more covalently bound GAG chains. The protein portion of a proteoglycan is referred to as the core protein. Proteoglycans differ from glycoproteins in the nature of the carbohydrate moieties, which are glycosaminoglycans in the case of proteoglycans and branched oligosaccharides in the case of glycoproteins. A proteoglycan can also be a glycoprotein if it carries oligosaccharides in addition to glycosaminoglycans. A number of excellent reviews of proteoglycan structure and biochemistry have appeared in recent years (16–18).

The GAGs are arbitrarily divided into four families on the basis of structure and function (19): the heparins and

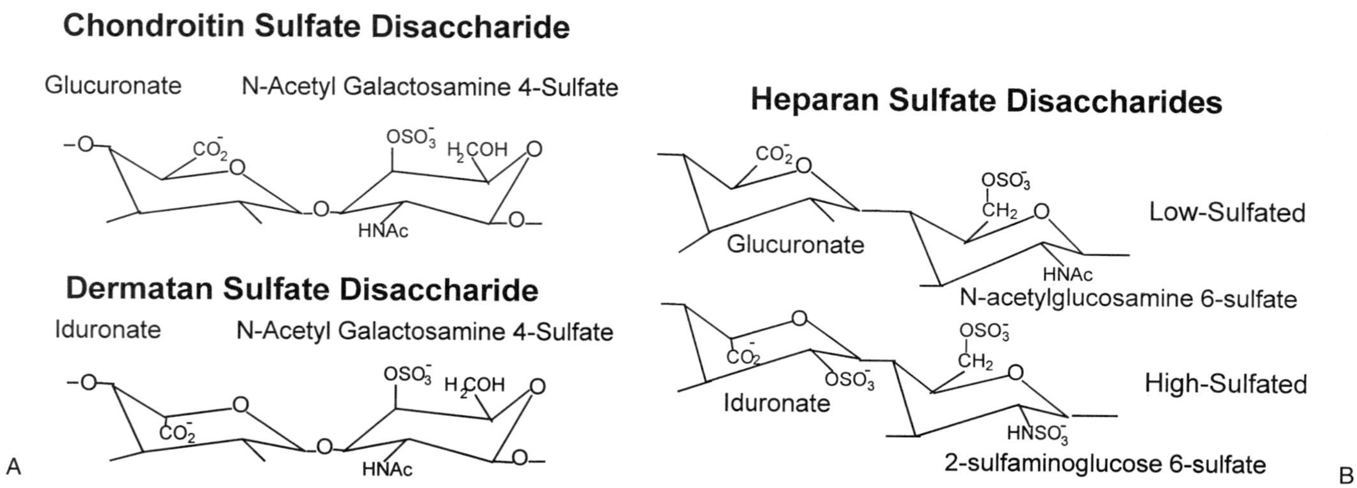

FIG. 1. Structures of major disaccharides comprising glycosaminoglycans. Keratan sulfate and hyaluronate disaccharides are not shown. **(A)** Chondroitin- and dermatan-sulfate-type disaccharides. In addition to those shown, chondroitin sulfate disaccharides can also be 6-sulfated rather than 4-sulfated; 4,6-disulfated residues are occasionally found. Most chondroitin sulfate molecules are composed of predominately 4- or 6-sulfated disaccharides. Dermatan sulfate can also contain 2-sulfoiduronate (up to 15% of residues) and occasional chondroitin-sulfate-type residues. **(B)** Heparin and heparan sulfate disaccharides. N-Acetylglucosamine and glucuronate are always paired, as are N-sulfaminoglucosamine and iduronate. The high-sulfated disaccharides predominate in heparins whereas the low-sulfated type disaccharides predominate in heparan sulfates. Also found are 2-sulfoiduronate and sulfaminoglucosamine 3,6-disulfate, an essential monosaccharide in the antithrombin binding site. Heparan sulfates seem to consist of blocks of high-sulfated and blocks of low-sulfated residues rather than random copolymers.

heparan sulfates, the chondroitin and dermatan sulfates, hyaluronate, and the keratan sulfates. Structures of the major disaccharides found in the first two families are shown in Fig. 1, and Table 1 summarizes the major constituents, glycosidic bonds, and important structural features of the glycosaminoglycans. This chapter concentrates on the first two families because these are found as the constituents of cell-surface proteoglycans, whereas hyaluronate and keratan sulfate are constituents of connective tissue.

Examination of the structures in Fig. 1 reveals several factors of importance in relating structure and function with the chemistry of GAGs. The negative charge of the carboxylate and sulfate moieties confers a strong negative charge on glycosaminoglycans, which tends to dominate the chemistry of these molecules. In general, at the ionic strengths commonly found in tissue, these polymers exist as fairly rigid rods (20). Close examination of Fig. 1 shows that 4- and 6-sulfation place the sulfate on different sides of the molecule, and admixing 4- and 6-sulfation produces discontinuities in charge distribution that may relate to function. An α-L-iduronate and a β-D-glucuronate place the carboxylate on different sides of the molecule as well. Thus, the overall shape of glycosaminoglycans is linear with bulky, highly charged sulfate and carboxylate moieties distributed in a regular pattern over the surface, with the exact geometric details being dependent on the particulars of bonds and sulfation.

The structural chemistry of glycosaminoglycans is much more complex than is usually presented in textbooks, which generally describe the structure of a GAG as being composed of a single repeating disaccharide unit such as the archetypal disaccharides shown in Fig. 1. Nowhere is this complexity more evident than in the heparin–heparan sulfate family. At a structural level, 17 different saccharide components were identified in heparin using gas chromatography/mass spectrometry (21). At a functional level, a pentasaccharide sequence containing an unusual 3-sulfated 2-deoxy-2-sulfaminoglucose (synonymous with sulfaminoglucosamine) is necessary for high activity in enhancing the thrombin–antithrombin reaction of heparin (22), and even small differences in the charge density of heparins results in large differences in activity (23). Recently, as the role of cell-surface heparan sulfates in regulation of cell growth and binding of growth factors has begun to be understood, structural motifs necessary for biological activity have been identified in these molecules (24).

The high charge density of the sulfated glycosaminoglycans is crucial to their function because the strength of many protein–glycosaminoglycan interactions is governed by charge density and distribution. The strength of the interaction between heparin and thrombin is directly related to heparin charge density and governs the enhancement of the thrombin–antithrombin reaction rate by heparin (23,25). Model studies of the interactions of

TABLE 1. *Saccharide constituents and bonds of glycosaminoglycans*

Glycosaminoglycan	Uronate/Hexose	Bond	Hexosamine	Bond
Hyaluronate	β-D-Glucuronate	(1→3)	β-D-N-Acetylglucosamine	(1→4)
Chondroitin sulfate	β-D-Glucuronate	(1→3)	β-D-N-Acetylgalactosamine 4/6-sulfate	(1→4)
Dermatan sulfate	α-L-Iduronate	(1→3)	β-D-N-Acetylgalactosamine 4-sulfate	(1→4)
Keratan sulfate	β-D-Galactose	(1→4)	β-D-N-Acetylglucosamine 6-sulfate	(1→4)
Heparin/heparan sulfate				
High-sulfated	α-L-Iduronate	(1→4)	α-D-N-Sulfoglucosamine 6-sulfate	(1→4)
Low-sulfated	β-D-Glucuronate	(1→4)	α-D-N-Acetylglucosamine 6-sulfate	(1→4)

glycosaminoglycans with organic cations shows that the high charge of the glycosaminoglycan produces an ordering of water molecules (26). In fact, many reactions of glycosaminoglycans are entropy-driven by the ordering and disordering of this water layer (27). Because each charged group can order several water molecules, an individual glycosaminoglycan chain can be hydrated by several hundred water molecules (28), producing a highly hydrophilic environment in the direct vicinity of the glycosaminoglycans.

The biology of proteoglycans is a composite of both the core protein and of the attached GAG chains. Proteoglycans vary in composition from 90% or more GAG by weight, containing a hundred or more glycosaminoglycan chains (cartilage proteoglycan), to those that are predominately protein and may contain only a single glycan chain (18,19,29). The GAG chains are covalently attached to serine residues on the proteoglycan core protein through a specialized linkage oligosaccharide (ser-xyl-gal-gal-glcUA) (19). Digestion of the glycosaminoglycan with special lyases leaves this linkage oligosaccharide as a "stub" with the uronate residue having an unsaturated double bond. This stub produced from chondroitin and dermatan sulfates is antigenic and can be detected by an antibody (30). A corresponding antibody for stubs derived from heparan sulfate chains has not been reported.

Improvements in structural knowledge and immunologic reagents are beginning to support classification by the structure of the core protein, which is replacing classification according to size and the kind of glycosaminoglycan chains (e.g., large chondroitin sulfate proteoglycan). Increasingly, proteoglycans are being named (16–18). The core proteins can vary widely in size, from as small as 11 kDa to well over 300 kDa (16,19). On electrophoresis, proteoglycans tend to migrate as broad bands, which indicates considerable heterogeneity in size and sulfation of the proteoglycan chains.

Fueled by discoveries that proteoglycans play major roles in growth, differentiation, and maintenance of epithelial structure and are major mediators in stromal–epithelial interactions (31), interest in proteoglycans has exploded in recent years. The matrix seems to exist in growth-promoting and differentiation-promoting forms, but the regulation of the matrix seems, in part, to involve events occurring in the epithelium. A biochemical loop between matrix and epithelium, with each affecting the properties of the other, seems to be present. This phenomenon probably underlies tumorigenesis in the genitourinary tract (32).

In regard to epithelial structure, three functional cellular surfaces can be identified—the basal lamina or basement membrane contact surface, the cell–cell contact surface within the epithelium, and the luminal surface, if present. Each of these surfaces may well have its own unique proteoglycan complement related to its distinct role.

Basal lamina or basement membranes underlie all epithelia and endothelia and play an active role in the biology of the overlying cellular layer. Heparan sulfate proteoglycans in basement membrane and extracellular matrix bind and apparently store heparin-binding growth factors, from which they can be released by other heparan sulfate molecules or by heparan-sulfate-degrading enzymes, thereby stimulating growth of the overlying cell layer (33). Syndecan, a large heparan sulfate proteoglycan, mediates interactions with a variety of extracellular matrix molecules such as fibronectin and communicates with the cell interior (34,35). Biglycan, although homologous to another small chondroitin sulfate proteoglycan, decorin, which is found in the extracellular matrix, is a distinct proteoglycan distributed mainly on cell–cell contact surfaces (36). Biglycan is postulated to play a role in maintaining these surfaces and possibly in regulating cell growth in the epithelium.

PROTEOGLYCANS OF THE BLADDER LUMINAL SURFACE

Relatively little is known concerning the proteoglycans of the luminal layer of the bladder, even though they were implicated many years ago as being important to the bladder defenses against bacterial adherence, and more recent evidence has suggested a role in maintaining bladder surface impermeability. The main evidence for a role in antiadherence is from animal model studies by Parsons and colleagues, who have shown not only that treatment of the bladder with dilute acid (10 mM HCl) removes some components of the luminal proteoglycans and glycoproteins and thereby damages the bladder's defenses against bacterial and microcrystal adherence but also that treatment of the damaged bladder with exogenous sulfated polysaccharides such as heparin and pentosanpolysulfate restores the antiadherence activity (2,10,12,14,37,38). Recently, Parsons has shown an increased bladder permeability to urea and potassium ions in some 70% of interstitial cystitis patients, which is relieved in many patients by treatment with exogenous glycosaminoglycan with concomitant symptomatic relief in at least 50% of patients with interstitial cystitis (12–14). Moreover, treatment of the normal bladder with protamine, a substance that binds ionically to glycosaminoglycans, almost instantly produces urgency and pain in normals and causes the bladder to become permeable to urea, both in patients and in animal models; however, treatment with exogenous glycosaminoglycan restores impermeability to urea and alleviates the symptoms (9,10).

Recent studies with a mouse autoimmune cystitis model of interstitial cystitis has shown that permeability changes accompany the development of cystitis (39). A similar increase in the epithelial permeability was found in a guinea pig model in which mast cell activation perturbed the membrane (40). It is therefore possible that, regardless of the cause, permeation of the deeper tissues of the bladder leads to chronic injury, irritation, pain, and degeneration of the bladder musculature and that this mechanism is at least one important pathophysiological basis for interstitial cystitis.

Additional, indirect evidence was derived from clinical studies of the levels of glycosaminoglycan in the urine of normals, interstitial cystitis patients, and spinal cord injury patients (41). The latter were chosen as a positive control in that they are known to have chronic bladder damage. As a group, interstitial cystitis patients excreted half the glycosaminoglycan found in urine of normals. The urine glycosaminoglycan levels of the cord injury patients were only slightly higher than those of the interstitial cystitis patients. If urinary glycosaminoglycan levels are used as a diagnostic marker, a sensitivity of 58% with a specificity of 80% is achieved. The wide distribution of values could reflect heterogeneity in the patient population in that patients with low and high values for glycosaminoglycan excretion could represent either different clinical entities or differences in the metabolism of surface proteoglycans. Based on earlier studies with an animal model (42), the authors speculated that the deficit in glycosaminoglycan levels in a substantial portion of interstitial cystitis patients probably reflects the presence of a damaged urothelium. Microscopic examination of bladder biopsies from 108 interstitial cystitis patients showed a loosely adherent urothelium with frequent patches that have been peeled off, suggesting that fragility of the urothelium from frequent damage is a feature of interstitial cystitis (43). As reviewed above, proteoglycan–matrix interactions are major factors in epithelial structure, and these findings are consistent with a failure or inhibition of proteoglycan synthesis in the urothelium. It should be noted that a recent study of glycosaminoglycan excretion that used different methods concluded that the difference between controls and IC patients was due to differences in urine dilution (44).

Recent work in our laboratories has sought to isolate and characterize the proteoglycans of the luminal surface (45) and to determine whether a demonstrable deficit in luminal proteoglycans could be identified in interstitial cystitis. A method was first developed to specifically extract the luminal layer of proteoglycans using a 1-hr extraction with guanidinium chloride in the presence of protease inhibitors. The extraction was applied to large-scale biochemical isolation and characterization of proteoglycans from the bovine bladder and to small-scale analytic studies of human bladder. Subsequent to the extraction, proteoglycans were partially purified and characterized by separation by DEAE ion exchange and then by size on Sepharose CL-4B column chromatography. Table 2 shows the results. Four proteoglycan species comprised 98% of the total. It is possible that each of these proteoglycans may be heterogeneous because they were identified only on the basis of a distinct peak on Sepharose chromatography. A more complex pattern of chondroitin-sulfate-containing proteoglycans was identified from a mixture of the peaks pooled after Sepharose chromatography. The proteoglycans were partially deglycosylated with chondroitinase ABCase to liberate the antigenic stub. Six separate chondroitin-sulfate-containing proteoglycan core proteins were identified by Western blot analysis after electrophoretic separation (Table 3). Of these, one is clearly a hybrid proteoglycan containing both heparan and chondroitin sulfate chains because its mobility was shifted to 45 kDa by heparitinase digestion. Also of interest is the 29-kDa core protein. The sharpness of the band indicates less charge heterogeneity than the other proteoglycans.

Additional biochemical evidence supporting the importance of luminal surface proteoglycans in bladder defenses and as a factor in interstitial cystitis is the observation of a deficit of chondroitin sulfate proteoglycans on the luminal surface of the interstitial cystitis bladder (46). Immunohistochemical studies using the antistub antibody showed that 14 of 24 (58%) of non-IC controls showed a distinct pink to purple layer indicative of chondroitin sulfate proteoglycans on the bladder surface. In contrast, only five of 31 (16%) unselected interstitial cystitis patients showed positive staining on the surface (p = 0.0001). In addition, seven of 12 (58%) controls and five of 19 (26%) (p = 0.032) showed a distinct layer underlying the urothelium as well. These data provide irrefutable evidence for a deficit of chondroitin sulfate on the bladder surface in interstitial cystitis. Clinical evidence also suggests a leaky epthelium in a high proportion of interstitial cystitis patients. The natural question is how these observations are related.

TABLE 2. *K_{av} and molecular weights of bovine bladder lumen proteoglycans eluted from Sepharose CL-4B[a]*

Peak	K_{av}	MW (kDa)	Relative abundance
1	0.42	380	0.01
2	0.45	240	0.71
3	0.48	190	0.91
4	0.51	135	1.00
5	0.55	85	0.89
6	0.61	42	0.01

[a]K_{av} represents the position of the peak between the void volume and the retained volume. Molecular weights were assessed from K_{av} values of known standard proteins. Relative abundance was calculated with respect to uronate content.

TABLE 3. *Molecular weights of partially deglycosylated core proteins determined by electrophoresis and visualized by Western blotting with "antistub" antibody*

Band	MW (kDa)	Comments
1	>180	
2	84	
3	60	Shifted to 45 kDa after heparitinase treatment
4	45	
5	29	Sharp band
6	27	

That the dense layer of glycosaminoglycan on the bladder surface acts as a permeability barrier by maintaining a bound water layer at the cell surface was first proposed many years ago (2). Recently, however, studies have shown that the lipid bilayer membrane itself is highly impermeable, which has brought into question the concept of the proteoglycans acting as a permeability barrier. In fact, these two sets of observation are probably not in conflict. We present a new hypothesis below to describe the relationship of the proteoglycan layer and membrane permeability.

We first address the question of how much of a water layer the observed density of proteoglycans will produce and then consider whether, if it is diminished in interstitial cystitis, the physical chemical model will provide a reasonable model for reality. The amount of proteoglycan on the bladder surface was directly measured at 16 nmol uronate/cm^2 of bladder surface (44). This density can be converted to a local concentration to use in a physical model by making several assumptions: that the actual surface area is much larger, perhaps by an order of magnitude, and that the depth of this layer is perhaps 10 μm (0.001 cm) (7). Then, (16 nmol/cm^2) × (1/10) × (0.01 cm^{-1}) = 1.6 M. This is an enormous concentration of a charged polysaccharide and will result in a strongly bound water layer (8), which is thermodynamically equivalent to exclusion of other solutes. If the charged species is bound to the membrane surface, it is nondiffusible and therefore formally equivalent to being separated from the bulk solution by a semipermeable membrane. The Donnan membrane equilibrium model can be used to mathematically describe the bladder surface.

If primed values refer to those outside the layer containing the glycosaminoglycan, and unprimed values to those outside the layer, if Z is the charge on the glycosaminoglycan (approximately -2 per uronate residue), and m refers to the molality of a species, with +, -, and G subscripts referring to the positive, negative, and glycosaminoglycan ions, respectively, the concentration of the negative counterion is obtained by solving the quadratic (47):

$$(m_-)^2 - Zm_G(m_-) - (m'_-)^2 = 0$$

If the concentration of negative co-ion, e.g., chloride, is 0.15 m in the bulk solution, then with Z = -2 and m_G = 1.6 as calculated above, the concentration of negative ion and, hence, NaCl within the bound water layer is 0.007 m versus 0.15 m outside the layer. With such a high surface density, solute exclusion is independent of salt concentration. Only when 90% of the total glycosaminoglycan is lost does the solute exclusion effect diminish. With m_G = 0.16, the salt concentrations within the layer would fall to 0.1 m if the bulk concentration were 0.15 m and 0.35 at 0.10 m in the bulk solution. This is consistent with the observation that symptoms are diminished if urine is kept dilute.

However, solute exclusion is an equilibrium property, whereas membrane conductivity measured in Ussing chambers is related to a transport property. It is therefore not clear that the high impermeability of the lipid bilayer membrane itself excludes a role for the glycosaminoglycan layer. In fact, both are likely essential to the proper functioning of the bladder defenses, especially because impairment of cell surface GAG in both rodents and humans increases epithelial permeability *in vitro* (Ussing chamber) and *in vivo,* and this effect can be reversed with exogenous sulfated polysaccharides (9–11). Lewis has also shown that urinary proteases degrade epithelial sodium channels (48), and previous results show that trypsin is excluded from the vicinity of the bladder surface by the enormous density of proteoglycans (42). Moreover, the glycosaminoglycan layer will greatly enhance the functionality of the ion pumps by decreasing or even reversing the concentration gradient of solutes in the region of the membrane. In interstitial cystitis, however, the deficit of proteoglycan upsets this arrangement. The cell membrane is, in effect, in more direct contact with the urine, unbuffered by the proteoglycan layer and unprotected from urinary proteases and other proteins. This lack of exclusion of proteins is graphically seen in the depth of penetration of the GP51 glycoprotein into the urothelium of interstitial cystitis patients (49). Figure 2 illustrates this model of the bladder surface in schematic form.

It is not known whether the membrane itself is also more permeable in interstitial cystitis than is the normal

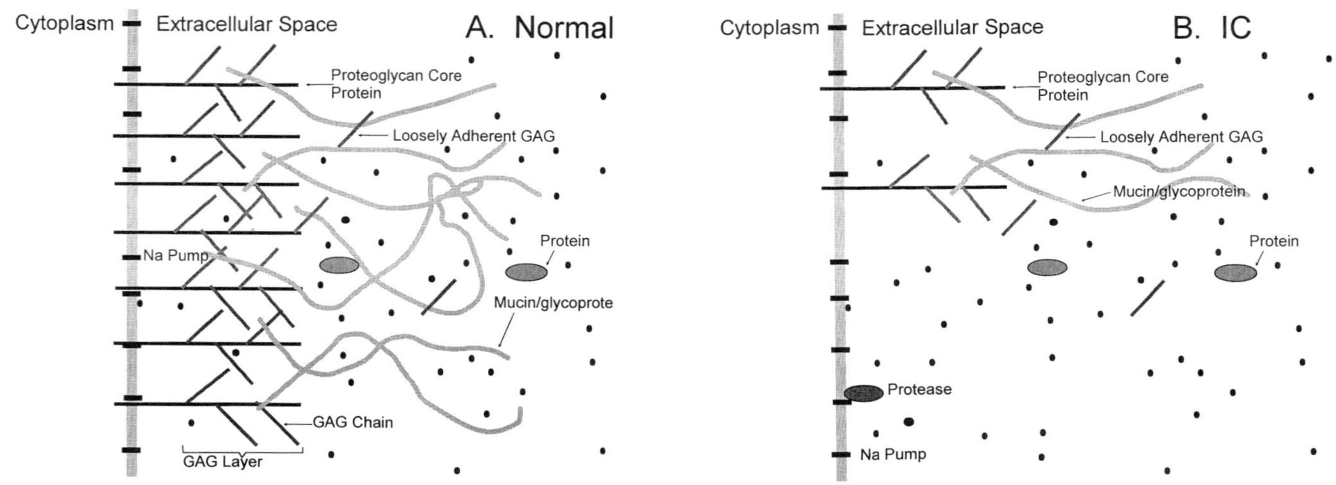

FIG. 2. Schematic structure of bladder surface showing the function of the glycosaminoglycan layer in conjunction with the ion pumps on the bladder surface to maintain bladder surface impermeability. **(A)** The extremely dense layer of proteoglycans serves to exclude most ionic and protein solutes from the bladder surface. Also shown are loosely adherent glycoproteins that probably function in bacterial antiadherence as well as urinary glycosaminoglycans weakly bound to proteins of the bladder surface. **(B)** The absence or deficit of proteoglycan no longer protects the bladder surface. Proteases molecules in the urine attack ion pumps and other surface proteins. The higher concentration of salt also may overwhelm ionic pumps. Urine is toxic to cultured urothelial cells that lack the boundary protection of the glycosaminoglycan layer.

membrane. The possibility definitely exists, particularly because increasing evidence also suggests that the bladder uroepithelium is exhibiting altered differentiation (46,49–51). Such altered differentiation is further indicated by the findings of a deficiency of chondroitin sulfate proteoglycans in the lamina propria, because the differentiation and proliferation of epithelia are controlled by the underlying stroma (44). Proteoglycans, particularly those containing chondroitin sulfate, are major actors in this process (52–56). One possibility is that the alterations at the bladder surface represent alterations in the pattern of gene expression, possibly involving failure to synthesize proteoglycans in normal amounts. If the synthesis of other proteins is altered by the interstitial cystitis process, the bladder surface may well express other deficits in the normal barrier functions.

A number of possibilities exist to explain how such a situation might arise. An acute injury to the urothelium will normally heal rapidly as the basal cells rapidly divide and differentiate. However, this normal healing may not occur. Possibly bacteria become established in the injury and produce substances that prevent reestablishment of the normal differentiation program (57–59). Alternatively, injury to deeper tissues, nerves, muscle, and vascular elements may result from chronic penetration of urinary solutes, producing much the same result (51,60,61). In any event, a chronic injury or irritative situation becomes established, and the normal pattern of urothelial differentiation may not redevelop, with long-lasting consequences for the underlying stroma and muscularis. Long-term treatment with intravesical heparin or Elmiron, either intravesically, orally, or subcutaneously administered, may allow the urothelium to heal by providing an artificial barrier. During the healing phase, muscle, nerves, and the vascular supply may improve as reflected in slowly progressive recovery of patients often seen on chronic heparin therapy (13).

CONCLUSIONS

Several facts suggest a role for bladder surface glycosaminoglycans in normal bladder physiology and in the pathophysiology of interstitial cystitis. These include the high density of proteoglycan actually measured, the deficit in these molecules in interstitial cystitis patients, increased permeability of the bladder, and the positive clinical response of many patients to treatment with exogenous glycosaminoglycan. Physical chemical modeling suggests a mechanism by which the permeability of the bladder surface is maintained through a combination of the exclusion of ionic solutes by the concentrated negative charges of the proteoglycan layer and the impermeability of the bladder surface itself.

Acknowledgments

This work was supported, in part, by the Interstitial Cystitis Database Project from the National Institutes of Health (to J.B.R. and C.L.P.).

REFERENCES

1. Parsons CL, Greenspan C, Moore SW, Mulholland SG. Role of surface mucin in primary antibacterial defense of bladder. *Urology* 1977;9: 48–52.
2. Parsons CL, Stauffer C, Schmidt JD. Bladder-surface glycosaminoglycans: an efficient mechanism of environmental adaptation. *Science* 1980;208:605–607.
3. Kanwar YS, Linker A, Farquahar MG. Increased permeability of the glomerular basement membrane to ferritin after removal of glycosaminoglycans (heparan sulfate) by enzyme digestion. *J Cell Biol* 1980;86:688–693.
4. Hicks MR, Ketterer B, Warren RC. The ultrastructure and chemistry of the luminal plasma membrane of the mammalian urinary bladder: a structure with low permeability to water and ions. *Phil Trans R Soc Lond B* 1974;268:23–38.
5. Jost SP, Gosling JA, Dixon JS. The morphology of normal human bladder urothelium. *J Anat* 1989;167:103–115.
6. Lewis SA, Berg JR, Kleine TJ. Modulation of epithelial permeability by extracellular macromolecules. *Physiol Rev* 1995;75:561–589.
7. Nickel JC, Cornish J. Ultrastructural study of an antibody-stabilized bladder surface: a new perspective on the elusive glycosaminoglycan layer. *World J Urol* 1994;12:11–14.
8. Hurst RE, Zebrowski R, Young JL, Roy JB, Parsons CL. Structure and function of proteoglycans and glycosaminoglycans in bladder epithelium. *J Urol* 1994;152:1641–1645.
9. Lilly JD, Parsons CL. Bladder surface glycosaminoglycans is a human epithelial permeability barrier. *Surg Gynecol Obstet* 1990;171:493–496.
10. Parsons CL, Boychuk D, Jones S, Hurst RE, Callahan H. Bladder surface glycosaminoglycans: an epithelial permeability barrier. *J Urol* 1990;143:139–142.
11. Parsons CL, Stein PC, Bidair M, Lebow D. Abnormal sensitivity to intravesical potassium in interstitial cystitis and radiation cystitis. *Neurourol Urodyn* 1994;13:515–520.
12. Mulholland SG, Hanno P, Parsons CL, Sant GR, Staskin DR. Pentosan polysulfate sodium for therapy of interstitial cystitis. A double-blind placebo-controlled clinical study. *Urology* 1990;35:552–558.
13. Parsons CL, Housley T, Schmidt JD, Lebow D. Treatment of interstitial cystitis with intravesical heparin. *Br J Urol* 1994;73:504–507.
14. Parsons CL, Schmidt JD, Pollen JJ. Successful treatment of interstitial cystitis with sodium pentosanpolysulfate. *J Urol* 1983;130:51–53.
15. Parsons CL. The therapeutic role of sulfated polysaccharides in the urinary bladder. *Urol Clin North Am* 1994;21:93–100.
16. Hassell JR, Kimura JH, Hascall VC. Proteoglycan core protein families. *Annu Rev Biochem* 1986;55:539–567.
17. Ruoslahti E. Structure biology of proteoglycans. *Annu Rev Cell Biol* 1988;4:229–255.
18. Kjellen L, Lindahl U. Proteoglycans: structures and interactions. *Annu Rev Biochem* 1991;60:443–475.
19. Hook M, Kjellen L, Johansson S. Cell-surface glycosaminoglycans. *Annu Rev Biochem* 1984;53:847–869.
20. Tanaka K. Physicochemical properties of chondroitin sulfate. II. Molecular weight dependence of intrinsic viscosity sedimentation coefficient analysis as a semi-flexible coil. *J Biochem* 1978;83:655–659.
21. Barker SA, Hurst RE, Settine J, Fish FP, Settine RL. Structural analysis of heparin by methylation glc-ms: preliminary results. *Carbohydr Res* 1984;125:291–300.
22. Thunberg L, Backstrom G, Lindahl U. Further characterization of the antithrombin-binding sequence in heparin. *Carbohydr Res* 1982;100: 393–410.
23. Hurst RE, Poon MC, Griffith MJ. Structure–activity relationships of heparin. Independence of heparin charge density antithrombin-binding domains in thrombin inhibition by antithrombin heparin cofactor II. *J Clin Invest* 1983;72:1042–1045.
24. Turnbull JE, Gallagher JT. Distribution of iduronate 2-sulphate residues in heparan sulphate. Evidence for an ordered polymeric structure. *Biochem J* 1991;273:553–559.
25. Nordenman B, Bjork I. Influence of ionic strength and pH on the interaction between high-affinity heparin and antithrombin. *Biochim Biophys Acta* 1981;672:227–238.
26. Menter JM, Hurst RE, Nakamura NN, West SS. Thermodynamics of mucopolysaccharide–dye binding. III. Thermodynamics and cooperativity of the acridine orange–heparin system. *Biopolymers* 1979;18: 493–505.
27. Hurst RE. Thermodynamics of the partition of chondroitin sulfate–hexadecylpyridinium complexes in butanol/aqueous salt biphasic solutions. *Biopolymers* 1978;17:2601–2608.
28. Pass G, Phillips GO, Wedlock DJ, Morley RG. Interaction of sulfated polysaccharides with counter-ions. In: Schweiger RG, ed. *Carbohydrate Sulfates*. Washington, DC: American Chemical Society, 1978; 259–281.
29. Iozzo RV. Proteoglycans and neoplasia. *Cancer Metastasis Rev* 1988;7: 39–50.
30. Couchman JR, Caterson B, Christner JE, Baker JR. Mapping by monoclonal antibody detection of glycosaminoglycans in connective tissues. *Nature* 1984;307:650–652.
31. Nathan C, Sporn M. Cytokines in context. *J Cell Biol* 1991;113: 981–986.
32. Rao JY, Hemstreet GP, Hurst RE, Bonner RB, Jones PL, Min KW, Fradet Y. Alterations in phenotypic biochemical markers in bladder epithelium during tumorigenesis. *Proc Natl Acad Sci USA* 1993;90: 8287–8291.
33. Bashkin P, Doctrow S, Klagsbrun M, Svahn CM, Folkman J, Vlodavsky I. Basic fibroblast growth factor binds to subendothelial extracellular matrix and is released by hepatitinase and heparin-like molecules. *Biochemistry* 1989;28:1737–1743.
34. Bernfield M, Kokenyesi R, Kato M, Hinkes MT, Spring J, Gallo RL, Lose EJ. Biology of the syndecans: a family of transmembrane heparan sulfate proteoglycans. *Annu Rev Cell Biol* 1992;8:365–393.
35. Jalkanen M. Biology of cell surface heparan sulfate proteoglycans. *Med Biol* 1987;65:41–47.
36. Bianco P, Fisher LW, Young MF, Termine JD, Robey PG. Expression and localization of the two small proteoglycans biglycan and decorin in developing human skeletal and non-skeletal tissues. *J Histochem Cytochem* 1990;38:1549–1563.
37. Parsons CL. Prevention of urinary tract infection by the exogenous glycosaminoglycan sodium pentosanpolysulfate. *J Urol* 1982;127: 167–169.
38. Parsons CL, Danielson B, Feldstrom B. Inhibition of sodium urate crystal adherence to bladder surface by polysaccharide. *J Urol* 1985;134: 614–616.
39. Bullock AD, Becich MJ, Klutke CG, Ratliff TL. Experimental autoimmune cystitis: A potential murine model for ulcerative interstitial cystitis. *J Urol* 1992;148:1951–1956.
40. Saban R, Christensen M, Keith I, Graziano FM, Undem BJ, Aagaard J, Bjorling DE, Bruskewitz RC. Experimental model for the study of bladder mast cell degranulation and smooth muscle contraction. *Semin Urol* 1991;9:88–101.
41. Hurst RE, Parsons CL, Roy JB, Young JL. Urinary glycosaminoglycan excretion as a laboratory marker in the diagnosis of interstitial cystitis. *J Urol* 1993;149:31–35.
42. Hurst RE, Rhodes SW, Adamson PB, Parsons CL, Roy JB. Functional and structural characteristics of the glycosaminoglycans of the bladder luminal surface. *J Urol* 1987;138:433–437.
43. Johansson SL, Fall M. Pathology of interstitial cystitis. *Urol Clin North Am* 1994;21:55–62.
44. Erickson DR, Ordille S, Martin A, Bhavanandan VP. Urinary chondroitin sulfates, heparan sulfate and total sulfated glycosaminoglycans in interstitial cystitis. *Urology* 1997;157:61–64.
45. Hurst RE, Zebrowski R. Identification of proteoglycans present at high density on bovine and human bladder luminal surface. *J Urol* 1994; 152(Part 1):1641–1645.
46. Hurst RE, Roy JB, Min KW, Veltri RW, Marley G, Patton K, et al. Deficit of chondroitin sulfate proteoglycans on the bladder uroepithelium in interstitial cystitis. *J Urol* 1996;48:817–821.
47. Tanford C. *Physical Chemistry of Macromolecules*. New York: John Wiley & Sons, 1961.
48. Lewis SA, Clausen C. Urinary proteases degrade epithelial sodium channels. *J Membr Biol* 1991;122:77–88.
49. Moskowitz MO, Byrne DS, Callahan HJ, Parsons CL, Valderrama E, Moldwin RM. Decreased expression of a glycoprotein component of bladder surface mucin (GP1) in interstitial cystitis. *J Urol* 1994;151: 343–345.
50. Liebert M, Wedemeyer G, Stein JA, Washington R Jr, Faerber G, Flint A, Grossman HB. Evidence for urothelial cell activation in interstitial cystitis. *J Urol* 1993;149:470–475.
51. Elgavish A. Effects of *Escherichia coli* and *E. coli* lipopolysaccharides on the function of human ureteral epithelial cells cultured in serum-free medium. *Infect Immun* 1993;61:3304–3312.

52. Santra M, Skorski T, Calabretta B, Lattime EC, Iozzo RV. *De novo* decorin gene expression suppresses the malignant phenotype in human colon cancer cells. *Proc Natl Acad Sci USA* 1995;92: 7016–7020.
53. Iozzo RV, Cohen IR, Grässel S, Murdoch AD. The biology of perlecan: The multifaceted heparan sulphate proteoglycan of basement membranes and pericellular matrices. *Biochem J* 1994;302:625–639.
54. Milstone LM, Hough-Monroe L, Kugelman LC, Bender JR, Haggerty JC. Epican a heparan/chondroitin sulfate proteoglycan form of CD44, mediates cell–cell adhesion. *J Cell Sci* 1994;107:3183–3190.
55. Yamagata M, Kimata K. Repression of a malignant cell–substratum adhesion phenotype by inhibiting the production of the anti-adhesive proteoglycan, PG-M/versican. *J Cell Sci* 1994;107:2581–2590.
56. Bernfield M, Hinkes MT, Gallo RL. Developmental expression of the syndecans: Possible function and regulation. *Development* 1993;119 (Suppl):205–212.
57. Theoharides TC, Sant GR, El-Mansoury M, Letourneau R, Ucci AA Jr, Meares EM Jr. Activation of bladder mast cells in interstitial cystitis: A light and electron microscopic study. *J Urol* 1995;153:629–636.
58. Theoharides TC, Sant GR. Bladder mast cell activation in interstitial cystitis. *Semin Urol* 1991;9:74–87.
59. Sant GR, Theoharides TC. The role of the mast cell in interstitial cystitis. *Urol Clin North Am* 1994;21:41–53.
60. Elgavish A, Pattanaik A, Lloyd K, Reed R. Integrin-mediated adhesive properties of uroepithelial cells are inhibited by treatment with bacterial toxins. *Am J Physiol* 1994;266:C1552–C1559.
61. Domingue GJ, Ghoniem GM, Bost KL, Fermin C, Human LG. Dormant microbes in interstitial cystitis. *J Urol* 1995;153:1321–1326.

Interstitial Cystitis, edited by Grannum R. Sant.
Lippincott–Raven Publishers, Philadelphia ©1997.

CHAPTER 12

The Mast Cell as a Neuroimmunoendocrine Effector in Interstitial Cystitis

Theoharis C. Theoharides and Grannum R. Sant

Interstitial cystitis (IC) is a sterile bladder condition characterized by severe urinary urgency, frequency, nocturia, suprapubic pain and pressure, and dyspareunia (1,2). Diagnostic criteria recommended by the U.S. National Institutes of Health (NIH) include negative urine cultures, cystoscopic finding of ulcers or petechial mucosal hemorrhages (glomerulations) on bladder distention under anesthesia (general/spinal), and the absence of transitional carcinoma (2–4). There are an estimated 500,000 IC cases in the United States, 90% of whom are women (3,5), and fewer than 10% of whom are minority women (6).

Hunner's ulcers occur in fewer than 10% of IC patients, and the remainder have milder changes including mucosal breaks and suburothelial hemorrhages (7,8). The pathologic features of chronic IC include edema and vasodilation of the submucosa and detrusor layers of the bladder wall. Unlike earlier reports, there is little if any inflammatory infiltrate except in patients with classic IC characterized by Hunner's ulcers (9,10). Interestingly, the degree of cystoscopic and pathologic findings does not parallel the severity of symptoms (3,7).

The etiology of IC is multifactorial, and IC is better clarified as a clinical syndrome than as a specific disease. Etiologies include autoimmunity, infection, genetic, neurogenic, and hormonal factors as well as the effect of toxic substances in the urine (3,4,11–13). A significant number of premenopausal women with IC report perimenstrual worsening of their symptoms (1) suggestive of pelvic inflammatory disease or endometriosis, leading to unnecessary laparoscopy and hysterectomies (14,15).

T. C. Theoharides: Department of Pharmacology and Experimental Therapeutics, Tufts University School of Medicine and New England Medical Center, Boston, Massachusetts 02111.

G. R. Sant: Department of Urology, Tufts University School of Medicine and New England Medical Center, Boston, Massachusetts 02111.

Patients with IC experience a higher incidence of allergies, irritable bowel syndrome (IBS), fibromyalgia, migraines, chronic fatigue syndrome, and certain autoimmune diseases (Table 1) (15).

The two most prevalent etiologic theories of IC are that of a defect in bladder cytoprotection (16) and a pathophysiologic role for the mast cell (17), first suggested by Simmons (18). The bladder epithelium in IC has been thought to have defective surface glycosaminoglycans (GAGs) and increased permeability (19,20), even though the latter has recently been challenged (21). Nevertheless, such changes could allow potential mast cell secretagogues to penetrate the normally impermeable bladder lining and activate bladder mast cells (17,22). The factors responsible for the migration and proliferation of the mast cells in IC are unknown, even though stem cell factor (SCF, c-kit ligand) and cytokines (e.g. IL-3, IL-9) released by damaged urothelial cells have been implicated (23).

A number of neuroimmunoendocrine conditions occur more frequently in women than men (Table 2), including

TABLE 1. *Coexistence of IC and Other Syndromes*

Condition	Incidence[a] (approximate percentage of patients)
Allergies (drugs, food etc.)	50–60
Irritable bowel syndrome (IBS)	40
Migraines	20
Chronic fatigue syndrome	10–20
Endometriosis	10
Fibromyalgia	10–20
Autoimmune disorders (MS, SLE)[b]	5

[a]Much higher percentages have been reported in tertiary medical centers.
[b]MS, multiple sclerosis; SLE, systemic lupus erythematosus.

TABLE 2. *Neuroimmunoendocrine syndromes with mast cell activation or proliferation*

Condition	Female/male ratio
Interstitial cystitis (IC)	10:1
Irritable bowel syndrome (IBS)	6:1
Migraines	3:1
Multiple sclerosis	2:1
Systemic sclerosis	2:1
Neurofibromatosis	2:1

TABLE 3. *Triggers of mast cell secretion*

Anaphylatoxins (C3a and C5a)
Bacteria (adherent *E. coli*)
Chemicals (detergents; food additives/preservatives; xenoestrogens)
Contrast media used in radiology
Cytokines (IL-1, IL-2, IL-4, TNF-α)
Drugs (local anesthetics; neuromuscular junction blockers; opioids)
Free radicals
Hormones (adrenocorticotropic hormone, ACTH; corticotropin releasing hormone, CRH; estradiol; parathormone)
IgE and antigen
Neuropeptides (bradykinin; calcitonin gene-related peptide, CGRP; myelin basic protein, MBP; neurotensin, NT; somatostatin, SRIF; substance P, SP; vasoactive intestinal peptide, VIP)
Neurotransmitters (acetylcholine)
Physical conditions (cold; exercise; pressure)
Radiation
Toxins (bacterial; insect; jellyfish; plants; seafood)
Viruses (measles, parainfluenza, Sendai)

IC, irritable bowel syndrome (IBS), migraines, multiple sclerosis, scleroderma, and neurofibromatosis (24). A possible underlying feature of these syndromes is an increase in numbers and/or activation of a unique immunocyte, the mast cell. Activated mast cells release various cytokines and are known to participate in many neuroinflammatory disorders (25–27).

MAST CELL BIOLOGY

Mast cells were first recognized by Friedrich von Recklinghausen in 1863, were stained by Paul Erhlich using toluidine blue in 1887, and were later shown to participate in allergic reactions (28). Mast cells originate from the bone marrow as undifferentiated cells that enter the tissues and mature under the influence of microenvironmental factors such as stem cell factor (SCF or c-kit ligand) and interleukins (28). There are at least two mast cell subtypes that differ in their histochemical properties, type of granule-associated proteoglycans, neutral proteases, and cytokines as well as in their morphology, sensitivity to secretagogues, and susceptibility to inhibitory drugs: (a) the typical, connective tissue mast cell (CTMC), present in the skin and lungs, and (b) the atypical mucosal mast cell (MMC), found mostly in the bladder and the gastrointestinal tract (28,29). Human mast cell heterogeneity has also been demonstrated in other organs (30).

The MMC are susceptible to aldehyde fixation and are best fixed in isosmotic formaldehyde/acetic acid solution (IFAA; 0.6% formaldehyde, 0.5% glacial acetic acid) (31). The classic techniques for recognizing mast cells are histochemical staining with acidified toluidine blue or alcian blue counterstained with safranin (31). Toluidine blue binds to the negatively charged heparin located in CTMC secretory granules and changes its color from blue to violet, a process called metachromasia. However, MMCs contain sulfated proteoglycans other than heparin that do not show metachromasia. Alcian blue and safranin stain CTMC red and MMC light blue. Neither technique reliably identifies degranulated mast cells. Proper fixation is also critical for retaining mast cell ultrastructure for electron microscopy, and Karnovsky's fixative with the addition of tannic acid gives excellent results (32).

Mast cells are mandatory for the development of type I hypersensitivity in which immunoglobulin E (IgE) attaches to specific surface binding proteins (FcεRI) on mast cells and triggers a cascade of reactions that lead to compound exocytosis or degranulation (33,34). Fusion of the perigranular membrane with the plasma membrane results in the secretion of numerous biologically active molecules. In addition to IgE and antigen, other triggers of mast cell secretion (35) include anaphylatoxins, cytokines, lectins, drugs, radiation, various toxins, viruses, and certain adherent strains of *E. coli* (36), which also induce mast cell phagocytosis (37) (Table 3). Mast cells can also be triggered by kinins (38), the neuropeptides neurotensin (NT), somatostatin (SRIF), and substance P (SP) (39,40), and the neurotransmitter acetylcholine (ACh) (32). Mast cell mediators may be granule-stored, preformed molecules such as heparin, histamine, proteases, phospholipases, chemotactic substances, and cytokines, or synthesized *de novo,* e.g., leukotrienes, prostaglandins (PGD), platelet-activating factor (PAF), and nitric oxide (NO) (41,42). Mast cells also release the potent vasodilators vasoactive intestinal peptide (VIP) and tumor necrosis factor (TNF) (42,43). Mast cell products have a variety of effects that are relevant to the clinical and pathologic findings in IC (Table 4).

MAST CELL ACTIVATION IN IC

A number of studies have demonstrated increased numbers of mast cells in the bladders of patients with IC (17,22,44–46). Mast cells have been recovered in the bladder washings from patients with classic IC (46), and it was proposed that >30 mast cells/mm^3 in the detrusor muscle could serve as a diagnostic criterion for IC (44). Conflicting reports in the literature indicate that mast cells are not uniformly increased in IC in the lamina pro-

TABLE 4. *Mast cell mediators*

Mediators	Possible effects in IC
Prestored	
Arylsulfatases	Lipid/proteoglycan hydrolysis
Chemotactic factors	Infiltration of leukocytes
Chymase	Tissue damage, pain
Cytokines (IL-1, -2, -3, -4, -5, -6, GM-CSF, interferon-γ, MIF, TNF-α)[a]	Tissue damage, leukocyte migration, pain
Heparin (CTMC), protean sulfate (MMC)	Angiogenesis, nerve growth factor stabilization
Histamine	Vasodilation, angiogenesis, mitogenesis, pain
5-Hydroxytryptamine (5-HT, serotonin)	Vasoconstriction, pain
Kinins (bradykinin)	Vasodilation, pain
Kinogenases	Synthesis of vasodilatory kinins, pain
Tryptase	Tissue damage, pain
Vasoactive intestinal peptide (VIP)	Vasodilation
De novo synthesized	
Leukotriene B_4	Leukocyte chemotaxis
Leukotriene C_4	Vasoconstriction, pain
Nitric oxide	Vasodilation
Platelet-activating factor (PAF)	Platelet activation; serotonin release
Prostaglandin D_2	Vasodilation, pain

[a]GM-CSF, granulocyte/monocyte colony-stimulating factor; MIF, macrophage inflammatory factor; TNF, tumor necrosis factor.

pria (LP), the detrusor layer, or both (2,4,47–50). The large standard deviations in the reported studies suggest that there may be subgroups of patients in whom bladder mastocytosis is more prevalent. The high number of bladder mast cells found in transitional carcinoma (51) may contribute to the high number of MC sometimes observed in "control" groups of patients (2).

Nevertheless, mast cells in nonulcer IC were shown to be highly activated by both ultrastructural criteria (4,51) and increased levels of urinary methylhistamine (52) and tryptase (53), a unique mast cell product. The increase in bladder mast cells in IC was recently related to possible high local levels of corticotropin-releasing factor (CRF) (23). Bladder mast cells secrete more in response both to ACh and to IgE and antigen and SP (17). Thus, it appears that the mast cell has a pathogenetic role in at least a subset of patients with interstitial cystitis (54,55).

ULTRASTRUCTURAL APPEARANCE OF MAST CELLS

Electron microscopic examination of bladder mast cells from control patients showed that over 70% to 80% contained numerous homogeneous, intact, electron-dense granules (Fig. 1, upper panel). In contrast, fewer than 30% of the granules in mast cells from IC patients were intact: some were entirely empty or contained electron-dense contents at different stages of dissolution (51,56) (Fig. 1, lower panel), indicating granule release of their contents.

The secretory granules of bladder mast cells in IC contain altered contents or appear empty, unlike the massive degranulation seen in allergic or anaphylactic conditions (17,56). Mast cell secretion in IC appears to be slow and gradual with differential (possible selective) release of secretory mediators, a process shown to involve secretion without compound exocytosis (57,58). Secretion without degranulation as observed in IC patients (51) has been termed "piecemeal degranulation" or "intragranular activation" (59,60). Mast cells that have totally released their granular contents do not stain with routine histochemistry, thus leading to an erroneously low number of appar-

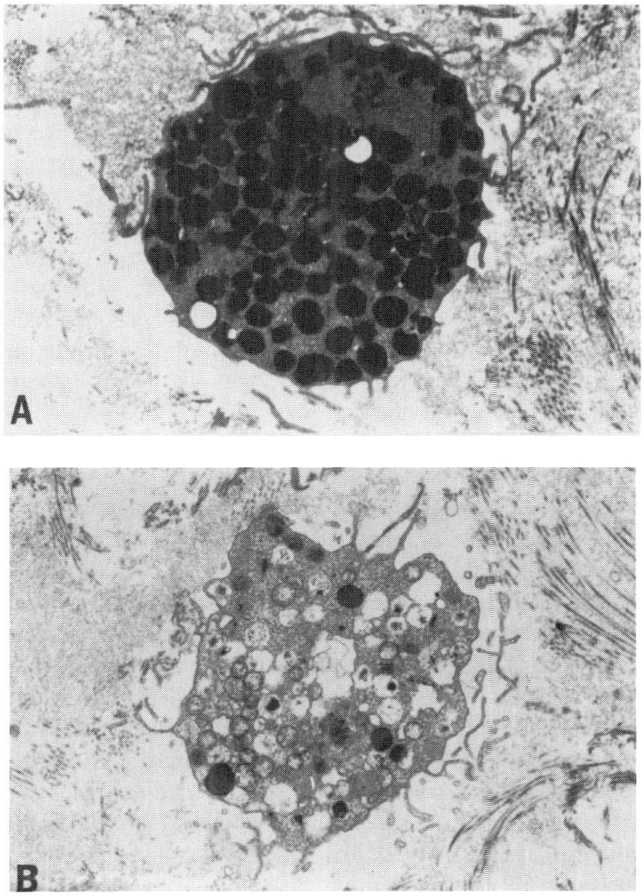

FIG. 1. Ultrastructural appearance of human bladder mast cells. **(A)** Mast cell from control patient with numerous round, homogeneous, and intact electron-dense secretory granules. Magnification ×12,500. **(B)** Mast cell from a patient with IC in which most of the secretory granules have swollen and appear to have a clear ring at their periphery; other granules contain granular material in a state of dissolution, and still others are entirely empty, indicating secretion. Magnification

TABLE 5. *Bladder mastocytosis and activation in IC*[a]

Condition	Mean mast cell count (no./mm^2)	Activation[b] (% total)	Patients with ↑ mast cells (% total)
Control (10)	10	15	—
Transitional cell CA (9)	40	20	100
Interstitial cystitis (20)	35	80	65

[a]In mucosa and submucosa; detrusor was not examined.
[b]Defined by electron microscopy as electron-dense content alteration in >10% of secretory granules.

ent mast cells unless electron microscopy or measurement of urine mast cell mediators is used concurrently. This problem has been described in mast cells associated with scleroderma, i.e., "phantom" mast cells (61). In patients with bladder carcinoma, electron microscopy identified an increased number of mast cells, but 80% of these were normal with intact electron-dense granules (51). In contrast, IC patients also had increased mast cells, of which 80% were activated (17,51) (Table 5).

MAST CELL–NEURON INTERACTIONS

Functional interactions have been proposed between mast cells and neurons in the central (24) and peripheral (62,63) nervous systems. Mast cell–neuronal association is currently being invoked in the pathophysiology of certain inflammatory diseases (64–66). Electron microscopic studies have shown mast cells to be intimately related to sensory nerve fibers containing neuropeptides (60,67,68). Moreover, direct nerve stimulation results in mast cell activation (69), and endogenous histamine can stimulate peripheral nerves (70).

A proliferation of sympathetic bladder nerve fibers containing neuropeptide Y and calcitonin gene-related peptide has been noted in IC (71,72). Substance-P-containing nerve fibers adjacent to mast cells are increased in the bladder submucosa of IC patients (73), and a close anatomic relationship between bladder neurons and mast cells has been demonstrated by electron microscopy (56,60), as had been previously shown in Crohn's disease (74). Rat bladder mast cells can be activated *in vitro* by the neurotransmitters ACh and SP (17), molecules known to stimulate hypothalamic mast cells *in vitro* (75). Bladder distention reduces IC symptoms and depletes SP-positive nerves in the rat urinary bladder (76), whereas intravesical capsaicin, which acutely stimulates neuronal release of SP, relieves pain in patients with hypersensitive bladder disorders (77).

The fact that 60% of IC patients report that their symptoms are exacerbated by stress (15) is interesting because immobilization stress results in rat bladder (78) and intestinal (79) mast cell activation. Mast cells have been reported close to increased numbers of SP fibers in the colon and the bladder of a patient with both IC and irritable bowel syndrome (IBS) (80). The latter is exacerbated by stress and occurs in almost 40% of IC patients (24). Mast cells are also increased in the terminal ileum of patients with IBS (81). IBS is in many ways similar to IC in that it occurs more often in women, is characterized by abdominal pain, and is associated with urinary frequency, dyspareunia, and fatigue (82). Not only are symptoms of IBS clearly exacerbated by stress, but patients with IBS show hypersensitivity selectively to visceral but not somatic stimuli, a process that is also selectively activated by the sympathetic nervous system (83). Stress is known to affect the development of inflammation, and the contribution of the nervous system to the regulation of immune and inflammatory processes is now accepted (84,85), possibly through corticotropin-releasing hormone (CRH), which has peripheral proinflammatory actions, including mast cell activation (86).

FEMALE SEX HORMONES AND MAST CELLS

Many premenopausal IC patients report symptom exacerbations perimenstrually or at the time of ovulation. This frequently leads to gynecologic evaluation and diagnosis of endometriosis, etc.

Estradiol augments rat peritoneal mast cell histamine secretion *in vivo* (87) and that triggered by SP *in vitro* (88) as well as bladder mast cell secretion *in situ*. Bladder mast cells in IC have increased expression of high-affinity estrogen receptors (89) but only few progesterone receptors. Furthermore, estrogens induce proliferation of bladder mast cells in guinea pigs (90). These findings support the role of the female sex hormones in the regulation of the immune processes (91,92). Furthermore, the changing hormone levels may explain why the prevalence of autoimmune disorders changes in adolescence from a male to female predominance (93) and why allergic problems worsen in association with the menstrual cycle (94).

TABLE 6. *Neuroimmunoendocrine findings in IC*

Emotional or physical stressors worsen IC symptoms
Psychological stress activates bladder mast cells
Estrogens induce CRH release[a]
Bladder mast cells are estrogen-receptor positive
Acetylcholine stimulates bladder mast cell activation
Proliferation of SP-positive bladder nerve endings
Substance P stimulates bladder mast cell activation
Neural activation of mast cells is augmented by estrogens

[a]CRH, corticotropin-releasing hormone.

The effects of the female sex hormones on mast cells may explain the high incidence of IC in women and the worsening of IC symptoms perimenstrually (95). The latter group of patients may benefit from treatment with the antiestrogen tamoxifen or gonadotropin-releasing hormone (GnRH) agonists (e.g., lupron). Thus, IC has many of the characteristics of a neuroimmunoendocrine disorder (Table 6).

POSSIBLE DIAGNOSIS OF IC

Some of the symptoms and cystoscopic findings in IC may be caused by the release of vasodilatory, proinflammatory (Table 4), and nociceptive (Table 7) mast cell mediators, especially TNF and tryptase, which could cause direct tissue damage and pain (96). Skin epithelium participates in immune reactions by releasing cytokines on stimulation or injury (97). A similar mechanism may be present in IC whereby damaged urothelial cells produce cytokines (IL-1, IL-8) that then stimulate and activate tissue mast cells. Even though elevated histamine was demonstrated in bladders of IC patients (22,49), there was no difference in the histamine content of either spot or 24-hr urine between control and IC patients; histamine, however, was elevated in IC following bladder hydrodistention (98). Moreover, the urinary excretion of the major histamine metabolite 1,4-methylimidazoleacetic acid (1,4-MIAA) was elevated in IC patients with detrusor mastocytosis (99), and methylhistamine was also significantly elevated in 24-hr urine of IC patients (52). Likewise, the unique mast cell marker tryptase was also elevated (53).

Other immune molecules are not increased in the urine of IC patients, e.g., urine prostaglandin E_2 (PGE_2) measured by radioimmunoassay (49). In another study of "nonulcer" IC, neither PGE_2, PGD_2, PGF_2, thromboxane B_2, nor TNF was significantly different between IC patients and controls (100). A small increase of interleukin-6 has been reported in IC patients (100), and IL-6 is known to be secreted from mast cells (42).

Eosinophils are increased in IC patients with detrusor mastocytosis, and this increase is paralleled by elevated levels of ECP in urine (101), which are reduced by subcutaneous heparin administration (102). Heparin has been reported to inhibit mast cell secretion, and mast cells secrete an eosinophilic chemotactic factor that mobilizes eosinophils to the site of inflammation (96). Eosinophils, in turn, secrete eosinophil cationic protein (ECP), major basic protein (MBP), and eosinophil-derived neurotoxin, which are known to activate mast cells (35).

TABLE 7. *Nociceptive mast cell mediators*

ATP
Chymase
Histamine
Interleukins
Kinins
Leukotrienes
Prostaglandins
Serotonin
Substance P
TNF-α
Tryptase
VIP

MAST CELL INHIBITORS FOR TREATMENT

No therapy is uniformly successful in IC (3). Partial remissions are achieved with pentosanpolysulfate (103), heparin (104), and intravesical dimethylsulfoxide (DMSO) (105). Dimethylsulfoxide is sometimes associated with an initial worsening of symptoms, which could result from the fact that the 50% concentration used clinically may increase mast cell secretion (106). A similar explanation may hold true for the initial symptom exacerbation following hydrodistention, which results in histamine release (98), possibly via osmotic lysis of bladder mast cells.

The tricyclic antidepressant amitriptyline reduces the symptoms of IC in about 30% of patients (107), an action that may be caused by its ability to inhibit histamine secretion from mast cells (57). Unfortunately, a considerable number of patients do not tolerate amitriptyline because of sedation and weight gain. Another tricyclic antidepressant, doxepin, may be beneficial in these patients (1). The antiallergic mast cell "stabilizer" drug disodium cromoglycate (cromolyn) had been tried in chemical cystitis, and pretreatment appeared to reduce the inflammatory response. Unfortunately, intravesical cromolyn was recently shown to have no significant results in IC (108), probably because it is not very soluble and does not inhibit MMC (109).

Antihistamines (H_1-receptor blockers), first used by Simmons to treat IC, are not effective, and their sedative side effects further limit their use (18). The heterocyclic piperazine H_1-receptor antagonist hydroxyzine was reported to have considerable benefit when given at 75 mg/day for more than 3 months (110,111). This effect is attributed to its ability to block neurogenic stimulation of bladder mast cells in addition to its anticholinergic, anxiolytic, and sedative properties. The beneficial effect of hydroxyzine is more pronounced in IC patients with a history of allergies, increased numbers of bladder mast cells, or elevated urine levels of mast cell mediators.

It is particularly difficult for IC patients, as well as their physicians, to deal with IC and other coexisting syndromes. This problem is compounded by the fact that drugs likely to be administered could have unwanted effects on IC or other accompanying symptoms. Table 8 summarizes the effects of commonly used drugs for IC with respect to their ability to inhibit or block mast cell secretion.

TABLE 8. *Drugs used for the treatment of interstitial cystitis*

Drug	Effect on bladder mast cell secretion
Amitriptyline	↓[a]
Dimethyl sulfoxide	±
Doxepin	↓
Elmiron (pentosanpolysulfate)	±
Gastrochrome (cromolyn)	→
Heparin	↓
Hydroxyzine	↓
Nalmefene	±
Nifedipine	±

[a]↑, increased; ↓, decreased; →, no change; ±, variable.

SUMMARY

Interstitial cystitis (IC) is a sterile bladder inflammatory condition that occurs primarily in women and is characterized by irritative voiding symptoms and pain. It is a syndrome of multifactorial etiology. However, the predominant pathogenetic mechanisms appear to be an altered bladder lining and increased number of activated bladder mast cells.

A defective bladder glycosaminoglycan (GAG) layer could allow mast cell secretagogues to penetrate and activate bladder mast cells with release and secretion of numerous vasoactive, nociceptive, and proinflammatory molecules in response to allergic triggers, drugs, neuropeptides, stress, trauma, toxins, and adherent bacteria. These molecules, in turn, can sensitize sensory bladder neurons, which can further activate mast cells by releasing neurotransmitters or neuropeptides. Additionally, the mast cell can directly cause tissue damage and attract immune cells, thus participating in neurogenic vasodilation and immune cell infiltration.

The fact that IC symptoms are exacerbated during various phases of the female menstrual cycle and stress further implicate mast cells, the activation of which is augmented by estrogens and by nontraumatic restraint stress in rats. Urine methylhistamine and tryptase levels are elevated in IC, and this could be utilized as a possible diagnostic tool in conjunction with cystoscopy, biopsy, etc.

Interstitial cystitis is a syndrome with neural, immune, and endocrine components, and activated mast cells may play a central role in its pathogenesis. Treatment options should focus on underlying causes by the combined use of bladder surface protectors and mast cell degranulation blockers. The two major theories of causation in IC—a GAG deficiency and bladder mast cell activation—may well operate in concert to cause bladder inflammation and the symptoms of IC. An individual IC patient may be exposed to multiple mast cell triggers with release of various mast cell moderators. Specific mast cell mediators and their inhibitors should be evaluated in an effort to improve the pharmacologic treatment of interstitial cystitis.

Acknowledgments

This work was supported in part by grants DK42409 and DK44816 from the U.S. National Institutes of Health and a pilot grant from the Interstitial Cystitis Association. Thanks are due to Ms. Linda Tamulaites and Ms. Susan Mayo for their word-processing skills.

REFERENCES

1. Sant GR. Interstitial cystitis. *Monogr Urol* 1991;12:37–63.
2. Hanno PM, Levin RM, Monson FC, et al. Diagnosis of interstitial cystitis. *J Urol* 1990;143:278–281.
3. Sant GR. Inflammatory diseases of the bladder. In: Gillenwater J, Grayhack J, Howards S, Duckett J, eds. *Adult and Pediatric Urology*, 3rd ed. St Louis: CV Mosby, 1995;1327–1354.
4. Thompson AC, Christmas TJ. Interstitial cystitis—an update. *Br J Urol* 1996;78:813–820.
5. Held PJ, Hanno PM, Wein AJ, et al. Epidemiology of interstitial cystitis: In: Hanno PM, Staskin DR, Krane RJ, Wein AJ, eds. *Interstitial Cystitis*. London: Springer-Verlag, 1990;29–48.
6. Sant GR. Interstitial cystitis in minority women. *J Assoc Acad Minority Physicians* 1993;4:89–92.
7. Messing EM, Stamey TA. Interstitial cystitis: early diagnosis, pathology and treatment. *Urology* 1978;12:381–392.
8. Parivar F, Bradbrook RA. Interstitial cystitis. *Br J Urol* 1986;58: 239–244.
9. Johansson SL, Fall M. Clinical features and spectrum of light microscopic changes in interstitial cystitis. *J Urol* 1990;143:1118–1124.
10. Elbadawi A, Light JK: Distinctive ultrastructural pathology of nonulcerative interstitial cystitis. *Urol Int* 1996;56:137–162.
11. Mattila J. Vascular immunopathology in interstitial cystitis. *Clin Immunol Immunopathol* 1982;23:648–655.
12. Bullock AD, Becich MJ, Klutke CG, Ratliff TL. Experimental autoimmune cystitis: a potential murine model for ulcerative interstitial cystitis. *J Urol* 1992;148:1951–1956.
13. Fall M, Johansson SL, Aldenborg F. Chronic interstitial cystitis: a heterogenous syndrome. *J Urol* 1987;137:35–38.
14. Ratner V, Slade D, Whitmore KE. Interstitial cystitis: A bladder disease finds legitimacy. *J Women's Health* 1992;1:63–68.
15. Koziol JA, Clark DC, Gittes RF, Tan EM. The natural history of interstitial cystitis: a survey of 374 patients. *J Urol* 1993;149: 465–469.
16. Parsons CL, Stauffer C, Schmidt JD. Bladder-surface glycosaminoglycans: an efficient mechanism of environmental adaptation. *Science* 1980;208:605–607.
17. Sant GR, Theoharides TC. The role of the mast cell in interstitial cystitis. *Urol Clin North Am* 1994;21:41–53.
18. Simmons JL, Bunce PL. On the use of an antihistamine in the treatment of interstitial cystitis. *Am Surg* 1958;24:664–667.
19. Hurst RE, Parsons CL, Roy JB, Young JL. Urinary glycosaminoglycan execution as a laboratory marker in the diagnosis of interstitial cystitis. *J Urol* 1993;149:31–35.
20. Parsons CL, Stein PC, Bidair M, Lebow D. Abnormal sensitivity to intravesical potassium in interstitial cystitis and radiation cystitis. *Neurourol Urodyn* 1994;13:515–520.
21. Erickson DR, Ordille S, Martin A, Bhavanandan VP. Urinary chondroitin sulfates, heparin sulfate and total sulfated glycosaminoglycans in interstitial cystitis. *J Urol* 1997;157:61–64.
22. Kastrup J, Hald J, Larsen L, Nielsen VG. Histamine content and mast cell count of detrusor muscle in patients with interstitial cystitis and other types of chronic cystitis. *Br J Urol* 1983;55:495–500.
23. Pang X, Sant GR, Theoharides TC. Mast cell (MC) growth factor receptor (c-kit) expression in IC bladders. NIH-NIDDK/ICA Interstitial Cystitis Scientific Workshop, San Diego, 1995;43.
24. Theoharides TC. Mast cell: a neuroimmunoendocrine master player. *Int J Tissue React* 1996;18:1–21.
25. Church MK, Lowman MA, Rees PH, Benyon RC. Mast cells, neuropeptides and inflammation. *Agents Actions* 1989;27:8–16.
26. Holgate ST. The human lung mast cell: Morphology, biochemistry and role in allergic asthma. *Adv Neurol* 1983;19:287–299.

27. Metcalfe DD. Mast cell mediators with emphasis on intestinal mast cells. *Ann Allergy* 1984(part 2);53:563–575.
28. Galli SJ. New insights into "the riddle of the mast cells": microenvironmental regulation of mast cell development and phenotypic heterogeneity. *Lab Invest* 1990;62:5–33.
29. Shanahan F, Denburg JA, Fox J, Bienenstock J, Befus D. Mast cell heterogeneity: effects of neuroenteric peptides on histamine release. *J Immunol* 1985;135:1331–1337.
30. Schwartz LB. Mediators of human mast cells and human mast cell subsets. *Ann Allergy* 1987;58:226–235.
31. Enerbäck L, Miller HRP, Mayrhofer G. Methods for the identification and characterization of mast cells by light microscopy. In: Befus AD, Bienenstock J, Denburg JA, eds. *Mast Cell Differentiation and Heterogeneity*. New York: Raven Press, 1986;405–417.
32. Dimitriadou V, Lambracht-Hall M, Reichler J, Theoharides TC. Histochemical and ultrastructural characteristics of rat brain perivascular mast cells stimulated with compound 48/80 and carbachol. *Neuroscience* 1990;39:209–224.
33. Dvorak AM. Human mast cells. *Adv Anat Embryol Cell Biol* 1989; 114:1–107.
34. Beaven MA, Metzger H. Signal transduction by Fc receptors: the FcεRI case. *Immunol Today* 1993;14:222–226.
35. Lagunoff D, Martin TW, Read G. Agents that release histamine from mast cells. *Annu Rev Pharmacol Toxicol* 1983;23:331–351.
36. Malaviya R, Ross E, Jakschik BA, Abraham SN. Mast cell degranulation induced by type 1 fimbriated *Escherichia coli* in mice. *J Clin Invest* 1994;93:1645–1653.
37. Malaviya R, Ross EA, MacGregor JI, et al. Mast cell phagocytosis of FimH-expressing enterobacteria. *J Immunol* 1994;152:1907–1914.
38. Johnson AR, Erdös EG. Release of histamine from mast cells by vasoactive peptides. *Proc Soc Exp Biol Med* 1973;142:1252–1256.
39. Theoharides TC, Douglas WW. Somatostatin induces histamine secretion from rat peritoneal mast cells. *Endocrinology* 1978;102: 1637–1640.
40. Fewtrell CMS, Foreman JC, Jordan CC, Oehme P, Renner H, Stewart JM. The effects of substance P on histamine and 5-hydroxytryptamine release in the rat. *J Physiol* 1982;330:393–411.
41. Serafin WE, Austen KF. Mediators of immediate hypersensitivity reactions. *N Engl J Med* 1987:317:30–34.
42. Gordon JR, Burd PR, Galli SJ. Mast cells as a source of multifunctional cytokines. *Immunol Today* 1990;11:458–464.
43. Cutz E, Chan W, Track NS, Goth A, Said SI. Release of vasoactive intestinal polypeptide in mast cells by histamine liberators. *Nature* 1978;275:661–662.
44. Larsen S, Thompson SA, Hald T, et al. Mast cells in interstitial cystitis. *Br J Urol* 1982;54:283–286.
45. Aldenborg F, Fall M, Enerbäck L. Proliferation and transepithelial migration of mucosal mast cells in interstitial cystitis. *Immunology* 1986;58:411–416.
46. Enerbäck L, Fall M, Aldenborg F. Histamine and mucosal mast cells in interstitial cystitis. *Agents Actions* 1989;27:113–116.
47. Sant GR, Kilaru P, Ucci AA,Jr. Mucosal mast cell (MMC) contribution to bladder mastocytosis in interstitial cystitis. *J Urol* 1988;139:276.
48. Feltis JT, Perez-Marrero R, Emerson LE. Increased mast cells of the bladder in suspected cases of interstitial cystitis: a possible disease marker. *J Urol* 1987;138:42–43.
49. Lynes WL, Flynn SD, Shortliffe LD, et al. Mast cell involvement in interstitial cystitis. *J Urol* 1987;138:746–752.
50. Christmas TJ, Rode J. Characteristics of mast cells in normal bladder, bacterial cystitis and interstitial cystitis. *Br J Urol* 1991;68:473–478.
51. Theoharides TC, Sant GR, El-Mansoury M, Letourneau RJ, Ucci AA Jr, Meares EM Jr. Activation of bladder mast cells in interstitial cystitis: a light and electron microscopic study. *J Urol* 1995;153:629–636.
52. El-Mansoury M, Boucher W, Sant GR, Theoharides TC. Increased urine histamine and methylhistamine in interstitial cystitis. *J Urol* 1994;152: 350–353.
53. Boucher W, El-Mansoury M, Pang X, Sant GR, Theoharides TC. Elevated mast cell tryptase in urine of interstitial cystitis patients. *Br J Urol* 1995;76:94–100.
54. Frenz AM, Christmas TJ, Pearce FL. Does the mast cell have an intrinsic role in the pathogenesis of interstitial cystitis? *Agents Actions* 1994;41:C14–C15.
55. Dundore PA, Schwartz AM, Semerjian H: Mast cell counts are not useful in the diagnosis of non-ulcerative interstitial cystitis. *J Urol* 1996;155:885–887.
56. Ratliff TL, Klutke CG, Hofmeister M, He F, Russell JH, Bechich MJ. Short analytical review: Role of the immune response in interstitial cystitis. *Clin Immunopathol* 1995;74:209–216.
57. Theoharides TC, Bondy PK, Tsakalos ND, Askenase PW. Differential release of serotonin and histamine from mast cells. *Nature* 1982;297: 229–231.
58. Kops SK, Theoharides TC, Cronin CT, Kashgarian MG, Askenase PW. Ultrastructural characteristics of rat peritoneal mast cells undergoing differential release of serotonin without histamine and without degranulation. *Cell Tissue Res* 1990;262:415–424.
59. Dvorak AM, McLeod RS, Onderdonk A, et al. Ultrastructural evidence for piecemeal and anaphylactic degranulation of human gut mucosal mast cells in vivo. *Int Arch Allergy Immunol* 1992;99:74–83.
60. Letourneau RJ, Pang X, Sant GR, Theoharides TC. Intragranular activation of bladder mast cells and their association with nerve processes in interstitial cystitis. *Br J Urol* 1996;77:41–54.
61. Claman HN, Choi KL, Sujansky W, Vatter AE. Mast cell "disappearance" in chronic murine graft-vs-host disease (GVHD)—ultrastructural demonstration of "phantom mast cells." *J Immunol* 1986;137: 2009–2013.
62. Foreman JC. Peptides and neurogenic inflammation. *Brain Res Bull* 1987;3:386–398.
63. Payan DG, Levine JD, Goetzl EJ. Modulation of immunity and hypersensitivity by sensory neuropeptides. *J Immunol* 1984;132: 1601–1604.
64. Goetzl EJ, Cheng PPJ, Hassner A, Adelman DC, Frick OL, Speedharan SP. Neuropeptides, mast cells and allergy: novel mechanisms and therapeutic possibilities. *Clin Exp Allergy* 1990;20:3–7.
65. McKay DM, Bienenstock J. The interaction between mast cells and nerves in the gastrointestinal tract. *Immunol Today* 1994;15:533–538.
66. Marshall JS, Waserman S. Mast cells and the nerves—potential interactions in the context of chronic disease. *Clin Exp Allergy* 1995;25: 102–110.
67. Newson B, Dahlström A, Enerbäck L, Ahlman H. Suggestive evidence for a direct innervation of mucosal mast cells. *Neuroscience* 1983;10: 565–570.
68. Stead RH, Dixon MF, Bramwell NH, Riddell RH, Bienenstock J. Mast cells are closely apposed to nerves in the human gastrointestinal mucosa. *Gastroenterology* 1989;97:575–585.
69. Dimitriadou V, Buzzi MG, Moskowitz MA, Theoharides TC. Trigeminal sensory fiber stimulation induces morphologic changes reflecting secretion in rat dura mast cells. *Neuroscience* 1991;44:97–112.
70. Christian EP, Undem BJ, Weinreich D. Endogenous histamine excites neurones in the guinea-pig superior cervical ganglion in vitro. *J Physiol* 1989;409:297–312.
71. Hohenfellner M, Nunes L, Schmidt RA, Lampel A, Thuroff JW, Tanagho EA. Interstitial cystitis: increased sympathetic innervation and related neuropeptide synthesis. *J Urol* 1992;147:587–591.
72. Christmas TJ, Rode J, Chapple CR, Milroy EJ, Turner-Warwick RT. Nerve fibre proliferation in interstitial cystitis. *Virchows Arch [A]* 1990;416:447–451.
73. Pang X, Marchand J, Sant GR, Kream RM, Theoharides TC. Increased number of substance P positive nerve fibers in interstitial cystitis. *Br J Urol* 1995;75:744–750.
74. Dvorak AM, McLeod RS, Onderdonk AB, et al. Human gut mucosal mast cells: ultrastructural observations and anatomic variation in mast cell–nerve associations *in vivo*. *Int Arch Allergy Immunol* 1992;98: 158–168.
75. Lambracht-Hall M, Konstantinidou AD, Theoharides TC. Serotonin release from rat brain mast cells *in vitro*. *Neuroscience* 1990;39: 199–207.
76. Lasanen LT, Tammela TLJ, Liesi P, et al. The effect of acute distension on vasoactive intestinal polypeptide (VIP), neuropeptide Y (NPY)- and substance P (SP)-immunoreactrive nerves in the female rat urinary bladder. *Urol Res* 1992;20:259–263.
77. Barbanti G, Maggi C, Beneforti P, et al. Relief of pain following intravesical capsaicin in patients with hypersensitive disorders of the lower urinary tract. *J Urol* 1993;71:686–691.
78. Spanos C, Pang X, Ligris K, et al: Stress-induced bladder mast cell activation: implications for interstitial cystitis. *J Urol* 1997; 157:669–672.
79. Castagliuolo I, Bhaskar KR, Kirmani IA, LaMont JT, Pothoulakis C. Acute psychologic stress stimulates mast cell degranulation, prostaglandin E_2 and mucin release from rat colon. *Gastroenterology* 1994;106:A474.

80. Pang X, Boucher W, Triadafilopoulos G, Sant GR, Theoharides TC. Mast cell and substance P-positive nerve involvement in a patient with both irritable bowel syndrome and interstitial cystitis. *Urology* 1996;47:436–438.
81. Weston AP, Biddle WL, Bhatia PS, Miner PB Jr. Terminal ileal mucosal mast cells in irritable bowel syndrome. *Dig Dis Sci* 1993;38:1590–1595.
82. Farthing MJG. Irritable bowel, irritable body, or irritable brain? *Br Med J* 1995;310:171–175.
83. Iovino P, Azpiroz F, Domingo E, Malagelada J-R. The sympathetic nervous system modulates perception and reflex responses to gut distention in humans. *Gastroenterology* 1995;108:680–686.
84. Sternberg EM, Chrousos GP, Wilder RL, Gold PW. The stress response and the regulation of inflammatory disease. *Ann Intern Med* 1992;117:854–866.
85. Ader R, Cohen N, Felten D. Psychoneuroimmunology: interactions between the nervous system and the immune system. *Lancet* 1995; 345:99–103.
86. Theoharides TC, Spanos CP, Pang X, et al: Stress-induced intracranial mast cell degranulation. A corticotrophin releasing hormone-mediated effect. *Endocrinology* 1995;136:5774–5750.
87. Conrad MJ, Feigen GA. Sex hormones and kinetics of anaphylactic histamine release. *Physiol Chem Phys* 1974;6:11–16.
88. Vliagoftis H, Dimitriadou V, Boucher W, et al. Estradiol augments while tamoxifen inhibits rat mast cell secretion. *Int Arch Allergy Immunol* 1992;98:398–409.
89. Pang X, Cotreau-Bibbo MM, Sant GR, Theoharides TC. Bladder mast cell expression of high affinity estrogen receptors in patients with interstitial cystitis. *Br J Urol* 1995;75:154–161.
90. Patra PB, Tibbitts FD, Westfall DP. *Endocrine status and urinary mast cells: possible relationship to interstitial cystitis.* Paper presented at NIH IC Symposium, Jan 9–11, 1995.
91. Grossman CJ. Regulation of the immune system by sex steroids. *Endocr Rev* 1984;5:435–455.
92. Schuurs AH, Verheul HA. Effects of gender and sex steroids on the immune response. *J Steroid Biochem* 1990;35:157–172.
93. Wormald PJ. Age–sex incidence in symptomatic allergies: an excess of females in the child-bearing years. *J Hyg* 1977;79:39–42.
94. Gibbs CJ, Coutts II, Lock R, Finnegan OC, White RJ. Premenstrual exacerbation of asthma. *Thorax* 1984;39:833–836.
95. Spanos C, El-Mansoury M, Letourneau RJ, et al. Carbachol-induced activation of bladder mast cells is augmented by estradiol—implications for interstitial cystitis. *Urology* 1996;48:809–816.
96. Galli SJ. New concepts about the mast cell. *N Engl J Med* 1993;328: 257–265.
97. Luger TA, Wirth U, Kock A. Epidermal cells synthesize a cytokine with interleukin 3-like properties. *J Immunol* 1985;134:915–927.
98. Yun SK, Laub DJ, Weese DL, Lad PM, Leach GE, Zimmern PE. Stimulated release of urine histamine in interstitial cystitis. *J Urol* 1992;148:1145–1148.
99. Holm-Bentzen M, Søndergaard I, Hald T. Urinary excretion of a metabolite of histamine (1,4-methyl-imidazole-acetic-acid) in painful bladder disease. *Br J Urol* 1987;59:230–233.
100. Felsen D, Frye S, Trimble LA, et al. Inflammatory mediator profile in urine and bladder wash fluid of patients with interstitial cystitis. *J Urol* 1994;152:355–361.
101. Lose G, Frandsen B, Holm-Bentzen M. Urine eosinophil cationic protein in painful bladder disease. *Br J Urol* 1987;60:39–42.
102. Lose G, Frandsen B, Hojemsgard JC. Chronic interstitial cystitis: increased levels of eosinophil cationic protein in serum and urine and an ameliorating effect of subcutaneous heparin. *Scand J Urol Nephrol* 1983;17:159–161.
103. Mulholland SG, Hanno PM, Parsons CL, Sant GR, Staskin DR. Pentosan polysulfate sodium for therapy of interstitial cystitis. A double-blind placebo-controlled clinical study. *Urology* 1990;35: 552–558.
104. Parsons CL, Housley T, Schmidt JD, Lebow D. Treatment of interstitial cystitis with intravesical heparin. *Br J Urol* 1994;73:504–507.
105. Sant GR. Intravesical 50% dimethyl sulfoxide (RMSO-50) in treatment of interstitial cystitis. *Urology [Suppl]* 1987;29:17–21.
106. Candussio L, Klugmann FB, Decorti G, Bevilacqua S, Baldini L. Dimethyl sulfoxide inhibits histamine release induced by various chemicals. *Agents Actions* 1987;20:17–21.
107. Hanno PM, Buehler J, Wein AJ. Use of amitriptyline in the treatment of interstitial cystitis. *J Urol* 1989;141:846–848.
108. Kennelly MJ, Konnak JW. *Intravesical cromolyn sodium for treatment of interstitial cystitis—a double blind placebo controlled pilot study.* Paper presented at 1995 Interstital Cystitis Symposium, p 64.
109. Pearce FL, Befus AD, Gauldie J, Bienenstock J. Mucosal mast cells. II: Effects of anti-allergic compounds on histamine secretion by isolated intestinal mast cells. *J Immunol* 1982;128:2481–2486.
110. Theoharides TC. Hydroxyzine for interstitial cystitis. *J Allergy Clin Immunol* 1993;91:686–687.
111. Theoharides TC. Hydroxyzine in the treatment of interstitial cystitis. *Urol Clin North Am* 1994;21:113–119.

Interstitial Cystitis, edited by Grannum R. Sant.
Lippincott–Raven Publishers, Philadelphia ©1997.

CHAPTER 13

Interstitial Cystitis and Diet

Larrian M. Gillespie

The concept of treating urologic disorders through dietary management has gained increasing acceptance as medical science has made advances in understanding the complexities of the interaction between the gastrointestinal (GI) and urinary tracts, e.g., irritable bowel syndrome. Since the discovery that the gastrointestinal tract contains large amounts of serotonin (5-HT), intense research has been focused on the role of 5-HT as a neurotransmitter released from enteric nerves in addition to its function as a paracrine substance released from the enterochromaffin cells in the mucosa. As a result, new therapeutic agents have been developed that successfully treat propulsive or motility disorders of the GI tract.

The hypersensitive bladder disorder interstitial cystitis has offered clinicians an excellent *in vivo* model in which to explore the effect of diet, gastrointestinal absorption, and related functions on urinary contents. From improved understanding of the effect of diet, hormones, and pharmacologic agents on gastric emptying, new insight has been gained on the resultant by-products found in urine that may increase cellular permeability (1). As a result, dietary modification of the symptoms of interstitial cystitis can be accomplished in the motivated patient. In order to understand the role of diet in interstitial cystitis (IC), it is important to review the significance of serotonin in the manipulation of gastric motility and digestion by the autonomic nervous system and draw potential parallels between the GI and genitourinary (GU) tracts.

SEROTONIN AND GASTROINTESTINAL TRANSPORT

It has been estimated that up to 10 mg of the total amount of 5-HT in the body is in the gastrointestinal tract (2,3). The amount of 5-HT in the tissue is a dynamic function of synthesis, release, and metabolism, each of which can be influenced by drugs and physiology, especially stress. Tryptophan is necessary for the formation of the transmitter amine serotonin (5-hydroxytryptamine) in the central nervous system, through the sequential action of the rate-limiting enzyme tryptophan-5-hydrolase and 5-hydroxytryptophan decarboxylase. Mucosal 5-HT levels are modulated by dietary tryptophan (4,5). The levels are increased by antibiotics, especially sulfonamides, and by ACTH administration and decreased after nicotine, bradykinin, α-methyldopa, reserpine, and steroids (6–14). Mast cell 5-HT is stored bound to heparin and histamine (15).

Serotonin receptors are located in the central nervous system, alimentary canal (including the intestinal tract and enterochromaffin cells), the heart, the adrenal glands, and the urinary tract (16–20). Serotonin can be released by food ingestion, vagal or sympathetic adrenergic stimulation, a lowering of intraluminal pH, circulating catecholamines, sucrose solutions, and amino acids (3,21–25). Mechanical distension, ischemia, and obstruction of normal motility can also release 5-HT (26–29). The half-life of intestinal serotonin has been estimated to be 7 to 12 hr in man (30). Calcitonin gene-related peptide (CGRP) has been reported to be secreted by some primary afferent neurons excited by mucosal stimulation (31). The peristaltic reflex can be blocked by serosal application of 5-HT, implying that 5-HT receptors are critical for maintenance as well as initiation of the reflex (32). Understanding 5-HT-mediated neural mechanisms in the bowel is of considerable importance, as many patients are taking medications to affect mood, appetite, or other mental functions. Serotonergic neural transmission is the target of many of these compounds, e.g., fluoexitine (Prozac).

BICARBONATE SECRETION

Bicarbonate secretion occurs from the surface epithelial cells and is equivalent to about 5% to 10% of the acid output in the stomach and 20% to 30% in the duodenum

L. M. Gillespie: Beverly Hills, California 90212.

(33,34). Studies suggest that extracellular fluid is a major source of secreted HCO_3^- even in the pancreas, where cellular metabolism is sufficient to supply CO_2 for maximal rates of secretion (35,36). The secretion of HCO_3^- in the stomach and duodenum maintains a nearly neutral pH in the mucous gel adherent to the surface despite acidity as high as pH 1.5 to 3 in the lumen, resulting in a pH gradient across the mucous gel at the surface of the mucosa. This indicates that HCO_3^- secretion, along with the mucous gel, provides the first line of protection in the stomach and forms the main defense mechanism in the duodenum (37). Prostaglandins stimulate HCO_3^- secretion, whereas nonsteroidal antiinflammatory agents decrease HCO_3^- secretion by inhibiting the mucosal prostaglandin generation (38–42). The gastroduodenal mucosa is kept intact by multiple protective mechanisms despite exposure to acid and other chemical hazards.

Bicarbonate secretion is one of the mechanisms that plays an important role in protection of the mucosa against acid. This is best seen by the finding that the mucosa responds to acid by a significant increase of HCO_3^- secretion. Because the proximal duodenum is continuously exposed to acid emptied from the stomach, its physiological importance may be even higher than that of the stomach. Agents such as indomethacin and other prostaglandin inhibitors significantly reduce the acid-neutralizing capacity in the duodenum, increase the mucosal susceptibility to acid, and induce duodenal ulcers or inflammation when gastric hypersecretion is concomitant (39,43,44). Surface glycosaminoglycans (GAGs) are thought to play a similar protective role in the bladder, and a defect or deficiency of GAGs is felt to be a cause of IC.

ENZYMATIC DIGESTION

Unlike carbohydrates and lipids, a considerable amount of protein digestion occurs in the stomach, where gastrin stimulates the release of tissue factors such as serotonin and histamine in conjunction with acetylcholine and hydrochloric acid. The proteolytic enzyme pepsin preferentially hydrolyzes those linkages involving the amino group of the aromatic amino acids tryptophan, phenylalanine, and tyrosine. Although pepsin mainly degrades proteins into polypeptides of varying lengths, some short-chain peptides and even some free amino acids, notably phenylalanine and tryptophan, may be released. Chymotrypsin then cleaves peptide bonds involving the carboxyl group of tyrosine, phenylalanine, and tryptophan, while secretin stimulates the secretion of pancreatic juice rich in bicarbonate without further enzymatic activity. Any residual tryptophan is metabolized to indoxyl by bowel bacteria, where excessive amounts may be reabsorbed from the large bowel, conjugated with sulfate from the liver, and excreted in urine as indicans. This gives a rancid, putrefying odor to urine if present in any significant quantity. Indoleamines enhance electrically stimulated cholinergic "twitch" contractions in longitudinal and circular smooth muscle (45–47).

STRESS

Stress, either physical or psychological, is an important mediator of peptic ulcer disease and other GI disease, e.g., IBS. Under these conditions, the neuronal activity of the sympathetic in addition to the parasympathetic nerves is increased, leading to an increase in acid secretion and a decrease in mucosal blood flow. Stress reduces HCO_3^- secretion by a decrease in the mucosal blood flow secondary to activation of sympathetic nerves and a decrease in prostaglandin production, probably caused by the enhanced release of glucocorticoids. Increased sympathetic activity decreases HCO_3^- secretion via increased splanchnic nerve activity. Several types of experiments show that sympathetic nerves to the duodenum inhibit bicarbonate secretion, whether the nerves are electrically activated or stimulated by elicited reflexes (48,49). Hemlin and Sjovall reported that norepinephrine controlled the size of the pores in tight junctions between epithelial cells. The adrenergic influence through the sympathetic nerves decreased the pore size and thus the hydraulic conductivity of the epithelium (50). Dilations of tight junctions also occur during organic molecule absorption, and these dilations have been suggested as a mechanism whereby solvent drag couples additional absorption to active transport (51).

The transport of glucose and amino acids increases epithelial conductance through a specific effect of increasing tight junctional permeability. Altered bladder permeability has been reported in IC. Ischemia may reduce mucosal permeability through tight junctions (52). Loss of tight junctional resistance or integrity may affect secretion by increasing the absorption of secretory agents. L-Tryptophan (1 to 10 mM) causes a marked disruption of the tight junctions and inhibits absorption *in vivo* (53,54). As a result, smaller peptides can enter the pericellular path through dilated tight junctions during physiological glucose absorption (55). The disruptions may allow entrance of food proteins into the mucosa and initiate immunologic reactions that can cause secretion, such as by N-formyl-methionyl-leucyl-phenylalanine (56). Similarly, in IC, an altered bladder surface permeability may allow toxic substances in the urine to elicit bladder inflammation.

Any response of the intestine that increases fluid entry into the interstitial space, such as increased mucosal fluid absorption or increased capillary pressure, will wash out tissue colloids and reduce interstitial colloid osmotic pressure. This effect will act as a compensatory mechanism to reduce the rate of entry of fluid into the interstitium and limit interstitial hydration. Loss of fluid from the plasma will concentrate plasma proteins at the same time that it dilutes interstitial proteins. This will limit further losses of fluid into the interstitium. Sympathetic denervation increases blood flow and reduces absorption. Sympathetic stimulation has the opposite effect. It has been well established that autonomic nerve fibers control smooth muscles in vessels and in various hollow organs such as the gastrointestinal tract and the urinary bladder. Less well known is the autonomic nervous control of epithelia.

The enteric nervous system (ENS) represents one of the major parts of the autonomic nervous system (ANS). Discovery of this system is not new, however, as evidenced by the classic monograph by Langley (1921) in which he divides the ANS into three major parts: the sympathetic, the parasympathetic, and the enteric nervous systems (57). This view is again gaining popularity as histochemical reports as well as morphologic and functional studies of the ENS clearly suggest that the ENS can function as an independent part of the ANS.

THE EFFECTS OF DIETARY MODIFICATION ON THE SYMPTOMS OF INTERSTITIAL CYSTITIS

The Women's Clinic for Interstitial Cystitis was established in 1984 in order to study patients who complained of irritative bladder symptoms in the absence of infection. These patients reported that a variety of foods and medications could initiate an attack of urgency and frequency and cause a flare-up of their IC symptoms. Uniformly, patients described an unusual odor that heralded the onset of pain, typically stating that their urine smelled of "rancid pineapple" or like a "dead mouse in their bladder (58)." Slowly, a list was compiled that broke down into two main categories of foods: those that stimulate histamine and serotonin release from the stomach and those with the highest amounts of the biogenic amines: tryptophan, phenylalanine, tyrosine, and tyramine (Table 1). Selective metabolites of this family of amino acids have been shown to bind to the sulfate groups of the polysaccharides in the glycosaminoglycan (GAG) layer of the bladder epithelium and inactivate their hydrophilic property. Electron microscopy and histologic staining of bladder tissue demonstrated breaks in the mucous layers in addition to wide open junctional gaps (59–61). Because numerous patients related that dietary control resulted in significant pain relief, a study was designed to attempt to identify some of the metabolic factors contributing to the symptoms of interstitial cystitis and to determine if the concentrations of certain metabolites and amino acids were altered in patients with hypersensitive bladders and interstitial cystitis.

Two hundred fifty patients (237 women, 13 men) with the clinical, histologic, and immunofluorescent diagnosis of interstitial cystitis were selected for dietary evaluation (1). Ten individuals with no urinary symptoms served as controls, eating an identical diet to their partners. Competition for a transluminal carrier occurs in amino acid absorption during gastric and pancreatic metabolism (62). Some of the membrane transport systems are antiporters; i.e., they transport two amino acids in opposite directions at the same time. Consequently, oral (not intravenous) ingestion of the arylalkylamines was utilized in this study. All medications and vitamin supplements were discontinued for 72 hr before testing, with the exception of antidepressants, steroids, H_2 blockers, and asthmatic medications, which were discontinued 7 days before the study.

In order to accomplish "stress" dietary testing, patients were required to ingest as many of the foods in Table 1 as possible during the following 24 hr. During the same time period, 24-hr urine collection was done after discarding the first morning void. The samples were pooled in a preservative-free container and were tested for the following metabolites: indicans, 3-methoxy-4-hydroxyphenylglycol (MHPG), xanthurenic acid, kynurenic acid, tryptophan, urinary ammonia, and pH. Each patient kept a voiding log (time, volume) annotated with comments on symptoms. The log was handed in the following morning. The first morning void at the end of the 24-hr period ended the collection. Following this, blood was drawn for histamine, serotonin, prolactin, tryptophan,

TABLE 1. *Foods to be avoided in the pain-control diet*[a]

Acid foods	
All alcoholic beverages	Guava
Apple juice; red and green apples	Lemon juice
	Nectarines
Apricots	Peaches
Cantaloupes	Pineapple
Carbonated drinks	Plums
Chilis; spicy foods	Strawberries
Citrus fruits	Tea
Coffee	Tomatoes
Cranberries	Vinegar
Grapes	
Foods high in tyrosine, tyramine, tryptophan, aspartate, and phenylalanine	
Avocados	Nutrasweet (aspartame)
Bananas	Nuts
Beer	Onions
Brewer's yeast	Pickled herring
Canned figs	Pineapple
Champagne	Prunes
Cheeses	Raisins
Chicken livers	Rye bread
Chocolate	Saccharine
Corned beef	Sour cream
Cranberries	Soy sauce
Fava beans	Vitamins buffered with aspartate
Lima beans	
Marmite	Wines
Mayonnaise	Yogurt

[a]From Gillespie (58), with permission.

TABLE 2. *Results of stress testing*

	Control (*n* = 10)	Interstitial cystitis (*n* = 250)
Blood		
Histamine (5–15 μg/dl)	10 ± 3	28 ± 4
Serotonin (90–340 μg/liter)	210 ± 28	127 ± 31
Prolactin (112.8 μg/liter)	11 ± 2	4 ± 1
Ammonia (nitrogen) (5–69 μg/dl)	17 ± 8	49 ± 22
Tryptophan (≤73 μmol/liter)	53 ± 5	54 ± 7
24-hr Urine		
Ammonia (0.14–1.5 g)	0.92 ± 18	0.1 ± 0.3
MHPG (1,027–1,647 μg)	1,246 ± 174	982 ± 114
Kynurenine (0–3 mg)	0.64 ± 0.24	3.8 ± 0.19
Xanthurenine (0–3 mg)	0.73 ± 0.19	4.1 ± 0.16
Indicans (1–20 mg)	14 ± 3	28 ± 10
pH (5–6.3)	5.3 ± 2	6.9 ± 0.3
Tryptophan (≤200 μmol/24 hr)	91 ± 17	Trace

and ammonia as nitrogen. Serum for ammonia was immediately frozen, and the blood for serotonin was iced following inversion four times to stimulate platelet release. The total pH of the volume was measured before the addition of preservatives. The same procedure was done for each of the ten controls.

The results of this study are documented in Table 2. In the control group of patients the values were within the normal range, indicating that excessive ingestion of the biogenic amines does not result in abnormal production of metabolites in those with normal digestion. Individuals with the clinical picture of interstitial cystitis did not demonstrate this response. Low levels of prolactin and serotonin were found despite normal levels of tryptophan in the blood. Phenylalanine or tyrosine is required for the synthesis of catecholamines, dopamine, norepinephrine, and epinephrine, as are the thyroid hormones thyroxine and triiodothyronine. Increased activation of dopamine (D_2) receptors in the pituitary can result in low prolactin levels, which may explain the findings in these patients. In contrast, high levels of ammonia and histamine were found in the serum. High levels of histamine increase cAMP in postsynaptic cells and thereby modify the function of other neural networks. Axelrod further demonstrated that stress increases tyrosinase neural activity (63).

In the central nervous system, tryptophan is necessary for the formation of the transmitter amine serotonin (5-hydroxytryptamine or 5-HT). The inability of tryptophan to be converted to serotonin can result in the appearance in urine of indicans, xanthurenic acid, and kynurenic acid, which have the ability to impair the hydrophilic activity of the bladder mucosal surface. Increased excretion of indicans, xanthurenic acid, and kynurenic acid was found in urine in the face of an alkaline pH. As previously discussed, indicans can stimulate cholinergic smooth muscle contractions such as those found in the interstitium of the bladder. These same compounds could account for the peculiar odor reported by patients before a severe attack of pain.

The MHPG is formed during the metabolism of norepinephrine from peripheral sympathetic nerves, and 89% of urinary MHPG is contributed by these nerves. Levels of MHPG were low in IC patients, and this supports the hypothesis that interstitial cystitis may represent a form of sympathetic dystrophy. Schildkraut and Keeler reported that urinary excretion levels of MHPG were significantly lower during depression, and low levels of serotonin were associated with lower pain thresholds in addition to depression (64). The findings of low serotonin and MHPG may provide a physiological explanation for the psychological profile of interstitial cystitis patients.

Many diverse biological effects have been attributed to the arylalkylamines and histamine, in particular on the cardiovascular and intestinal systems. The metabolism of amino acids is in a dynamic state, as the body's "metabolic pool," derived either endogenously from expended tissue protein or exogenously from dietary food proteins, is in a constant state of flux.

Blood ammonia levels were elevated in IC patients, indicating a problem with protein metabolism. However, urinary ammonia was quite low, in addition to a near absence of tryptophan in urine despite normal serum levels. The urinary bladder has been shown to absorb physiological components of urine, and the apparent lack of both ammonia and tryptophan supports the concept that interstitial cystitis represents a membrane leak (65). The alkaline urinary pH is also consistent with this hypothesis based on the Donnan effect, a mechanism by which opposite charges across a membrane will strive to achieve equilibrium (66). The normal intracellular pH is approximately 7.38, but if there is a leak through the cell junction or glycosaminoglycan layer, the intracellular pH will become acidic, triggering the release of lysosomal enzymes within the epithelial cells, which causes a shutdown of all alkaline-pH-dependent enzymes, coenzymes, and nucleic acids. Cellular degradation ensues. It is not surprising that 83% of patients reported increased frequency and pelvic pain during the study, and most required pain medication.

TABLE 3. *Results of nutritional limitation in ten patients*

Histamine (5–15 μg/dl)	12 ± 21 μg/dl
Serotonin (90–340 μg/dl)	139 ± 28 μg/dl
Prolactin (1–12.8 μg/liter)	3.8 ± 7 μg/liter
Ammonia (serum) (5–69 μg/dl)	38 ± 11 μg/dl
pH (5–6.3)	5.8 ± 0.1
Kynurenine (0–3 mg)	0.9 ± 0.3 mg
Xanthurenine (0–3 mg)	1.2 ± 0.8 mg
Indicans (10–20 mg)	16 ± 5 mg
Ammonia (urine) (0.14–1.5 g)	0.09 ± 0.5 g
MHPG (1,027–1,647 μg)	987 ± 92 μg
Tryptophan (urine) (≤200 μmol/24 hr)	4 ± 1 μmol/24 hr
Tryptophan (serum) (≤73 μmol/liter)	51 ± 8 μmol/liter

In order to demonstrate that dietary restriction resulted not only in symptomatic relief but also in changes in the serum and urine levels of these individuals, ten patients were restudied in an identical manner, this time eliminating the foods listed in Table 1. Serum levels of histamine and ammonia and urinary levels of indicans and of xanthurenic and kynurenic acid normalized (Table 3). However, serotonin, MHPG, prolactin, urinary ammonia, and tryptophan levels remained abnormal in the absence of triggered pain. I have used tricyclic antidepressant therapy since 1983 to treat IC patients, as it raises prolactin, serotonin, and norepinephrine levels, resulting in less depression and pain.

Heparin increases the negative electric potential of the vascular wall and confers increased electronegativity to cell membranes and surfaces. The anionic charge of heparin can be neutralized by histamine, basic dyes, alkaloids, quaternary ammonium drugs, and the biogenic amines (67). Tissue from patients with interstitial cystitis shows a loss of this acid mucopolysaccharide from the urothelium (61). In addition, the presence of antigenic staining for IgM within the endothelium of the subepithelial capillaries is consistent with damage to the endothelial lining. Endothelium modulates the release and destruction of norepinephrine and serotonin from the adrenergic endings, which is enhanced in the absence of endothelium (68). Abnormal proliferation of small blood vessels has been identified as a hallmark of the endoscopic appearance of interstitial cystitis. Rapid generation of capillaries, defined as angiogenesis, can be triggered by intracellular hypoxia, acidosis, hypercarbia, hypokalemia, and hypoglycemia, resulting in ischemic vasodilation and increased capillary permeability (69). Even mild changes in blood flow cause large changes in shear, which are directly related to flow velocity and viscosity and inversely related to the internal diameter of the vessel. Pulsatile changes in the intrinsic blood supply, therefore, would result in reperfusion injury (70). The appearance of petechial hemorrhaging after passive distension and decompression of the bladder in patients with interstitial cystitis is an example of such vascular perfusion alterations.

SUMMARY

The response of patients to dietary management offers a simple therapeutic approach for clinicians who are frustrated with current pharmaceutical and surgical options for IC. Patients who are willing to participate in their own care need little encouragement to utilize "pain control diet," as negative reinforcement serves as the best motivator. The use of medication as an adjunct to pain management has a rational physiological basis, as demonstrated in this chapter. By gaining further understanding of the interaction between the gastrointestinal and urinary tract, clinicians and their patients will benefit from advancing pharmaceutical research in both fields.

Clearly, further studies of the role of diet and dietary modifications in IC are needed. Carefully controlled dietary studies in large groups of patients (IC, controls) may well require sophisticated nutritional assessment techniques and measurements. Patients who note symptom exacerbation in association with various foods, beverages, etc. would be an ideal study population for the above studies.

It is not known at present whether dietary or urinary diet metabolites initiate or aggravate bladder inflammation in IC. The bladder urothelial interface between the urine, with its dietary substances, and the bladder wall is obviously a critical barrier to inflammation. Continued research in this area should lead to a better understanding of the role of diet in IC and to improved treatments.

REFERENCES

1. Gillespie L. Metabolic appraisal of the effects of dietary modification on hypersensitive bladder symptoms. *Br J Urol* 1993;72:293–297.
2. Thompson J. Serotonin in the alimentary tract. *Res Commun Chem Pathol Pharmacol* 1971;2:687–691.
3. Sjolund K, Sanden G, Kakanson R, Sundler F. Endocrine cells in human intestine: An immunohistochemical study. *Gastroenterology* 1984;85:1120–1129.
4. Sullivan T. The effect of diet on the 5-hydroxytryptamine content of the small intestine and other organs in rats and mice. *Br J Pharmacol* 1960;15:513–515.
5. Gal E, Drewes P. Studies on the metabolism of 5-hydroxytryptamine (serotonin). II. Effect of tryptophan deficiency in rats. *Proc Soc Exp Biol Med* 1962;110:368–372.
6. Thompson J, Campbell LB. Influence of sulphamerazine on gastrointestinal serotonin in the normal Sprague–Dawley rat. *Nature* 1966; 212:850.
7. Sullivan T. Effect of antibiotics on the 5-hydroxytryptamine content of the small intestine and other organs in rats and mice. *Br J Pharmacol* 1961;16:90–95.
8. Beaver M, Wostmann BS. Histamine and 5-hydroxytrytamine in the intestinal tract of the germ-free animals, animals harbouring one microbial special and conventional animals. *Br J Pharmacol* 1962;19: 385–389.
9. Glick O, Von Redlich D. Quantitative histological distribution of serotonin in the rat stomach. *Gastroenterology* 1969;57:390–392.
10. Burks T, Long JP. Release of 5-hydroxytryptamine from isolated dog intestine by nicotine. *Br J Pharmacol Chemother* 1967;30:229–233.
11. Peltola P. Release of serotonin during bradykinin infusion. *Scand J Clin Lab Invest [Suppl]* 1969;107:81–84.
12. Smith S. The pharmacological actions of 3,4-dihydroxyphenyl-*o*-methylalanine (*o*-methyldopa), an inhibitor of 5-hydroxytryptophan decarboxylase. *Br J Pharmacol* 1960;15:319–324.

13. Erspamer V. Occurrence of indolealkyl amines in nature. In: Eichler OFA, ed. *Handbuch der Experimentellen Pharmakologie.* Berlin: Springer, 1966;132–140.
14. Telford J, West GB. The effects of corticosteroids and related compounds on the histamine and 5-hydroxytryptamine content of rat tissues. *Br J Pharmacol* 1960;15:532–537.
15. Green J. Synthesis, uptake and binding of histamine and 5-hydroxytryptamine in mast cells. In: von Euler US, Ulvans E, eds. *Mechanisms of Release of Biogenic Amines.* London: Pergamon, 1966;125–134.
16. Grossman C, Kilpatrick G, Bunce K. Development of a radioligand binding assay for the 5-HT_4 receptors in guinea-pig and rat brain. *Br J Pharmacol* 1993;109:618–625.
17. Craig D, Clarke DE. 5-Hydroxytryptamine and cholinergic mechanisms in guinea-pig ileum. *Br J Pharmacol* 1989;96:247–251.
18. Gebauer H, Racke K, Kiblinger H. Modulation by 5-HT_3 and 5-HT_4 receptors of the release of 5-hydroxytryptamine from the guinea-pig small intestine. *Naunyn-Schmiedebergs Arch Pharmacol* 1993;347: 347–350.
19. Bockaert J, Fozard J, Dumuis A, Clarke D. The 5-HT_4 receptor: A place in the sun. *Trends Pharmacol Sci* 1992;13:141–145.
20. Ford A, Clarke DE. The 5-HT_4 receptors. *Med Res Rev* 1993;13: 633–640.
21. Resnick R, Gray SJ. Chemical and histologic demonstration of hydrochloric acid-induced release of serotonin from intestinal mucosa. *Gastroenterology* 1962;42:48–51.
22. Burks T, Long JP. Catecholamine-induced release of 5-hydroxytryptamine (5-HT) from perfused vasculature of isolated dog intestine. *J Pharm Sci* 1966;55:1383–1389.
23. O'Hara R, Fox RO, Cole JW. Serotonin release mediated by intraluminal sucrose solutions. *Surg Forum* 1959;10:215–222.
24. Drapanas T, MacDonald J, Stewart JD. Serotonin release following instillation of hypertonic glucose into the proximal intestine. *Ann Surg* 1962;156:528–531.
25. Zimmerman I, Alvestrand A, Bergstrom J. Elevated concentration of 5-hydroxytryptamine in ultrafiltrate of human liver vein plasma after infusion of amino acids. *Acta Physiol Scand* 1988;134:399–344.
26. Cole J, Schneider J, McKalen A. Effect of intraluminal pressure on enterochromaffin cells in the rat duodenum. *Proc Soc Exp Biol Med* 1961;107:58–63.
27. Bennett A, Bucknell A, Dean A. The release of 5-hydroxytryptamine from the rat stomach *in vitro. J Physiol* 1966;182:57–59.
28. Strauss R, Rubin K, Newman F, Strauss RD, Stuckey J. Serotonin levels in portal vein plasma after occlusion of the superior mesenteric artery in dogs with intact and divided vagus nerves. *Surgery* 1973;74: 333–337.
29. Warner R, Feldman M, Warner G, Parnes I, DiGiorgi F. Changes in blood serotonin concentration in mechanical obstruction of the small intestine II. Findings in patients with intestinal obstruction. *Surgery* 1966;59:758–762.
30. Erspamer V, Testini A. Observations on the release and turnover rate of 5-hydroxytryptamine in the gastrointestinal tract. *J Pharm Pharmacol* 1959;11:618–620.
31. Grider J. CGRP as a transmitter in the sensory pathway mediating peristaltic reflex. *Am J Physiol* 1994;266:G1139.
32. Bulbring E, Lin RC. The effect of 5-hydroxytryptamine and 5-hydroxytryptophan on peristalsis; the local production of 5-HT and its release in relation to intraluminal pressure and propulsive activity. *J Physiol* 1958;140:381–386.
33. Flemstrom G, Garner A. Gastroduodenal HCO_3 transport: characteristics and proposed role in acidity regulation and mucosal protection. *Am J Physiol* 1982;242:G183(abst).
34. Flemstrom G. Gastric and duodenal mucosal bicarbonate secretion. In: Johnson L, Cristensen J, Grossman MI, Jacobson ED, Schultz SG, eds. *Physiology of the Gastrointestinal Tract.* New York: Raven Press, 1987:1011–1026.
35. Burgen A. Secretory processes in salivary glands. *Handbook of Physiology, Alimentary Canal.* Bethesda, MD: American Physiology Society, 1976;561–574.
36. Raawls J, Wostrand PJ, Maren TH. Effects of acid–base changes and carbonic anhydrase inhibition on pancreatic secretion. *Am J Physiol* 1963;205:651–658.
37. Flemstrom G, Turnberg LA. Gastroduodenal defence mechanisms. *Clin Gastroenterol* 1984;13:327–435.
38. Takeuchi K, Tanaka H, Furukawa O, Okabe S. Gastroduodenal HCO_3 secretion in anesthetized rats: effects of 16,16-dimethyl PGE_2, topical acid, and acetazolamide. *Jpn J Pharmacol* 1986;41:87–90.
39. Takeuchi K, Furukawa O, Tanaka H, Okabe S. A new model of duodenal ulcers induced in rats by indomethacin plus histamine. *Gastroenterology* 1986;90:636–641.
40. Garner A, Flemstrom G, Heylings JR. Effects of anti-inflammatory agents and prostaglandins on acid and bicarbonate secretions in the amphibian-isolated gastric mucosa. *Gastroenterology* 1979;77: 457–463.
41. Takeuchi K, Furukawa O, Tanaka H, Okabe S. Determination of acid-neutralizing capacity in rat duodenum: influences of 16,16-dimethyl prostaglandin E_2 and nonsteroidal antinflammatory drugs. *Dig Dis Sci* 1986;31:631–637.
42. Okabe S, Takeuchi K, Niida H, Takinami Y. Effects of TY-10975, a stable PGI_2 derivative, on gastroduodenal lesions and secretory responses in the rat. *Digestion* 1990;45:61–65.
43. Furukawa O, Nishiwaki H, Takeuchi K, Okabe S. Effects of prostaglandin biosynthesis inhibitors and ouabain on duodenal mucosa and HCO_3 secretion in rats. *Jpn J Pharmacol* 1987;43: 449–455.
44. Takeuchi K, Furukawa O, Okada M, Okabe S. Duodenal ulcers induced by indomethacin plus histamine in the dog: involvement of the impaired duodenal alkaline secretion in their pathogenesis. *Digestion* 1988;39:230–234.
45. Rizzi C, Coccini T, Onori L, Manzo L, Tonini M. Benzimidazolone derivatives: A new class of 5-$hydroxytryptamine_4$ receptor agonists with prokinetic and acetylcholine releasing properties in the guinea pig ileum. *J Pharmacol Exp Ther* 1992;261:412–417.
46. Schiavone A, Giraldo E, Giudici L, Turconi M, Sagrada A. DAU 6285: A novel antagonist at the putative 5-HT_4 receptors. *Life Sci* 1992;51:583–586.
47. Tonini M, Candura S, Onori L, Coccini T, Manzo L, Rizzi C. 5-$Hydroxytryptamine_4$ agonists facilitate cholinergic transmission in the circular muscle of guinea pig ileum: Antagonism by tropisetron and DAU 6285. *Life Sci* 1992;50:PL173.
48. Fandricks L, Jonson C, Nylander O. Effects of splachnic nerve stimulation and of clonidine on gastric and duodenal HCO_3 secretion in the anaesthetized cat. *Acta Physiol Scand* 1987;130:251–257.
49. Jonson C, Fandricks L. Bleeding-induced decrease in duodenal HCO_3 secretion in the rat is mediated via alpha-2 adrenoceptors. *Acta Physiol Scand* 1987;130:387–392.
50. Hemlin M, Sjovall H. Evidence for sympathetic regulation of the hydraulic conduction of rat jejunal mucosa *in vivo. Acta Physiol Scand* 1989;135:459–464.
51. Madara J. Loosening tight junctions. Lessons from the intestine. *J Clin Invest* 1989;83:1089–1093.
52. Pappenheimer J, Volpp K. Transmucosal impedance of small intestine: correlation with transport of sugars and amino acids. *Am J Physiol* 1992;263:C480(abst).
53. Teichberg SR, Zdanowicz M, Roberts B, Ribeiro H, Lifshitz F. Morphologic and functional alterations in absorptive epithelial cells during L-tryptophan induced inhibition of net sodium and fluid absorption in the rat ileum. *Lab Invest* 1989;60:88–93.
54. Madara J, Carlson S. Supraphysiologic L-tryptophan elicits cytoskeletal and macromolecular permeability alterations in hamster small intestinal epithelium *in vitro. J Clin Invest* 1991;87:454–457.
55. Altisook K, Madara J. An oligopeptide permeates intestinal tight junctions at glucose-elicited dilations. *Gastroenterology* 1991;100: 719–722.
56. Von Ritter C, Sekizuka E, Grisham M, Granger D. The chemotactic peptide N-formyl-methionyl-leucyl-phenylalanine increases mucosal permeability in the distal ileum of the rat. *Gastroenterology* 1988;95: 651–655.
57. Langley J. *The Autonomic Nervous System.* London: Heffner, 1921.
58. Gillespie L. *You Don't Have to Live with Cystitis!* New York: Rawson Associates, 1996.
59. Kaufman J, Stauffer C, Schmidt JD, et al. *The effect of tryptophan metabolites on the anti-adherence nature of the bladder surface sulfonated glycosaminoglycan.* Paper presented at proceedings of the 75th Annual Meeting of the American Urological Association, San Diego, 1980.
60. Said J, Van de Velde R, Gillespie L. Immunopathology of interstitial cystitis. *Mod Pathol* 1989;2:593–601.
61. Gillespie L, Said J, Sostrin S, et al. Immunofluorescent and histo-

chemical staining confirm the identification of the many diseases called interstitial cystitis. *Br J Urol* 1990;66:265–273.
62. Kalser M. Physiology of the small intestine. In: Bockus H, ed: *Gastroenterology*, 2nd ed. Philadelphia: WB Saunders, 1964;21–39.
63. Axelrod J. Noradrenaline: fate and control of its biosynthesis. *Science* 1971;173:598–606.
64. Schildkraut J, Keeler BA. MHPG excretion in depressive disorders: relation to clinical subtypes and desynchonized sleep. *Science* 1973;181:762–764.
65. Morris C, Bryan GT. Absorption of C^{14}-labeled tryptophan, its metabolites, glycine, and glucose by the urinary bladder of the mouse. *Invest Urol* 1966;3:577–585.
66. Ganong W. *Review of Medical Physiology.* San Francisco: Lange Medical Publications, 1969.
67. Jaques L. Heparin: a unique misunderstood drug. *Trends Pharmacol Sci* 1982;3:289–291.
68. Cohen RA, Weisbrod RM. Endothelium inhibits norepinephrine release from adrenergic nerves of rabbit carotid artery. *Am J Physiol* 1988; 254:H871–H878.
69. Knighton D, Schumerth S, Fliegel V. Environmental regulation of macrophage angiogenesis. In: Rifkin D, Klagsbrun M, eds. *Current Communications in Molecular Biology: Angiogenesis Mechanisms and Pathobiology*. New York: Cold Spring Harbor Laboratory, 1987;150–154.
70. Stein B, Israel D, Cohen M. Pathogenesis of coronary occlusion. *Hosp Pract* 1988;April:87–99.

Interstitial Cystitis, edited by Grannum R. Sant.
Lippincott–Raven Publishers, Philadelphia ©1997.

CHAPTER 14

Bladder Cell Activation and Mucosal Immunity in Interstitial Cystitis

Monica Liebert

Urothelial cells, which form the transitional epithelium that lines the urinary tract from the renal pelvis through the ureters, into the bladder, and through the internal portion of the urethra, serve important protective functions in the body. Urothelial cells serve as a barrier between the urine and the rest of the body. Toxic materials as well as bacteria are sometimes present in the urine and would have dire effects on the bladder and the body if allowed to enter the body. The surface of the bladder is lined by this urothelial cell barrier, which prevents these potentially damaging materials from reaching the body. Besides this barrier function, urothelial cells, like many other epithelial cells in the body, are also a part of a mucosal immune system.

Interstitial cystitis (IC) is a disease of the urinary bladder characterized by pain, frequency, and urgency in the absence of a known infectious etiology (1,2). There is evidence for defective barrier functioning of urothelial cells in at least some patients with IC (3–5). The focus of this chapter is to review the literature on mucosal immunity in the bladder and to explore the role of urothelial mucosal immunity in IC.

MUCOSAL IMMUNITY IN THE NORMAL SKIN

Local immune/irritant/allergic reactions have been studied extensively in skin, and the local action of cytokines has been implicated in these reactions. Cytokines are a group of small-molecular-weight proteins that have potent and profound biological effects on the cells sensitive to them (6). Cytokines often act locally, either in an autocrine fashion (that is, acting on the cell that produces it) or paracrine fashion (acting on nearby cells; 6). In the skin, many cytokines are produced or released by the keratinocyte (7–13), including interleukins (IL) IL-1α, IL-1β, IL-3, IL-6, IL-8, granulocyte/macrophage colony-stimulating factor (GM-CSF), macrophage colony-stimulating factor (M-CSF), and tumor necrosis factor α (TNF-α). Cytokines are thought to act in a "network," with one cytokine stimulating or inhibiting the production of others; the net effect on any cell results from the local concentration of various cytokines and other stimuli in the environment (6,14,15).

A paradigm of the cytokine-mediated responses in skin is the response of skin to urushiol, the active component in poison ivy (7,8). Initial exposure activates expression of adherence receptors in the endothelium, induces expression of chemotactic cytokines such as IL-8 by keratinocytes, ad causes white blood cell margination in vessels and leukocyte migration into the tissue. Later, these migratory immune cells are retained at the site as a result of the action of TNF-α and interferon-γ (IFN-γ), which cause the expression of "activation" antigens such as HLA class II (or HLA-DR) and intercellular adherence molecule-1 (ICAM-1) on keratinocytes. These antigens serve to activate and bind leukocytes, especially lymphocytes, within the lesion. At this point, keratinocytes may also produce other cytokines, such as IL-1, IL-6, and/or TNF-α, that increase the leukocyte response (9,10). As the reaction resolves, the levels of keratinocyte ICAM-1 fall, followed by a reduction in the infiltrating inflammatory cells (7,8). Keratinocyte activation and cytokine generation are central to these events.

Cytokines themselves may modulate the cytokine cascade. For example, transforming growth factor β (TGF-β) is known to have immunosuppressive activity (16) and to inhibit IL-1 stimulation of IL-6 monocyte production (17). However, TGF-β and IL-1 both stimulate production of IL-6 in chondrocytes (18). The TGF-β inhibits the expression of the IL-1 receptor in murine leukocytes (19).

M. Liebert: Department of Urology, The University of Texas M.D. Anderson Cancer Center, Houston Texas 77030.

A recently identified cytokine, IL-10, has broad inhibitory activities similar to those of TGF-β: IL-10 inhibits the synthesis and production of IFN-γ, IL-2, IL-3, and GM-CSF production by lymphocytes (20). Furthermore, IL-10 has profound inhibitory effects the antigen-presenting functions of macrophages and dendritic cells as a result of inhibiting cytokine generation and alterations in the surface antigen displays of these cells (20–25). Expression of IL-10 appears to regulate itself, possibly by feedback inhibition (20). Thus, the cytokine cascade is a complex response that can include both enhancing and suppressive actions. The local response at any given time is likely to depend on the overall effect of the local cytokine concentrations (6,11,14,15).

MUCOSAL IMMUNITY IN NORMAL BLADDER

Normal urothelial cells also respond via a cytokine cascade when appropriately stimulated. Using cultured normal urothelial cells, we have shown that urothelial cells respond to cytokine stimulation by cell surface expression of the activation antigens HLA-DR and ICAM-1 (26,27). Similar results of ICAM-1 and HLA-DR expression were observed following stimulation of intact ureteral samples in short-term tissue culture (26). Furthermore, cultured urothelial cells produce cytokines such as IL-1α and IL-8 in response to IFN-γ and TNF-α stimulation (26,28). A model for urothelial activation in shown in Fig. 1.

Activation antigens and cytokine generation by normal urothelial cells have also been observed in patients. In a series of papers, Svanborg and her colleagues have shown that urinary levels of IL-6 and IL-8 are associated with bacterial cystitis (29–34). Furthermore, urothelial cells were implicated as the source of cytokine production (29,32–34). One study in which bacteria were introduced into the bladders of normal women showed that urinary IL-8 levels were coincident with pyuria (29). *In vitro* experiments from the same workers showed that human bladder cancer cell lines were induced to produce IL-8 in response to stimulation by *Escherichia coli* (34).

The clinical use of Bacillus Calmette-Guérin (BCG) for the treatment of bladder cancer also has provided information on urothelial responses to bacterial stimulation. Increased HLA-DR expression after BCG administration has been reported not only on bladder tumor cells but also on surrounding normal cells (35–37). A more recent study also reported increased expression of ICAM-1 on both bladder cancer cells and normal urothelial cells after BCG treatment (38). Because the levels of both HLA-DR and ICAM-1 are low on tumor cells and normal urothelial cells before treatment, induction of antigen expression on these cells is related to the treatment. Furthermore, cytokines IFN-γ (39), IL-1, IL-2, and TNF-α (40,41) are found in the urine shortly after BCG administration. Consistent with the existence of a homeostatic regulation of cytokines, an inhibitor of IL-2 was also detected in urine in response to BCG treatment (41). Although infiltrating leukocytes will contribute to cytokine generation, it is clear that initial responses are mediated by urothelial cells and that urothelial cells may continue to contribute to the cytokine response throughout treatment.

MUCOSAL IMMUNITY IN INTERSTITIAL CYSTITIS

As noted in the previous discussion, urothelial cells are normally HLA-DR- and ICAM-1-negative but can express both of these antigens in response to appropriate stimulation. Consequently, expression of HLA-DR or ICAM-1 on urothelial cells suggests that a stimulus is present. Christmas and Bottazzo observed expression of HLA-DR on urothelial cells in 20 of 22 patients with interstitial cystitis (42). In our own studies, we also observed that 13 of 16 patients with interstitial cystitis expressed HLA-DR on urothelial cells (27). However, only three of these patients expressed ICAM-1, in marked contrast to our previous studies of urothelial activation in response to cytokine stimulation using short-term culture of ureteral samples (26) or cultured normal urothelial cells (27), and in contrast to the observation of expression of both ICAM-1 and HLA-DR on urothelial cells of patients treated with BCG (35-38). A graph demonstrating this contrasting expression is shown in Fig. 2. These data suggest that urothelial activation is present in interstitial cystitis but that this response is different from the response observed after IFN-γ and TNF-α treatment or after BCG treatment.

Many investigators have searched for urinary mediators that may be involved in the urothelial activation in interstitial cystitis. The results have been contradictory and confusing. Martins and her co-workers were able to detect urinary IL-1 in patients with bacterial cystitis but not in patients with interstitial cystitis (43). Urinary IL-6 was detected in a group of self-identified patients with interstitial cystitis (44), in whom IL-6 levels correlated with pain scores. In this study, the investigators performed *in situ* hybridization for IL-6 mRNA and were able to show urothelial expression of IL-6 mRNA in at least one sample. However, in another study using National Institutes of Arthritis, Diabetes, and Digestive and Kidney Diseases (NIDDK) diagnostic criteria (1,2) to identify eligible patients, urinary IL-6 was observed in only six of 54 interstitial cystitis patients (45). In addition, we were also unable to identify IL-6 mRNA by reverse-transcriptase polymerase chain reaction in specimens from patients with interstitial cystitis (28). Elgebaly and her co-workers reported the presence of a chemotactic factor in the urine of patients with intersti-

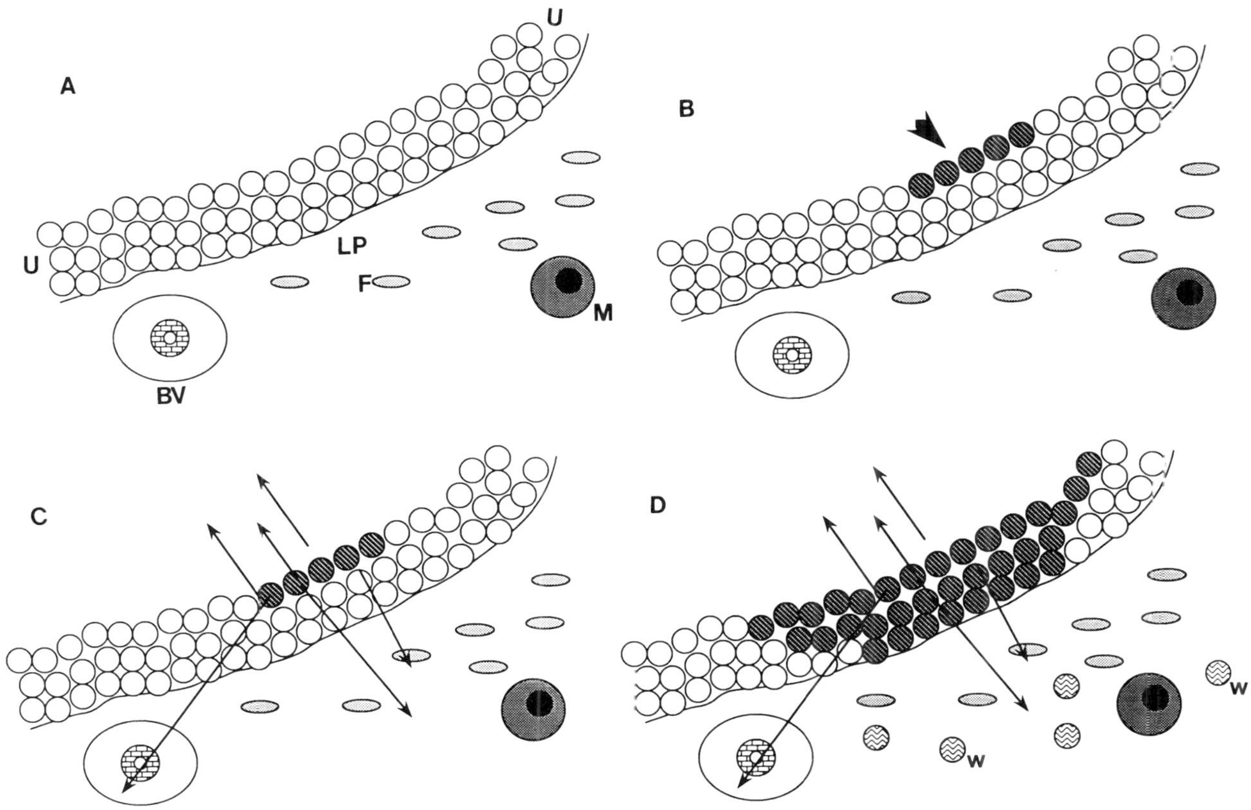

FIG. 1. A model for the mucosal immune cascade within the urinary bladder. **(A)** The normal bladder, marking urothelial cells (U); lamina propria (LP); interstitial fibroblasts (F); resident mast cells (M); and blood vessels (BV). **(B)** Initial activation. Stimulus *(arrowhead)* activates surface urothelial cells *(shaded)*. Such activated urothelial cells will express activation antigens (HLA-DR and ICAM-1). **(C)** Activated urothelial cells produce and release cytokines that diffuse into the local environment *(arrows)*. **(D)** High local concentrations of cytokines activate other local urothelial cells *(shading)* and stimulate cytokine production by other cells such as fibroblasts and release of granules by mast cells; activate endothelial cells in blood vessels causing them to express their own activation antigens and release cytokines; and cause influx of white blood cells (w) into the area. Over time, with reduction in the stimulus, this cascade should resolve (7, 8, 10, 12, 13, 26–41).

tial cystitis (46); however, Felsen and her collaborators were unable to reproduce this finding (45). Felsen's results are consistent with our studies using reverse transcriptase polymerase chain reaction to detect mRNA for cytokines, in which fewer specimens from patients with interstitial cystitis were positive for IL-8 (a major chemotactic cytokine) than were control specimens (28). The presence of an IL-2 inhibitor was noted in the urine of interstitial cystitis patients (52). The levels of IL-2 inhibitor were not useful diagnostically because they did not differ from those found in patients with other types of cystitis.

Other inflammatory mediators in the urine of interstitial cystitis patients have also been evaluated. Lynes and his co-workers described increased levels of prostaglandin E_2 in the urine of patients with interstitial cystitis (47). However, Felsen and her colleagues were unable to reproduce this finding (45). Urinary levels of eosinophilic cationic protein, a product of mast cells, were reported to be increased in patients with interstitial cystitis (48,49); however, a more recent study failed to reproduce these findings (50). More recent studies have utilized the NIDDK criteria for diagnosis of interstitial cystitis (1,2). These stricter diagnostic criteria may result in stricter patient selection than those in previous studies.

Finally, an enzymatically active protease, kallikrein, was detected in higher levels in the urine of patients with interstitial cystitis than in controls (51). Active proteases may disturb the integrity of urothelial cells and lead to urothelial activation. Alternatively, active proteases may enzymatically activate other molecules contributing to urothelial activation. No consistent urinary mediator of inflammation has been identified in interstitial cystitis to explain the unusual urothelial cell antigenic profile (high expression of HLA-DR with little expression of ICAM-1) (27) that has been described.

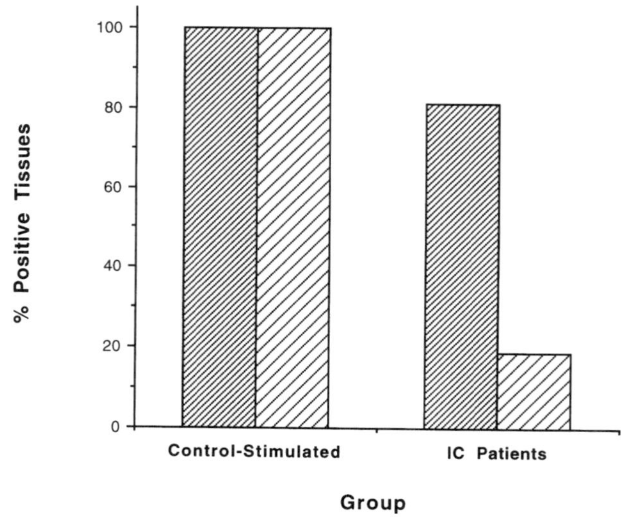

FIG. 2. Expression of activation antigens on urothelial cells. This figure represents the expression of HLA-DR (heavy cross-hatching) and ICAM-1 (light cross-hatching) on normal control urothelial cells after cytokine stimulation either in culture (26,27) or after BCG treatment (36–38). In contrast, the expression of HLA-DR is frequently observed, but the expression of ICAM-1 is reduced in interstitial cystitis specimens. (Adapted from reference 27, with permission.)

SUMMARY

Urothelial cells are part of the larger epithelial mucosal immune system and are capable of responding to various stimuli by the expression of cell surface activation markers (HLA-DR and ICAM-1) and the generation of cytokines (26–40). The cytokine cascade induced by activation of the urothelial cells leads to a protective leukocyte response in the bladder and, if necessary, in the rest of the body. The function of urothelial HLA-DR and ICAM-1 is less well understood, although a recent report indicates that bladder cancer cells are able to present antigens to immune cells in a further induction of the specific immune system (53). Normal urothelial cells may have the same or similar capability under specific circumstances. Antigen presentation is facilitated by functioning HLA-DR and ICAM-1, so the unusual phenotype in IC patients (expression of HLA-DR without ICAM-1 expression; 27) may result in abnormal function.

The expression of the HLA-DR activation antigen but not the ICAM-1 activation antigen on urothelial cells from patients with interstitial cystitis indicates that an unusual, if not abnormal, urothelial activation is present in interstitial cystitis (27). Our preliminary finding, using reverse transcriptase polymerase chain reaction for cytokine mRNA in bladder biopsies, that fewer patients with interstitial cystitis have detectable IL-8 than do normal controls, also supports an unusual, if not abnormal, urothelial cytokine response in interstitial cystitis (28).

Autoimmunity has long been suspected as a contributing, if not causal, factor in interstitial cystitis (54,55). Interstitial cystitis has been associated with some other autoimmune disorders, such as lupus (56) and Sjögren's syndrome (57). Several animal models have been explored based on an autoimmune response (reviewed in 55). In spite of the active research and interest in this hypothesis, no clear indication of an autoimmune cause of interstitial cystitis has been observed. Autoimmunity in IC is extensively reviewed in Chapter 6.

The concept that interstitial cystitis is a group of disorders with multiple etiologies has been emerging. The introduction of the NIDDK diagnostic criteria (1,2) may have resulted in a stratification of patients that did not exist previously. For example, Erickson and her colleagues have identified some stratification variables for patients with interstitial cystitis based on bladder volume, presentation, presence of inflammation, and response to therapeutic hydrodistention (58). Although this study included a small number of patients, these observations are encouraging in that specific subgroups may be identified that have common pathologic features and potentially common etiology.

Finally, the role of bacteria and the urothelial responses to bacteria in interstitial cystitis must be explored. Although the diagnosis of interstitial cystitis requires the exclusion of bacterial or viral cystitis (1,2), low levels of bacteria and fungi can be found in greater frequency in urine from patients with interstitial cystitis than in that from controls (59). As shown by Svanborg, the response to bacterial challenge is genetically influenced in mice (60) and humans (61). Thus, the unusual urothelial response observed in interstitial cystitis (27) may be a reflection of a genetically controlled aberrant immune response to small numbers of normally nonpathogenic bacteria or other stimuli.

Although many questions remain to be answered, research on interstitial cystitis has significantly increased our understanding of the role of the urothelial cell in mucosal immunity.

Acknowledgments

The author thanks Sunita Patterson for her editorial assistance. This work was supported in part by grant R01-DK44804 from the National Institutes of Arthritis, Diabetes, Digestive and Kidney Diseases, National Institutes of Health.

REFERENCES

1. Gillenwater JY, Wein AJ. Summary of the National Institute of Arthritis, Diabetes, Digestive and Kidney Diseases Workshop on Interstitial Cystitis, National Institutes of Health, Bethesda, Maryland, August 28–29, 1987. *J Urol* 1988;140:203–206.
2. Hanno P, Levin RM, Monson FC, Teuscher C, Zhou ZZ, Ruggieri M,

Whitmore K, Wein AJ. Diagnosis of interstitial cystitis. *J Urol* 1990; 143:278–281.
3. Parsons CL, Lilly JD, Stein P. Epithelial dysfunction in nonbacterial cystitis (interstitial cystitis). *J Urol* 1991;145:732–735.
4. Chelsky MJ, Rosen SI, Knight LC, Maurer AH, Hanno PM, Ruggieri MR. Bladder permeability in interstitial cystitis is similar to that of normal volunteers: Direct measurement by transvesical absorption of 99m-technicium-diethylenetriaminepentaacetic acid. *J Urol* 1994;151: 346–349.
5. Parsons CL, Boychuk D, Jones S, Hurst R, Callahan H. Bladder surface glycosaminoglycans: an epithelial permeability barrier. *J Urol* 1990; 143:139–142.
6. Balkwill FR, Burke F. The cytokine network. *Immunol Today* 1989;10:299–304.
7. Griffiths CE, Barker JN, Kunkel S., and Nickoloff, B.J. Modulation of leucocyte adhesion molecules, a T-cell chemotaxin (IL- 8) and a regulatory cytokine (TNF-alpha) in allergic contact dermatitis (*Rhus* dermatitis). *Br J Dermatol* 1991;124:519–526.
8. Nickoloff BJ, Griffiths CE, Barker JN. The role of adhesion molecules, chemotactic factors, and cytokines in inflammatory and neoplastic skin disease—1990 update. *J Invest Dermatol* 1990;94(Suppl): 151S–157S.
9. Norris DA. Cytokine modulation of adhesion molecules in the regulation of immunologic cytotoxicity of epidermal targets. *J Invest Dermatol* 1990;95(Suppl):111S–120S.
10. Kupper TS. The activated keratinocyte: a model for inducible cytokine production by non-bone marrow-derived cells in cutaneous inflammatory and immune responses. *J Invest Dermatol* 1990;94(Suppl): 146S–150S.
11. Ansel J, Perry P, Brown J, Damm D, Phan T, Hart C, Luger T, Hefeneider S. Cytokine modulation of keratinocyte cytokines. *J Invest Dermatol* 1990;94(Suppl):101S–107S.
12. Luger TA, Schwarz T. Evidence of an epidermal cytokine network. *J Invest Dermatol* 1990;95:100S–104S.
13. McKenzie RC, Sauder DN. The role of keratinocyte cytokines in inflammation and immunity. *J Invest Dermatol* 1990;95(Suppl): 105S–107S.
14. Arai KI, Lee F, Miyajima A, Miyatake S, Arai N, Yokota T. Cytokines: coordinators of immune and inflammatory responses. *Annu Rev Biochem* 1990;59:783–836.
15. Arend WP, Dayer JM. Cytokines and cytokine inhibitors or antagonists in rheumatoid arthritis. *Arthritis Rheum* 1990;33:305–315.
16. Wahl SM, McCartney-Francis N, Mergenhagen SE. Inflammatory and immunomodulatory roles of TGF-beta. *Immunol Today* 1989;10: 258–261.
17. Musso T, Espinoza-Delgado I, Pulkki K, Gusella GL, Longo DL, Varesio L. Transforming growth factor beta downregulates interleukin-1 (IL-1)-induced IL-6 production by human monocytes. *Blood* 1990; 76:2466–2469.
18. Guerne PA, Carson DA, Lotz M. IL-6 production by human articular chondrocytes. Modulation of its synthesis by cytokines, growth factors, and hormones *in vitro*. *J Immunol* 1990;144:499–505.
19. Dubois CM, Ruscetti FW, Palaszynski EW, Falk LA, Oppenheim JJ, Keller JR. Transforming growth factor beta is a potent inhibitor of interleukin 1 (IL-1) receptor expression: proposed mechanism of inhibition of IL-1 action. *J Exp Med* 1990;172:737–744.
20. Moore KW, O'Garra A, de Waal Malefyt R, Vieira P, Mosmann TR. Interleukin-10. *Annu Rev Immunol* 1993;11:165–190.
21. de Waal Malefyt R, Yssel H, Roncarolo MG, Spits H, de Vries JE. Interleukin-10. *Curr Opin Immunol* 1992;4:314–320.
22. Fiorentino DF, Zlotnik A, Mosmann TR, Howard M, O'Garra A. IL-10 inhibits cytokine production by activated macrophages. *J Immunol* 1991;147:3815–3822.
23. Spits H, de Waal Malefyt R. Functional characterization of human IL-10. *Int Arch Allergy Immunol* 1992;99:8–15.
24. Howard M, O'Garra A, Ishida H, de Waal Malefyt R, de Vries J. Biological properties of interleukin 10. *J Clin Immunol* 1992;12: 239–247.
25. Howard M, O'Garra A. Biological properties of interleukin 10. *Immunol Today* 1992;13:198–200.
26. Liebert M, Wedemeyer G, Abruzzo LV, Kunkel SL, Hammerberg C, Cooper KD, Grossman HB. Stimulated urothelial cells produce cytokines and express an activated cell surface antigenic phenotype. *Semin Urol* 1991;9:124–130.
27. Liebert M, Wedemeyer G, Stein JA, Washington R, Faerber G, Flint A, Grossman HB. Evidence for urothelial cell activation in interstitial cystitis. *J Urol* 1993;149:470–475.
28. Liebert M, Wedemeyer G, Stein J, Chung M, Hubbel A, Faerber G, Grossman HB. Cytokine profiles in interstitial cystitis. *J Urol* 1994; 151:283A.
29. Agace WW, Hedges SR, Ceska M, Svanborg C. Interleukin-8 and the neutrophil response to mucosal gram-negative infection. *J Clin Invest* 1993;92:780–785.
30. Hedges S, Stenquist K, Lidin-Janson G, Martinell J, Sandberg T, Svanborg C. Comparison of urine and serum concentrations of interleukin-6 in women with acute pyelonephritis of asymptomatic bacteriuria *J Infect Dis* 1992;166:653–656.
31. Benson M, Jodal U, Andreasson A, Karlsson A, Rydberg J, Svanborg C. Interleukin 6 response to urinary tract infection in childhood. *Pediatr Infect Dis J* 1994;13:612–616.
32. Svanborg C, Agace W, Hedges S, Lindstedt R, Svensson ML. Bacterial adherence and mucosal cytokine production. *Ann NY Acad Sci* 1994; 730:162–181.
33. Hedges S, Agace W, Svensson M, Sjogren A-C, Ceska M, Svanborg C. Uroepithelial cells are part of a mucosal cytokine network. *Infect Immun* 1994;62:2315–2321.
34. Agace W, Hedges S, Andersson U, Andersson J, Ceska M, Svanborg C. Selective cytokine production by epithelial cells following exposure to *Eschericia coli*. *Infect Immun* 1993;61:602–609.
35. Prescott S, James K, Busuttil A, Hargreave TB, Chisholm GD, Smyth JF. HLA-DR expression by high grade superficial bladder cancer treated with BCG. *Br J Urol* 1989;63:264–269.
36. Leong AS, Wannakrairot P, Jose J, Milios J. Bacillus Calmette-Guerin-treated superficial bladder cancer: correlation of morphology with immunophenotyping. *J Pathol* 1990;162:35–41.
37. Bohle A, Gerdes J, Ulmer AJ, Hofstetter AG, Flad HD. Effects of local Bacillus Calmette-Guerin therapy in patients with bladder carcinoma on immunocompetent cells of the bladder wall. *J Urol* 1990;144:53–58.
38. Jackson AM, Alexandroff AB, McIntyre M, Esuvaranathan KE, James K, Chisholm GD: Induction of ICAM-1 expression on bladder tumors by BCG immunotherapy. *J Clin Pathol* 1994;47:309–312.
39. Prescott S, James K, Hargreave TB, Chisholm GD, Smyth JF. Radioimmunoassay detection of interferon-gamma in urine after intravesical Evans BCG therapy. *J Urol* 1990;144:1248–1251.
40. Bohle A, Nowc C, Ulmer AJ, Musehold J, Gerdes J, Hofstetter AG, Flad HD. Elevations of cytokines interleukin-1, interleukin-2 and tumor necrosis factor in the urine of patients after intravesical Bacillus Calmette-Guerin immunotherapy. *J Urol* 1990;144:59–64.
41. Fleischmann JD, Toossi Z, Wentworth DB, Ratliff TL, Imbembo AL. Urinary interleukin production in patients receiving intravescial BCG therapy. *Cancer* 1989;64:1447–1454.
42. Christmas TJ, Bottazzo GF. Abnormal urothelial HLA-DR expression in interstitial cystitis. *Clin Exp Immunol* 1993;87:450–454.
43. Martins SM, Darlin DJ, Lad PM, Zimmern PE. Interleukin-1B: A clinically relevant urinary marker. *J Urol* 1994;151:1198–1201.
44. Lotz M, Villiger P, Hugli T, Koziol J, Zuraw BL. Interleukin-6 and interstitial cystitis. *J Urol* 1994;152:869–873.
45. Felsen D, Frye S, Trimble LA, Bavendam TG, Parsons CL, Sim Y, Vaughan ED. Inflammatory mediator profile in urine and bladder wash fluid of patients with interstitial cystitis. *J Urol* 1994; 152:355–361.
46. Elgebaly SA, Allam ME, Walzak MP, Oselinsky D, Gillies C, Ymasae H. Urinary neutrophil chemotactic factors in interstitial cystitis patients and a rabbit model of bladder inflammation. *J Urol* 1992;147: 1382–1387.
47. Lynes WL, Flynn SD, Shortliffe LD, Lemmers M, Zipser R, Roberts LJ, Stamey TA. Mast cell involvement in interstitial cystitis. *J Urol* 1987;138:746–752.
48. Lose G, Fradsen R, Holm-Bentzen M, Larsen S, Jacobsen F. Urine eosinophilic cationic protein in painful bladder disease. *Br J Urol* 1987;60:39–42.
49. Larsen S, Thompson SA, Hald T, Barnard RJ, Gilpin C, Dixon JS, Gosling JA. Mast cells in interstitial cystitis. *Br J Urol* 1982;54: 283–286.
50. Steinert BW, Diokno AC, Robingson JE, Mitchell BA. Complement C3, eosinophili cationic protein and symptom evaluation in interstitial cystitis. *J Urol* 1994;151:350–354.
51. Zuraw BL, Sugimoto S, Parsons CL, Hugli T, Lotz M, Koziol J. Acti-

vation of urinary kallikrein in patients with interstitial cystitis. *J Urol* 1994;152:874–878.

52. Shingleton WB, Fleischmann J. Urinary interleukin-2 inhibitor and the voiding symptoms in women patients with interstitial cystitis. *Semin Urol* 1991;9:120–123.
53. Lattime EC, Gomella LG, McCue PA. Murine bladder carcinoma cells present antigen to BCG-specific CD4[+] T-cells. *Cancer Res* 1992;52: 4286–4290.
54. Anderson JB, Parivar F, Lee G. The enigma of interstitial cystitis—an autoimmune disease? *Br J Urol* 1989;63:58–63.
55. Ratliff TL, Klutke CG, Hofmeister M, He F, Russel JH, Becich MJ. Role of the immune response in interstitial cystitis. *Clin Immunol Immunopathol* 1995;74:209–216.
56. De La Serna AR, Alarcon-Sogovia D. Chronic interstitial cystitis as an initial manifestation of systemic lupus erythematosis. *J Rheumatol* 1981;8:808–810.
57. Van De Merwe J, Kamerling R, Arendsen E, Mulder D, Hooijkaas H. Sjögren's syndrome in patients with interstitial cystitis. *J Rheumatol* 1993;20:962–966.
58. Erickson DR, Simon LJ, Belchis DA. Relationships between bladder inflammation and other clinical features in interstitial cystitis. *Urology* 1994;44:655–659.
59. Keay S, Schwalbe RS, Trifillis AL, Lovchik JC, Jacobs S, Warren JW. A prospective study of microorganisms in urine and bladder biopsies from interstitial cystitis patients and controls. *Urology* 1995;45: 223–229.
60. Agace W, Hedges S, Svanborg C. Lps genotype in the C57 black mouse background and its influence on the interleukin-6 response to *E. coli* urinary tract infection. *Scand J Immunol* 1992;35:531–538.
61. Lomberg H, Jodal U, Leffler H, De Man P, Svanborg C. Blood group non-secretors have an increased inflammatory response to urinary tract infection. *Scand J Infect Dis* 1992;24:77–83.

Interstitial Cystitis, edited by Grannum R. Sant.
Lippincott–Raven Publishers, Philadelphia ©1997.

CHAPTER 15

Urinary Markers of Interstitial Cystitis

Deborah R. Erickson

Interstitial cystitis (IC) is a multifactorial syndrome characterized by pelvic/perineal pain with urinary frequency/urgency. This chapter describes research in identifying urinary markers for IC. Markers may be considered for three different purposes: (a) to diagnose IC, (b) to support a certain theory of pathophysiology, (c) to predict or follow response to different treatments.

DIAGNOSTIC MARKERS OF IC

It is unlikely that a single marker to diagnose or exclude IC will be identified. One reason is that IC is a multifactorial syndrome that probably has several different etiologies. It is unlikely that a single marker would identify them all. A second reason is that, even if such a marker did exist, there is currently no "gold standard" by which to evaluate the marker's accuracy (1). The closest approximation to a gold standard is the National Institute of Diabetes, Digestive and Kidney Diseases (NIDDK) criteria (for the original criteria see ref. 2; the revised criteria are listed in refs. 1 and 3). However, the purpose of these criteria is to improve uniformity among patients in IC research studies. Uniformity requires stringent criteria, which may exclude a significant number of patients with true IC. For both of these reasons, identifying a diagnostic marker for the entire spectrum of IC does not seem feasible at this time.

MARKERS TO SUPPORT SPECIFIC PATHOPHYSIOLOGICAL THEORIES

The various pathophysiological theories for IC are described elsewhere in this book. For several of these theories, specific urinary markers can be predicted. If the predicted markers are found in a subset of IC patients, then further research can be focused on that subset. This chapter includes several markers with relevance to different etiologic theories.

MARKERS OF TREATMENT RESPONSE

Successful identification of these markers would be quite useful. Because many different treatments for IC are available, a marker with good predictive value for response to a specific treatment would be extremely helpful. Also, markers that change in response to individual treatments can be valuable for research studies on specific pathophysiologic theories. The current knowledge of markers for treatment response is summarized in this chapter.

MAST CELL RELATED MARKERS

Background

Mast cells are well known to participate in allergic reactions by releasing the contents of their cellular granules. The classic stimulus for degranulation is binding of antigen to IgE antibody on the mast cell surface. However, a variety of other stimuli can also cause degranulation. These include acetylcholine, bradykinin and other peptides, iodinated contrast and other drugs, hormones, and trauma (4,5). The granules contain many substances relevant to the symptoms of IC. A partial list includes histamine, serotonin, prostaglandins (especially D), leukotrienes, lymphokines, and chemotactic factors (especially for eosinophils).

Mast cells are found in bladder biopsies of some patients with IC. The detrusor muscle is the most commonly described location, but the lamina propria and epithelium may also be involved. Mast cells are not specific for IC and can also be found in other bladder dis-

D. R. Erickson: Division of Urology, The Milton S. Hershey Medical Center, Pennsylvania State University College of Medicine, Hershey, Pennsylvania 17033-0850.

eases (6). An important consideration for IC research is that routine tissue fixation and staining do not provide a complete assessment of mast cell activity. One reason is that the granules are the targets for histochemical stains, so degranulated mast cells are often missed. Another reason is that the mucosal type of mast cell requires special fixation and staining techniques to be visualized. Therefore, in reading reports of mastocytosis in IC, it is essential to know what techniques were used (for reviews see refs. 4 and 5).

Several mast cell-related urinary markers have been studied. These include histamine, its metabolites methylhistamine and 1,4-methylimidazoleacetic acid (1,4-MIAA), and prostaglandin D_2. Also, because mast cells secrete an eosinophil chemotactic factor, eosinophil products (including eosinophil cationic protein and major basic protein) have also been evaluated.

Mast Cell Mediator Research

Yun et al. compared random-voided urine histamine levels in healthy controls and IC patients who met the original NIDDK criteria (7). Histamine levels were similar for the two groups, whether expressed as histamine concentration or normalized to creatinine. However, after bladder distention, the IC patients had a significant increase in urinary histamine/creatinine ratio relative to predistention values. In healthy controls, pre- and postdistention histamine/creatinine ratios were similar. These results suggest that distention stimulated histamine release in the IC patient group.

El-Mansoury et al. compared IC and control urine for both histamine and methylhistamine, its major metabolite (8). Subjects avoided foods containing bioactive amines for 24 hr before urine collection. Both methylhistamine and histamine concentrations were increased in the urine of IC patients relative to those in controls. However, the increase was much greater for methylhistamine than for histamine. Neither marker correlated with overall disease severity in IC patients, but these may be useful markers for indentification and further research on a specific subset of IC patients.

Felsen et al. compared IC patients (one group meeting the NIDDK criteria and another group that met the criteria except for glomerulations) and healthy controls for urinary prostaglandin D_2, the major prostaglandin from mast cells (9). Prostaglandin $F_{2\alpha}$ (a metabolite of D_2) was also assayed. Prostaglandin levels (normalized to urinary creatinine) were similar for both groups of IC patients and healthy controls.

Other investigators have sought correlations between the number of mast cells on bladder biopsy and various urinary markers. Lynes et al. found that patients with pyuria had higher counts of degranulated mast cells in the detrusor than patients without pyuria (10). Holm-Bentzen et al. compared IC patients on the basis of the number of detrusor mast cells (more than or fewer than 28 mast cells/mm^2). The high-mast cell group had increased 24-hr urinary 1,4-MIAA excretion (11) and increased urine eosinophil cationic protein concentration (12,13).

Because mast cells secrete a chemotactic factor for eosinophils, eosinophil products have been evaluated in IC. One product, major basic protein, was evaluated in urine and serum of IC patients and healthy controls. Urine levels were barely detectable in both groups, and the serum levels for IC patients were within the normal range (10). Another product of interest is eosinophil cationic protein. Lose et al. found that urine eosinophil cationic protein concentration decreased, along with symptoms, when patients were treated with subcutaneous heparin (14). In contrast, Steinert et al. reported that eosinophil cationic protein concentration did not correlate with symptom severity in IC and, in fact, did not differ significantly for IC patients and healthy controls (15). One reason for this difference may be that Lose's patients all had severe detrusor mastocytosis (>50 cells/mm^2), which is found in a minority of IC patients overall. Future studies may reveal that elevated urinary eosinophil cationic protein and/or severe detrusor mastocytosis can predict a positive response to subcutaneous heparin treatment.

OTHER INFLAMMATORY MEDIATORS

Arachidonic Acid Metabolites

Each of the several arachidonic acid metabolites (prostaglandins, thromboxanes, leukotrienes) has a variety of effects on different tissues. In many cases two prostaglandins will have opposing effects. Several of these effects could be relevant to IC, but a complete review is beyond the scope of this chapter. Concerning eicosanoids as urinary markers for IC, Felsen et al. assayed urine and bladder wash fluid for prostaglandins E_2, D_2, and $F_{2\alpha}$ as well as thromboxane B_2. Subjects were IC patients who met the NIDDK criteria, a separate group who met the criteria except for glomerulations, and healthy controls. All of the urinary eicosanoid levels (normalized to creatinine) were similar for the three subject groups (9). In contrast, Lynes et al. found that IC patients had higher urinary prostaglandin E_2 (expressed per hour in timed first-morning specimens) than healthy controls (10). Also, among IC patients, those who responded well to bladder distention with oxychlorosene instillation had higher urinary prostaglandin E_2 levels than nonresponders. The difference between Lynes's and Felsen's results may be related to the methods of urine collection and normalization; another possibility is that Lynes's patient population may have included a larger proportion of patients with severe bladder inflammation. At this time, the role of prostoglandin E_2 as a marker in IC is still undetermined.

Interleukins

Interleukins are a family of cytokines that have integral roles in inflammatory/immune responses. A complete review of interleukin types and effects is beyond the scope of this chapter. The interleukins studied as urinary markers for IC are described below.

Interleukin-1β (IL-1β) is the first cytokine produced in the antigen recognition immune cascade (16). Martins et al. evaluated IL-1β in the urine of ten IC patients (NIDDK criteria), 40 healthy controls, and 33 patients with urologic diseases other than IC (16). They found that IL-1β levels (normalized to creatinine) were similar for IC patients and healthy controls but elevated in patients with bacterial cystitis and bladder tumors. After treatment of bacterial cystitis, urinary IL-1β levels returned to normal. These results suggested that IL-1β was a marker for infection or tumor rather than IC. Infection with fastidious organisms or low-count bacteriuria may have a role in some cases of IC, although routine urine cultures are by definition sterile (17–19). Urinary IL-1β may be useful as a marker for further studies on infection in a subset of IC patients.

Interleukin-2 (IL-2) is produced by activated T cells. It promotes growth and activation of several inflammatory cell types. Shingleton and Fleischmann tested IC patients' urine for an IL-2 inhibitor after observing that this inhibitor was present in the urine of patients with bacterial cystitis and bladder tumors (20). They found that 24 of 34 IC patients had elevated IL-2 inhibitor levels (normalized to creatinine). Among all patients considered as a group, there was no correlation between IL-2 inhibitor level and symptom score. However, when six individual patients were followed over time, IL-2 inhibitor levels tended to correlate with symptom scores. In a subsequent prospective study of ten IC patients, the same investigators followed symptom scores and urinary IL-2 inhibitor levels before and during treatment with nifedipine (21). Nine patients were evaluable after 4 months of nifedipine therapy, and all had urinary IL-2 inhibitor levels of zero or near zero. However, some patients continued to be symptomatic and even to have symptom score increases in spite of zero IL-2 inhibitor levels. This suggests that these patients' symptoms were not related to an IL-2-mediated immune response.

Interleukin-6 (IL-6) is expressed by many cell types including macrophages, lymphocytes, epithelial cells, and fibroblasts. It has a variety of proinflammatory effects. Felsen et al. used both bioassay and enzyme-linked immunosorbent assay (ELISA) techniques and found elevated urinary IL-6 levels in six of 54 patients who met the revised NIDDK criteria (9). Bladder wash fluid was negative for IL-6 in all subjects. Lotz et al., using a different bioassay, found that IC patients had significantly higher urinary IL-6 levels (normalized to creatinine) than healthy controls (22). They also found a significant positive correlation between urinary IL-6 levels and pain scores. Interleukin-6 was confirmed to be bladder derived by comparing voided and ureteral catheter-obtained urine in IC patients and by *in situ* hybridization for IL-6 mRNA on IC bladder tissue. Thus, IL-6 may be useful as a marker of active bladder inflammation. Comparison of urinary IL-6 levels and symptom scores before and after IC treatments may help to elucidate the mechanisms of specific treatments.

Tumor Necrosis Factor

Tumor necrosis factor (TNF) has several proinflammatory effects and also kills tumor cells. Felsen et al. measured urinary TNF by ELISA and bioassay (9). Most IC patients and controls had positive bioassay (cell kill). Interestingly, the group that lacked glomerulations but otherwise met the NIDDK criteria had the highest cytotoxic activity. The ELISA results were different from the bioassay results. With ELISA, many subjects were negative for TNF, and the positive subjects were clustered in the IC patients (both with and without glomerulations) rather than the healthy controls. Thus, the TNF immunogenic and urine cytotoxic properties in this study did not correlate with each other.

Neutrophil Chemotactic Activity

A variety of neutrophil chemotactic factors can be released from injured tissues. Walzak et al. studied urinary neutrophil chemotactic activity in (a) healthy controls, (b) controls with urologic disease other than IC, and (c) IC patients before and after dimethylsulfoxide (DMSO) treatment (23,24). There was no neutrophil chemotactic activity in the urine of healthy or non-IC diseased controls. Untreated IC patients had high urinary neutrophil chemotactic activity, which decreased to zero after treatment with DMSO. The DMSO alone did not alter neutrophil migration. A formal symptom evaluation was not performed, but patients were described as symptomatically improved after DMSO treatment (23). Thus, urinary neutrophil chemotactic activity was specific to untreated IC in these studies. An interesting question is whether this urinary marker also decreases after other types of IC treatment; if not, this would suggest a specific mechanism of action for DMSO.

Kallikrein

Kallikrein is a protease that cleaves kininogen, releasing bradykinin. Bradykinin has several effects that may be relevant to IC symptoms including pain, edema, and smooth muscle contraction. Zuraw et al. investigated urinary kallikrein in IC patients and normal controls (25). Mean urinary kallikrein activity (normalized to creatinine) was significantly higher for IC patients. Among the

IC patients, urinary kallikrein activity was associated with higher pain scores.

Kallikrein also was evaluated for ten IC patients before and after bladder distention. Five patients had symptomatic improvement 30 days after distention, and five had no improvement. The improved patients had high predistention urinary kallikrein activity, which decreased significantly after bladder distention. The unimproved patients had lower predistention urinary kallikrein activity, which did not change significantly after distention. Thus, in this study, urinary kallikrein activity was both a marker of disease activity and a predictive marker for symptom response to bladder distention. Because kallikrein tends to increase with inflammation, the predictive value for high urinary kallikrein activity is consistent with our report that patients with severe bladder inflammation had better symptom relief after distention than patients with mild inflammation (26).

MARKERS OF EPITHELIAL ABNORMALITIES

Background

Several investigators have focused on the role of the bladder epithelium in IC. A main theory is that the bladder epithelium is abnormally permeable, allowing urinary constituents to penetrate the bladder wall. The urinary factors may be normal (for example, hydrogen or potassium ions) or abnormal (allergens, toxins, etc.). It is unknown whether altered epithelial permeability is a primary cause of IC or an effect of one or more inflammatory mediators. It may turn out that both of these explanations are true for different subsets of IC patients.

Research to date on bladder permeability in IC has given varying results. For example, Tamm–Horsfall protein (which should be excluded by the epithelium) was identified within the epithelium by some investigators (27) but not by others (28,29). Patients with IC were reported to have increased absorption of intravesically instilled urea (30) but not of ^{99m}Tc-technetium diethylenetriaminepentaacetic acid (31,32). Parsons et al. described a clinical test in which patients had intravesical instillation of water followed by instillation of 0.4 M KCl (33). Water instillation was not painful, but KCl instillation was painful for 70% of IC patients. Intravesical KCl also caused pain for subjects with radiation cystitis but not for healthy controls, which suggests that this test may be identifying patients with epithelial dysfunction.

In regard to the structural aspects of bladder permeability, epithelial glycoconjugates have received the most attention. Negatively charged glycoconjugates (including glycosaminoglycans, mucins, and other glycoproteins) absorb water onto the bladder surface and maintain a permeability barrier. Epithelial glycoconjugates of IC and control bladders have been compared in several studies. The electron microscopic appearance was similar for IC and controls (34,35). On the other hand, biochemical analysis of glycosaminoglycans (GAGs) in epithelial scrapings showed different GAG types in IC than in controls (men with benign prostatic hyperplasia) (36). Moskowitz et al. raised a mouse antibody against a 51-kDa bladder epithelial glycoprotein and showed that normal human bladder epithelium stained strongly, whereas IC bladders had weak or absent staining (37). These results, as well as the urinary studies discussed below, suggest that bladder epithelial glycoconjugates are abnormal in at least a subset of IC patients. This is discussed in detail in Chapter 11.

Urinary Markers of Epithelial Dysfunction

A urinary marker for epithelial dysfunction *per se* has not been established. Gillespie found that IC patients had lower urinary tryptophan excretion (normalized to time in 24-hr collections) than healthy controls (38). She suggested that tryptophan is reabsorbed by the permeable bladder epithelium in IC. However, other mechanisms such as altered tryptophan production, metabolism, or absorption from the GI tract are also possible.

Several studies have investigated urinary glycoconjugate levels in IC. Parsons and Hurst compared IC patients, healthy controls, and spinal-cord-injured controls for urinary GAG and macromolecular uronate concentrations (39,40). The IC patients had lower concentrations of both substances than healthy controls. Spinal-cord-injured patients had an interesting result: their urinary GAG levels were similar to those of normal controls, but their macromolecular uronate levels were similar to those of IC patients. The differences between IC patients and healthy controls were significant when expressed either as concentration or normalized to creatinine. However, in most groups the data were more variable when normalized to creatinine (40).

In addition to GAGs, mucin glycoproteins are also decreased in the urine of interstitial cystitis patients. Shupp-Byrne et al. found that urinary excretion of a 51-kDa epithelial glycoprotein was lower in IC patients than in healthy controls (41). Consistently, we found that IC patients had lower urinary levels of a MUC-1 glycoprotein than healthy controls. The difference was significant both for glycoprotein concentration and when normalized to creatinine. Unlike the GAG results described above, normalizing the mucin glycoprotein concentrations to creatinine decreased variability (42).

For all of the above studies, mean urinary glycoconjugate levels were lower in IC patients than in healthy controls. It is currently unknown whether the changes in glycoconjugates are a cause or an effect of IC. These markers would not be useful for diagnosing IC because there is significant overlap between IC and control val-

TABLE 1. *Urinary markers in IC and their associations*

Marker (reference)	Association
1,4-MIAA[a] (11)	Positive association with detrusor mastocytosis
Eosinophil cationic protein (12,13)	Positive association with detrusor mastocytosis
Prostaglandin E_2 (10)	High levels before bladder distention were associated with symptom relief after distention and oxychlorosene instillation
Interleukin-1β (16)	High levels in bacterial cystitis, not IC
Interleukin-2 inhibitor (20,21)	Decreased after nifedipine treatment
Interleukin-6 (22)	Positive association with pain scores
Neutrophil chemotactic activity (23,24)	Decreased after DMSO[b] treatment
Kallikrein (25)	Positive association with pain scores; high levels before bladder distention were associated with symptom relief after distention

[a]1,4-Methylimidazoleacetic acid.
[b]Dimethylsulfoxide.

ues. However, they may be useful for identification and further research on a specific subset of IC patients with epithelial abnormalities.

BACTERIURIA

Bacterial cystitis is an exclusion criterion for IC (1–3). However, infection may be relevant for the pathophysiology in some cases. Patients with IC may be infected by a fastidious organism (19), or they may have an abnormal immune/allergic response to low levels of bacteria (including "normal" flora), bacterial fragments, or toxins. Thus, bacteriuria may be a useful marker to identify a subset of patients for further research studies including directed antibiotic therapy.

Wilkins et al. cultured urine (both catheterized and midstream specimens), urethral swab, and bladder biopsies in ten IC patients and six patients with similar symptoms but no glomerulations (18). Routine urine cultures for aerobic pathogens had been negative. Seven IC patients grew either *Gardnerella vaginalis* or *Lactobacillus* in the catheterized and midstream urine specimens. Five of these patients had identical organisms grown from their bladder biopsies. Of the six patients with IC-like symptoms but no glomerulations, four grew *Gardnerella vaginalis* in the midstream urine and urethral swab cultures. However, the significance of these positive cultures remained uncertain because the study did not include asymptomatic control women.

Keay et al. cultured urine (suprapubic aspiration or urethral catheterization) and bladder biopsies from 11 IC patients and seven controls undergoing cystoscopy for other urologic diseases (17). Six of the IC patients had positive urine cultures for various bacteria, cytomegalovirus, or *Torulopsis glabrata,* but none of the seven controls did. Results were similar when acridine orange staining was used to identify bacteriuria. Bladder biopsies were positive for two IC patients and grew the same organism found in the urine. Three controls (with negative urine cultures) had positive bladder biopsies for *Pseudomonas* or *Staphylococcus epidermidis.* The increased incidence of positive urine cultures in IC could be explained by two different mechanisms. First, infection may be the cause of IC in these patients. Alternatively, infection may reflect a damaged epithelium, which becomes colonized more easily than healthy epithelium.

SUMMARY

At this time, identification of a single diagnostic marker for IC does not seem feasible, primarily because IC is a spectrum of conditions rather than a single disease. However, several urinary markers have been identified that support specific etiologic theories. Markers have also been found to associate with other features or correlate with response to specific treatments. The presently known associations are summarized in Table 1. Urinary markers, both those presently known and those yet to be discovered, will be valuable for identifying specific subsets of IC patients and focusing future research on specific pathophysiologies and treatments.

REFERENCES

1. Hanno PM. Diagnosis of interstitial cystitis. *Urol Clin North Am* 1994;21:63–66.
2. Gillenwater JY, Wein AJ. Summary of the National Institute of Arthritis, Diabetes, Digestive and Kidney Diseases Workshop on Interstitial Cystitis, National Institutes of Health, Bethesda, Maryland, August 28–29, 1987. *J Urol* 1988;140:203–206.
3. Stryker GE. Special communication: KUH notes. *J Urol* 1989;142:139.
4. Theoharides TC, Sant GR. Bladder mast cell activation in interstitial cystitis. *Semin Urol* 1991;9:74–87.
5. Sant GR, Theoharides TC. The role of the mast cell in interstitial cystitis. *Urol Clin North Am* 1994;21:41–53.
6. Hanno PM, Levin RM, Monson FC, et al. Diagnosis of interstitial cystitis. *J Urol* 1990;143:278–281.
7. Yun SK, Laub DJ, Weese DL, Lad PM, Leach GE, Zimmern PE. Stimulated release of urine histamine in interstitial cystitis. *J Urol* 1992;148: 1145–1148.

8. El-Mansoury M, Boucher W, Sant GR, Theoharides TC. Increased urine histamine and methylhistamine in interstitial cystitis. *J Urol* 1994;152:350–353.
9. Felsen D, Frye S, Trimble LA, et al. Inflammatory mediator profile in urine and bladder wash fluid of patients with interstitial cystitis. *J Urol* 1994;152:355–361.
10. Lynes WL, Flynn SD, Shortliffe LD, et al. Mast cell involvement in interstitial cystitis. *J Urol* 1987;138:746–752.
11. Holm-Bentzen M, Sondergaard I, Hald T. Urinary excretion of a metabolite of histamine (1,4-methyl-imidazole-acetic-acid) in painful bladder disease. *Br J Urol* 1987;59:230–233.
12. Lose G, Frandsen B, Holm-Bentzen M, Larsen S, Jacobsen F. Urine eosinophil cationic protein in painful bladder disease. *Br J Urol* 1987; 60:39–42.
13. Frandsen B, Lose G, Holm-Bentzen M. Autorosette inhibition factor: a positive acute phase reactant in interstitial cystitis. *Eur Urol* 1988;14: 309–312.
14. Lose G, Frandsen B, Hojensgard JC, Jespersen J, Astrup T. Chronic interstitial cystitis: increased levels of eosinophil cationic protein in serum and urine and an ameliorating effect of subcutaneous heparin. *Scand J Urol Nephrol* 1983;17:159–161.
15. Steinert BW, Diokno AC, Robinson JE, Mitchell BA. Complement C3, eosinophil cationic protein and symptom evaluation in interstitial cystitis. *J Urol* 1994;151:350–354.
16. Martins SM, Darlin DJ, Lad PM, Zimmern PE. Interleukin-1β: a clinically relevant urinary marker. *J Urol* 1994;151:1198–1201.
17. Keay S, Schwalbe RS, Trifillis AL, Lovchik JC, Jacobs S, Warren JW. A prospective study of microorganisms in urine and bladder biopsies from interstitial cystitis patients and controls. *Urology* 1995;45: 223–229.
18. Wilkins EGL, Payne SR, Pead PJ, Moss ST, Maskell RM. Interstitial cystitis and the urethral syndrome: a possible answer. *Br J Urol* 1989; 64:39–44.
19. Domingue GJ, Ghoneim GM, Bost KL, Fermin C, Human LG. Dormant microbes in interstitial cystitis. *J Urol* 1995;153:1321–1326.
20. Shingleton WB, Fleischmann J. Urinary interleukin-2 inhibitor and the voiding symptoms in women patients with interstitial cystitis. *Semin Urol* 1991;9:120–123.
21. Fleischmann JD, Huntley HN, Shingleton WB, Wentworth DB. Clinical and immunological response to nifedipine for the treatment of interstitial cystitis. *J Urol* 1991;146:1235–1239.
22. Lotz M, Villiger P, Hugli T, Koziol J, Zuraw B. Interleukin-6 and interstitial cystitis. *J Urol* 1994;152:869–873.
23. Walzak MP, Elgebaly SA, Allam ME, Oselinsky D. Leukocyte chemotactic factors in interstitial cystitis: a possible biological marker of the disease. *Semin Urol* 1991;9:131–135.
24. Elgebaly SA, Allam ME, Walzak MP, Oselinsky D, Gillies C, Yamase H. Urinary neutrophil chemotactic factors in interstitial cystitis patients and a rabbit model of bladder inflammation. *J Urol* 1992;147:1382–1387.
25. Zuraw BL, Sugimoto S, Parsons CL, Hugli T, Lotz M, Koziol J. Activation of urinary kallikrein in patients with interstitial cystitis. *J Urol* 1994;152:874–878.
26. Erickson DR, Simon LJ, Belchis DA. Relationships between bladder inflammation and other clinical features in interstitial cystitis. *Urology* 1994;44:655–659.
27. Fowler JE, Lynes WL, Lau JLT, Ghosh L, Mounzer A. Interstitial cystitis is associated with intraurothelial Tamm–Horsfall protein. *J Urol* 1988;140:1385–1389.
28. Stone AR, Vogelsang P, Miller CH, MacDermott JP. Tamm–Horsfall protein as a marker in interstitial cystitis. *J Urol* 1992;148:1406–1408.
29. Stein PC, Santamaria PJ, Kurtz SB, Parsons CL. Evaluation of urothelial Tamm–Horsfall protein and serum antibody as a potential diagnostic marker for interstitial cystitis. *J Urol* 1993;150:1405–1408.
30. Parsons CL, Lilly JD, Stein P. Epithelial dysfunction in nonbacterial cystitis (interstitial cystitis). *J Urol* 1991;145:732–735.
31. Chelsky MJ, Rosen SI, Knight LC, Maurer AH, Hanno PM, Ruggieri MR. Bladder permeability in interstitial cystitis is similar to that of normal volunteers: direct measurement by transvesical absorption of 99m-technetium-diethylenetriaminepentaacetic acid. *J Urol* 1994;151: 346–349.
32. Hohlbrugger G. Re: Bladder permeability in interstitial cystitis is similar to that of normal volunteers (Letter). *J Urol* 1994;152:2105–2106.
33. Parsons CL, Stein PC, Bidair M, Lebow D. Abnormal sensitivity to intravesical potassium in interstitial cystitis and radiation cystitis. *Neurol Urodyn* 1994;13:515–520.
34. Dixon JS, Holm-Bentzen M, Gilpin CJ, et al. Electron microscopic investigation of the bladder urothelium and glycocalyx in patients with interstitial cystitis. *J Urol* 1986;135:621–625.
35. Nickel JL, Emerson L, Cornish J. The bladder mucus (glycosaminoglycan) layer in interstitial cystitis. *J Urol* 1993;149:716–718.
36. Holm-Bentzen M, Ammitzboll T, Hald T. Glycosaminoglycans on the surface of the human urothelium: a preliminary report. *Neurol Urodyn* 1986;5:519–523.
37. Moskowitz M, Byrne DS, Callahan HJ, Parsons CL, Valderrama E, Moldwin RM. Decreased expression of a glycoprotein component of bladder surface mucin (GP1) in interstitial cystitis. *J Urol* 1994;151:343–345.
38. Gillespie L. Metabolic appraisal of the effects of dietary modification on hypersensitive bladder symptoms. *Br J Urol* 1993;72:293–297.
39. Parsons CL, Hurst RE. Decreased urinary uronic acid levels in individuals with interstitial cystitis. *J Urol* 1990;143:690–693.
40. Hurst RE, Parsons CL, Roy JB, Young JL. Urinary glycosaminoglycan excretion as a laboratory marker in the diagnosis of interstitial cystitis. *J Urol* 1993;149:31–35.
41. Shupp-Byrne DE. Urinary glycoprotein (GP51) may be a laboratory marker in the diagnosis of interstitial cystitis. *AUA Today* 1995;8:1.
42. Erickson DR, Mast S, Ordille S, Bhavanandan VP. Urinary epitectin (MUC-1 glycoprotein) in the menstrual cycle and interstitial cystitis. *J Urol* 1996;156:938–942.

Interstitial Cystitis, edited by Grannum R. Sant.
Lippincott–Raven Publishers, Philadelphia ©1997.

CHAPTER 16

Interstitial Cystitis: The Neurovascular Perspective

Paul P. Irwin and Niall T.M. Galloway

At the heart of the interstitial cystitis (IC) enigma is its unknown etiology. The attractive hypotheses that have been explored in recent decades have often tended to focus too sharply on isolated histologic, immunologic, and biochemical aspects of IC in the hope that these phenomena might yield a specific etiologic cause. Unfortunately, none of these popular hypotheses can explain all of the clinical, cystoscopic, and histologic features that make up the disease entity we know as interstitial cystitis (IC). The glycosaminoglycan (GAG) layer theory, for instance, provides possible explanations for the presence of bacteria and potentially toxic substances in the bladder wall, which in turn might provide a stimulus for bladder inflammation. But why is the GAG layer deficient in the first place? How does increased bladder wall permeability tie in with autonomic nerve fiber proliferation in the suburothelial layer? Is there a link between the presence of bacteria in the bladder wall and detrusor mastocytosis?

Although the minutiae of these hypotheses are dealt with elsewhere in this book, a brief overview is warranted in order to highlight certain aspects that are pertinent to the neurovascular hypothesis. For the purpose of clarity, the salient points are reviewed under two broad categories: immunologic mechanisms and deficient urothelial defenses.

IMMUNOLOGIC MECHANISMS IN IC

Oravisto and Jokinen provided the first serious challenge to the belief that IC was an immunologic disorder (1,2). They failed to find any association with systemic diseases, and none of their patients had elevated levels of antithyroid or anti-parietal-cell antibodies or of bladder-specific antibodies. The tissue antibody levels that were raised in their patient population were directed against non-organ-specific antigens (i.e., cell nuclei and unidentified cytoplasmic components). Therefore, IC is not a local variant of an autoimmune disease but rather is a separate clinical entity in which the disease is confined to one organ and in which the tissue antibodies are not organ specific. These antibody levels fall after cystectomy, suggesting that the stimulus to antibody production in IC is situated within the bladder (3). Andersson and associates suggested that the nonspecific nature of the immunologic response in IC is more likely to represent a secondary phenomenon associated with damage to the bladder by other causes (4).

McDermott et al. demonstrated that the nonspecific inflammatory changes in the bladder wall in IC (suburothelial inflammation, mastocytosis, edema, and fibrosis) are similar to those seen in the bowel wall submucosa of enterocystoplasties and that this reaction is independent of the bladder disorder for which the cystoplasty was performed (5). It was proposed that this histologic response is the normal reaction of a nonwaterproof epithelial surface to exposure to urine. This suggests that the inflammatory changes in the bladder in IC are provoked by the presence of urine or its constituents within the bladder wall, an event that could only occur if the bladder's normal defensive barrier to urine is deficient.

DEFICIENT BLADDER UROTHELIAL DEFENSES

The importance of the glycosoaminoglycans (GAG) layer in providing both an antiadherence and an impermeability barrier has been extensively demonstrated

P.P. Irwin: Department of Urology, University of Manchester and Manchester Royal Infirmary, Manchester M13 9WL United Kingdom.
N. T. M. Galloway: Department of Urology, Emory University School of Medicine, Atlanta, Georgia 30133.

(6–8). The GAG layer hypothesis proposes that defects in the structural integrity or composition of the GAG layer might be important in the etiology of the condition. The hypothesis was first tested by Hurst and associates, who found that the production of GAGs by the bladder urothelium is defective in IC and suggested that the ability to bind GAG produced by the upper urinary tract might also be impaired (9). To our knowledge, this is the only study in which such quantitative differences have been demonstrated, and to date neither ultrastructural (10,11) nor biochemical studies (12,13) have revealed any significant differences between the bladder GAG layers of IC and healthy control subjects. Nonetheless, the finding of unusual microorganisms in the bladder wall of patients with IC would suggest that the defect in the "impermeable barrier" is real (14–16). Wilkins and co-workers suggested that such bacteria might provide the initiating stimulus for the disease. It is equally possible, however, that the presence of microorganisms in the bladder wall is an abnormal phenomenon in itself, reflecting a weakness in the bladder's ability to combat infection. Such a loss of integrity of the bladder's defenses could only result from a pathologic process already in progress.

The neurovascular hypothesis proposes that the features we associate with IC are but secondary manifestations of an ongoing bladder-damaging process. We have proposed that the primary underlying pathology is a neurovascular process remote from the bladder but the sequelae of which have a deleterious effect on the structure and function of that organ. There are striking similarities in the clinical features and disease course between IC and the neurovascular disorder reflex sympathetic dystrophy (RSD) (17).

REFLEX SYMPATHETIC DYSTROPHY

Reflex sympathetic dystrophy is a neurovascular syndrome in which pain is accompanied by loss of function and evidence of autonomic dysfunction (18). It usually affects an extremity and is characterized by chronic pain and dystrophic tissue changes (19–21). The changes that develop in the affected limb are the result of a combination of pain-provoked disuse and ischemia, both of which are believed to be mediated by prolonged inappropriate sympathetic autonomic efferent activity. The severity of the patient's pain is usually disproportionate to the original injury. It is aggravated by movement of the affected part, and even light touch or vibrations may induce agonal paroxysms of pain. Patients may develop behavioral and personality traits aimed at protecting the affected limb and often withdraw from normal daily activities in order to obtain seclusion and rest (19–21).

Although it is widely accepted that sympathetic autonomic overactivity has an important role to play, the precise pathophysiology of RSD is still unclear and a full account is beyond the scope of this book. A greatly simplified summary of the proposed neurologic events is as follows:

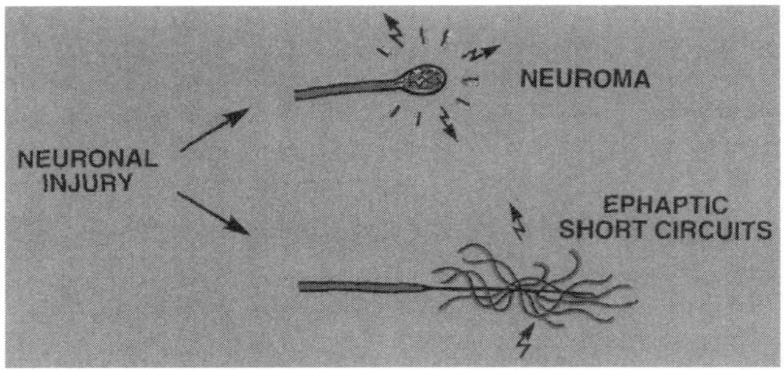

FIG. 1. The possible consequences of abnormal neuronal healing following injury include the development of a neuroma and the formation of ephaptic short circuits between the somatic sensory and autonomic nervous systems.

Initial Neuronal Injury

The onset of symptoms in RSD usually dates from an episode of end-organ injury causing partial damage to a peripheral nerve (21–23). It is postulated that failure of the normal neuronal healing process after injury sets up an abnormal cascade of neurologic events (Fig. 1). Damage to a peripheral nerve occasionally results in the formation of a neuroma, and in a small percentage of such patients this becomes painful (24). Traumatic neuromata may become the seats of abnormal spontaneous discharges, producing increased activity at the posterior root ganglion (25). Neuromata may fire spontaneously or in response to pressure and movement and are often hypersensitive to norepinephrine (22). Neuroma development is not a common sequel to nerve injury, as only a small percentage of RSD patients have histologic evidence of neuroma (26). Nerve fiber proliferation may occur, but incomplete neuronal repair, partial atrophy or degeneration, and nerve fiber proliferation are more commonly found. Demyelinated segments capable of generating spontaneous ectopic impulses may result (24). In fact, even brief periods of ischemia may convert normal peripheral nerves into spontaneous ectopic generators (27). It is plausible, therefore, that demyelinated segments of damaged nerves result in the formation of ephapses, or artificial synapses, between damaged sensory afferent and sympathetic efferent neurons (28,29). Roberts and Janig proposed that ephaptic transmission between unmyelinated sympathetic efferent fibers and demyelinated segments of sensory afferent fibers may create a short circuit between the two systems (Fig. 1) (29,30).

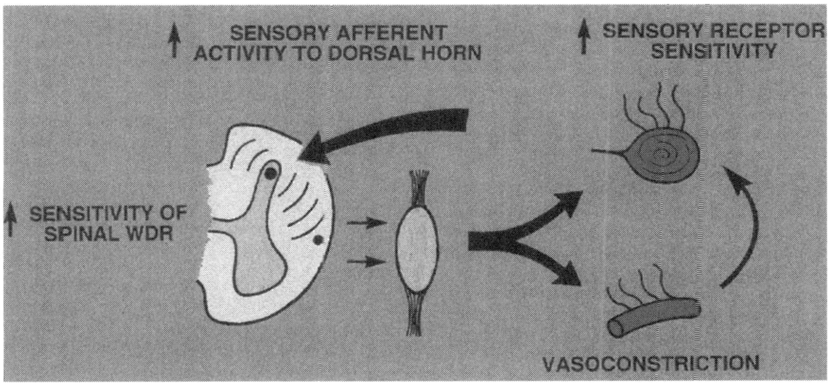

FIG. 2. As a result of continuous bombardment of the dorsal horn with sensory afferent stimuli, the sensitivity of multireceptive WDR neurons is heightened. Afferent stimuli of many kinds maintain this hypersensitivity. Adjacent areas of the same spinal segment, and in adjacent segments above and below the affected part of the cord, are recruited to an internuncial pool, with increased activity in the lateral horns of the cord culminating in enhanced sympathetic autonomic efferent output to the periphery.

Bombardment of the Dorsal Horn by Afferent Stimuli

Roberts proposed that activity in the sympathetic efferent nerve would stimulate myelinated mechanoreceptor afferents via the ephapse and create a continuous afferent input on a group of multireceptive wide-dynamic-range neurons (WDRs) in the spinal cord. Whatever the mechanism, chronic soft tissue injury results in bombardment of the spinal cord with afferent impulses (Fig. 2). This hyperactivity in turn excites multireceptive WDR neurons in the dorsal horn of the spinal cord, thereby greatly increasing their sensitivity to a wide range of afferent stimuli, including those that are not normally associated with pain (30). The evidence to support this hypothesis comes from animal studies that show that activity in C-fiber pain receptors can sensitize spinal WDR neurons (31,32). Surgical injury can produce a similar and longer-lasting hypersensitivity (33). As a result, spinal WDRs may increase their responsiveness or "gain" to both mechanical and painful stimulation (32–34). This huge increase in neurologic activity excites an "internuncial pool" of neurons in the anterior and lateral horns of the affected spinal cord segment, creating a continuous reflex increase in the activity of motor and sympathetic efferents.

The "Vicious Circle"

The effect of increased sympathetic efferent activity is twofold (Fig. 2). First, it may increase the sensitivity of peripheral sensory receptors, so that the affected part becomes hypersensitive (35). Sympathetic efferent stimulation has been shown to activate slowly adapting mechanoreceptors in cats, and these receptor afferents are known to make excitatory monosynaptic connections with WDR neurons (36). Second, by increasing vasomotor tone, microcirculatory blood flow through the affected part is altered. End-organ hypersensitivity is therefore maintained by both ischemia and persistent sympathetic autonomic efferent activity, and a "vicious circle of pain," altered blood flow, and ischemic injury result (Fig. 3) (37).

With time, dystrophic features (muscle wasting and osteoporosis in particular) become more pronounced and are accompanied by serious alterations in microcirculatory dynamics and tissue perfusion. The normal vasomotor responses to cooling and to changes in posture, which are dependent on an intact sympathetic nerve supply, are lost (38). The limb may become pale, cold, and fixed as a result of chronic loss of function and immobility, and specialized epithelial functions are lost.

NEUROLOGIC ASPECTS OF IC

Although the etiologic trigger in IC is unknown, it is possible that a severe urinary infection or trauma from pelvic or spinal surgery might initiate the disease process. More than 50% of IC patients report at least one episode of urinary infection before the onset of IC symptoms (39). Many more report previous pelvic operations, the most common being hysterectomy, an operation that is well recognized as being a common cause of bladder dysfunction (40). Although most of the damage was sus-

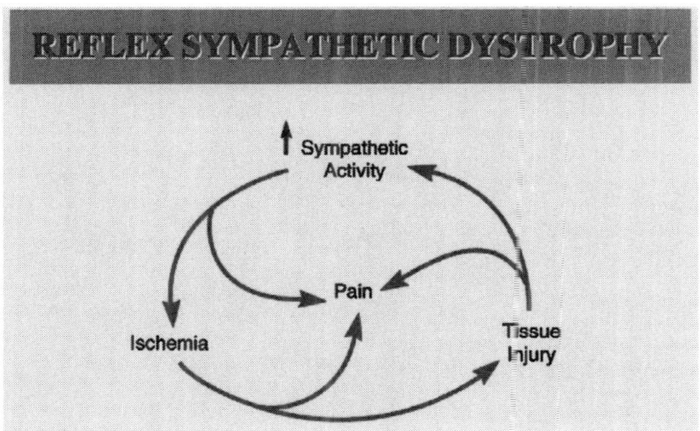

FIG. 3. The "vicious circle" proposed by Livingston.

tained by the parasympathetic nerves in Pary's study, such injury could theoretically damage either group of nerves, sympathetic or parasympathetic, and result in the formation of ephaptic short circuits between demyelinated injured nerve segments and unmyelinated sympathetic fibers. In Koziol's epidemiologic study in the United States, 44% of IC women had undergone hysterectomy before the onset of IC symptoms (the hysterectomy rate for controls being 17.5%) (41).

Pain is a central feature of IC. Typically, it is worse when the bladder is filled and is eased by voiding, possibly reflecting heightened sensitivity of stretch receptors in the bladder wall. It is well known that amputation of the painful limb in RSD/causalgia can be complicated by phantom limb pain, and it is noteworthy that cystourethrectomy does not provide a guarantee of relief of bladder pain in IC (42–44).

An intriguing aspect of recent IC research has been the rediscovery of nerve fiber proliferation in the suburothelial and detrusor layers of the bladder (45,46). Many of these new neurons contain vasoactive intestinal peptide (VIP) and neuropeptide Y, neuropeptides that elsewhere are found mainly in sympathetic-like nerve fibers (46). The precise significance of these findings is not known, but it is highly likely that these autonomic nerves have an intimate anatomic and functional relationship with bladder mast cells. The final common path in the pathophysiology of IC may well reside at this level.

The evidence for increased spinal sympathetic efferent activity in interstitial cystitis is indirect. We used an isolated cold stress test to study pedal skin temperature in 19 patients with IC (all of whom satisfied the NIDDK diagnostic criteria) and in 11 healthy controls (47). No patient in either group was taking antihypertensive medication, and patients with evidence of peripheral vascular disease or of Raynaud's phenomenon were excluded. The IC group had a lower mean base-line temperature ($p = 0.01$) and a more rapid fall in skin temperature during the cooling phase of the study (Fig. 4). Mean temperature remained lower in the IC group throughout the test. Although the rate of rewarming was similar in both groups, 16 feet (42%) in the IC group failed to return to within 2° of base-line temperature within the 20-min recovery period. In contrast, only five (23%) of the 22 control feet failed to return to the base-line temperature. In the absence of clinical evidence of vascular insufficiency, these results may only be explained by differences in vasomotor regulation. Rapid skin cooling and slow rewarming would be expected in the setting of excessive sympathetic efferent outflow. This is the pattern that was observed in the feet of most of our IC patients, which contrasted with the "warmer" pattern seen in the control group.

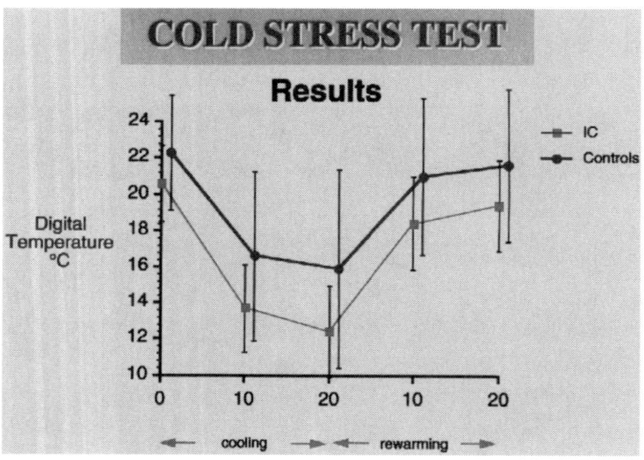

FIG. 4. Mean pedal skin temperatures (±SD) for IC and control subjects. (From Irwin et al., ref. 47, reproduced with permission from Wiley-Liss Publishers.)

The sympathetic autonomic supply to the feet and to the pelvic organs emanates from almost adjacent regions of the spinal cord. That to the feet comes from the lumbar region (L_1 to L_3), whereas the pelvic organs obtain their sympathetic supply from the lower thoracic and upper lumbar segments (T_8 to L_2) via the hypogastric plexus. Livingston proposed that abnormally increased activity in the lateral horns of the spinal cord spreads to involve adjacent segments, thereby recruiting their respective sensory dermatomes to the pathologic process (37). If the same process were to occur in IC, sympathetic dysfunction in adjacent neurologic fields might be expected. Thus, the finding of significant vasomotor disturbance in our group of IC patients would suggest that increased spinal sympathetic reflex activity is a feature of the disorder.

If the sympathetic nervous system has a role to play in the pathophysiology of IC, sympathetic blockade should have an impact on its clinical presentation. This is not a new concept; indeed, sympathectomy was a popular treatment for a wide variety of painful bladder disorders in the early part of this century (48–55). The physiological premise on which the operation was based was that section of the sympathetic nerve supply produced bladder neck relaxation, decreased bladder sensation, and increased vesical blood supply.

At Emory University, we treated a large number of patients with painful bladder disorders using lumbar sympathetic blocks (56). Epidural injections of 0.25% bupivacaine at the L_1–L_2 interspace were used. In one series we administered 55 injections to 13 patients with IC over an 18-month period. Mean follow-up was 6.5 months. Immediate relief of pain was obtained following 49 of these injections, and it lasted more than 24 hr in 41. The duration of significant pain relief ranged from 2 days to 75 days (mean 15.1 days). With successive injections the duration of pain remission tended to increase. In most instances the improvement in pelvic pain symptoms was accompanied by significant improvements in quality of life and sleep habit. Eight patients reported discomfort at

A
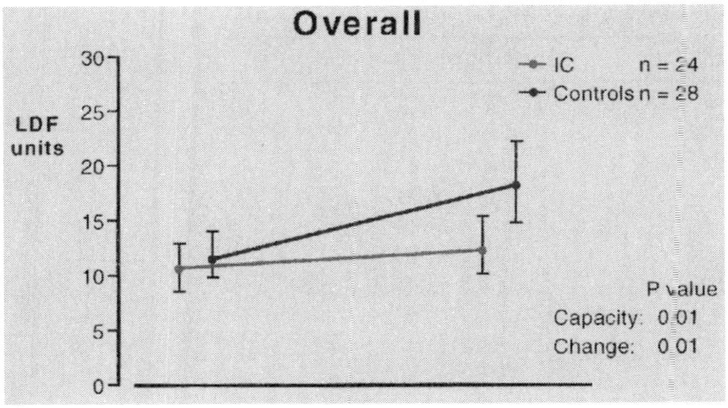

B
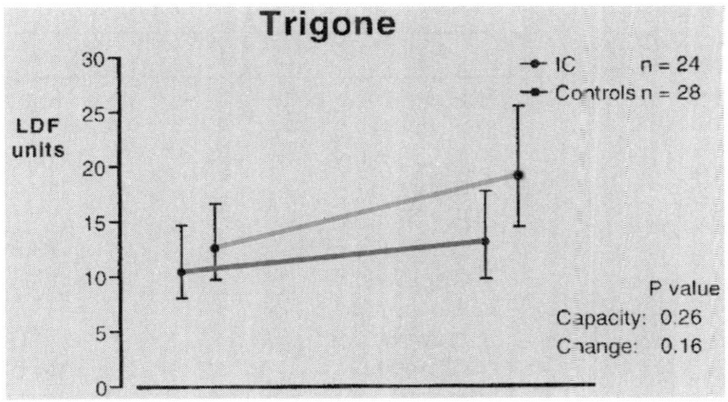

C
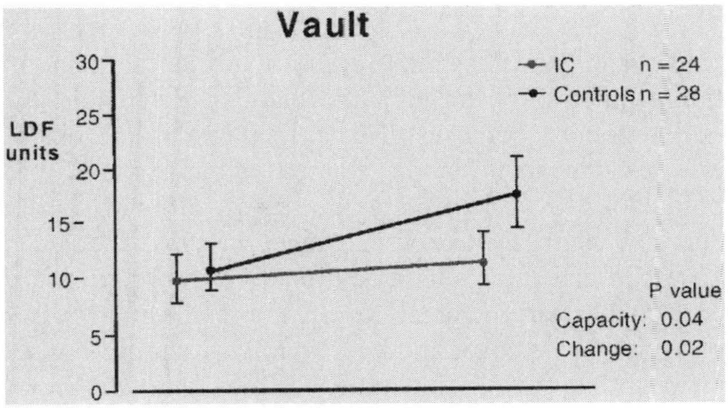

FIG. 5. Mean overall bladder perfusion (LDF units) was similar for the IC and control groups when the bladder was almost empty. The significant increase in bladder perfusion following distention in the control group was not observed in the IC group.

the site of injection lasting from 1 to 3 weeks. Apart from this, there were no adverse reactions or complications from the treatment.

For logistic and financial reasons, it was possible to treat patients with only a single epidural injection at each visit. It might have been preferable to deliver the anesthetic agent by infusion through a cannula inserted in the epidural space, which would have provided a more prolonged block. Hampson and associates reported good results with such a technique (57).

VASCULAR ASPECTS OF IC

As early as the 1930s, researchers had suggested a possible link between bladder ischemia and interstitial cystitis (58,59). The hypothesis was never challenged, largely because of the lack of a satisfactory method of measuring bladder blood flow in humans. However, with continued refinements in laser Doppler flowmetry (LDF) technology, a safe and relatively noninvasive means of obtaining continuous real-time measurements of microcirculatory blood flow is now available (60,61). Although the measurements obtained with LDF are not absolute, linear correlations between the LDF signal from single sites and tissue blood flow as measured by established methods have been documented (61–63).

We used LDF to compare bladder perfusion between a group of 24 IC patients (who satisfied the NIDDK diagnostic criteria) and a control group of 28 patients who underwent cystoscopy for clinical indications other than IC or malignancy (64). Cystoscopies were performed under general anesthesia, and the irrigating fluid was set at a height of 80 cm above the level of the patient. Measurements were obtained from several sites with the bladder almost empty and again with the bladder filled to capacity.

Perfusion to the bladder as a whole and to its separate portions, trigone and vault, was similar in both groups when the bladder was almost empty ($p = 0.7$). However, when the bladder was filled to capacity, perfusion increased in all but three patients in the control group (89%) but in only ten patients (38%) in the IC group. In contrast, whereas bladder perfusion decreased following distention in 11 IC patients (42%), this occurred in only three (10%) of the control subjects. Mean overall bladder perfusion increased by a mean of 7.6 LDF units in the control group but by only 3.4 units in the IC group, a magnitude of change that was significantly different ($p = 0.04$) (Fig. 5A). Changes in trigonal perfusion following distention were not statistically different between the two groups (Fig. 5B). The data are shown in Table 1 and illustrated in Fig. 5.

These differences in bladder perfusion at capacity might well have been explained by differences in bladder capacity alone. Mean bladder capacity under anesthesia was 751 ml in the control group and 606 ml in the IC group. However, the differences remained significant following covariant analysis controlling for anesthetic capacity.

TABLE 1. *Perfusion measurements (mean LDF units ± SD) for IC and control groups*

	IC (*n* = 26)	Controls (*n* = 29)
Maximum capacity (ml)	606.9 ± 187.0	751.3 ± 273.0
LDF (Overall)		
Low volume	12.06 ± 5.8	12.8 ± 7.0
Capacity	15.48 ± 8.6	20.4 ± 11.1
LDF (Trigone)		
Low volume	13.8 ± 9.8	16.3 ± 13.0
Capacity	17.5 ± 14.2	24.8 ± 21.2
LDF (Vault)		
Low volume	11.3 ± 4.9	12.2 ± 6.9
Capacity	14.5 ± 8.7	19.3 ± 9.7

Why is there such a marked difference in LDF changes following distention between the vault and the trigone (Fig. 5B,C)? It might well be explained by the relative lack of dispensability of the trigone compared to the vault. It is noteworthy, however, that the cystoscopic features of IC are most prominent in the vault, whereas the trigone is usually spared. A more likely explanation for both the relative lack of morphologic change in the trigone in IC and the lack of a significant perfusion deficit in the trigone following distention is that the latter probably receives a collateral blood supply from ureteral and urethral vessels.

The finding that bladder perfusion fails to increase with distention suggests an ischemic basis for the IC patient's pain, which is characteristically worse when the bladder is full and is somewhat eased by voiding. Chronic ischemia might be expected to result in the development of a fibrotic, small capacity bladder (Fig. 6). It is easy to imagine how the production of glycosaminoglycans by the bladder urothelium or its capacity to bind GAGs produced elsewhere in the urinary tract might be impaired by chronic vascular insufficency. The attenuation of the GAG layer as well as the overall impairment in the nutritional blood flow through the bladder wall could also undermine its defenses. This might render the bladder less resistant to infection by microorganisms and more permeable to such proteins as Tamm–Horsfall protein and to potentially toxic substances in urine that, when absorbed into the bladder wall, could provoke an inflammatory reaction characterized by mononuclear cells, lymphocytes, mast cells, and eosinophils. A similar nonspecific inflammatory infiltrate is found in the bowel segments of enterocystoplasties, where urinary constituents are absorbed into a tissue that lacks the waterproof properties of the normal bladder wall.

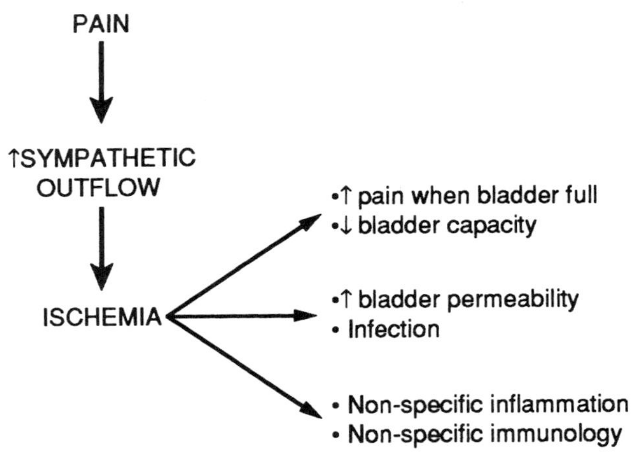

FIG. 6. Many of the clinical and laboratory findings associated with IC may be explained by the neurovascular hypothesis.

SUMMARY AND CONCLUSIONS

These studies provide indirect support for the hypothesis that interstitial cystitis might be a neurovascular disorder. However, although the results may be exciting in their own right, their precise significance remains speculative and should remain so until challenged and corroborated by further studies.

Could it be that IC—this crippling "bladder disease"—is not a primary bladder disorder at all? Only continued research into the neurologic and vascular aspects of IC in tandem with ongoing studies of bladder wall neurophysiology will provide the answer.

REFERENCES

1. Oravisto K, Alfthan OS, Jokinen EJ. Interstitial cystitis: clinical and immunological findings. *Scand J Urol Nephrol* 1970;4:37–42.
2. Jokinen EJ, Alfthan OS, Oravisto KJ. Antitissue antibodies in interstitial cystitis. *Clin Exp Immunol* 1972;11:333–339.
3. Jokinen EJ, Oravisto KJ, Alfthan OS. The effect of cystectomy on antitissue antibodies in interstitial cystitis. *Clin Exp Immunol* 1973;15: 457–460.
4. Anderson JB, Parviar F, Lee G, Wallington TB, MacIver AG, Bradbrook RA, Gingell JC. The enigma of interstitial cystitis: an autoimmune disease? *Br J Urol* 1989;63:58–63.
5. MacDermott JP, Charpied GL, Tesluk H, Stone AR. Recurrent interstitial cystitis following cystoplasty: fact or fiction? *J Urol* 1990;144:37–40.
6. Parsons CL, Schmidt JD, Pollen JJ. Bladder surface glycosoaminoglycans: an efficient mechanism of environmental adaptation. *Science* 1980;208:605.

7. Parsons CL, Schmidt JD, Pollen JJ. Successful treatment of interstitial cystitis with sodium pentosan-polysulfate. *J Urol* 1983;130:51–53.
8. Gill WB, Jones KW, Ruggiero KJ. Protective effects of heparin and other sulfated glycosoaminoglycans on crystal adhesion to injured urothelium. *J Urol* 1892;127(1):152–154.
9. Hurst R. The mechanisms for low glycosaminoglycans excretion in interstitial cystitis and mechanisms for the protection of bladder from urine. *J Urol* 1986;135:189A.
10. Dixon JS, Holm-Bentzen M, Gilpin CJ, Gosling JA, Bostofte E, Hald T, Larsen S. Electron microscopic investigation of the bladder urothelium and glycocalyx in patients with interstitial cystitis. *J Urol* 1986; 135:621–625.
11. Anderstrom CRK, Fall M, Johansson SL. Scanning electron microscopic findings in interstitial cystitis. *Br J Urol* 1989;63:270–275.
12. Sant GR, Ucci AA, Alroy J. Bladder surface glycosaminoglycans (GAGs) in interstitial cystitis. *J Urol* 1986;135:287A.
13. Holm-Bentzen M, Ammitzboll T, Hald T. Glycosaminoglycans on the surface of the human urothelium: a preliminary report. *Neurol Urodyn* 1986;5:519–523.
14. Wilkins EG, Payne SR, Pead PJ, Moss ST, Maskell RM. Interstitial cystitis and the urethral syndrome: a possible answer. *Br J Urol* 1989; 64:39–43.
15. Fugazzotto P. Urinary tract infections: the need for pure culture technology in clinical laboratory diagnosis. *Br J Urol* 1991;68:557.
16. Domingue GJ, Ghoniem GM, Bost KL, Fermin C, Human LG. Dormant microbes in interstitial cystitis. *J Urol* 1995;153:1321–1326.
17. Galloway NTM, Gabale D, Irwin P. Interstitial cystitis or reflex sympathetic dystrophy of the bladder? *Semin Urol* 1991;9(2):148–152.
18. Amadio PC, Mackinnon SE, Merritt WH, Brody GS, Terzis JK. RSDS: Consensus report of an *ad hoc* committee of the American Association of Hand Surgery on the definition of RSDS. *Plast Reconstruct Surg* 1991;87:371–375.
19. Rowlingson JC. The sympathetic dystrophies. *Int Anesthesiol Clin* 1983;21:117–129.
20. Schwartzmann R, McLellan T. Reflex sympathetic dystrophy—a review. *Arch Neurol* 1987;44:555–561.
21. Payne R. Reflex sympathetic dystrophy syndrome: diagnosis and treatment. In: Fields HL, ed. *Pain Syndromes in Neurology.* London: Butterworths, 1990;107–129.
22. Bonica JJ. In: Bonica JJ, Liebskind JC, Albe-Fessard DG, eds. *Advances in Pain Research and Therapy.* New York: Raven Press, 1979; 141–166.
23. Sunderland S. *Nerves and Nerve Injuries.* Edinburgh: Churchill Livingstone, 1978.
24. Wynn Parry CB. Pain in avulsion lesions of the brachial plexus. *Pain* 1980;9:41–53.
25. Wall PD, Gutnick M. Properties of afferent nerve impulses originating from a neuroma. *Nature* 1974;248:740–743.
26. Withrington RH, Parry CBW. The management of painful peripheral nerve disorders. *J Hand Surg* 1984;9B:24–28.
27. Ochoa JL, Torebjork HE. Paresthesiae from ectopic impulse generation in human sensory nerves. *Brain* 1980;103:835–853.
28. Schutzer S, Gossling H. Current concepts review: The treatment of reflex sympathetic dystrophy syndrome. *J Bone Joint Surg* 1984;66A: 625–629.
29. Janig W, Kollmann W. The involvement of the sympathetic nervous system in pain. *Drug Res* 1984;34(2):1066–1073.
30. Roberts WJ. A hypothesis on the physiological basis for causalgia and related pains. *Pain* 1986;24:297–311.
31. Chung JM, Kenshalo DR, Gerhart KD, Willis WD. Excitation of primate spinothalamic neurons by cutaneous C-fiber volleys. *J Neurophysiol* 1979;42:1354–1369.
32. Schouenborg J, Sjolund BH. Activity evoked by A- and C-afferent fibers in rat dorsal horn neurons and its relation to a flexion reflex. *J Neurophysiol* 1983;54:513–520.
33. Price DD, Browe AC. Spinal cord coding of graded non-noxious and noxious temperature increases. *Exp Neurol* 1975;48:201–221.
34. Kenshalo DR, Leonard RB, Chung JM, Willis WD. Facilitation of the responses of primate spinothalamic cells to cold and mechanical stimuli by noxious heating of the skin. *Pain* 1982;12:141–152.
35. Wallin G, Torebjork E, Hallin R. Preliminary observations on the pathophysiology of hyperalgesia in the causalgic pain syndrome. In: Zotterman Y, ed. *Sensory Function of the Skin in Primates.* Oxford: Pergamon Press, 1976.
36. Roberts WJ, Elardo SM, King KA. Sympathetically induced changes in the responses of slowly-adapting type I receptors in cat skin. *Somatosens Mot Res* 1985;2:223–236.
37. Livingston WK. A physiologic interpretation of causalgia and its related states. *Pain Mechanisms.* New York: Macmillan, 1943;83–127.
38. Rosen J, Ostergren B, Fagrell B. Skin microvascular circulation in the sympathetic dystrophies evaluated by videophotometric capillaroscopy and laser Doppler fluxmetry. *Eur J Clin Invest* 1988;18:305–308.
39. Held PJ, Hanno PM, Wein AJ, Pauly MV, Cahn MA. Epidemiology of interstitial cystitis. In: Hanno PM, Staskin DR, Krane RJ, Wein AJ, eds. *Interstitial Cystitis,* Vol 2. London: Springer-Verlag, 1990;29–48.
40. Parys BT, Woolfenden KA, Parsons KF. Bladder dysfunction after simple hysterectomy: urodynamic and neurological evaluation. *Eur Urol* 1990;17:129–133.
41. Koziol JA. Epidemiology of interstitial cystitis. *Urol Clin North Am* 1994;21(1):7–20.
42. Baskin LS, Tanagho EA. Pelvic pain without pelvic organs. *J Urol* 1992;147(3):683–686.
43. Irwin P, Galloway NTM. Pelvic pain without pelvic organs (letter). *J Urol* 1992;148(4):1265.
44. Webster GD, MacDiarmaid SA, Timmons SL, Perez L. Impact of urinary diversion procedures in the treatment of interstitial cystitis and chronic bladder pain. *Neurol Urodyn* 1992;11(4):76A.
45. Christmas TJ, Rode J, Chapple CR, Milroy EJG, Turner-Warwick RT. Nerve fibre proliferation in interstitial cystitis. *Virchows Arch [A] Pathol Anat* 1990;416:447–451.
46. Hohenfellner M, Nunes L, Schmidt RA, Lampel A, Thuroff JW, Tanagho EA. Interstitial cystitis: increased sympathetic innervation and related neuropeptide synthesis. *J Urol* 1992;147:587–591.
47. Irwin P, James S, Watts L, Fleming LL, Galloway NTM. Abnormal pedal thermoregulation in interstitial cystitis. *Neurol Urodyn* 1993; 12(2):139–144.
48. Jacobson CE, Braasch WF, Love JG (1944). Presacral neurectomy for vesical pain. *Surg Gynecol Obstet* 1944;79:21–26.
49. Douglas HL. Excision of the superior hypogastric plexus in the treatment of intractable interstitial cystitis. *Am J Surg* 1934;25(2):249–257.
50. Jaboulay M. Le traitment de la neuralgia pelvienne par la paralysie due sympathique sacre. *Lyon Med* 1899;90:102.
51. Pieri G. Enervation ou ramisection? *Presse Med* 1926;34:141–142.
52. Rochet V. Traitement chirugical des cystites douloureuses. *Lyon Chir* 1921;18:462–480.
53. Pearl F, Strauss B. Presacral neurectomy and sacral ganglionectomy. *J Urol* 1939;39:645.
54. Learmonth JR, Braash WF. Resection of the presacral nerve for disease of the bladder: experience in 24 cases. *Trans Am Assoc Genitourinary Surg* 1932;25:313–333.
55. Nesbit RM, McLellan FC. Sympathectomy for the release of physical spasm and pain resulting from intractable bladder infection. *Surg Gynecol Obstet* 1939;68:540–546.
56. Irwin P, Hammonds WD, Galloway NTM. Lumbar epidural blockade in the management of pain in interstitial cystitis. *Br J Urol* 1993;71: 413–416.
57. Hampson SJ, Bowen-Wright M, Worth PH. Epidural anaesthesia in the management of the painful bladder. *Br J Urol* 1992;70:503–505.
58. Meads AM. Hunner's ulcer. *Urol Cutan Rev* 1934;38:631–634.
59. Engle WJ. Interstitial cystitis. *Cleve Clin Quart* 1939;6:307–312.
60. Shepherd AP, Reidel GL, Kiel JN, Hammschild DJ, Maxwell LC. Evaluation of an infrared laser Doppler blood flowmeter. *Am J Physiol* 1987;252:G832–G839.
61. Oberg PA, Tenland T, Nilsson GE. Laser Doppler flowmetry—a non-invasive and continuous method for blood flow evaluation in microvascular studies. *Acta Med Scand* 1983;687:17–24.
62. Ahn H, Lindhagen J, Nilsson GE, Salerud EG, Jodal M, Lundgren O. Evaluation of laser Doppler flowmetry in the assessment of intestinal blood flow in cat. *Gastroenterology* 1985;88:951–957.
63. Kvietys PR, Shepherd AP, Granger DN. Laser Doppler, H_2 clearance and microsphere estimates of mucosal blood flow. *Am J Physiol* 1985;249:G221–G227.
64. Irwin P. *Neurovascular mechanisms in interstitial cystitis.* MCh thesis, University College Dublin, 1995.

Interstitial Cystitis, edited by Grannum R. Sant.
Lippincott–Raven Publishers, Philadelphia ©1997.

CHAPTER 17

Interstitial Cystitis: Clinical and Endoscopic Features

Denise A. Nigro and Alan J. Wein

Very few areas of medical diagnosis remain where the art of medicine is so apparent as in the diagnosis of interstitial cystitis (IC). Despite the intensive amount of research being done on the etiology and treatment of IC, the diagnosis is still implicitly dependent on physician awareness and suspicion (1). There are few if any pathognomonic findings in interstitial cystitis. Thus, much of the workup entails ruling out other likely causes of the patient's symptomatology. There are some controversies as to the value of specific individual tests in the treatment decisions and overall outcome for the patient, but generally, it is agreed that the diagnosis rests on a thorough history and physical exam combined with a lack of another identifiable cause to explain the patient's symptoms, and the presence of certain cystoscopic findings.

Hunner supplied the urologic community with what can be viewed by some as a blessing and by others as a curse when he described the endoscopic finding of a cracked and bleeding area in the bladders of several women who suffered with pelvic pain and urinary urgency and frequency (2). Since the original description, it has been found that this elusive ulcer (3) is a very rare finding in light of the number of patients who suffer with the symptoms of interstitial cystitis. Messing and Stamey conjecture that no other single criterion has been more detrimental to the diagnosis of IC (4). In the past, urologists have diligently sought the Hunner's ulcer to clinch the diagnosis of IC. Unfortunately, it has been realized that this single criterion does not define the disorder. As a matter of fact, the findings of a reduced bladder capacity under anesthesia and Hunner's ulcer are exceedingly rare (4–7). Thus, many cases have gone undiagnosed.

In August 1987, the NIDDK developed a set of criteria for accrual of patients in NIH-sponsored studies on IC. A list of the guidelines is shown in Table 1 (8). The original intention was only to specify and standardize criteria for entrance into research protocols on IC, to ensure that the patient population was homogeneous and similar from one site to another. The criteria quickly became a *de facto* list for the symptomatic diagnosis of IC. Many felt these criteria were too restrictive in the clinical setting (9), and later, in November 1988, the cri-

D. A. Nigro and A. J. Wein: Division of Urology, University of Pennsylvania School of Medicine, Philadelphia, Pennsylvania 19104.

TABLE 1. *Original NIDDK consensus criteria for inclusion in IC studies*[a]

Automatic exclusions
Age <18 years
Benign or malignant bladder tumors
Radiation cystitis
Tuberculous cystitis
Bacterial cystitis
Vaginitis
Cyclophosphamide cystitis
Symptomatic urethral diverticulum
Uterine, cervical, vaginal, or urethral cancer
Active herpes
Bladder or lower ureteral calculi
Waking frequency less than five times in 12 hr
Nocturia less than two times
Symptoms relieved by antibiotics, urinary antiseptics, urinary analgesics (for example, phenazopyridine hydrochloride)
Duration <12 months
Involuntary bladder contractions (urodynamics)
Capacity >400 cc, absence of sensory urgency
Automatic inclusions
Hunner's ulcer
Positive factors (two required for inclusion in study population)
Pain on bladder filling, relieved by emptying
Pain (suprapubic, pelvic, urethral, vaginal, or perineal)
Glomerulations on endoscopy
Decreased compliance on cystometrogram

[a]From refs. 8–11.

teria were revised (Table 2) (10,11). For the present time, any research studies should be conducted with these restrictions in mind. However, it must be kept in mind that these criteria do not represent a least common denominator of symptoms and signs and that there are patients who are clinically considered to have IC but who would be excluded from studies on IC if this checklist comprised the study entrance criteria.

Diagnosis of the disorder in practice is subject to a different set of recommendations. In assessing a potential IC patient, it is helpful to keep in mind that this is a symptom complex and that there are no pathognomonic findings associated with the disease (12). The revised NIDDK criteria are still helpful in the clinical setting as an outline and checklist for the history and physical exam and cystoscopic examination.

TABLE 2. *Revised NIDDK consensus criteria for inclusion in IC studies[a]*

The presence of any one of the following criteria will exclude the diagnosis of interstitial cystitis for study purposes:

- Bladder capacity greater than 350 ml on awake cystometry using either gas or liquid as a filling medium
- Absence of an intense urge to void with the bladder filled to 100 ml of gas or 150 ml of water during cystometry, using a fill rate of 30 to 100 ml/min
- The demonstration of phasic involuntary bladder contractions on cystometry using the fill rate described above
- Duration of symptoms less than 9 months
- Absence of nocturia
- Symptoms relieved by antimicrobials, urinary antiseptics, anticholinergics, or antispasmodics (musculotropic relaxants)
- A frequency of urination, while awake, less than eight times per day
- A diagnosis of bacterial cystitis or prostatitis within a 3-month period
- Bladder or lower ureteral calculi
- Active genital herpes
- Uterine, cervical, vaginal, or urethral cancer
- Urethral diverticulum
- Cyclophosphamide or any type of chemical cystitis
- Tuberculous cystitis
- Radiation cystitis
- Benign or malignant bladder tumors
- Vaginitis
- Age less than 18 years

[a]To be diagnosed with IC, patients must have either glomerulations on cystoscopic examination or a classic Hunner's ulcer, and they must have either pain associated with the bladder or urinary urgency. An examination for glomerulations should be undertaken after distention of the bladder under anesthesia to 80 to 100 cm of water pressure for 1 to 2 min. The bladder may be distended up to two times before evaluation. The glomerulations must be diffuse—present in at least three quadrants of the bladder—and there must be at least ten glomerulations per quadrant. The glomerulations must not be located along the path of the cystoscope (to avoid artifact from instrumentation contact).

DIAGNOSIS

History

The diagnosis of any medical disorder begins with a thorough history. The majority (90%) of patients are female (13–15). A disproportionate majority of patients are Caucasian (15). The onset of symptoms generally occurs between 30 and 50 years of age (13). Typically, the IC patient complains of unremitting urinary frequency and urgency (2,4,14,15). There may be suprapubic pain and pressure only when the bladder is full, and voiding may relieve the pelvic discomfort (14,15). A few patients will describe irritation at the end of voiding (13). Dysuria is less common; still, 33% to 56% of patients report burning (4,15). Nocturia has long been considered one of the hallmarks of IC. Patients are awakened multiple times with a strong and/or painful desire to void. This pattern of diurnal and nocturnal voiding differs from that of psychosomatic voiding dysfunction, in which nocturia is disproportionately minimal or conspicuously absent. Male patients, in addition to the urgency and frequency, often describe perineal, scrotal, and groin discomfort (13). Although patients often describe the combination of abnormal voiding patterns and pelvic pain, one of the two symptom complexes tends to predominate.

Dyspareunia is a common finding in women with IC (1,12,13). In Koziol's review of 347 patients, 50% reported discomfort with sexual intercourse (15). Parsons reported that over 74% of 200 patients had painful intercourse (12). Some of the women experience such severe discomfort that they abstain from sexual intercourse altogether. Clearly, this is an issue that needs to be addressed in the initial evaluation and subsequent treatment of the patient.

Incontinence is rare but, when present, is generally of the urgency type (16). There is a suggestion that in some cases of mixed incontinence, the urgency component may actually be caused by IC (13). Gross hematuria is also uncommon.

The onset of symptoms is acute, and most patients can pinpoint an exact date or period when the problem began (17). Some can associate the initiation of their difficulty with some exact cause such as a specific urinary tract infection or bladder or pelvic surgery (5,13). Because of the similarity in presentation to an acute cystitis, many patients are treated with one or multiple courses of antibiotics before referral (17).

In general, patients will suffer with the symptoms for anywhere from 3 to 7 years before the correct diagnosis is made (4,18,19). A significant number of these patients endure several evaluations and consults and perhaps surgeries before actually being given a diagnosis of IC. The average IC patient has seen three to five physicians before arriving at the proper diagnosis (20).

Interstitial cystitis symptomatology is characterized by the periods of exacerbations followed by spontaneous remissions. The exacerbations may occur in association with dietary indiscretions (usually patient specific), other illnesses or stress, or they may be unassociated with any obvious precipitating factor. Some investigators have noted a plateau and stabilization of the symptoms after a period of time (15,18), although there may be some variation on a day-to-day basis (17).

Allergies, autoimmune disorders, and gynecologic and gastrointestinal problems appear to be more common in IC patients than among controls (21) and the general population (22). A number of patients do report prior gynecologic surgery (13). There are reportedly three times as many hysterectomies and twice as many suspensions and oophorectomies in IC patients as in controls (5). Many patients experience fluctuation of their symptoms relative to their ovulatory cycle (5,13,23). Pregnancy does not affect symptoms in a consistent manner. The incidence of IC is unrelated to marital status, number of sexual partners, or parity (24). Family history and genetics do not appear to have a significant role in this symptom complex (12).

Physical Examination

Abdominal, pelvic, and neurologic examinations are nonspecific and often unremarkable (13,17,25). Women may have tenderness over the bladder base and/or urethra on a vaginal examination (14,26). Vaginitis, urethral diverticulum, and vestibular adenitis or vulvitis/vulvodynia must be excluded, as these can cause the symptoms of IC but require different therapy (27). Focal vulvitis with inflammation of the vestibular glands at the introitus of the vagina, if present, can be the source of significant dyspareunia (13). Suprapubic tenderness or bladder tenderness may be elicited on bimanual examination (14). Male patients usually have a normal prostate and genitalia on examination.

Laboratory

Urinalysis is usually normal. Microscopic hematuria and pyuria are present in a minority of patients (4). By definition, the urine culture must be negative. Urethral and vaginal cultures must also be negative for pathologic organisms such as gonorrhea, *Chlamydia,* fungus, and *Trichomonas* (1). Certain laboratory studies such as voided urine or bladder lavage cytology are suggested more to rule out the other diagnoses and do not show any characteristic findings in IC. There is no serologic testing to diagnose IC. The value of assays for urinary and serologic substances such as stress protein genes, uronic acid and glycosaminoglycans, mast cell tryptase, Tamm–Horsfall protein autoantibody, etc. is as yet speculative. These are used purely for investigational purposes and do not yet have a defined role in the diagnosis of IC (28–31). Tests of immune function also have minimal value in the diagnosis of IC (4). In men, expressed prostatic secretions have no typical findings relative to IC, but localization cultures and microscopic exams should be performed to exclude bacterial or abacterial prostatitis (13).

Radiographic Studies

Unless specifically indicated to rule out concurrent diagnoses, there are no radiographic studies to define IC. Many clinicians routinely order pelvic ultrasounds to screen for a pelvic mass or other abnormality that might cause symptoms through compression or adjacent inflammation, for example. Because most patients are evaluated by several physicians before being diagnosed with IC, they frequently have undergone full uroradiologic evaluation including voiding cystourethrogram, intravenous pyelogram, CT scan, and even MRI.

Urodynamic Studies

To date there are no specific urodynamic findings in IC. On cystometry (see Table 2), most IC patients have a hypersensitive bladder with a small volume at first sensation to void and at capacity. Patients with urethral tenderness on exam tend to have lower volumes at first sensation to void, whereas patients with bladder base tenderness tend to have lower volumes at severe urge to void (32). Overall, patients with lower volumes have more severe endoscopic disease (33). The detrusor should be quiescent during filling (i.e., no involuntary contractions), and the compliance is generally normal, although in fibrotic bladders, the compliance may be decreased. After filling, the patient should empty to completion at a normal detrusor pressure (no obstruction) (34,35).

CYSTOSCOPY

Aside from a thorough history and physical exam, cystoscopy (Table 2) has been described as the most important diagnostic tool in assessing the potential IC patient (17). Endoscopy is used as much to rule out other disorders as to rule in IC. Cystoscopy under local anesthesia can be helpful in that an awake patient who can tolerate several hundred milliliters of fluid in the bladder most probably does not have IC (25). Generally, however, cystoscopy is performed under anesthesia to allow for sufficient distention to afford visualization of glomerulations and/or Hunner's ulcers. After the diagnostic examination (hydrodistentions followed by refilling and observation), anesthesia further affords the opportunity to carry out a therapeutic hydrodistention as well. An initial urethroscopy and cystoscopy is performed before hydraulic distension to exclude pathology such as tumors or stones. The urethra should be normal in appearance and caliber

(13). In the absence of a Hunner's ulcer or scarring, the bladder also has a normal appearance (17). Bladder barbotage for cytology should be done at the time of cystoscopy. It is recommended that this be done following the diagnostic distention to prevent mistaking bladder wall trauma for glomerulations (25).

Diagnostic hydrodistention is performed with the irrigation fluid at 80 to 100 cm above the patient's bladder (27). The fluid is allowed to run into the bladder until it slows to a drip at capacity. Manual compression of the urethra, achieved by applying pressure on the anterior vaginal wall on either side of the cystoscope, is usually required to prevent leakage of the fluid and to obtain an accurate volume. The anterior, superior portion of the bladder should be continuously observed for possible rupture during filling. This is a rare occurrence but should be suspected when the capacity seems too large and the rate of filling shows no sign of decreasing. At capacity, no abnormality is usually apparent other than faint trabeculation (25). The diagnostic distention is held for 1 to 2 min, the bladder is drained, and the volume of the effluent is measured. Typically, the fluid is clear and then becomes blood-tinged for the last 50 to 100 cc (25). Bloody effluent, however, does not necessarily indicate the presence of glomerulations (33). The capacity is reduced in the classic or ulcer variety of IC, whereas it is normal or only slightly reduced in the nonulcer variety (27,33).

The bladder is reinspected in a slightly distended state. The classic description of IC is a reddened bladder with a reduced capacity and fissures and scars that crack and bleed after distention (4). Despite the severity of symptoms, the presence of this "Hunner's patch" on endoscopy is extremely rare. It is probably present only in more extreme or severe cases of IC. The classic "patch" or ulcer does seem to be more prevalent in postmenopausal women and in European women (36). Over the years, controversy has developed as to the actual existence of this "patch." Badenoch speculated that this lesion was produced by the endoscopist (14). Most clinicians now use the phrase "Hunner's patch," although there are a variety of pictures and descriptions that are presented as true ulcers (8). The most constant endoscopic finding following hydrodistention in patients with IC are the small, bleeding, raspberry-like spots called glomerulations (4,17). These are pinpoint petechial hemorrhages. In typical IC patients, they are present in at least three quadrants of the bladder and not just in the path of the endoscope. The appearance can be a lattice- or checkerboard-type pattern, or they may appear as splotchy areas over a whole section of the bladder (4). Even though the quantity and exact locations are variable, the trigone is usually spared, and predominantly the posterior wall, dome, and side walls are affected (4). The appearance is graded as mild, moderate, or severe. A range of mild to severe glomerulations along with a Hunner's patch is depicted in Figs. 1–4.

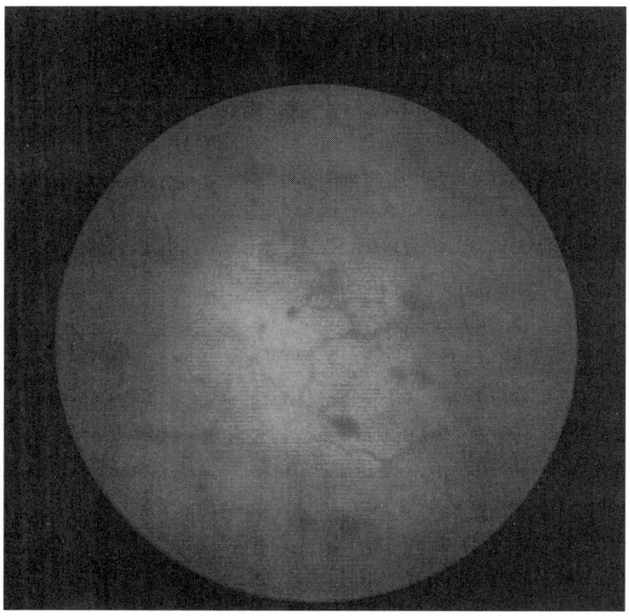

FIG. 1. Mild glomerulations. (Photo courtesy of C. Lowell Parsons, M.D., UCSD, San Diego.) See color plate 3.

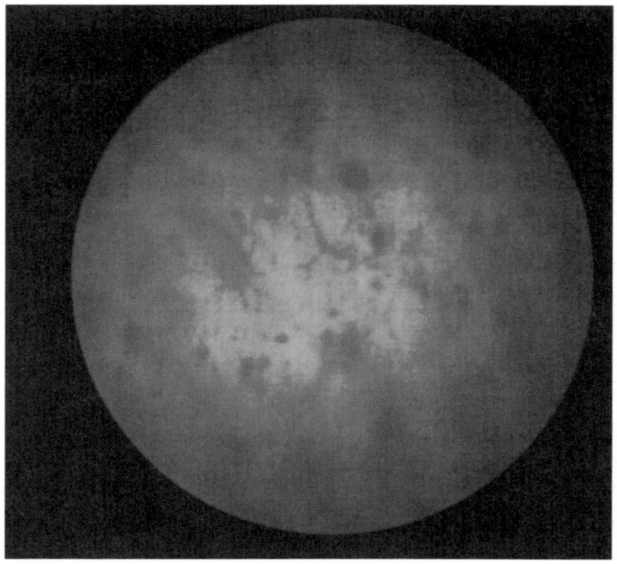

FIG. 2. Moderate glomerulations. (Photo courtesy of C. Lowell Parsons, M.D., UCSD, San Diego.) See color plate 4.

Although Messing and Stamey (4) stated that gomerulations do not occur in the normal bladder, glomerulations are not specific for IC. They can be seen in various types of inflammatory bladder disease: after treatment with intravesical chemotherapy and radiation, with infectious (tuberculosis, fungus), toxic (cyclophosphamide, formalin), and neoplastic (especially carcinoma *in situ*) disorders of the bladder. They may also simply be a result of stretching the bladder several hundred cubic centime-

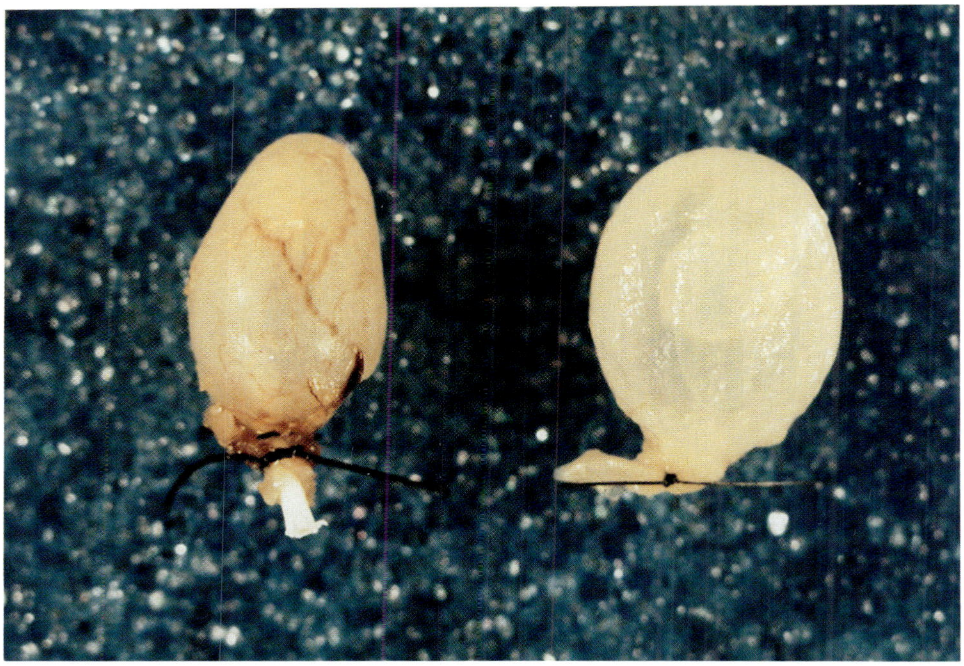

COLOR PLATE 1. The experimental autoimmune cystitis (EAC) bladder **(left)** is fibrotic and contracted with increased vascularity compared to the thin-walled normal bladder. See Chapter 5, Fig. 1.

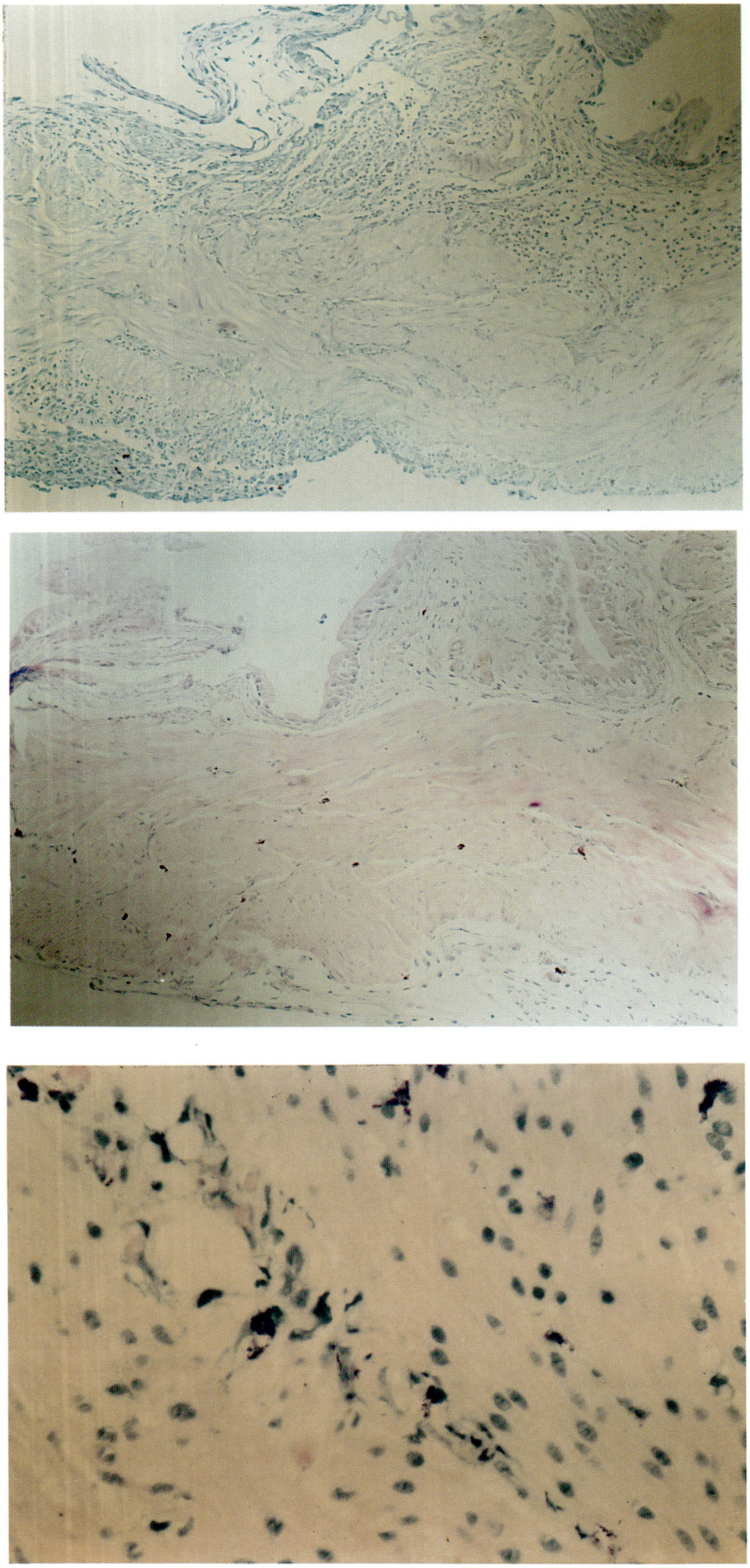

A

B

C

COLOR PLATE 2. (A) Bladder with bacterial cystitis displays small numbers of connective tissue mast cells with few in the detrusor muscle. **(B)** Bladder with EAC shows numerous mast cells concentrated in the detrusor muscle layer. **(C)** The mast cells in EAC are often degranulated. See Chapter 5, Fig. 7.

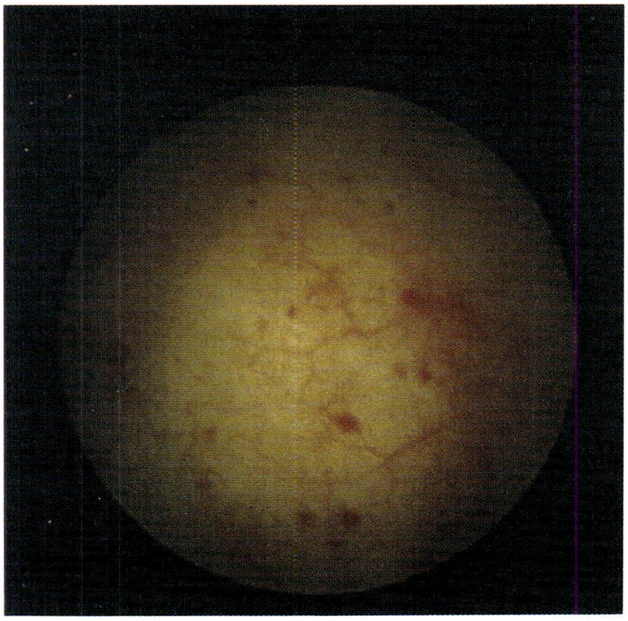

COLOR PLATE 3. Mild glomerulations. (Photo courtesy of C. Lowell Parsons, M.D., UCSD, San Diego.) See Chapter 17, Fig. 1.

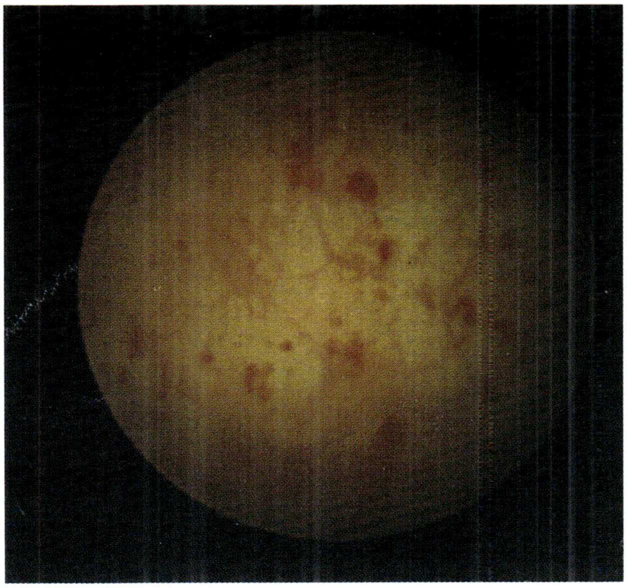

COLOR PLATE 4. Moderate glomerulations. (Photo courtesy of C. Lowell Parsons, M.D., UCSD, San Diego.) See Chapter 17, Fig. 2.

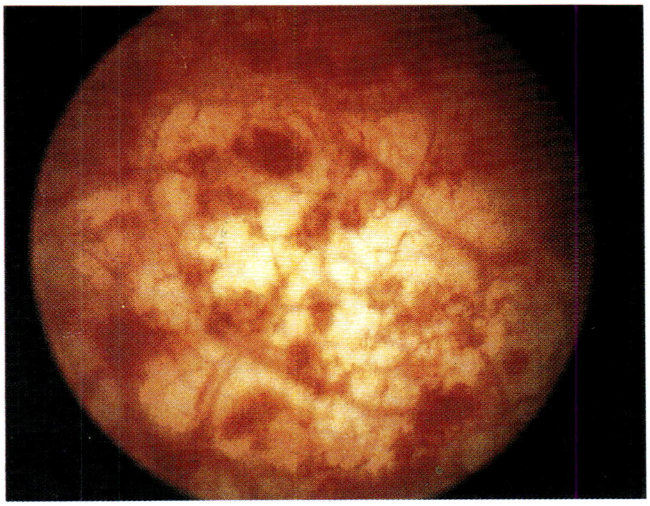

COLOR PLATE 5. Severe glomerulations. (Photo courtesy of C. Lowell Parsons, M.D., UCSD, San Diego.) See Chapter 17, Fig. 3.

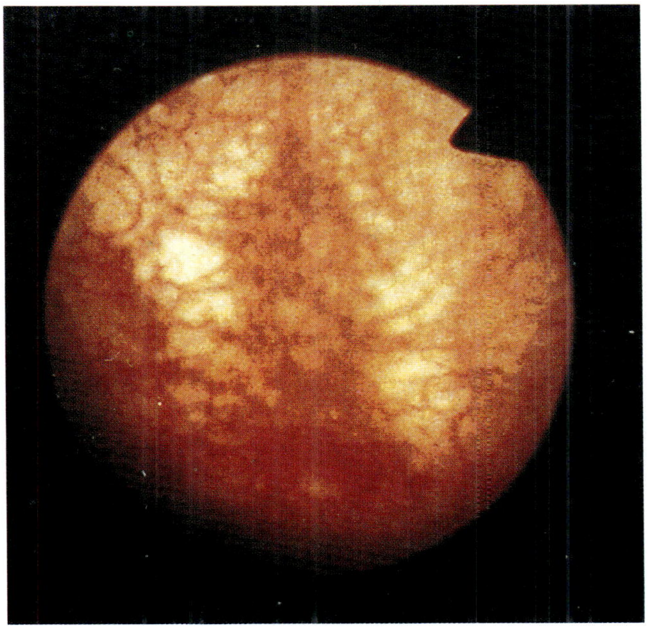

COLOR PLATE 6. Hunner's patch. (Photo courtesy of C. Lowell Parsons, M.D., UCSD, San Diego.) See Chapter 17, Fig. 4.

ters beyond its usual capacity, especially after a prolonged period of chronic underfilling, as in patients with defunctionalized bladders or in those with sensory urgency and resultant frequency (37). Nevertheless, glomerulations are not usually found in completely normal bladders.

A second or therapeutic distention may be carried out at this point. This distention is held at least 8 to 10 min, after which the bladder is drained.

Biopsies may be taken of abnormal areas and should include deep and superficial specimens. The specimens must be deep enough to include the detrusor and may be taken from two different sites (1,38). Unfortunately, there are no pathognomonic histologic findings for IC. Biopsy is done largely to rule out other varieties of cystitis or malignant or premalignant (CIS) conditions (25). Biopsy must be done after hydrodistention. If deep biopsies are done, catheter drainage should be instituted, in our opinion, to reduce the chance of perforation/extravasation.

It is well known that the severity of findings on cystoscopy, including the density of glomerulations and the amount of bleeding, do not necessarily parallel the symptom state (4,9,25,27). Few studies have been done on changes in endoscopic capacity and appearance after treatment of IC. This is understandable because once some significant measure of relief is obtained, patients with IC generally refuse any unnecessary manipulation. Messing (39) suggested that the cystoscopic appearance does not change after treatment. Prophylactic treatment of patients on the basis of endoscopic findings is not advised. Finally, it should be noted that there are patients who seem to fulfill the symptomatic and urodynamic diagnosis of IC but who do not exhibit the characteristic cystoscopic findings (40).

A few centers (41) have limited the routine use of cystoscopy in the workup of patients with suspected IC

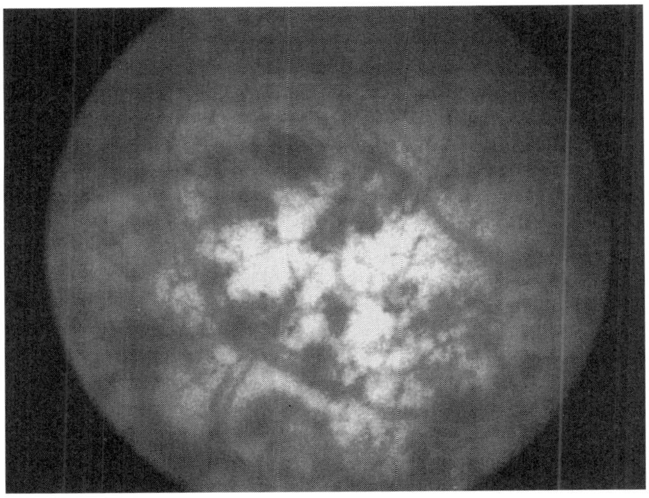

FIG. 3. Severe glomerulations. (Photo courtesy of C. Lowell Parsons, M.D., UCSD, San Diego.) See color plate 5.

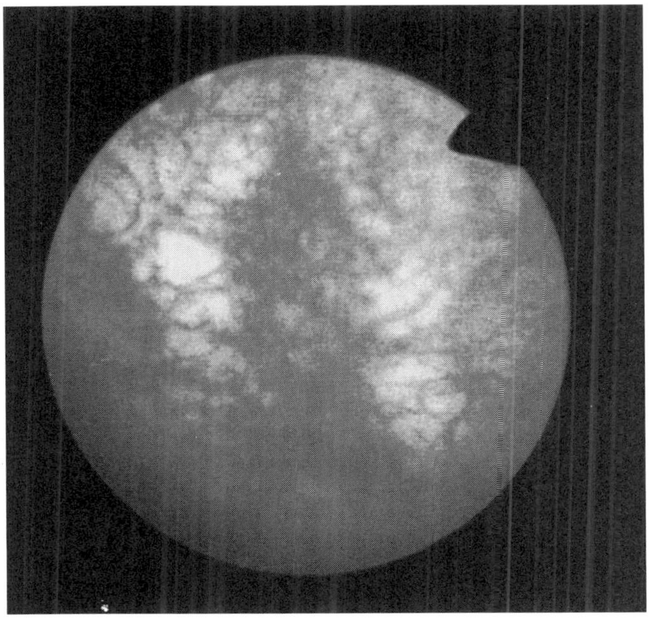

FIG. 4. Hunner's patch. (Photo courtesy of C. Lowell Parsons, M.D., UCSD, San Diego.) See color plate 6.

because of the glaring lack of conclusive diagnostic criteria. It is still necessary to rule out the possibility of other disorders such as carcinoma *in situ* or bladder cancer. Thus, cystoscopy is still a necessary tool in the workup of interstitial cystitis.

SUMMARY

The diagnosis of IC was one of exclusion in 1915 (2) and remains so today. Thus, arriving at a final diagnosis of IC is not a concise or rapid process and requires a well-informed physician and patient who are willing to commit the time and necessary effort. As the medical awareness of the general public is increasing, patients and their families are demanding more exact diagnoses accompanied by a description of exact findings. On the other hand, a final diagnosis of IC may be a difficult conclusion for everyone involved to accept because of the limitations of current treatment regimens.

Acknowledgments

This work was supported by the National Institutes of Health and the American Foundation of Urologic Disease through grant K12DK02196, a physician-scientist training grant.

REFERENCES

1. Resnick MI, Thompson S. Update of urological advances and controversies. *Infect Urol* 1990;31:8–13.

2. Hunner GL. A rare type of bladder ulcer in women: Report of cases. *J Boston Med Surg* 1915;172:660–665.
3. Benson GS. Interstitial cystitis. In: Hanno PM, Staskin DR, Krane RJ, Wein AJ, eds. *Interstitial Cystitis*. London: Springer-Verlag, 1990;131.
4. Messing EM, Stamey TA. Interstitial cystitis. Early diagnosis, pathology, and treatment. *Urology* 1978;XII:381–392.
5. Hand JR. Interstitial cystitis: report of 223 cases (204 women and 19 men). *J Urol* 1949;61:291–310.
6. Oravisto KJ, Alfthan OS. Treatment of interstitial cystitis with immunosuppression and chloroquine derivatives. *Eur Urol* 1976;2:82–84.
7. Walsh A. Interstitial cystitis. Observations on diagnosis and on treatment with anti-inflammatory drugs, particularly benzydamine. *Eur Urol* 1977;3:216–217.
8. Gillenwater JY, Wein AJ. Summary of the National Institute of Arthritis, Diabetes, Digestive and Kidney Diseases Workshop on Interstitial Cystitis, National Institutes of Health, Bethesda, MD, August 28–29. *J Urol* 1988;140:203–206.
9. Hanno PM, Levin RM, Monson FC, Teuscher C, Zhou ZZ, Ruggieri MR, Whitmore K, Wein AJ. Diagnosis of interstitial cystitis. *J Urol* 1990;143:278–281.
10. Wein AJ, Hanno PM, Gillenwater JY. Interstitial cystitis: An introduction to the problem. In: Hanno PM, Staskin DR, Krane RJ, Wein AJ, eds. *Interstitial Cystitis*. London: Springer-Verlag, 1990;13–14.
11. Parsons CL. Interstitial cystitis: Clinical manifestations and diagnostic criteria in over 200 cases. *Neurourol Urodyn* 1990;9:241–250.
12. Sant GR. Interstitial cystitis. *Monogr Urol* 1991;12:37–63.
13. Badenoch AW. Chronic interstitial cystitis. *Br J Urol* 1971;43:718–721.
14. Koziol JA, Clark DC, Gittes RF, Tan EM. The natural history of interstitial cystitis—a survey of 374 patients. *J Urol* 1993;149:465–469.
15. Leach GE, Raz S. Interstitial cystitis. In: Raz S, ed. *Female Urology*. Philadelphia: WB Saunders, 1983;351–356.
16. Parivar F, Bradbrook RA. Interstitial cystitis. *Br J Urol* 1986;58:239.
17. Oravisto KJ. Epidemiology of interstitial cystitis. *Ann Chir Gynecol Fenn* 1975;64:75–77.
18. Leach GE, Raz S. Interstitial cystitis. In: Raz S, ed. *Female Urology*. Philadelphia: WB Saunders, 1983;351–356.
19. Held PJ, Hanno PM, Wein AJ, Pauly MV, Cahn MA. Epidemiology of interstitial cystitis: 2. In: Hanno PM, Staskin DR, Krane RJ, Wein AJ, eds. *Interstitial Cystitis*. London: Springer-Verlag, 1990;35.
20. Keene FB. Elusive ulcer of the bladder. *Am J Obstet Gynecol* 1925;10:380–382.
21. Rosin RD, Griffiths T, Sofras F, James DC, Edwards L. Interstitial cystitis. *Br J Urol* 1979;51:524–527.
22. Jokinen EJ, Oravisto KJ, Alfthan OS. Antitissue antibodies in interstitial cystitis. *Clin Exp Immunol* 1972;11:333–339.
23. Pool TL. Interstitial cystitis: clinical considerations and treatment. *Clin Obstet Gynecol* 1967;10:185–191.
24. Held PJ, Hanno PM, Wein AJ, Pauly MV, Cahn MA. Epidemiology of interstitial cystitis: 2. In: Hanno PM, Staskin DR, Krane RJ, Wein AJ, eds. *Interstitial Cystitis*. London: Springer-Verlag, 1990;38.
25. Messing EM. The diagnosis of interstitial cystitis. *Urology* 1987;29 (4 Suppl):4–7.
26. Lapides J. Observations on interstitial cystitis. *Urology* 1975;5:610–611.
27. Sant GR, Meares EM Jr. Interstitial cystitis: Pathogenesis, diagnosis, and treatment. *Infect Urol* 1990;31:24–30.
28. Neal DE Jr., Dilworth JP, Kaack MB. Tamm–Horsfall autoantibodies in interstitial cystitis. *J Urol* 1991;145:37–39.
29. Parsons CL, Boychuk D, Jones S, Hurst R, Callahan H. Bladder surface glycosaminoglycans: an epithelial permeability barrier. *J Urol* 1990;143:139–142.
30. Boucher W, El-Mansoury M, Pang X, Sant GR, Theoharides TC. Elevated mast cell tryptase in the urine of patients with interstitial cystitis. *Br J Urol* 1995;76:94–100.
31. Zhao Y, Whitmore KE, Gordon D, Wein AJ, Levin RM. Detection of stress gene mRNAs in bladder biopsies, exfoliated cells in urine, and cells in bladder barbotage obtained from interstitial cystitis patients. *J Urol* 1995;153:329A.
32. Kirkemo A. *Associations between urodynamic findings and symptoms in females with interstitial cystitis*. Paper presented at the Interstitial Cystitis Association meeting, October 6, 1995.
33. Nigro DA. *Associations among cystoscopic and urodynamic findings for women with interstitial cystitis*. Paper presented at the Interstitial Cystitis Association meeting, October 6, 1995.
34. Stone AR. Editorial comment: The clinical evaluation of patients with painful bladder disease. In: Hanno PM, Staskin DR, Krane RJ, Wein AJ, eds. *Interstitial Cystitis*. London: Springer-Verlag, 1990;35.
35. Kerr WS Jr. Interstitial cystitis: treatment by transurethral resection. *J Urol* 1971;105:664–666.
36. Herbst RH, Baumrucker GO, German KL. Elusive ulcer (Hunner) of the bladder with an experimental study of the etiology. *Am J Surg* 1937;38:152–156.
37. Fall M, Johansson SL, Aldenborg F. Chronic interstitial cystitis: a heterogeneous syndrome. *J Urol* 1987;137:35–38.
38. Hanno PM. Diagnosis of interstitial cystitis. *Urol Clin North Am* 1994;21:63–66.
39. Slade DKA. Interstitial cystitis: a challenge to urology. *Urol Nurs* 1989;9:5–7.
40. Messing EM. Interstitial cystitis and related syndromes. In: Walsh PC, Gittes RF, Perlmutter AD, Stamey TA, eds. *Campbell's Urology*. Philadelphia: WB Saunders, 1985;1070–1092.
41. Chaiken DC, Blaivas JG, Blaivas ST. Behavioral therapy for the treatment of refractory interstitial cystitis. *J Urol* 1993;149:1445–1448.

Interstitial Cystitis, edited by Grannum R. Sant.
Lippincott–Raven Publishers, Philadelphia ©1997.

CHAPTER 18

The Pathology of Interstitial Cystitis

Sonny L. Johansson, Kumiko Ogawa, and Magnus Fall

Interstitial cystitis (IC) was described more than 100 years ago, and in spite of significant research efforts, the statement made by Hanash and Pool in 1969 that "the cause is unknown, the diagnosis is difficult, and the treatment is temporary and palliative" is still very much valid (1). Although IC is likely to be a syndrome rather than a specific disease, two subgroups of patients with urgency, frequency, and bladder-associated pain have been identified.

The separation into the two groups is done by cystoscopic examination with bladder distention with a pressure of at least 70 to 80 cm H_2O with the patient under general or spinal anesthesia. This procedure allows identification of two categories of patients, the ulcer (classic) and nonulcer (so-called early) type. Hunner's ulcers are present in the ulcer category of patients, whereas the nonulcer patient shows multiple petechial hemorrhages generally referred to as glomerulations. For reasons that are unknown (possibly related to the embryology of the bladder), the trigone is generally spared in IC. The nonulcer type was described by Messing and Stamey in 1978 (2). More systematic histopathologic studies were later published (3,4). Still, there are different opinions as to the value of biopsies with histopathologic evaluation in patients with interstitial cystitis. It has been said that light microscopic findings in IC are nonspecific and of little or no value, perhaps with the exception of ruling out carcinoma *in situ* (2,5). However, individuals other than ourselves have expressed the view that the histopathologic features identified may play a supportive role in the diagnosis of IC (6).

S. L. Johansson and K. Ogawa: Department of Pathology and Microbiology, The Eppley Institute for Research in Cancer and Allied Diseases, University of Nebraska Medical Center, Omaha, Nebraska 68198.

M. Fall: Division of Urology, Department of Surgery, Sahlgrenska University Hospital, University of Göteborg, Göteborg, Sweden.

PATIENT MATERIAL

All patients with a clinical suspicion of IC or verified IC and treated at Sahlgrenska University Hospital, Göteborg, Sweden, between 1976 and 1988 were evaluated clinically and cystoscopically by one of us (M.F.). The patients underwent cystoscopy, and their bladders were distended with a pressure of up to 70 cm H_2O. All patients were subjected to biopsies, generally by means of transurethral resection of the bladder (TURB). Material was taken from the ulcer(s) as well as from areas of hemorrhage and often from normal-appearing mucosa. The nonulcer patients' biopsies were generally taken from areas showing glomerulations. A total of nine patients with ulcer disease as well as one patient with nonulcer disease were subjected to partial or total cystectomy. The material included 210 interstitial patients, of whom 146 had ulcer-type IC, whereas 64 had nonulcer disease. A total of six individuals were men in the ulcer group, and 140 were women. The average age was 57 years. This agrees with the observation that nonulcer patients are as a group younger, although symptoms may be as chronic as in classic IC (7). In the group of nonulcer patients, five were male, and 59 were female, with an average age of 38 years. The results of the histopathologic examination of part of the material and of the total material have been reported previously (4,8). The high proportion of ulcer patients is partly related to the referral pattern and to the fact that we were not aware of the existence of nonulcer IC until the early 1980s. However, at the present time, the ratio of ulcer to nonulcer patients is approximately 1:1, which is different from that in the U.S. experience, where ulcer IC is said to account for only approximately 10% of all IC cases.

HISTOPATHOLOGIC FINDINGS

Most patients with ulcer disease showed striking light microscopic findings dominated by ulcerations associ-

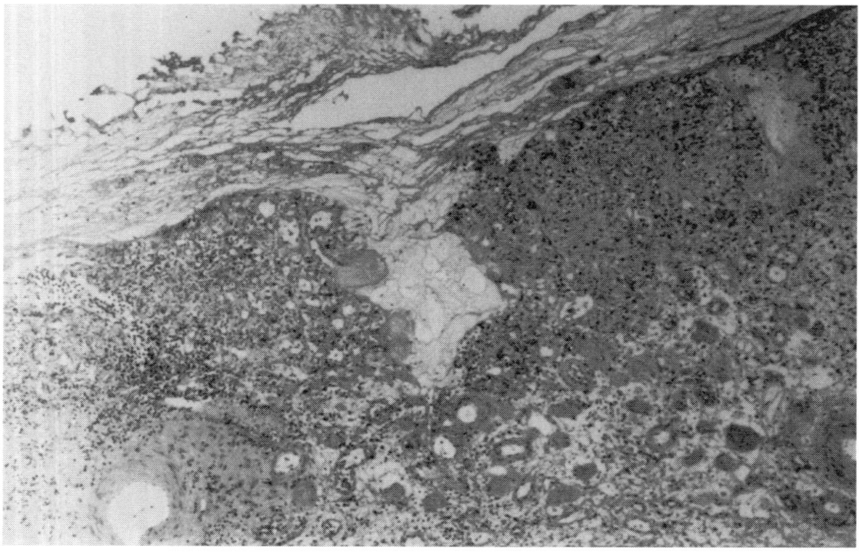

FIG. 1. A TURB specimen from an ulcer patient. Note the fibrin-covered ulceration surrounded by granulation tissue and marked mononuclear inflammatory infiltrate. Hematoxylin and eosin (H&E), original magnification ×28.

ated with marked inflammatory changes. An additional significant finding was the presence of granulation tissue in the lamina propria, which was found in almost 90% of the patients (Fig. 1; Table 1). This reparative tissue is likely to be generated by the rupture of the bladder mucosa during normal filling, and the area is likely a *locus minoris resistentie.* Cystoscopically, it probably corresponds to the area looking like a thin scar frequently covered by a small coagulum or fibrin deposit. This area easily ruptures during cystoscopy and bladder distention (4).

We are convinced that the formation of granulation tissue has taken place continuously in the ulcer-type lesions (classic IC) and is not a result of a previous transurethral resection of the bladder biopsy. However, such measures sometimes result in abundant local scar formation. Bladder tissue responds to different types of biopsy procedures with the formation of collagenized scar, foreign body granuloma, necrotizing granuloma (rheumatoid type), or pseudosarcoma of the bladder (also called postoperative spindle-cell nodule) (9). Histologically, the appearance of these types of lesions is different from that of the granulation tissue seen in ulcer-type interstitial cystitis patients. Mucosal hemorrhage was generally more extensive than in non-IC patients and was seen in 86% of ulcer patients (Fig. 2). The inflammatory changes were dominated by mononuclear cells (lymphocytes, plasma cells, and mast cells), with fewer neutrophils. Germinal center formation was often present. Inflammatory changes were generally limited to the lamina propria, a striking analogy with the histologic findings in ulcerative colitis (10,11). Perineural inflammatory lymphocytic infiltrates were present in 80% of patients below the lamina propria. Significant fibrosis of the detrusor muscle was present in only 15 of the cases, including all of the nine patients subjected to partial or complete cystectomy, who all had symptoms of a contracted bladder. A characteristic fibrosis with collagen distribution inside the muscle fascicles was described by Larsen et al. in their group of IC patients (12). We were unable to verify this type of fibrosis in our patients. In our relatively large series of ulcer patients, only 10% had significant fibrosis, and fibrosis was virtually absent in the nonulcer patients. The ulcers are often wedge-shaped and often covered by fibrin (Fig. 1). The ulcers for the most part did not extend deeper than to the level of the muscularis mucosa. The surface of the bladder often displayed absence of urothelium, the mucosa was frequently completely denuded, a finding also reported by Lynes et al. (6) (Fig. 2). This occurred in both ulcer and nonulcer patients but almost never in control patients (8). Sometimes urothelium was present, "floating" above

TABLE 1. *Histopathologic findings in interstitial cystitis patients*[a]

Patient category	Ulcer	Granulation tissue	Mucosal hemorrhage	Mucosal rupture	(+)	Mononuclear infiltrate +	++	+++	Perineural infiltrate
Ulcer (classic; 146 patients)	140 (96%)	130 (89%)	126 (86%)	0	0	16 (11%)	70 (48%)	60 (41%)	118 (81%)
Nonulcer (early; 64 patients)	0	0	57 (89%)	53 (83%)	49 (77%)	9 (14%)	6 (9%)	0	0

[a]From Johansson and Fall (8), with permission.

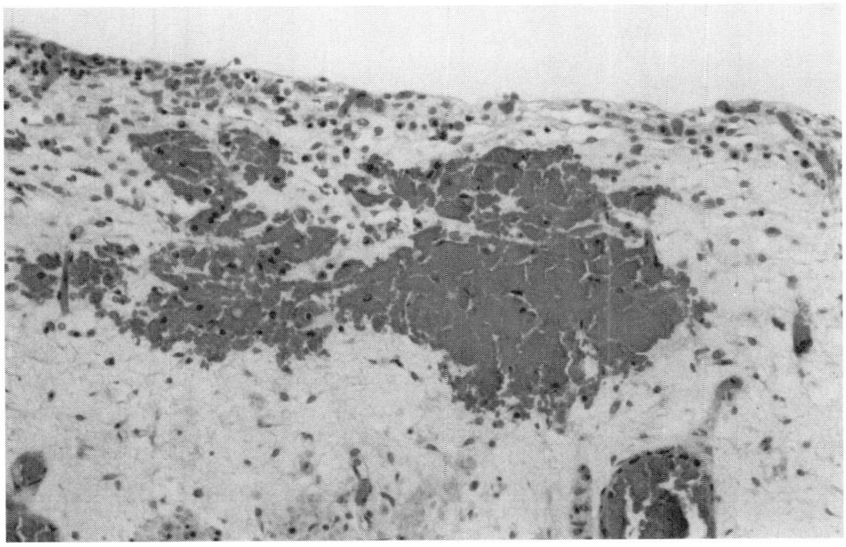

FIG. 2. A TURB specimen from an ulcer patient showing denudation of mucosa with lamina propria hemorrhage. H&E, original magnification ×140.

the surface of ulcer patients (Fig. 3). The denudation is most likely the result of the cystoscopic examination, instrumentation, and biopsy procedures. The IC bladder seems to be more vulnerable and sensitive to this type of manipulation, which results in easier detachment of the urothelium. Another fairly consistent finding is the presence of relatively marked edema of the lamina propria with dilated vascular channels, especially venules. These vessels often contain neutrophils showing margination and, in one-third of the cases, involvement of the wall of the vein.

In spite of the fact that all our IC patients had virtually identical symptoms of frequency, urgency, and pain, the histopathologic findings in the nonulcer patients were strikingly meager compared to the ulcer patients. The majority displayed suburothelial hemorrhage corresponding to glomerulations, and the hemorrhage was generally limited (Fig. 4). However, in some cases, it was more prominent even with involvement of the urothelium. Some 80% of the patients displayed mucosal ruptures, which are tears in the urothelium only superficially involving the lamina propria. Interestingly, there was no significant inflammation associated with these tears (Fig. 5). Overall, the inflammatory response did not differ significantly from that of control patients. The ruptures are unlikely to be artifact because in a total of 30 control patients subjected to the same bladder manipulation, ruptures were not identified. As a matter of fact, they may be a sign of weakness of the urothelial lining or poor adhesion between urothelial cells.

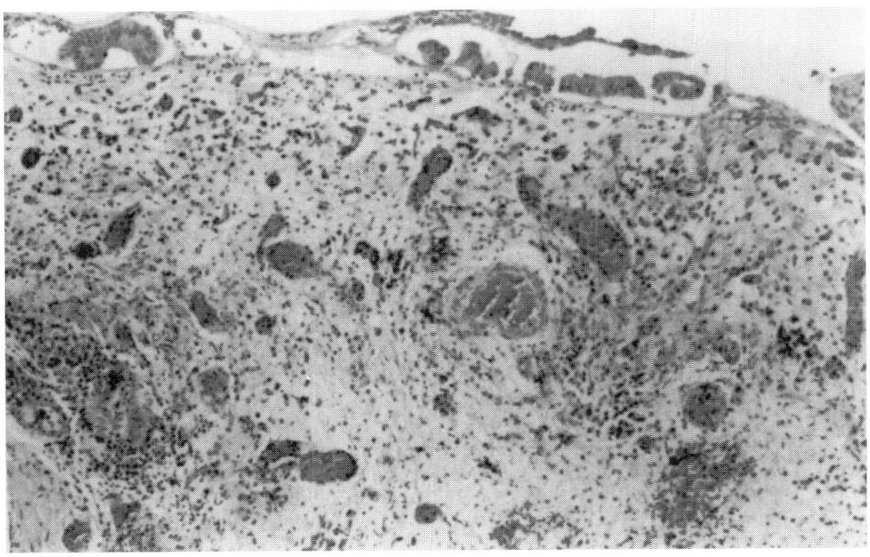

FIG. 3. A TURB specimen from an ulcer patient from an area without ulceration. Note the detached urothelium. H&E, original magnification ×140.

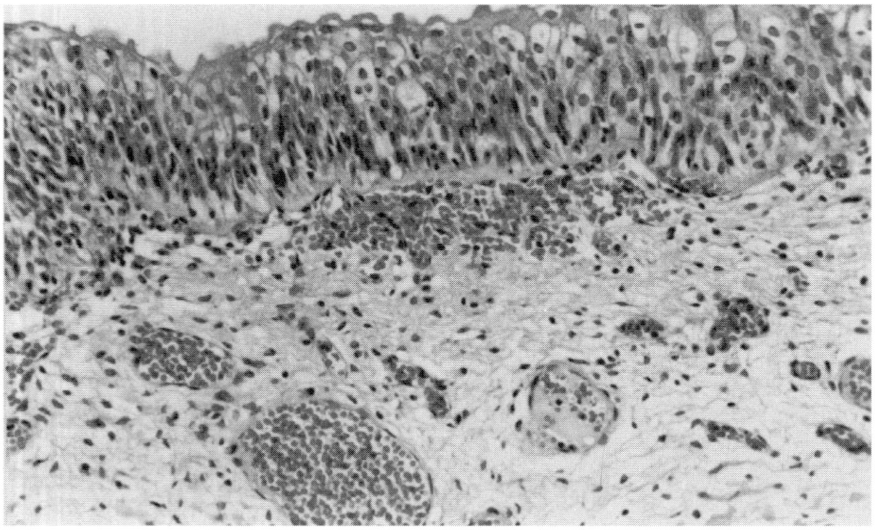

FIG. 4. A TURB specimen from a nonulcer patient showing normal urothelium associated with suburothelial hemorrhage corresponding to glomerulation. H&E, original magnification ×280.

HISTOPATHOLOGIC FINDINGS IN BLADDER TISSUE IN U.S. PATIENTS

The transurethrally resected material from the Swedish patients included large strips of bladder, generally including half the depth of the detrusor muscle, which made the light microscopic evaluation easier. In contrast, in the United States, this type of biopsy material is not generally obtained because of 1-day surgery limitations. The majority of patients in the United States undergo cold cup or forceps biopsies rather than transurethral resection biopsies. During the last 5 years, 82 patients with a clinical diagnosis of IC or a clinical suspicion of IC have been seen at The University of Nebraska Medical Center or had biopsy material sent in consultation to one of us (S.L.J.) (Table 2). Seventy-four patients underwent forceps or cold cup biopsies, whereas eight underwent partial or total cystectomy. Of these patients, 21 had the characteristic features of the ulcer type of disease, and 41 had features consistent with nonulcer interstitial cystitis. In 20 patients, the biopsies were either completely normal or the patients were found to have other conditions (Table 3). The nine patients with normal findings may or may not have had nonulcer IC, but it is interesting to notice that the mean age was 10 years higher than that of the patients having both clinical and light microscopic findings of nonulcer type of IC.

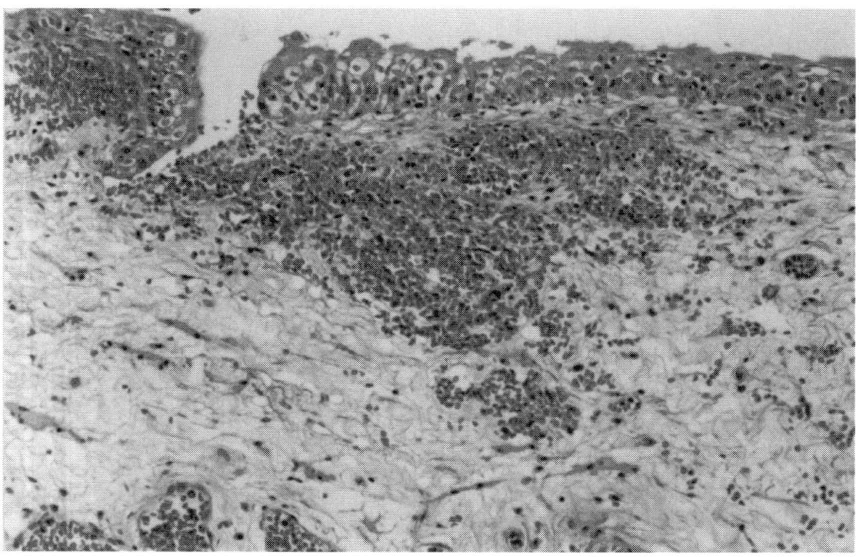

FIG. 5. A TURB specimen from a nonulcer patient showing mucosal rupture and glomerulation. Note the lack of significant inflammation. H&E, original magnification ×140.

TABLE 2. *Age, gender, and diagnostic procedure/treatment in the different patient categories*

	Swedish patients		U.S. patients		
	Ulcer (n = 146)	Nonulcer (n = 64)	Ulcer (n = 21)	Nonulcer (n = 41)	Nondiagnostic (n = 20)
Mean age	57	38	56	38	55
Age range	27–84	19–71	22–86	19–73	22–81
Men	6	5	2	2	3
Women	140	59	19	39	17
Diagnostic treatment procedure					
Biopsy	-	-	17	38	17
TURB[a]	137	63	-	-	2
Partial/total cystectomy	9	1	4	3	1

[a]TURB, transurethral resection of the bladder.

The main differential diagnosis in IC seems to be eosinophilic cystitis, and six patients were diagnosed with this condition, three men and three women. Clinically, the symptoms may be indistinguishable from those of IC. However, eosinophilic cystitis is a true pancystitis in contrast to ulcer IC. Muscle necrosis is typically present, and the inflammatory infiltrate "spills over" into the perivesical fat and contains a significant number of eosinophils (13,14). Two patients had bacterial cystitis, and one of them, an 81-year-old woman, died of urosepsis 2 days after the biopsy. One patient had severe dysplasia or carcinoma *in situ.* One female patient with a history of bladder cancer and intravesical chemotherapy developed marked urgency and frequency 2 years after the final treatment and was suspected to have IC. However, the only significant biopsy finding was marked fibrosis of the lamina propria. Although some authors have reported increased eosinophils in IC patients, we do not share that experience.

TABLE 3. *Patients with clinical diagnosis or suspicion of IC in whom the diagnosis could not be verified or was different*

	Sex	Age	Urgency/frequency	Pain	Clinical diagnosis	Pathology diagnosis[a]
1	F	40	+	+	IC	NPA
2	F	67	+	+	IC	NPA
3	F	39	+	+	IC	NPA
4	F	57	+	+	IC	NPA
5	F	58	+	+	IC	NPA
6	F	22	+	+	IC	NPA
7	F	34	+	+	IC	NPA
8	F	44	+	+	IC	NPA
9	F	63	+	-	IC?	NPA
10	M	42	+	+	IC	EOC
11	M	55	+	+	IC	EOC
12	F	71	+	+	IC?	EOC
13	M	81	+	-	IC?	EOC
14	F	39	+	+	IC?	EOC
15	F	47	+	+	IC?	EOC
16	F	81	+	(+)	IC?	Bacterial cystitis
17	F	47	+	+	IC	Bacterial cystitis
18	F	74	+	-	IC?	Severe dysplasia CIS
19	F	70	+	-	IC?	Fibrosis of LP[b]
20	F	46	+	-	IC?	Cystitis glandularis

[a]NPA, no pathologic abnormality; EOC, eosinophilic cystitis; LP, lamina propria.
[b]Status following intravesical treatment for bladder cancer.

ULTRASTRUCTURAL STUDIES

Very few ultrastructural studies have been performed on patients with IC. In the first of these, Collan et al. did not report any pathologic abnormalities on transmission electron microscopy (15). In contrast, Eldrup et al., using colloid lanthanum, found differences in the permeability of the urothelium between IC patients and controls (16). This may be related to possibly defective tight junctions. In another study by Dixon and collaborators, some variations in the thickness of the glycocalyx (glycosaminoglycan layer) were identified (17). They used ruthenium red to visualize the glycocalyx. The differences, however, seem to be related to the surface topography of the luminal cells. Besides that, the investigators did not find any differences in the variability between interstitial cystitis patients and controls. Said et al., using transmission electron microscopy, reported widening of the intercellular spaces between transitional cells in all layers of the urothelium (18). They also were able to identify microvilli.

A study in our laboratory using scanning electron microscopy involved 13 patients with ulcer-type IC and nine controls (19). We found that the proportion of cells covered by round, uniform, and pleomorphic microvilli was higher in the IC patients than in the controls. Furthermore, it appeared that the IC patients had a reduced mucin layer. However, we have found in other studies that the presence of microvilli is seen not only in neoplastic conditions but also in reactive and reparative conditions such as catheter-associated polypoid cystitis (20). Therefore, the finding of increased microvilli was more likely to be a consequence of increased cell turnover than a surface-specific characteristic for the ulcer type of interstitial cystitis. It must be emphasized that none of the other reported ultrastructural studies defined the type of IC patients had, i.e., ulcer versus nonulcer.

Uroplakins are four distinct proteins (Ia, Ib, II, III) that have been isolated from the asymmetric unit membrane (AUM) of bovine urothelium. Monospecific polyclonal antibodies to these proteins have shown that all of them are AUM associated (21). The AUM is characteristic of the mammalian bladder and believed to play a role in strengthening the urothelial surfaces, thus preventing the bladder cells from rupturing during distention (22). In a preliminary study using immunoperoxidase, we have evaluated 16 ulcer patients with a mean age 61 years (range 32 to 77); 11 nonulcer patients, mean age 36 (range 20 to 59); and six controls with a mean age of 44 (26 to 52 years). The antibody used was a lyophilized rabbit anti-AUM antiserum, which has been shown to react strongly with uroplakin III, moderately with uroplakin Ia and Ib, and weakly with uroplakin II. This polyclonal antibody works on paraffin sections of human and bovine bladders.

Generally, the ulcer patients had negative staining, although sometimes a few positive cells could be found "floating" above the surface. Part of the explanation for the negative findings was the fact that ulceration and mucosal denudation were common, but even when residual mucosa was present, the staining was generally negative. In contrast, all nonulcer patients except one had positive staining. In all cases but one, it was discontinuous; this may have been related to the detachment of some umbrella cells or focal breakdown of AUM, which may be of etiologic importance in IC (Fig. 6). However, the possibility that discontinuous staining may be an artifact cannot be completely ruled out, and additional studies are needed. The six control patients were all positive, and half of them showed continuous staining (Fig. 7). The other three showed discontinuous staining similar to that in the nonulcer patients. It seems that uroplakins are expressed less in ulcer patients, which may be a result of the disease, but age may also be an additional factor

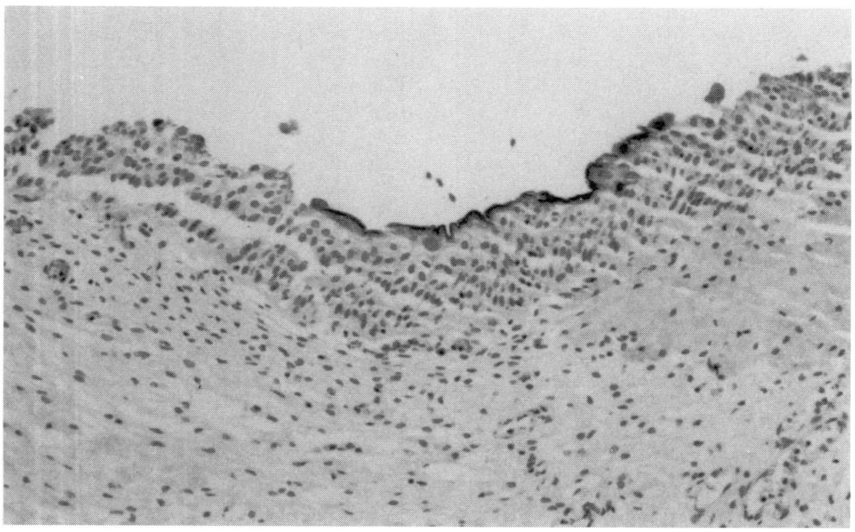

FIG. 6. Discontinuous superficial uroplakin staining in a 37-year-old nonulcer patient. Original magnification ×140.

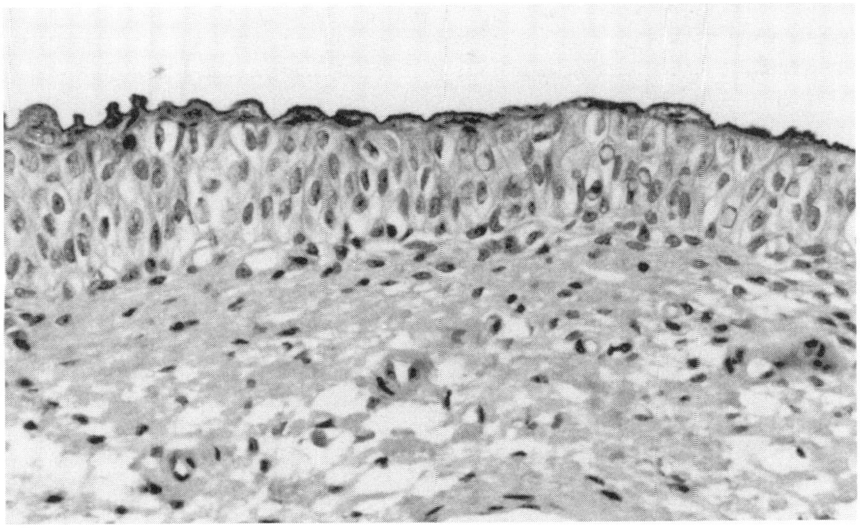

FIG. 7. Continuous superficial uroplakin staining of the umbrella cells in a 45-year-old control patient. H&E, original magnification ×280.

explaining the negative staining, as AUM seems to be reduced in number with increasing age, and the ulcer patients were significantly older than the nonulcer patients and controls.

IMMUNOLOGIC STUDIES

The fact that interstitial disease is a chronic, often relapsing condition and the majority of the patients are women has spawned the idea that immunologic mechanisms, especially autoimmunity, are involved in the etiology of interstitial cystitis. Findings by Mattila et al. tend to support this idea (23). Thus, in a study of 47 IC patients, 33 were found to have immune deposits in vessel walls. In a subsequent study using electron transmission electron microscopy, evidence of endothelial injury was found in 14 of 20 IC patients (24). Mattila and Linder demonstrated the presence of immunoglobulins, especially IgM, in vessel walls of over 50% of patients with IC usually associated with complement C_1q, C_3, and C_4 (25). In a similar study, Said et al. found that 50% of 308 patients with IC had strong IgM staining of the urothelium, whereas IgA was seen in only 6% of the patients (19). Approximately one-fourth of the patients had IgM deposits in blood vessels, and the majority of the lymphocytes revealed positive IgM surface membrane staining. All of these studies failed to separate ulcer and nonulcer patients and are therefore difficult to evaluate. The fact that interstitial cystitis symptoms generally disappear after urinary diversion without cystectomy as well as the occurrence of interstitial cystitic-like changes following enterocystoplasties speaks against an immune mechanism as the sole explanation (26).

In a study in our lab, immunohistochemistry was performed to evaluate cryostat sections of snap-frozen bladder biopsies. The study included 24 ulcer-type IC patients, nine nonulcer patients, and ten controls (27). Typically, the ulcer patients revealed aggregates of T cells as well as B-cell nodules with germinal centers. There was a decreased or normal helper/suppressor ratio, and suppressor cytotoxic cells were present in germinal centers. In contrast, the nonulcer group had only slightly increased numbers of lymphoid cells dominated by T-helper cells and with occasional T-cell aggregates. B-cell nodules were missing, and plasma cells were only rarely identified. As a matter of fact, the results of the nonulcer patients did not significantly differ from those of the control group. In a parallel study of peripheral blood by flow cytometry, an increased number of secretory IgM-positive B cells and activated lymphocytes were identified in the nonulcer group with a mildly abnormal κ/λ ratio as well as activated lymphocytes in the ulcer group. The control group revealed no such changes. These results suggest a partial role for immunologic mechanisms in the pathophysiology of interstitial cystitis.

CLINICOPATHOLOGIC CONSIDERATIONS

Although there is agreement that IC is a heterogeneous syndrome, there are still controversies about classification of this disease or diseases. It is noteworthy that in our blindly evaluated series, mast cells were found only in very low numbers equivalent to those in controls in the nonulcer patients. However, there was a marked increase of two phenotypes of mast cells in the classic type of IC (3). In contrast, in many U.S. studies, significant numbers of mast cells are identified in patients with the nonulcer category of IC (28). Interpretation of cystoscopic findings is crucial for the assignment to different categories. Ideally, in IC studies, cystoscopic pictures should be displayed visually, but this is, of course, not a practical pos-

TABLE 4. *Cystoscopic and histopathologic findings in patients with classic (ulcer-type) and nonulcer IC*

Classic IC	Nonulcer IC
Cystoscopic findings	
Circumscript lesion	Scattered glomerulations
Peripheral vascular injection	
Central scar with deposit	
Mucosal rupture at lesion site	Multiple small mucosal tears
Histopathologic findings	
Urothelial spongiosis and detachment	Submucosal hemorrhage
Granulation tissue	
Ulceration	Mucosal rupture
Focal perineural infiltrates of mononuclear cells	No or mild inflammation
Increase of connective tissue mast cells	
Presence of mucosal mast cells	

sibility. At the least, findings should be presented in some detail to allow comparison between different series of patients. The very marked difference in frequency of nonulcer to classic, the ratio being 9:1 in most U.S. centers compared to 1:1 in our series, is also puzzling. It might (at least partly) result from differences in interpretation of cystoscopic findings, although an alternative or additional explanation may be geographic differences in distribution. How to describe an "ulcer" may be a matter of variation. In fact, there is seldom a true ulcer but rather a circumscript, reddened area showing a characteristic vascular injection and a central scar with an attached small fibrin deposit or coagulum; the ulcer appears as a rupture of the central part of the lesion, but not until sufficient overdistention has occurred. In most cases, the lesions are typical, but they may sometimes be very discrete. Occasionally, in its most aggressive form, classic IC may appear as an almost generalized cystitis reaction including areas of mucosal scars. The appearance of glomerulations is less debatable, but the firmness of their link to IC is still not clearly evaluated. A major complication is that the description of cystoscopic findings is rather subjective. In this context, histopathology may support the diagnosis and subdivision. Table 4 lists the cystoscopic and histopathologic findings in ulcer (classic) and nonulcer IC.

The NIH-NIDDK guidelines (29), as currently used, are helpful by providing exclusion criteria to rule out IC-like conditions with different etiologies, e.g., bladder neoplasm (carcinoma *in situ*), radiation-induced or bacterial cystitis. These guidelines may, on one hand, still be too broad and sometimes permit inclusion of patients with other conditions, e.g., the urethral syndrome, where-as, on the other hand, there is no distinct subdivision into specific types of IC. We feel that, at this stage, in presenting clinical studies of IC patients, it is not enough to state that the patients meet the NIH criteria. More detailed clinical findings should also be presented in an attempt to establish firm and general criteria for the diagnosis.

Acknowledgments

The authors are grateful to Drs. Xue-Ru, Wu, and Tung-Tien Sun for providing the uroplakin antibody. The skillfull technical assistance by Karin Karlsson is recognized along with excellent secretarial help provided by Mary McAndrews.

REFERENCES

1. Hanash KA, Pool TL. Interstitial cystitis in men. *J Urol* 1969;102:427–428.
2. Messing EM, Stamey TA. Interstitial cystitis. Early diagnosis, pathology, and treatment. *Urology* 1978;12:381–392.
3. Fall M, Johansson SL, Aldenborg F. Chronic interstitial cystitis. A heterogeneous syndrome. *J Urol* 1987;137:35–38.
4. Johansson SL, Fall M. Clinical features and spectrum of light microscopic changes in interstitial cystitis. *J Urol* 1990;143:1118–1124.
5. Hanno P, Levin RM, Monson FC, Teuscher C, Zong Zhou Z, Ruggeri M, Whitmore K, Wein A. Diagnosis of interstitial cystitis. *J Urol* 1990;143:278–281.
6. Lynes WL, Flynn SD, Shortliffe LD, Stamey TA. The histology of interstitial cystitis. *Am J Surg Pathol* 1990;14:969–976.
7. Fall M. Transcutaneous electrical nerve stimulation in interstitial cystitis—update on clinical experience. *Urology* 1987;24(Suppl):40–42.
8. Johansson SL, Fall M. Pathology of interstitial cystitis. *Urol Clin North Am* 1994;21:55–62.
9. Johansson SL, Cohen SM. Diseases of the lower urinary tract. In: Damjanov I, Linder J, eds. *Anderson's Pathology,* 10th ed. St. Louis: Mosby, 1996.
10. Hand JR. Interstitial cystitis. Report of 223 cases (204 women and 19 men). *J Urol* 1949;61:291–310.
11. Bohne AW, Hodson JM, Rebuck JW, et al. An abnormal leukocyte response in interstitial cystitis. *J Urol* 1962;88:387–391.
12. Larsen S, Thompson SA, Hald T, et al. Mast cells in interstitial cystitis. *Br J Urol* 1982;54:283–286.
13. Hellstrom HR, Davis BK, Shonnard JW. Eosinophilic cystitis. A study of 15 cases. *Am J Clin Pathol* 1979;72:777–784.
14. Johansson SL, Smout MS, Taylor RJ. Eosinophilic cystitis associated with symptomatic ureteral involvement. A report of two cases. *J Urol Pathol* 1993;1:69–71.
15. Collan Y, Alfthan O, Kivilaakso E, Oravisto KJ. Electron microscopic and histological findings in urinary bladder epithelium in interstitial cystitis. *Eur Urol* 1976;2:242–247.
16. Eldrup J, Thorup J, Nielsen SL, et al. Permeability and ultrastructure of human bladder epithelium. *Br J Urol* 1983;55:488–492.
17. Dixon JS, Holm-Bentzen M, Gilpin CJ, et al. Electron microscopic

investigation of the bladder urothelium and glycocalyx in patients with interstitial cystitis. *J Urol* 1986;135:621–626.

18. Said JW, Van De Velde R, Gillespie L. Immunopathology of interstitial cystitis. *Mod Pathol* 1989;2:593.
19. Anderström CRK, Fall M, Johansson SL. Scanning electron microscopic findings in interstitial cystitis. *Br J Urol* 1990;63:270–275.
20. Anderström C, Ekelund P, Hansson HA, Johansson SL. Scanning electron microscopy of polypoid cystitis, a reversible lesion of the human urinary bladder. *J Urol* 1984;131:242–246.
21. Wu X-R, Manabe M, Yu J, Sun T-T. Large scale purification and immune localization of bovine uroplakins I, II and III. *J Biol Chem* 1990;265:1970–1979.
22. Wu X-R, Lin JH, Walz, T. Mammalian uroplakins, a group of highly conserved urothelial differentiation-related membrane proteins. *J Biol Chem* 1994;269:13716–13724.
23. Mattila J. Vascular immunopathology in interstitial cystitis. *Clin Immunol Immunopathol* 1982;23:648–655.
24. Mattila J, Pitkanen R, Vaalasti T. Fine-structural evidence for vascular injury in patients with interstitial cystitis. *Virchows Arch* 1983;398:347–355.
25. Mattila J, Linder E. Immunoglobin deposits in the bladder epithelium and vessels in interstitial cystitis. Possible relationship to circulating anti-intermediate filament autoantibodies. *Clin Immunol Immunopathol* 1984;3:81–89.
26. McGuire ES, Lytton B, Carnog SL. Interstitial cystitis following colocystoplasty. *Urology* 1973;2:28–29.
27. Harrington DS, Johansson SL, Fall M. Interstitial cystitis: An immune histological and cytofluorimetric analysis of bladder mucosa and peripheral blood. *J Urol* 1990;144:868–871.
28. Theoharides TC, Sant GR, El-Mansoury M, Letourneau R, Ucci AA Jr, Meares EM Jr. Activation of bladder mast cells in interstitial cystitis. A light and electron microscopic study. *J Urol* 1995;153:629–636.
29. Gillenwater JY, Wein AJ. Summary of the National Institute of Arthritis, Diabetes, Digestive and Kidney Diseases workshop on interstitial cystitis, National Institutes of Health, Bethesda, Maryland, August 28–29, 1987. *J Urol* 1988;140:203–206.

Interstitial Cystitis, edited by Grannum R. Sant.
Lippincott–Raven Publishers, Philadelphia ©1997.

CHAPTER 19

Gynecologic Aspects of Interstitial Cystitis

Neeraj Kohli, Eddie H.M. Sze, and Mickey M. Karram

Ninety percent of patients with interstitial cystitis are female. Many of the patients have seen as many as seven physicians, undergone multiple workups with normal findings, and endured symptoms for an average of 3 to 5 years before a diagnosis was made (1). It is also recognized that for every patient diagnosed with interstitial cystitis, there are at least five who remain undiagnosed. Although the gynecologist has not played an active role in diagnosing and managing this condition, there is no question that many of the symptoms of interstitial cystitis overlap with symptoms of gynecologic conditions. Unfortunately, most gynecologists have very little knowledge of interstitial cystitis, and most urologists know very little about gynecologic conditions that present with similar symptoms. It is not surprising to note that many patients with interstitial cystitis initially present to the gynecologist's office. Physicians, especially those within surgical subspecialties, have always been hesitant and insecure managing conditions in which no obvious etiologic agent is recognized and no standard therapy is available, a situation that has long existed in gynecologic circles in regard to chronic pain syndromes, premenstrual syndrome, endometriosis, recurring vulvar and vaginal pain disorders, and dyspareunia, to mention only a few. It is not difficult to understand why patients with chronic pelvic pain syndromes will commonly get passed back and forth between the gynecologist and the urologist.

The objective of this chapter is to review the differential diagnosis of interstitial cystitis, discuss gynecologic conditions that may commonly present with symptoms similar to those of interstitial cystitis, and, finally, include a discussion of the association between interstitial cystitis and certain gynecologic disorders.

DIFFERENTIAL DIAGNOSIS OF INTERSTITIAL CYSTITIS

Although the diagnosis of interstitial cystitis is made on the basis of symptomatology and cystoscopic findings, it is often a diagnosis of exclusion. This has been confirmed by several studies including Hanno et al. (2), who found that only 36% of patients with interstitial cystitis met the required diagnostic criteria set forth by the National Institute of Health workshop in 1987 (3). Because of the difficulty of accurately diagnosing this condition, the urologist must be aware of other conditions that may present in a similar fashion. Although the pelvis is often viewed on a compartmentalized basis by many subspecialists, it is important to remember that it represents a complex collection of various organ systems that are closely integrated on both an anatomic and physiological level. Various pathologic conditions of any of these systems may mimic the nonspecific symptoms of interstitial cystitis, and a multidisciplinary approach may achieve greater success in determining the correct diagnosis.

Irritable bladder symptoms such as urgency, frequency, and dysuria, often found in patients with interstitial cystitis, are common in a variety of other urologic disorders including urinary tract infection, detrusor instability, radiation cystitis, tuberculous involvement of the bladder, and bladder cancer (4). Gynecologic disorders such as pelvic infection, urogenital atrophy, and endometriosis involving the bladder may also have similar presenting symptoms because of the close proximity and possible involvement of the urinary tract.

Pelvic pain is a vague, nonspecific complaint reported by many patients with interstitial cystitis. Although the

N. Kohli: Division of Urogynecology and Reconstructive Pelvic Surgery, Good Samaritan Hospital, Cincinnati, Ohio 45220.

E. H. M. Sze: Department of Obstetrics and Gynecology, Medical Center of Central Georgia, Mercer University School of Medicine, Macon, Georgia 31201.

M. M. Karram: Division of Urogynecology and Reconstructive Pelvic Surgery, Good Samaritan Hospital, Department of Obstetrics and Gynecology, University of Cincinnati Medical Center, Cincinnati, Ohio 45220.

TABLE 1. *Causes of chronic pelvic pain*

Urologic
Interstitial cystitis
Urethral syndrome
Urethral diverticulum
Urolithiasis
Neoplasm
Detrusor sphincter dyssynergia
Gynecologic
Endometriosis
Vulvodynia
Pelvic infection
Urogenital atrophy
Pelvic adhesions
Leiomyoma
Gastroenterologic
Irritable bowel syndrome
Inflammatory bowel disease
Diverticular disease
Hernia
Ischemic bowel disease
Neoplasm
Musculoskeletal
Degenerative joint disease
Pelvic floor myalgia
Psychological

pain is generally described as suprapubic in location, it has also been reported deep in the pelvis, localized to the lower back, shooting to the vagina and perineum, and radiating to the upper abdomen or groin (5). Deep pelvic pain may result from a variety of acute and chronic conditions involving the gynecologic or gastrointestinal (GI) tract, and lower back pain may suggest musculoskeletal involvement or endometriosis. Pain localized to the vagina and perineum may indicate disorders of the lower urogenital tract, and radiation to the upper abdomen should alert the clinician to consider pathologic conditions of the upper abdominal organs such as the stomach, liver, gallbladder, and pancreas. A psychological component should also be considered with somatization or personality disorders in the differential diagnosis (Table 1). An increased prevalence of psychosocial stress factors and childhood sexual or physical abuse has been reported in patients with chronic pelvic pain syndrome (8).

Pelvic pressure, occasionally reported by patients with interstitial cystitis (5), is a common symptom in a variety of gynecologic and gastrointestinal conditions. Endometriosis, adenomyosis, urogenital atrophy, and pelvic relaxation all may initially present with symptoms of pelvic pressure. Disorders of the GI tract with a similar clinical picture include irritable bowel syndrome, inflammatory bowel disease, abdominal hernias, and neurogenic bowel. With the exception of pelvic relaxation, physical examination may be completely normal in all of these conditions.

Dyspareunia, which occurs in up to 40% to 60% of patients with interstitial cystitis (7), is a common symptom that may be caused by many gynecologic and urologic conditions. A careful history may categorize the symptom into one of three subsets: entrance dyspareunia, vaginal dyspareunia, and deep thrust dyspareunia. Although certain conditions may fall within more than one subset, entrance dyspareunia is typically seen when there is primary involvement of the vaginal introitus such as in vulvar disease, urogenital atrophy, urethritis, urethral syndrome, and interstitial cystitis. Vaginal dyspareunia is most commonly noted with inadequate lubrication, vaginismus, and vaginal strictures, whereas deep thrust dyspareunia suggests endometriosis or symptomatic uterine retroversion (Table 2). In addition to the pain component, many patients manifest emotional stress as a result of interference with sexual function and interpersonal relationships. Up to one-third of all patients with interstitial cystitis have been abandoned by their husband or sexual partner as a result of their illness. Similar to patients with pelvic pain, a psychological component may also be present and should be considered in the diagnosis and management of this type of chronic pain syndrome (8).

GYNECOLOGIC DISORDERS THAT MAY MIMIC INTERSTITIAL CYSTITIS

Interstitial cystitis is predominantly found in young to middle-aged women who present with nonspecific symptoms. Therefore, a variety of genital tract disorders must be considered in the differential diagnosis, and gynecologic consultation may be helpful in the diagnostic workup. Although a number of gynecologic conditions

TABLE 2. *Differential diagnosis of dyspareunia*[a]

Entrance dyspareunia
Urogenital atrophy
Vulvar dystrophy
Vulvovaginitis
Vulvar vestibulitis
Vulvodynia
Urethritis
Urethral syndrome
Interstitial cystitis
Vaginal dyspareunia
Inadequate lubrication
Levator floor dysfunction
Vaginismus
Vaginal strictures
Deep thrust dyspareunia
Endometriosis
Pelvic adhesions
Uterine retroversion
Adnexal pathology

[a]From Steege and Ling (8), with permission.

may present with symptoms suggestive of interstitial cystitis, the most common entities that should be considered by the urologist in the differential diagnosis include endometriosis, vulvodynia, urogenital atrophy, pelvic infection, and gynecologic malignancies.

Endometriosis

Endometriosis, defined as the presence of functioning endometrial tissue outside the uterine cavity, is a common cause of pelvic pain and infertility in women of childbearing age. Although it primarily involves organs of the female genital tract, the urinary tract may be involved in 1% to 2% of cases (9), with bladder involvement being most common (10,11). Bladder endometriosis, reported in over 170 patients (12), often presents with urologic symptoms including urgency, frequency, and dysuria. Bladder detrusor endometriosis mimicking interstitial cystitis has been reported in a young woman with voiding symptoms and an invasive endometrial lesion on cystoscopic evaluation (13).

Etiology

Various theories regarding the pathogenesis of endometriosis have been proposed (14). Sampson's original theory proposed that endometriosis was caused by peritoneal implantation of endometrial cells through retrograde menstruation (15). Although this theory seems to be supported by the presence of endometrial implants on predominantly dependent portions of the pelvis such as the uterosacral ligaments, cul-de-sac, and uterovesical peritoneum, endometriosis does not develop in all women with retrograde menstruation. Recent research suggests that additional factors such as alterations in cell-mediated and humoral immunity responses may also be involved (16). Findings of endometrial implants in remote locations beyond the abdominal cavity seem to suggest that transport of ectopic endometrial tissue may occur through embolization of vascular or lymphatic channels or through the open uterine cavity at the time of surgery (14,17).

An alternative theory of coelomic metaplasia, proposed to explain the reported finding of endometriosis in men, is based on the concept that both the endometrium and peritoneum are embryonic derivatives of coelomic-wall epithelium. Metaplastic transformation from peritoneal mesothelium to endometrial tissue is thought to be evoked by chronic irritants found in the retrograde menstrual fluid (18).

Another theory postulates the presence of endometrial implants as a result of remnant Mullerian cells left at ectopic sites in the pelvis during migration at the time of embryonic development. These cells lie dormant until they are stimulated by estrogen, causing differentiation into functioning endometrial tissue (19). This concept may explain the pathogenesis of endometriosis in male patients receiving high-dose estrogen treatment (20).

Although the pathogenesis of endometriosis is still unresolved, recent data seem to suggest a genetic component in the development of this condition. Simpson et al. have reported a 7% risk of developing endometriosis if a first-degree relative is affected (21). Women with a family history of endometriosis are predisposed to developing earlier and more severe disease than controls.

Epidemiology

Although the exact incidence of endometriosis is unknown, several studies have reported rates varying from 1% to 50% with a widely accepted prevalence rate of 5% to 10%. Many patients are diagnosed incidentally at the time of laparoscopy or laparotomy. Five percent to 15% of reproductive-age women are noted to have endometriosis at the time of surgery, with the rate increasing to 30% to 45% in infertile patients (22). Williams, in a prospective study of 1,000 women undergoing laparotomy for benign disease, reported a 50% incidence of endometriosis (23).

There is a general belief that the incidence of endometriosis has been increasing over the last 25 years. This is probably linked to several factors. First, increased understanding and clinical awareness of the condition on the part of both physician and patient has contributed to its increased reporting. Also, the trend toward increasing age of childbearing and the use of diagnostic laparoscopy as part of the infertility workup has allowed for more frequent diagnosis of the condition. Endometriosis is currently one of the most common causes of pelvic pain in women.

Diagnosis

Typically, patients with endometriosis are in their mid-30s and may present with pelvic pain or infertility. The clinical manifestations of this condition are diverse, and no single symptom or constellation of symptoms is pathognomonic. Although the classic triad of dysmenorrhea, dyspareunia, and dyschezia is occasionally seen, more often patients have a variety of presenting symptoms including chronic pelvic pain, abnormal bleeding, and infertility. Those with endometrial involvement of the gastrointestinal or urinary tract may also have complaints of abdominal pain, intermittent constipation, diarrhea, urinary frequency, dysuria, or hematuria.

Physical examination will often reveal a fixed retroverted uterus with tenderness on palpation of the posterior cul-de-sac. Characteristic nodular masses consistent with endometrial implants may be palpated in the pouch of Douglas and along the thickened uterosacral ligaments. Palpation of an adnexal mass, usually unilateral, may suggest ovarian involvement in the form of an endometrioma or "chocolate cyst" of the ovary. Occasionally, a speculum exam may reveal a small area of endometriosis on the cervix or upper vagina.

Alternative modalities such as serum cancer antigen (CA-125) and radiologic testing have also been used for diagnosis. Levels of CA-125, elevated in cases of epithelial ovarian cancer, have been noted to be increased in patients with endometriosis as well as other nonmalignant conditions such as menses, pelvic inflammatory disease, ovarian cysts, and fibroids (24). Although levels seem to correlate with the severity of disease (25), the role of CA-125 in screening for endometriosis or monitoring response to therapy requires further investigation. Radiologic testing such as ultrasound and magnetic resonance imaging (MRI) may be helpful in the investigation of a suspected pelvic mass. Although both ultrasound and MRI are helpful in the diagnosis of large endometriomas, neither modality can detect focal endometrial lesions or accurately distinguish between medium-sized endometriomas and other benign or malignant ovarian conditions. The role of routine ultrasound in the diagnosis of endometriosis has not been established.

Although diagnostic laparoscopy remains the "gold standard" in the diagnosis of endometriosis, accurate identification is dependent on the experience of the laparoscopist. Endometriotic implants, commonly found on the ovary, posterior cul-de-sac, and uterosacral ligaments, vary in appearance, ranging from the classic "powder-burn" lesion to subtle white fibrotic areas (26) (Fig. 1). In addition, laparoscopy allows evaluation of the extent of disease and surgical staging according to the American Fertility Society classification system. Although severity of symptoms does not often correlate with the extent of disease, accurate staging may be useful in determining treatment and prognosis (27).

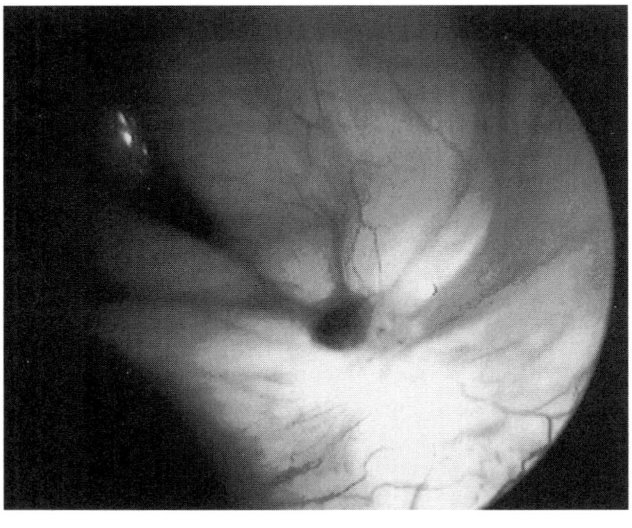

FIG. 1. Endometriotic implant noted on the bladder peritoneum at the time of diagnostic laparoscopy. Note the classic "powder-burn lesion" with the surrounding area of white fibrosis.

Management

The management of patients with endometriosis is based on several factors including the severity of symptoms, findings at the time of laparoscopy, and desire for future fertility. Treatment for stage I (minimal) and stage II (mild) endometriosis-associated infertility is generally expectant management. Patients with endometriosis-associated pain may initially be treated with nonsteroidal antiinflammatory agents with moderate success. For patients with persistent pain despite conservative measures, medical or surgical treatment is indicated.

Medical management of endometriosis is based on the concept that steroid hormones are responsible for growth and maintenance of ectopic endometrial tissue. Like the endometrial cells found in the uterine cavity, endometriotic implants contain receptors that react to estrogen, progesterone, and androgens produced by the gonads in response to stimulation of the hypothalamic–pituitary axis. Hypo- and hyperestrogenic conditions cause endometrial atrophy, whereas administration of progestins and androgens induces decidualization and subsequent degeneration of endometrial tissue (28).

Although unopposed estrogen was previously advocated for the treatment of endometriosis, current management involves the use of a combination estrogen–progesterone oral contraceptive in a continuous fashion for 6 to 12 months to induce a state of "pseudopregnancy." Although the actual effect of pseudopregnancy on endometrial implants is unknown, relief of pain has been reported in 75% to 89% of patients (29). Side effects of this therapeutic regimen are similar to those associated with cyclic oral contraceptives. Progestin-only therapy using oral or intramuscular medroxyprogesterone acetate has also been an effective mode of therapy. Side effects include menstrual irregularities, edema, breast tenderness, and depression.

Danazol, an androgenic derivative of 17α-ethynyltestosterone, has been used in the treatment of endometriosis since 1971 (30). Creating a state of chronic anovulation, danazol inhibits secretion of follicle-stimulating hormone (FSH) and luteinizing hormone (LH) and increases the level of free androgen by displacing testosterone from sex hormone-binding globulin (SHBG). Ninety percent of women with mild to moderate endometriosis reported significant improvement in pelvic pain after 6 months of danazol treatment (31), with the suppressive effects lasting up to 6 months following cessation of therapy (32). Unfortunately, danazol is not as effective at reducing dyspareunia or chronic pain associated with pelvic adhesions. Up to 80% of women taking danazol will experience some side effects, which include weight gain, hirsutism, decreased breast size, emotional lability, vaginal dryness, and menstrual irregularities (33).

Gonadotropin-releasing hormone (GnRH) agonists are the most recent advance in the medical management of endometriosis. When administered in a continuous fashion, either subcutaneously or intranasally, GnRH agonists cause down-regulation of the pituitary gland with a resulting decrease in the secretion of FSH and LH within 6 weeks of initial administration. This state of "pseudomenopause" subsequently leads to atrophy of the endometrial implants and improvement of pain-related symptoms. Several studies have confirmed that GnRH is as effective as danazol in the treatment of endometriosis-related pain (34,35), but up to 50% of women will have recurrence of symptoms to varying degrees within a year after cessation of therapy (36). Compared to the androgenic side effects seen with danazol, the side-effect profile of GnRH agonists is similar to that found in menopause and includes hot flushes, atrophic vaginitis, depression, fatigue, and joint stiffness. Use of GnRH agonists in the treatment of endometriosis has been limited to 6 months because of the osteoporosis effect of estrogen withdrawal, but current research with long-term "add-back" therapy, the use of GnRH with low-dose steroid hormone replacement, may provide alternative options in the future (37).

The surgical management of endometriosis often begins at the time of diagnostic laparoscopy. Conservative surgical therapy may be used to improve fertility potential and alleviate pain by destroying endometrial implants by excision, laser, or electrocautery. Although the extent of disease fails to correlate with severity of pain symptoms, studies have suggested a relationship between the depth of the implant and pain (38), recommending complete excision of the implant for pain alleviation (39). On the basis of numerous uncontrolled studies, the success rate of conservative surgical therapy in the improvement of pelvic pain varies between 60% and 100%. Adjunctive procedures such as adhesiolysis, uterine or ovarian suspension, tuboplasty, and presacral neurectomy have also been advocated with variable results. Although adhesiolysis may result in temporary alleviation of pelvic pain, adhesions may reform with recurrence of symptoms in up to 50% of patients (40). Polan and DeCherney have reported good success with presacral neurectomy in the treatment of endometriosis-related pain, with 75% of patients experiencing relief of symptoms during a mean follow-up of 2.3 years (41). Unfortunately, endometriosis has been shown to recur in up to 28% of patients within 18 months of ablation (42) and in 40% during 9 years of follow-up (43). This is often accompanied by recurrence of symptoms.

In the patient with endometriosis-related pain refractory to conservative surgical and medical treatments in whom loss of fertility potential is acceptable, definitive therapy in the form of total abdominal hysterectomy with bilateral salpingo-oopherectomy is indicated. It may also be an acceptable primary therapy for the woman with severe endometriosis-related symptoms who has completed childbearing and desires a permanent cure. Hysterectomy with bilateral oophorectomy and complete excision of abdominopelvic implants can achieve symptomatic resolution in over 90% of patients with good long-term results (44).

In patients with little to no ovarian involvement, preservation of the ovary may be considered. Although the risk of recurrence in stage III or IV disease may be as high as 40% without oophorectomy (45), the incidence of recurrent endometriosis requiring reoperation drops to 8% with preservation of one ovary in the presence of mild to moderate disease (46). A conservative approach may be an option dependent on intraoperative assessment of ovarian involvement, and this should be discussed with the patient preoperatively.

The role of estrogen therapy following definitive surgery is an important pre- and postoperative consideration. Most women undergoing hysterectomy with oophorectomy are premenopausal, and surgical castration will lead to a rapid decline in estrogen levels. Acute withdrawal symptoms, such as hot flushes, vaginal dryness, urogenital atrophy, and decreased libido, as well as long-term effects such as osteoporosis and increased risk of coronary disease, should be discussed with the patient preoperatively, and estrogen replacement therapy (ERT) postoperatively should be encouraged. With ERT, the risk of recurrence of endometriosis ranges from 0% to 5% in most women with disease confined to the pelvis, but it can be as high as 18% in women with endometriotic involvement of the bowel (46). The addition of a progestational agent after hysterectomy does not seem to provide any added benefit. The long-term benefits of estrogen replacement outweigh any small risk of recurrence, and patients should be continued on this regimen unless they experience recurrence of their symptoms.

Vulvodynia

Defined as chronic vulvar discomfort by the Seventh Congress for the International Society for the Study of Vulvar Disease (47), vulvodynia is characterized by a complex syndrome of vulvar pain including burning, stinging, irritation, and rawness of the external genitalia. This pelvic/perineal pain, along with dyspareunia and occasional urinary symptoms, make vulvodynia an important condition in the differential diagnosis of interstitial cystitis. Accurate diagnosis and management of this disorder have remained elusive, partially because of the varied terminology used to describe the condition.

TABLE 3. *Subsets of vulvodynia*[a]

Vulvar vestibulitis syndrome
Cyclic vulvovaginitis
Dysesthetic vulvodynia
Vulvar papillomatosis
Other causes
Cytolytic vaginitis
Lactobacillosis
Desquamative inflammatory vaginitis
Vulvar dermatoses

[a]From Paavonen (48), with permission.

Currently, vulvodynia can be divided into several well-defined subsets, which may vary in etiology, symptomatology, and treatment. Common subsets of vulvodynia include vulvar vestibulitis syndrome, cyclic vulvovaginitis, and dysesthetic vulvodynia. Less common entities may also present with vulvodynia (48) (Table 3).

Etiology

Although various etiologic theories have been proposed, the exact cause of vulvodynia remains unclear. However, it seems that focal irritation and subsequent inflammation of the vulvar tissue is the common pathway leading to the characteristic symptoms seen with vulvodynia. The various subsets may each have a different causative agent.

Vulvar vestibulitis syndrome (VVS), also known as vestibular adenitis or focal vulvitis, was defined by Friedrich in 1987 as a chronic disorder characterized by severe dyspareunia, point tenderness, and vulvar erythema (49). Early studies suggested a causal association between VVS and human papillomavirus (HPV) (50,51), but recent research has failed to support this hypothesis (52). Recurrent candidiasis has also been implicated in the development of VVS (53). Ashman and Ott have proposed that recurrent yeast infections cause the antigens of *Candida albicans* to cross-react with antigens of the vulvovaginal tissue, eventually resulting in inhibition of the normal immune response and causing hormonal or stress-induced "autoimmune" inflammation (54). Solomon et al. hypothesized that calcium oxalate crystals found in the urine may act as an irritant to the vulvovaginal tissue, leading to the development of vulvar vestibulitis (55). Chemicals and other irritants, history of destructive therapies such as laser therapy and cryosurgery, and allergic drug reactions have also been theorized as etiologic factors. Associated conditions such as inflammatory bowel disease and interstitial cystitis may support an autoimmune etiology in the pathogenesis of VVS (56). Further investigation is necessary for additional data, but a multifactorial etiology is most likely involved.

Cyclic vulvovaginitis (CVV), the second most common subset of vulvodynia, is associated with cyclic pain during the luteal phase of the menstrual cycle. Similar to VVS, cyclic vulvovaginitis may be caused by many factors, but a hypersensitivity reaction to *Candida* antigen is thought to be the most likely etiology (57). Dysesthetic vulvodynia (DV), also known as essential vulvodynia, is most common in perimenopausal or postmenopausal women. Dysesthetic vulvodynia is associated with less dyspareunia than VVS and is characterized by constant vulvar discomfort in contrast to CV. Diffuse hyperesthesia and neuralgias are common, leading to the theory that DV is caused by altered cutaneous perception secondary to a neuropathophysiological condition. These neurologic changes may be associated with menopause and its associated decrease in estrogen (58).

Epidemiology

Little is known about the epidemiology of vulvodynia, but it has been reported to be as high as 15% among women seen in a private gynecologic practice (59). Using a literature search to determine demographic characteristics, Baggish and Miklos have found women with vulvodynia to fall within a certain population profile: 90% of patients are white, and 62% are nulliparous; the mean age is 32 years with a range of 11 to 75 years. Similar to interstitial cystitis, many have seen multiple physicians for treatment after experiencing discomfort for 2 to 3 years (60). Patients with vulvodynia have also been reported to have a high incidence of physical or sexual abuse, allergies to various substances, and history of recurrent human papillomavirus or *Candida* infections (49,53,61).

Diagnosis

Patients with vulvodynia may present with a variety of symptoms depending on the subset involved, but most patients report pain of the external genitalia localized to the area of the vulva and vestibule (Fig. 2). The pain is usually described as a burning, stinging, or rawness (47) but is sometimes characterized as a deep, dull, continuous discomfort. Symptoms of dyspareunia, dysuria, and urinary frequency are also common. Physical examination often reveals the external genitalia to be normal on gross inspection, but they may present with edema and erythema of the vestibule. Superficial fissures and erosions may also be seen. Focal areas of tenderness elicited by gentle pressure using a moist cotton-tipped swab are characteristic. An internal pelvic exam, often poorly tolerated by the patient because of pain, may reveal a mild discharge but is frequently normal. A wet prep of any vaginal discharge, candidal cultures, and the application of 3% acetic acid to detect acetowhite changes may also be helpful in the diagnostic workup. Vulvodynia is often a diagnosis of exclusion based primarily on the patient's characteristic symptoms of localized pain rather than an abnormal exam.

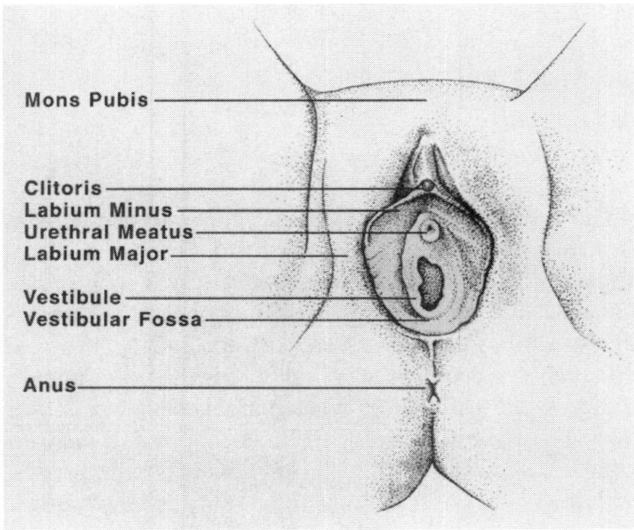

FIG. 2. Anatomy of the female external genitalia.

Management

The treatment of vulvodynia is based on the diagnostic subset determined by symptomatology, physical findings, colposcopy, and culture results. Because vulvodynia is thought to be related to irritation and inflammation of the vulvovaginal tissues, all patients should be instructed to discontinue any prior treatment regimens. Counseling and patient education before initiation of active therapeutic regimens are mandatory. A small set of patients may benefit from conservative therapy such as sitz baths, domoboro soaks, topical steroids, lubrication with coitus, antiinflammatory agents, antimycotics, and antibiotics. Some may also receive symptomatic relief with topical anesthetic agents. However, the majority of patients will require additional treatment based on accurate diagnosis of the specific condition.

Patients diagnosed with VVS have been treated with a variety of nonsurgical modalities. Intralesional and intramuscular interferon has been used with variable success. Although Horowitz reported complete relief in 80% of patients with vulvar vestibulitis treated with intralesional interferon (62), others have reported less promising results, with success rates ranging from 18% to 63% (61,63,64). Recently, the use of calcium citrate has been advocated on the basis of the postulated role of calcium oxalate crystals as a focal irritant to the vulvar tissues. This regimen, which consists of a low-oxalate diet with ingestion of calcium citrate tablets three or four times a day, theoretically inhibits the formation of calcium oxalate crystals (55). Further data regarding the long-term success rates of this regimen are needed.

According to the International Society for the Study of Vulvovaginal Disease Committee on vulvodynia, the best treatment results have been obtained by surgical resection of the vestibule (modified perineoplasty with vaginal advancement) (65). Mann et al. have reported that 66% of patients had improvement in their pain, and 78% had a significant decrease in dyspareunia following surgical resection (61). Marinoff and Turner have also demonstrated improved results, reporting a 90% to 95% short-term cure rate in selected patients following surgical correction (64). Our experience has shown that some patients with vulvodynia will experience resolution or significant improvement in their symptoms following bilateral excision of the Bartholin's glands. Studies regarding the efficacy of this surgical option are under way. Laser treatment of the vulva has also been reported. Unfortunately, results with the CO_2 laser have been disappointing, resulting not only in poor cure rates but in increased vulvar pain from thermal injury with associated scarring (66). However, Reid has reported good results with the pulsed dye laser, with 77% of patients reporting a compete or "major partial response" following one treatment (67). The mode of action of this technique seems to rely on selective destruction of the chronically inflamed blood vessels that lie adjacent to the painful sympathetic nerves (60). Further research in the use of the flashlamp-excited dye laser (FEDL) in the treatment of vulvodynia may prove this to be a safe and effective alternative to surgery.

The treatment of cyclic vulvovaginitis, thought to result from recurrent candidal infection, is prolonged maintenance therapy with antimycotics, topical or peroral, for 6 months or more. This regimen is effective at eradicating symptoms for most patients. On the basis of the neuropathic hypothesis of dysesthetic vulvodynia, McKay has reported significant improvement in the symptoms of DV using tricyclic antidepressants (68). Patients are usually begun on low-dose amitriptyline, 10 mg daily, for 1 to 2 weeks, at which time the dosage can be gradually increased to 50 mg daily if tolerated. Once symptomatic relief has been achieved, the peak dose should be maintained for 1 to 2 months, at which time a slow taper to a maintenance dose can be initiated. After a 3- to 6-month symptom-free interval, the patient is gradually taken off the drug. Many patients report good results with this regimen. Side effects of amitriptyline include palpitations, dry mouth, drowsiness, and weight gain. Imipramine, trazodone, and clonazepam can be used as alternatives in patients who tolerate amitriptyline poorly (48)

Urogenital Atrophy

Urogenital atrophy is a common finding among postmenopausal women who are not taking estrogen replacement therapy. In addition to the systemic manifestations of menopause such as hot flushes, depression, and fatigue, decreased estrogen production during the postmenopausal period results in atrophic changes of the female urogenital tract. Patients with urogenital atrophy often present with symptoms of dyspareunia, vulvar discomfort, vaginal spotting, dysuria, urinary urgency, and frequency. This constellation of symptoms makes urogenital atrophy an important consideration in the differential diagnosis of interstitial cystitis.

Etiology

Atrophy of the skin and mucosal surfaces is a normal part of the aging process but is accelerated in the urogenital tract during menopause by the synergistic effect of estrogen withdrawal. The urinary and genital tracts, both derived from the embryonic urogenital sinus, contain estrogen receptors that respond to local and systemic estrogen concentrations. Although estrogen receptors have been identified on the cervix, uterine corpus, fallopian tubes, and ovary, the primary symptoms of urogenital atrophy are related to degenerative changes of the vagina and urethra.

As a result of estrogen withdrawal, the vaginal mucosa loses its normal rugae and becomes thin and atrophic with a decrease in vaginal lubrication (69). Further estrogen deprivation may lead to decreased elasticity of the vagina as a consequence of an increase in connective tissue, resulting in shortening and narrowing of the vagina. These factors combined result in severe dyspareunia from atrophic vaginitis. Histologic loss of glycogen in the epithelial lining leads to a decrease in lactic acid production by lactobacilli and a subsequent rise in vaginal pH (70). The increased vaginal pH may encourage overgrowth of gram-negative uropathogens, resulting in an increased incidence of urinary tract infections. Because of the altered environment of the vagina, bacterial, fungal, or *Trichomonas* vaginitis may also develop. The thin vagina is easily traumatized and irritated and may be subject to lacerations or erosions, leading to postmenopausal bleeding (71).

The tissues of the urethra and bladder trigone also contain estrogen receptors and undergo degenerative changes during the menopause (72). Studying cytohormonal changes in the urethra of 123 postmenopausal women, Smith found that 85 patients had atrophic changes consistent with evidence of decreased estrogen response (73). Other investigators have suggested that this atrophic urethral mucosa is susceptible to infection and inflammation in the periurethral glands, leading to the onset of urethral syndrome (74), which is characterized by suprapubic discomfort, dysuria, frequency, nocturia, hesitancy, and urgency (72). The histologic changes associated with atrophic urethritis may also lead to an increased incidence in ascending urinary tract infection, worsening the already preexisting symptoms. Urethral atrophy and decreased periurethral vascularity may also cause stress urinary incontinence from intrinsic sphincter deficiency. End-stage atrophy may result in fibrosis and strictures of the distal urethra, converting it to a rigid tube with a friable mucosa and causing possible outflow obstruction (75).

Epidemiology

The average age of menopause in Western society is 51.4 years, whereas the average life expectancy for a woman is 78 years. Thus, many women will spend more than one-third of their lives in the menopause, experiencing the symptoms and risks that accompany estrogen withdrawal. According to a 1990 census, more than 35 million of the 127 million women in this country are over the age of 50, and this proportion is expected to increase with the aging population and improvements in medical technology (76). It is estimated that only one-fifth of the 75% of postmenopausal women who experience estrogen-deficiency-related symptoms seek medical care (77). However, this number is likely to improve with increased public awareness of the beneficial effects of hormone replacement therapy. The effects of estrogen on vasomotor symptoms, coronary heart disease, and osteoporosis have been well documented and highly publicized. However, it is difficult to ascertain the number of postmenopausal women actually on estrogen replacement therapy because of noncompliance and inherent sources of error in study data collection. Patient education and careful screening may be the cornerstones for initiating a successful long-term regimen of hormonal replacement in the postmenopausal patient.

Diagnosis

Most patients with menopausal symptoms will present in the fifth or sixth decade of life, but the occasional younger patient may present with estrogen withdrawal symptoms due to premature ovarian failure or complete surgical oophorectomy. Most often, patients will typically have complaints of vasomotor symptoms, emotional lability, decreased libido, or fatigue. Urogenital symptoms are often dismissed as a normal part of the aging process by many women. Symptoms suggesting atrophic vaginitis include dyspareunia, decreased vaginal lubrication, perineal pain, and vaginal spotting. Atrophic urethral syndrome is characterized by urgency, dysuria, frequency, and nocturia. Other less common symptoms such as postvoid fullness, urge or stress incontinence, and suprapubic discomfort have also been reported.

On pelvic exam, the mucosal surfaces of the vulva and vagina may appear pale and atrophic. Lacerations, erosions, and petechial hemorrhages may also be noted. A vaginal discharge may suggest an associated infectious vaginitis, and wet prep with cultures is recommended. Tenderness on palpation of the vestibule or vaginal vault may also be encountered. Pelvic relaxation is commonly seen as a result of decreased collagen content in the endopelvic fascial supports and reduced pelvic muscle strength, leading to descent of the uterus and anterior or posterior vaginal segments. Erythematous eversion of the urethral mucosa is sometimes seen in the postmenopausal patient and may be misdiagnosed as a tumor or caruncle. A vaginal smear may be used to determine the maturation index. Lack of superficial cells with an increase in intermediate and parabasal cells is diagnostic of estrogen deficiency (78). Urinalysis and urine culture should be obtained to exclude cystitis, and urine cytology may be helpful to rule out malignancy. Cystourethroscopy may reveal the urethral mucosa to be pale and atrophic, but it is often normal.

Management

The management of urogenital atrophy is based on adequate estrogen replacement therapy. Estrogen may be administered topically or orally with equal efficacy, but vaginal administration of estrogen results in irregular systemic absorption, and oral estrogen is recommended for long-term maintenance therapy. With reversal of the estrogen-deprived state, patients report symptomatic improvement over a short time period. Doses of 0.625 to 1.25 mg conjugated estrogen are required to produce significant reversal of the atrophic changes noted on cytologic examination. Signs of improvement are notable within 1 month of initiation of estrogen therapy (79). With estrogen replacement, proliferation of the epithelium occurs with a concomitant decrease in vaginal pH and increase in vaginal secretions. An increase in regional blood flow is also noted (80). The use of graduated vaginal dilators and Kegel exercises may also be recommended to improve elasticity and size of the vaginal canal, with resulting improvement in dyspareunia (8).

Urinary tract symptoms are also responsive to estrogen replacement. Salmon et al. reported significant improvement in symptoms of urgency, frequency, and dysuria in 12 of 16 postmenopausal women within 2 weeks of beginning estradiol therapy. Improvement in symptoms correlated with changes in the vaginal mucosa (81). Smith later correlated symptomatic improvement directly with changes in urethral cytology (82). In a retrospective study of 300 postmenopausal patients, Schleyer-Saunders reported a 30% improvement in urgency and dysuria and a 70% improvement in overall urinary symptoms following estrogen implant therapy (83). Estrogen treatment has also been effective in reducing the incidence of recurrent urinary tract infections. In a randomized double-blind placebo-controlled trial of 93 postmenopausal women using intravaginal estrogen cream, Raz and Stamm found a significant reduction in the incidence of urinary tract infection in the treatment group (84). Similar findings have been confirmed by several other investigators (85,86).

TABLE 4. *Sexually transmitted pathogens*[a]

Bacterial agents
Neisseria gonorrhoeae
Chlamydia trachomatis
Mycoplasma hominis
Ureaplasma urealyticum
Gardnerella vaginalis
Haemophilus ducreyi
Calymmatobacterium
Shigella sp.
Group B *Streptococcus*
Treponema pallidum
Fungal agents
Candida albicans
Candida glubrata
Viral agents
Herpes simplex virus
Hepatitis B virus
Human immunodeficiency virus
Cytomegalovirus
Human papilloma virus
Molluscum contagiosum virus
Protozoan agents
Trichomonas vaginalis
Entamoeba histolytica
Giardia lamblia

[a]From Landers and Sweet (87), with permission.

Pelvic Infection and Genital Malignancies

Although a comprehensive review of pelvic infections and genital malignancies that may present with symptoms similar to interstitial cystitis is beyond the scope of this chapter, the frequency and severity of these conditions warrant a brief discussion as an introduction for the practicing urologist. These conditions are an important part of the gynecologic differential diagnosis of interstitial cystitis.

Pelvic infection is a broad-based term referring to a variety of infectious agents that may involve any part of the female genital tract and present with a wide spectrum of clinical symptoms. The causative agents are often sexually transmitted organisms (87) (Table 4). Common pathogens of the lower genital tract causing vulvovaginitis include *Candida, Gardnerella, Trichomonas,* herpes simplex virus, and human papillomavirus. Patients with vulvovaginitis often present with vulvar itching or irritation, acute pelvic pain, and a vaginal discharge, but dysuria, dyspareunia, and irritable urinary symptoms are also often seen. On examination, the external genitalia may be erythematous or inflamed, and there is often tenderness on bimanual exam. A vaginal discharge may or may not be present. Diagnosis is based on clinical presentation and identification of the causative organism by appropriate testing such as a wet prep, Gram stain, culture, or DNA probe. Antibiotic therapy specific for the isolated organism is usually curative. Infections of the lower genital tract may predispose patients to ascending urinary infection because of the shortness of the female urethra and its close proximity to the heavily colonized vaginal vestibule. Pelvic infection of the upper genital tract in the form of cervicitis, endometritis, and pelvic inflammatory disease (PID) can be caused by multiple organisms including *Chlamydia, Neisseria gonorrhoeae, Bacteroides, E. coli,* and *Mycoplasma* (88). Patients with acute PID will often have abdominal tenderness, significant cervical motion and/or adnexal tenderness, and a fever, but chronic PID and cervicitis may present in a more limited manner with mild localized clinical findings. Chlamydial urethritis may often present with symptoms of urgency, frequency, dysuria, and suprapubic pain. As with infections of the lower genital tract, accurate identification and treatment of the causative organism is the cornerstone of effective therapy. However, broad-spectrum antibiotics may be useful in cases of polymicrobial infections or abcess development. Severe infections unresponsive to medical management may necessitate surgical intervention. Pelvic infection must be considered in the diagnostic workup, especially if the patient is sexually active and presents with acute onset of symptoms. When PID is found in the postmenopausal woman, the presence of genital malignancies, diabetes, or coexisting intestinal disease must be investigated (89).

Genital malignancies that may present with symptoms similar to those found in interstitial cystitis are rare and include cancerous conditions of the vulva and vagina. Although malignant conditions of the cervix, uterus, and overies should also be considered in the differential diagnosis of pelvic pain, these malignancies often present with abnormal vaginal bleeding, an obvious lesion on inspection or mass on palpation, and generalized constitutional symptoms such as weight loss and fatigue. Contrary to these tumors of the upper genital tract, cancer of the vulva or vagina usually presents with localized irritation or itching, vaginal discharge, and occasionally vaginal bleeding. Urinary frequency and dyspareunia may also be present. On exam, the vulva/vagina may appear inflamed or demonstrate an obvious lesion. Inguinal lymphadenopathy may also be noted. Definitive diagnosis is made on biopsy, and a delay in diagnosis is often associated with a worse prognosis. Treatment for vulvar cancer is primarily surgical, whereas radiation remains the mainstay for treatment of squamous cell carcinoma of the vagina. Consideration of these diagnoses in the woman with irritative pelvic/urinary symptoms and early biopsy of any suspected areas of involvement will help to rule out genital malignancies in the diagnostic workup of interstitial cystitis.

THE ASSOCIATION BETWEEN INTERSTITIAL CYSTITIS AND GYNECOLOGIC DISORDERS

There is little data regarding the association between interstitial cystitis and the various gynecologic disorders. This paucity of information is primarily a result of the difficulty of clearly identifying the patient with interstitial cystitis. Accurate and definitive diagnosis of this condition can be challenging, even for the experienced clinician, and many may disregard coexisting conditions that may contribute to genitourinary pain once the primary diagnosis is made. Despite these limitations, recent literature has begun to explore the relationship between interstitial cystitis and certain gynecologic conditions.

The close proximity of the urethra and bladder to the female genital tract and their common embryologic origin suggest that certain pathologic conditions of each system may be related. In a group of 46 young women with urogenital pain, McCormack found 11 (24%) to have both interstitial cystitis and focal vulvitis (90). Fitzpatrick et al. have also reported three cases of women with coexisting interstitial cystitis and vulvar vestibulitis (91). The possible etiologic association between these two disorders is based on the common embryologic origins of the urethra, bladder, and vestibule from the urogenital sinus. The etiology of this "urogenital sinus syndrome" is unknown. It may involve an autoimmune process directed at the epithelium derived from the urogenital sinus. Alternatively, both interstitial cystitis and vestibulitis have been associated with hypersensitivity to allergens and chemical irritants, and this may be a contributing factor. A psychological component, although never proven to be an etiologic factor, has also been recognized in both conditions and may be involved in this syndrome. We anticipate that further clinical and laboratory research will provide more data to explain this possible association.

Little is known about the relationship of interstitial cystitis to pregnancy. No data regarding a possible etiologic association or the effects of pregnancy on the course and symptomatology of interstitial cystitis exist. It is difficult to postulate the effects of physiological and hormonal changes that occur during pregnancy on the pathophysiology of preexisting interstitial cystitis. However, a relationship between changes in the female hormonal milieu and symptoms of interstitial cystitis has been proposed. Pang et al. have demonstrated the presence of high-affinity estrogen receptors on bladder mast cells, which are found in higher numbers in patients with interstitial cystitis than in normal controls. This finding may help to explain why interstitial cystitis and other associated symptoms are worst at midcycle (92). With increased understanding of this condition and improved diagnostic modalities, further research should be conducted in this area.

CONCLUSION

To progress further in understanding the etiology of these pelvic pain conditions and assess treatment options, collaborative efforts between different subspecialties will be necessary. It may be that the local changes that we see and treat are simply end-organ effects of a systemic process that could group painful bladder syndromes with such other pelvic pain conditions as vulvodynia.

The urologist who evaluates and treats painful bladder disorders must become familiar with gynecologic conditions that can simulate or coexist with interstitial cystitis. This should result in a more precise and directed approach to the evaluation and management of women with interstitial cystitis.

REFERENCES

1. Levine DZ. Interstitial cystitis: an overlooked cause of pelvic pain. *Postgrad Med* 1990;88:101–109.
2. Hanno P, Levin RM, Monson FC. Diagnosis of interstitial cystitis. *J Urol* 1990;143:278–281.
3. Gillenwater JY, Wein AJ. Summary of the National Institute of Arthritis, Diabetes, Digestive, and Kidney Disease Workshop on Interstitial Cystitis, National Institute of Health, Bethesda, MD, August 28–29, 1987. *J Urol* 1988;140:203.
4. Bowen LW, Sand PK, Ostergard DR. Interstitial cystitis. In: Ostergard DR, Bent AE, eds. *Urogynecology and Urodynamics: Theory and Practice,* 3rd ed. Baltimore: William & Wilkins, 1991;329–351.
5. Koziol JA. Epidemiology of interstitial cystitis. *Urol Clin North Am* 1994;21:7–71.
6. Walker E, Katon W. Relationship of chronic pelvic pain to psychiatric diagnosis and childhood sexual abuse. *Am J Psychiatry* 1988;145:75.
7. Ku JC, Lowe FC. Current approaches to interstitial cystitis. *Female Patient* 1996;21:39–50.
8. Steege JF, Ling FW. Dyspareunia: a special type of chronic pelvic pain. *Obstet Gynecol Clin North Am* 1993;20:779–793.
9. Kerr WS Jr. Endometriosis involving the urinary tract. *Clin Obstet Gynecol* 1966;9:331.
10. Aldridge KW, Burns JR, Singh B. Vesical endometriosis: a review and 2 case reports. *J Urol* 1985;134:539.
11. Stillwell TJ, Kramer SA, Lee RA. Endometriosis of the ureter. *Urology* 1986;28:81.
12. Fianu S, Ingelman-Sundberg A, Nasiell K, Rosen J, Vaclavinkova V. Surgical treatment of *post abortum* endometriosis of the bladder and postoperative bladder function. *Scand J Urol Nephrol* 1980;14:151–155.
13. Sircus SI, Sant GR, Ucci AA Jr. Bladder detrusor endometriosis mimicking interstitial cystitis. *Urology* 1988;33:339–342.
14. Boyd ME. Endometriosis. *Can J Surg* 1985;28:471.
15. Sampson JA. Perforating hemmorhagic (chocolate) cysts of the ovary: their importance and especially their relation to pelvic adenomas of the endometrial type ("adenomyoma" of the uterus, rectovaginal septum, sigmoid, etc.). *Arch Surg* 1921;3:245–323.
16. Halme J, Becker S, Haskill S. Altered maturation and function of peritoneal macrophages: possible role in pathogenesis of endometriosis. *Am J Obstet Gynecol* 1987;156:783–789.
17. Vermesh M, Zbella EA, Menchaca A, Confino E, Lipshitz S. Vesical endometriosis following bladder injury. *Am J Obstet Gynecol* 1985;153:894–895.
18. Gruenwald P. Origin of endometriosis form the mesenchyme of the celomic walls. *Am J Obstet Gynecol* 1942;44:470.
19. Cullen TS. Adenomyoma of the rectovaginal septum. *JAMA* 1916;67:401–406.
20. Schrodt GR, Alcorn MO, Ibanez J. Endometriosis of the male urinary system: a case report. *J Urol* 1980;124:722–723.
21. Simpson JL, Elias S, Malinak LR, Buttram VC Jr. Heritable aspects of endometriosis. Genetic studies. *Am J Obstet Gynecol* 1980;137:327–331.
22. Wheeler JM. Epidemiology of endometriosis-associated infertility. *J Reprod Med* 1989;34:41–46.
23. Williams TJ, Pratt JH. Endometriosis in 1,000 consecutive celiotomies: incidence and management. *Am J Obstet Gynecol* 1977;129:245–250.
24. Barbieri RL, Niloff JM, Bast RC Jr., et al. Elevated serum concentrations of CA-125 in patients with advanced endometriosis. *Fertil Steril* 1986;45:630–634.
25. Pittaway DE, Fayez JA. The use of CA-125 in the diagnosis and management of endometriosis. *Fertil Steril* 1986;46:790.
26. Jansen RP, Russell P. Nonpigmented endometriosis: clinical, laparoscopic, and pathologic definition. *Am J Obstet Gynecol* 1986;155:1154–1159.
27. Olive DL, Haney AF. Endometriosis-associated infertility: a critical review of therapeutic approaches. *Obstet Gynecol Surv* 1986;41:538–555.
28. Barbieri RL, Hornstein MD. Medical therapy for endometriosis. In: Wilson EA, ed. *Endometriosis.* New York: Alan R Liss, 1987;111–140.
29. Olive DL. Medical treatment: alternatives to danazol. In: Schenken RS, ed. *Endometriosis: Contemporary Concepts in Clinical Management.* Philadelphia: Lippincott, 1989;189–211.
30. Greenblatt RB, Dmowski WP, Mahesh VB, Scholer HFL. Clinical studies with an antigonadotropin—danazol. *Fertil Steril* 1971;22:102–112.
31. Bayer SR, Seibel MM, Saffan DS, Berger MJ, Taymor ML. Efficacy of danazol treatment for minimal endometriosis in infertile women: a prospective, randomized study. *J Reprod Med* 1988;33:179–183.
32. Henzel MR, Corson SL, Moghissi K, et al. Administration of nasal naferelin as compared with oral danazol for endometriosis. *N Engl J Med* 1990;318:485–489.
33. Dlugi AM, Rufo S, D'Amico JF, Siebel MM. A comparison of the effects of buserelin versus danazol on plasma lipoproteins during treatment of pelvic endometriosis. *Fertil Steril* 1988;49:913–916.
34. Nafarelin European Endometriosis Trial Group (NEET). Naferelin for endometriosis: a large-scale, danazol-controlled trial of efficacy and safety, with 1 year follow-up. *Fertil Steril* 1992;57:514–522.
35. Rock JA, Truglia FA, Caplan RJ, Zoladex Endometriosis Study Group. Zoladex (goserelin acetate implant) in the treatment of endometriosis: a randomized comparison with danazol. *Obstet Gynecol* 1993;82:198–205.
36. Fedele L, Fedele L, Parazzini F, et al. Buserelin acetate versus expectant management in the treatment of infertility associated with minimal to mild endometriosis: a randomized clinical trial. *Am J Obstet Gynecol* 1992;166:1345–1350.
37. Hurst BS, Schlaff WD. Treatment options for endometriosis: medical therapies. *Infertil Reprod Clin North Am* 1992;3:645–655.
38. Koninckx PR, Mueleman C, Demeyere S, et al. Suggestive evidence that pelvic endometriosis is a progressive disease, whereas deeply infiltrating endometriosis is associated with pelvic pain. *Fertil Steril* 1991;55:759–765.
39. Martin DC, Hubert GD, Levy BS. Depth of infiltration of endometriosis. *J Gynecol Surg* 1989;51:63–67.
40. Vancaille T, Schenken RS. Endoscopic surgery. In: Schenken RS, ed. *Endometriosis: Contemporary Concepts in Clinical Management.* Philadelphia: Lippincott, 1989;249–266.
41. Polan ML, DeCherney A. Presacral neurectomy for pelvic pain in infertility. *Fertil Steril* 1980;Vol 34:557–560.
42. Gordst S, Boechx W, Brosens I. Microsurgery of endometriosis in infertile patients. *Fertil Steril* 1984;42:520–525.
43. Wheeler JM, Malinak LR. Recurrent endometriosis: incidence, management, and prognosis. *Am J Obstet Gynecol* 1983;146:247–253.
44. Olive DL, Schwartz LB. Endometriosis. *N Engl J Med* 1993;328:1759–1769.
45. Colle ML, Greenblatt RB. Contraceptive properties of danazol. *J Reprod Med* 1976;17:98–101.
46. Walter MD. Definitive surgery. In: Schenken RS, ed. *Endometriosis: Contemporary Concepts in Clinical Management.* Philadelphia: Lippincott, 1989;267–278.
47. Burning vulvar syndrome: Report of the ISSVD. *J Reprod Med* 1984;29:457.
48. Paavonen J. Vulvodynia—a complex syndrome of vulvar pain. *Acta Obstet Gynecol Scand* 1995;74:243–247.
49. Friedrich EG Jr. Vulvar vestibulitis syndrome. *J Reprod Med* 1987;32:110–114.
50. Turner MLC, Marinoff SC. Association of human papillomavirus with vulvodynia and the vulvar vestibulitis syndrome. *J Reprod Med* 1988;33:533–537.
51. Umpierre SA, Kaufman RH, Adam E, Woods KV, Adler-Storz K

Human papillomavirus DNA in tissue biopsy specimens of vulvar vestibulitis patients treated with interferon. *Obstet Gynecol* 1991;78: 693–695.
52. Wilkinson EJ, Guerrero E, Daniel R, et al. Vulvar vestibulitis is rarely associated with human papillomavirus infection types 6, 11, 16, or 18. *Int J Gynecol Pathol* 1993;12:344–349.
53. Peckham BM, Maki DG, Patterson JJ, et al. Focal vulvitis: A characteristic syndrome and cause of dyspareunia. *Am J Obstet Gynecol* 1986; 154:855–864.
54. Ashman RB, Ott AK. Autoimmunity as a factor in recurrent vaginal candidiasis and the minor vestibular gland syndrome. *J Reprod Med* 1989;34:264–266.
55. Solomon CC, Melmed MH, Heitler SM. Calcium citrate for vulvar vestibulitis. *J Reprod Med* 1991;36:879–882.
56. Fulonge CB, Thin RN, Evans BE, McKee PH. Vulvar vestubulitis syndrome: a clinico-pathological study. *Br J Obstet Gynaecol* 1991;98: 701–706.
57. Witkin SS, Jeremiahs J, Ledger WJ. Recurrent vaginitis as a result of sexual transmission of IgE antbodies. *Am J Obstet Gynecol* 1988;159: 32–36.
58. Turner MLC, Marinoff SC. Pudendal neuralgia. *Am J Obstet Gynecol* 1991;165:1233–1236.
59. Goetsch MF. Vulvar vestibulitis: Prevalence and historic features in a general gynecologic practice population. *Am J Obstet Gynecol* 1991; 164:1609–1616.
60. Baggish MS, Miklos JR. Vulvar pain syndrome: A review. *Obstet Gynecol Surv* 1995;50:618–627.
61. Mann MS, Kaufman RH, Brown D, et al. Vulvar vestibulitis: Significant clinical variables and treatment outcomes. *Obstet Gynecol* 1992; 79:122–125.
62. Horowitz BJ. Interferon therapy for condylomatous vulvitis. *Obstet Gynecol* 1989;73:446–448.
63. Kent HL, Wisniewski PM. Interferon for vulvar vestibulitis. *J Reprod Med* 1990;35:1138–1140.
64. Marinoff SC, Turner ML, Hirsch RP, et al. Intralesional alpha-interferon: Cost-effective therapy for vulvar vestibulitis syndrome. *J Reprod Med* 1993;38:19–24.
65. McKay M, Frankman O, Horowitz BJ, et al. Vulvar vestibulitis and vestibular papillomatosis. Report of the International Society for the Study of Vulvar Disease Committee on Vulvodynia. *J Reprod Med* 1991;36:413–415.
66. Michlewitz H, Kennison RD, Turksoy RN, et al. Vulvar vestibulitis: Subgroup with bartholin gland duct inflammation. *Obstet Gynecol* 1989;73:410–413.
67. Reid R, Omoto KH, Precop SL, et al. Flashlamp-excited dye laser therapy of idiopathic vulvodynia is safe and efficacious. *Am J Obstet Gynecol* 1995;172:1684–1696.
68. McKay M. Dysesthetic ("essential") vulvodynia. *J Reprod Med* 1993; 38:9–13.
69. Notelovitz M. Gynecologic problems of menopausal women. I. Changes in genital tissue. *Geriatrics* 1978;33:24.
70. Semmens JP, Wagner G. Estrogen deprivation and vaginal function in postmenopausal women. *JAMA* 1982;248:445.
71. Voet RL. End organ response to estrogen deprivation. In: Buchsbaum HJ, ed. *The Menopause.* New York: Springer-Verlag, 1983.
72. Corlett RC. Urinary tract disorders. In: Buchsbaum HJ, ed. *The Menopause.* New York: Springer-Verlag, 1983.
73. Smith P. Age changes in the female urethra. *Br J Urol* 1972;44:667.
74. Brooks D, Mauder A. Pathogenesis of the urethral syndrome in women and its diagnosis in general practice. *Lancet* 1972;2:893.
75. Brown KH. Urogenital atrophy. *Obstet Gynecol Clin North Am* 1987; 15:13–32.
76. Mishell Jr DR. Menopause. In: Herbst AL, Mishell DR Jr, Stenchever MA, Droegemueller W, eds. *Comprehensive Gynecology,* 2nd ed. St Louis: Mosby Year Book, 1992;1245–1280.
77. Utian WH. Current status of menopause in postmenopausal estrogen therapy. *Obstet Gynecol Surv* 1977;32:193.
78. Blaustein RL. Cytology of the female genital tract. In: Blaustein A, ed. *Pathology of the Female Genital Tract.* New York, Springer-Verlag, 1982.
79. Geola FL, Frumar AM, Tataryn IV, et al. Biological effects of various doses of conjugated equien estrogens in postmenopausal women. *J Clin Endocrinol Metab* 1980;51:620.
80. Hammond CB, Maxson WS. Current status of estrogen therapy for the menopause. *Fertil Steril* 1982;37:5.
81. Salmon UJ, Walter RI, Geist SH. The use of estrogens in the treatment of dysuria and incontinence in postmenopausal women. *Am J Obstet Gynecol* 1941;42:845–851.
82. Smith PJB. The effect of oestrogens on bladder function in the female. In: Campbell S, ed. *The Management of the Menopause and Postmenopausal Years.* Lancaster: MTP Press, 1976;291–298.
83. Schleyer-Saunders E. Results of hormonal implants in the treatment of the climacteric. *J Am Geriatr Soc* 1971;32:221–223.
84. Raz R, Stamm WE. A controlled trial of intravaginal estriol in postmenopausal women with recurrent urinary tract infections. *N Engl J Med* 1993;329:753–756.
85. Kirkengen AL, Andersen P, Gjersoe E, et al. Oestriol in the prophylactic treatment of recurrent urinary tract infections in postmenopausal women. *Scand J Prim Health Care* 1992;10:139–142.
86. Privette M, Cade R, Peterson J, et al. Prevention of recurrent urinary tract infection in postmenopausal women. *Nephron* 1988;50:24–27.
87. Landers DV, Sweet RL. Sexually transmitted infections. In: Glass RH, ed. *Office Gynecology,* 4th ed. Baltimore: William & Wilkins, 1993;2.
88. Eschenbach DA, Buchanan T, Pollack HM, et al. Polymicrobial etiology of acute pelvic inflammatory disease. *N Engl J Med* 1975;293: 166.
89. Upper genital tract infections. In: Herbst AL, Mishell DR, Stenchever MA, Droegemueller W, eds. *Comprehensive Gynecology,* 2nd ed. St Louis: Mosby Yearbook, 1992;691–720.
90. McCormack WM. Two urogenital sinus syndromes: Interstitial cystitis and focal vulvitis. *J Reprod Med* 1990;35:873–877.
91. Fitzpatrick CC, DeLancey JOL, Elkins TE, McGuire EJ. Vulvar vestibulitis and interstitial cystitis: A disorder of urogenital sinus-derived epithelium. *Obstet Gynecol* 1993;81:860–862.
92. Pang X, Cotreau-Bibbo MM, Sant GR, Theoharides TC. Bladder mast cell expression of high affinity oestrogen receptors in patients with interstitial cystitis. *Br J Urol* 1995;75:154–161.

Interstitial Cystitis, edited by Grannum R. Sant.
Lippincott–Raven Publishers, Philadelphia ©1997.

CHAPTER 20

Interstitial Cystitis in Men

Jane L. Miller, Tamara G. Bavendam, and Richard E. Berger

Few men are included in most reports on interstitial cystitis (IC). The lack of published information specific to men is a result of the much lower prevalence of the diagnosis of interstitial cystitis syndrome in men than women. Most studies report an approximately 10:1 female-to-male patient ratio (1–5). The most recent article looking exclusively at male interstitial cystitis patients was Hanash and Pool's report in 1969 (6).

In the few studies that break down clinical symptoms by gender, male patients present with the classic irritative voiding symptoms (urinary urgency, frequency, nocturia) and pelvic/genital pain but more often localize their pain to their penis and perineum than to the suprapubic area (7). No published studies have evaluated differences in response to treatment between male and female patients. It is mainly in the differential diagnosis of interstitial cystitis that men and women differ.

The syndrome of interstitial cystitis is defined by chronic irritative voiding symptoms, pelvic pain, sterile, cytologically negative urine, and characteristic cystoscopic findings. The only objective positive criterion is the presence of petechial hemorrhages (glomerulations) seen on bladder hydrodistension under anesthesia. However, it is important to remember that the presence of petechial hemorrhages on hydrodistention is not pathognomonic for interstitial cystitis but is also associated with other conditions such as infectious cystitis, radiation cystitis, chemical cystitis, and carcinom *in situ* (CIS) of the bladder. In these latter conditions, there are usually endoscopic abnormalities on the initial cystoscopy before the hydrodistention, and the petechial hemorrhages of interstitial cystitis are apparent only after distention. It has been suggested that the glomerulations seen on hydrodistention may simply reflect changes seen when any bladder is stretched beyond its maximum functional capacity, determined when the patient is awake and the capacity is limited by the sensation of urge (8). Indeed, controlled studies are needed in normal men and in men with other urologic conditions to determine the significance of petechiae after hydrodistention. At this time, however, we consider the presence of moderate to severe petechiae after hydrodistention in men to be highly suggestive of interstitial cystitis.

Unfortunately, the clinical presentation of this syndrome—urinary frequency, urgency, nocturia, pelvic/genital pain—is not specific to interstitial cystitis. All patients, male and female, need to have conditions that may produce similar symptoms such as bacterial cystitis, tuberculosis, radiation cystitis, malakoplakia, and CIS of the bladder excluded. Unique to the differential diagnosis in men is the diagnosis of benign prostatic hyperplasia (BPH) with obstruction, prostatodynia (defined as a pelvic pain syndrome not associated with prostatic fluid inflammation), and nonbacterial prostatitis (defined as a genital pain syndrome associated with prostatic fluid inflammation but not infection with classic uropathogens) (9). Though not limited to men, carcinoma *in situ* of the bladder is of particular significance because of its higher incidence in men.

INTERSTITIAL CYSTITIS VERSUS PROSTATISM

In 1951, Emmett (10) noted that most cases of male interstitial cystitis are initially misinterpreted as vesical irritability from an obstructing prostate and are treated by transurethral prostatic resection (TURP). In Hanash and Pool's 1969 series of 123 male patients, 55% had undergone at least one transurethral resection before interstitial cystitis was diagnosed (6). Dejuana and Everett (3) reported that five of their 11 male patients had undergone TURP, and two had had open prostatectomy, and Hand (4) reported that three of 19 male interstitial cystitis patients had previously undergone TURP. As the criteria for prostatectomy to relieve bladder outlet obstruction

J. L. Miller, T. G. Bavendam, and R. E. Berger: Department of Urology, University of Washington, Seattle, Washington 98115.

become more standardized, and our awareness that interstitial cystitis does occur in men increases, fewer men with interstitial cystitis will undergo unnecessary prostatic surgery.

Differentiation of prostatism and interstitial cystitis can be difficult even with the current increased awareness of interstitial cystitis. Typically, when the man's primary complaints are of pain with vesical irritability, the diagnosis of interstitial cystitis should be seriously considered once bacterial infection and hematuria have been ruled out. However, many men with interstitial cystitis are predominantly bothered by irritative voiding symptoms with complaints of urinary frequency, nocturia, small voids, and slow stream. These symptoms without a pain component are consistent with prostatism and bladder outlet obstruction. These same symptoms can also be a result of sensory instability (11) and, on occasion, pelvic floor muscle spasm (12).

Multichannel urodynamic evaluation with fluoroscopy can differentiate among prostatic obstruction, sensory instability, and pelvic floor muscle spasm. This testing can document the presence or absence of obstruction, the level of obstruction (bladder neck, prostate, pelvic floor), and whether or not the pelvic floor is appropriately relaxed during voluntary voiding. When bladder outlet obstruction is confirmed on urodynamics (high voiding pressure and low flow), initial treatment can be directed at the obstruction. It is important to keep in mind that these two processes (IC and bladder outlet obstruction) may coexist. In patients who have severe frequency and pain as a part of their symptoms yet have a small postvoid residual, the urologist should consider hydrodistention before performing a prostatectomy. The patient should be forewarned that relief of obstruction may not resolve all of his symptoms.

INTERSTITIAL CYSTITIS VERSUS PROSTATODYNIA AND NONBACTERIAL PROSTATITIS

Messing suggested in 1987 that men with prostatodynia may represent a subset of patients with interstitial cystitis (13). Presenting symptoms in both conditions include pelvic or genital pain. Irritative voiding symptoms are usually a more predominant complaint of interstitial cystitis patients but can be a complaint of patients with nonbacterial prostatitis or prostatodynia (8). Siroky et al. (14) found that the pain of prostatitis was reproduced on bladder filling or with bladder contraction in 45% of men with prostatitis, suggesting that the bladder was the source of pain in these men. Patients of both sexes with interstitial cystitis classically report pain on bladder filling. Men with interstitial cystitis and prostatodynia complain of sexual dysfunction and psychological problems typical of any unexplained chronic pain syndrome (15,16). Urine cultures and cytology are negative in both patient groups. On urodynamic evaluation, sensory instability is often found in patients with interstitial cystitis (11) and patients with prostatodynia (17). Patients in both populations have been found to have a nonrelaxing or spastic pelvic floor (12,18).

One of us (R.B.) has performed hydrodistention on 38 men with the diagnosis of prostatitis or prostatodynia. Moderate to severe petechiae associated with terminal hematuria was found in 24 (63%) of the 38 men.

Men with moderate to severe petechial hemorrhage after hydrodistention had significantly shorter symptom histories, less testicular pain, fewer symptoms, a smaller bladder capacity, and fewer leukocytes in expressed prostatic secretions than men with no or few petechiae (Table 1). We found no significant differences in the incidence of perineal pain, suprapubic pain, back pain, rectal pain, frequency, or urgency between the groups. It is noteworthy that the men with more severe petechial hemorrhages more commonly had little prostatic inflammation and therefore were initially classified in the prostatodynia group. This association strongly suggests an overlap of prostatodynia with interstitial cystitis. It is our current belief that the overlap in clinical symptoms, urodynamic findings, and endoscopic findings strongly suggests an underlying similarity in the pathophysiology of prostatodynia and interstitial cystitis.

At the current time, the mainstay of treatment of nonbacterial prostatitis is antibiotics, although the efficacy is unproven. Initial treatment for both interstitial cystitis and prostatodynia is one of reassurance, behavior-oriented

TABLE 1. *Clinical correlates of severity of petechial hemorrhage after hydrodistention in 38 men with the diagnosis of nonbacterial prostatitis or prostatodynia*

Clinical data	Men with no or few petechiae (*n* = 14)	Men with moderate to severe petechiae (*n* = 24)	Statistical significance[a]
Years of symptoms	9.6 ± 10.1	3.4 ± 9	0.01*
Men with testicular pain (%)	9/14 (64%)	5/24 (21%)	0.01**
Mean no. of symptoms ± S.D.	4.64 ± 1.6	3.46 ± 1.18	0.01*
Leukocytes/mm^3 in prostatic secretions	2,723 ± 3,450	536 ± 664	0.02*
Bladder capacity under anesthesia (ml)	1,140 ± 306	919 ± 181	0.02*

[a]Significant according to *ANOVA or **chi-square test.

treatment regimens such as dietary modification, bladder retraining, stress management, relaxation, and physical therapy. Pharmacologic agents aimed at symptomatic relief such as low-dose tricyclic antidepressants, smooth and skeletal muscle relaxants, and antispasmodics are also helpful in many patients. Perhaps we should also be evaluating bladder-directed therapy such as DMSO instillations in men with proststodynia. We should either develop better diagnostic or treatment-related criteria to separate interstitial cystitis and prostatodynia or begin to look at these diagnoses as related disorders.

INTERSTITIAL CYSTITIS VERSUS BLADDER CARCINOMA

Bladder cancer, particularly carcinoma *in situ,* can mimic the clinical picture and endoscopic findings of interstitial cystitis. In 1944, Cristol et al. (19) reported that two of 113 men initially diagnosed with interstitial cystitis were subsequently found with bladder carcinoma. Hanash and Pool (6) reported that "vesical neoplasms were associated with interstitial cystitis in 5% of our cases." Twelve of 53 (23%) men who were initially diagnosed with interstitial cystitis were later found to have bladder cancer, versus three of 224 (1.5%) women in Utz and Zincke's 1974 series (20). In Dejuana and Everett's series, two of 11 male patients developed bladder cancer and died of their disease, whereas only three of their 99 female patients had cancers, which were small papillary tumors that did not progress (3). In Koziol's survey of 565 patients, bladder cancer did not appear to be a risk factor for interstitial cystitis (1). Whether these interstitial cystitis patients who were later found to have bladder cancer were initially misdiagnosed or subsequently developed bladder cancer is unclear from these reports. There is no evidence to suggest that interstitial cystitis patients have an increased risk of developing bladder cancer. However, when the diagnosis of interstitial cystitis is considered in male patients, bladder cancer/CIS must be ruled out with negative urine cytology and/or bladder biopsies. Men with significant smoking histories should be followed carefully even when the initial biopsies are negative, especially if the symptoms do not respond to treatment for interstitial cystitis. Repeat biopsies should be considered.

SUMMARY

At least 10% of patients diagnosed with interstitial cystitis are men. Significantly more may go undiagnosed or misdiagnosed with prostate-related conditions. Diagnosing interstitial cystitis in men begins with a high index of suspicion. Of particular importance to the male interstitial cystitis patient is the differential diagnosis. Three conditions—(a) prostatism with bladder outlet obstruction, (b) prostatodynia and its marked similarities, and (c) bladder carcinoma for its significant implications—need particular consideration for the men being diagnosed with interstitial cystitis.

REFERENCES

1. Koziol JA. Epidemiology of interstitial cystitis. *Urol Clin North Am* 1994;21:7–20.
2. Burford EH, Burford CE. Hunner ulcer of the bladder: A report of 187 cases. *J Urol* 1958;79:952–955.
3. DeJuana CP, Everett JC Jr. Interstitial cystitis: Experience and review of recent literature. *Urology* 1977;10:325–329.
4. Hand JR. Interstitial cystitis: Report of 223 cases (204 women and 19 men). *J Urol* 1949;61:291–310.
5. Oravisto KJ. Epidemiology of interstitial cystitis. *Ann Chir Gynaecol Fenn* 1975;64:57–58.
6. Hanash KA, Pool TL. Interstitial cystitis in men. *J Urol* 1969;102: 427–428.
7. Miller JL, Rothman I, Bavendam TG, Berger RE. Prostatodynia and interstitial cystitis: One and the same? *Urology* 1995;45:587–590.
8. Hanno PM, Levin RM, Manson FC, et al. Diagnosis of interstitial cystitis. *J Urol* 1990;143:278–281.
9. Orland SM, Hanno PM, Wein AJ. Prostatitis, prostatosis, and prostatodynia. *Urology* 1985;25:439–459.
10. Emmett JL. Discussion. *Trans Am Assoc Genitourin Surg* 1951;43:66.
11. Steinkohl WB, Leach GE. Urodynamic findings in interstitial cystitis. *Urology* 1989;34:399–401.
12. Schmidt RA, Vapnek JM. Pelvic floor behavior and interstitial cystitis. *Semin Urol* 1991;9:154–160.
13. Messing EM. The diagnosis of interstitial cystitis. *Urology* 1987; 29(Suppl 4):4–7.
14. Siroky MB, Golstein I, Krane RJ. Functional voiding disorders in men. *J Urol* 1981;126:200–204.
15. Keltikangas JL, Auvinen LA, Lehtonen T. Psychological factors related to interstitial cystitis. *Eur Urol* 1988;15:69–72.
16. Ireton RC, Berger RE. Prostatitis and epididymitis. *Urol Clin North Am* 1984;11:83–94.
17. Murnagham GF, Millard RJ. Urodynamic evaluation of bladder neck obstruction in chronic prostatitis. *Br J Urol* 1984;56:713–716.
18. Segura JW, Opitz JL, Greene LF. Prostatitis, prostatosis or pelvic floor muscle tension myalgia? *J Urol* 1979;122:168–169
19. Cristol DS, Greene LF, Thompson GJ. Interstitial cystitis of men: A review of seventy-eight cases. *JAMA* 1944;126:825–828.
20. Utz DC, Zincke H. The masquerade of bladder cancer *in situ* as interstitial cystitis. *J Urol* 1974;111:160–161.

Interstitial Cystitis, edited by Grannum R. Sant
Lippincott–Raven Publishers, Philadelphia ©1997.

CHAPTER 21

Urodynamic Evaluation in Interstitial Cystitis

Jerzy B. Gajewski and Said A. Awad

Urodynamic evaluation is a valuable study in patients with interstitial cystitis (IC). It is difficult, however, to estimate how often it is utilized. A European study showed that 55% of urologists from The Netherlands perform urodynamic tests for the investigation of interstitial cystitis (1). There are no similar studies from North America.

URODYNAMIC EVALUATION OF THE BLADDER

Standard cystometrogram (CMG) fluid or gas is predominantly used. This test documents bladder sensation, maximum cystometric capacity (MCC), detrusor compliance (DC), and the presence or absence of instability (DI). In patients with interstitial cystitis, a CMG with medium fill water at 50 ml/min usually finds volume at first sensation (VFS) and maximum cystometric capacity to be significantly decreased. Perez-Marrero et al. found VFS to be <100 ml and mean MCC of 287 ml (range 50 to 615) (2). Awad et al. (3) reported a mean MCC of 184 ml in a supine position and 169 ml standing. In our recent review, where 155 patients with interstitial cystitis were studied, we found the mean VFS to be 188 ml, and MCC was 292 ml (Table 1). Parsons (4), using a gas cystometrogram at 30 ml/min, reported lower values of VFS (<125 ml) and MCC (220 ml), with 90% of the patients having volumes of MCC <350 ml. It has been shown that the lower MCC correlates with the duration of the symptoms (2,4). The MCC appears to be larger than the functional cystometric capacity obtained from voiding diaries (106 ml) (4) but smaller than the cystoscopic capacity under anesthesia [561 ml (4) and 486 ml (3)]. The MCC was also used as a parameter of treatment results in several studies (2,5–8). For example, Perez-Marrero et al. (2) found that VFS and MCC are the most useful urodynamic values in predicting response to DMSO treatment. In patients undergoing augmentation cystoplasty (7), MCC was reported to be <100 ml. However, there were no urodynamic parameters that correlated well with the success of the surgery. Allusie et al. (8) used urodynamics in combination with a selective reversible nerve blockade to differentiate interstitial cystitis from the idiopathic urge syndrome. In patients with interstitial cystitis, there were only negligent increases in MCC from a mean of 114 to a mean of 215 ml after a blockade, whereas in patients with idiopathic urge syndrome, mean MCC increased from 124 ml to 604 ml.

Several reports have indicated the presence of detrusor instability (DI) in a number of patients with IC (2,3,7). Perez-Marrero et al. found instability in 13 of 50 (26%) (2) and seven of 30 (23%) (9). Awad et al. (10) reported 26% instability in patients with interstitial cystitis and voiding dysfunction. Parsons (4) had 5% instability in his interstitial cystitis population. Our recent review of 155 patients with interstitial cystitis showed instability in 19%. Perez-Marrero et al. (2) found more instability in patients with longer disease duration. Only 13% of those with less than 5 years' duration of symptoms had instability, whereas 47% with interstitial cystitis history of more than 5 years did have instability. Similar findings were reported by Hald et al. (11). Patients with DI tended to have lower MCCs than those without DI: 229 ml versus 287 ml (2). Similarly, our recent review showed VFS of 136 ml and MCC of 198 ml in patients with DI and values of 200 ml and 313 ml, respectively, in those without DI. According to NIH guidelines (12), bladder instability is an exclusion criterion for diagnosis of interstitial cystitis. The rationale for such exclusion is not clear, and it is controversial.

Perez-Marrero et al. (13) showed that patients with DI did not respond to DMSO treatment (none of seven) and hence should not be included in the diagnosis of interstitial cystitis. Parson (4) and NIH (12) followed the same logic. Our experience has been different. The response to

J.B. Gajewski and S.A. Awad: Department of Urology, Dalhousie University, Halifax, Nova Scotia B3H 3A7, Canada.

TABLE 1. *Urodynamic and cystoscopic findings of 155 patients with interstitial cystitis*[a]

	Male	Female	Total
Number	13	142	155
Age (years)	43	44	44
Volume first sensation	208 ml	186 ml	188 ml
Maximum cystometric capacity	306 ml	290 ml	292 ml
Detrusor instability	15%	19%	19%
Voided volume	232 ml	266 ml	263 ml
MFR	14.8 ml/sec	16.9 ml/sec	16.7 ml/sec
Residual	74 ml	24 ml	29 ml
UPP MUCP	113 cm H_2O	116 cm H_2O	116 cm H_2O
Abnormal EMG (*n*)	0	5	5
Cystoscopic capacity	490 ml	560 ml	554 ml
IC grade (0–3)	1.8	1.7	1.7

[a]CMG, water, medium fill, 50 ml/min; UPP, 8F balloon catheter; EMG, perianal skin electrodes.

DMSO treatment was 33% in patients with interstitial cystitis and DI, whereas it was 11% in those without DI. On the other hand, both groups responded equally to anticholinergic therapy: 18% with DI and 22% without DI. Also, both groups had similar cystoscopic findings after bladder distention by our grading method (Fig. 1), with a mean grade of 1.7. There was also no difference in pathologic findings in patients with interstitial cystitis and DI versus no DI in a previous study (3). Webster and Maggio (7) had three patients with instability in their cystoplasty group of 19 patients, and they considered the instability to be a secondary event. Moore et al. (14) even suggested that some cases of intractable idiopathic instability can be classified as undiagnosed interstitial cystitis. We feel that DI can be present with interstitial cystitis as an associated abnormality or possibly a secondary event and should not be an exclusion criterion in the study of patients with IC.

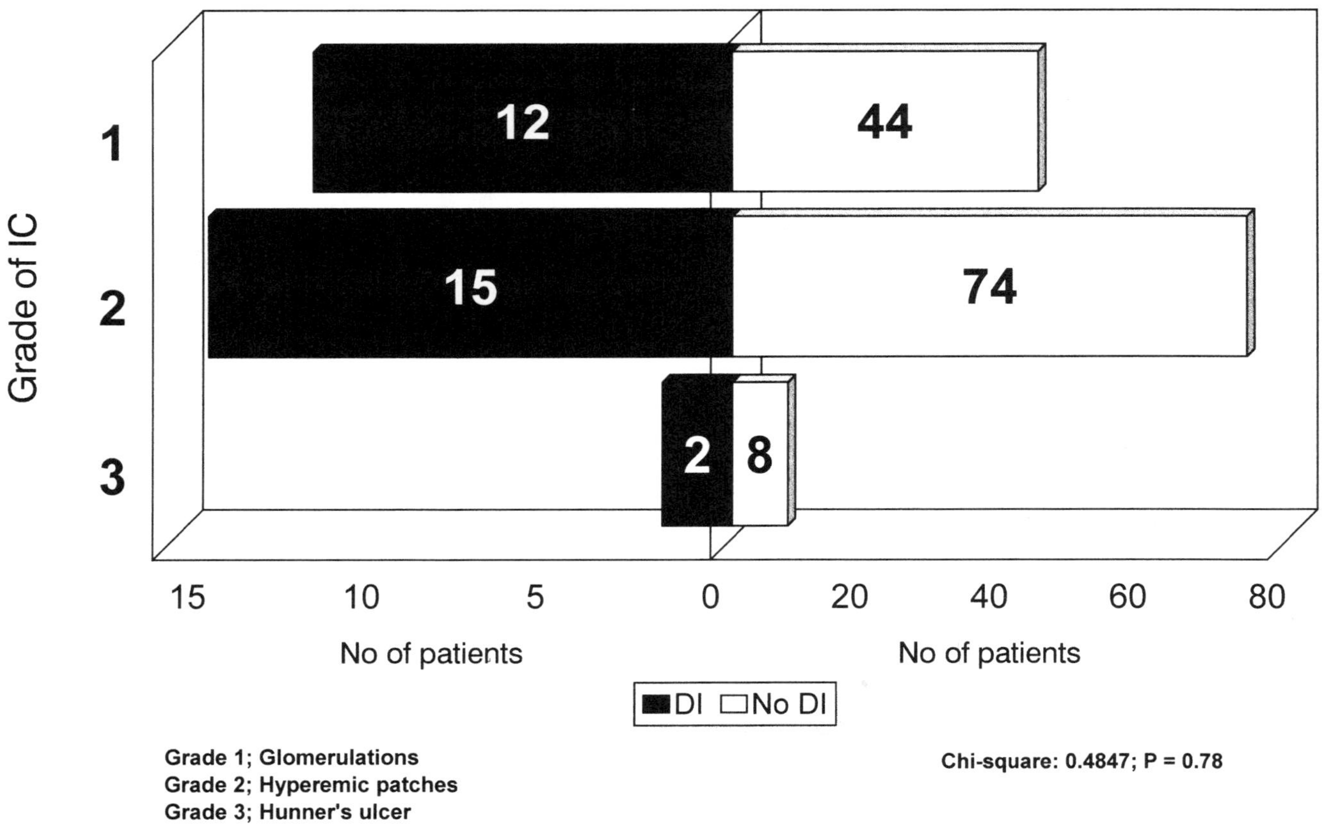

FIG. 1. Grade of interstitial cystitis (IC) at cystoscopy versus detrusor instability (DI) in 155 patients.

A small number of the patients with interstitial cystitis have been reported to have detrusor failure. This was first described by Holm-Bentzen et al. (15) in 1985 in 25 of 101 patients with nonbacterial cystitis. Parsons (2) found what he called detrusor myopathy in 11 of 225 patients. These patients had high residual volume (>50 ml), low detrusor contraction strength (<30 ml H_2O), and large capacity >750 ml. Webster and Maggio (7) described two of 19 patients in their ileocystoplasty group as having detrusor failure. In our population of 155 patients with interstitial cystitis, we found 16 (11%) patients who had maximum flow rates (MFR) <15 ml/sec, urinary residual volume >50 ml, normal sphincteric activity on EMG, and no cystoscopic evidence of obstruction. We consider these to be indirect criteria of detrusor failure. Obviously, only a pressure–flow study would answer this question, but as yet there are no published data. A finding of detrusor failure may have diagnostic and therapeutic implications.

Reports regarding bladder compliance vary from study to study, reflecting differences in patient population. Awad et al. (3) showed that detrusor compliance was lower but not significantly so in patients with interstitial cystitis than in those with reduced bladder storage and negative cystoscopy for interstitial cystitis (26.2 versus 32.8 ml/cm H_2O). Other studies reported decreased compliance in 26% (7) to 80% (16) of patients without specifying the criteria for decreased compliance. Decreased compliance may reflect bladder fibrosis in an end-stage disease or increased sympathetic input to the bladder (17).

URODYNAMIC EVALUATION OF THE OUTLET

There are only scarce reports in the literature regarding evaluation of the bladder outlet and urethra in interstitial cystitis patients. Urethral pressure profilometry (UPP) has been used only rarely in patients with interstitial cystitis. In our recent review of 155 patients with interstitial cystitis, we found increased values of maximum urethral closure pressure (MUCP) in female patients (116 cm H_2O versus our normal values for the same age group of 70 cm H_2O) using 8F balloon urodynamic catheters for investigation. Fifteen percent of the women had MUCP >150 cm H_2O. In male patients, such an increase was not as evident. An increase in sympathetic innervation to the area or altered metabolism of VIP and neuropeptide Y in interstitial cystitis as postulated by Hohenfellner (17) can possibly explain some of these findings. Schmidt and Vapnek (18) studied urethral and bladder pressure simultaneously during water cystometry with medium fill at 50 ml/min in 16 patients with interstitial cystitis (15 women and one man). Static maximum closure pressure was 64 cm H_2O (range 30 to 110). However, abnormal urethral activity was found in the filling, prevoid, and voiding phases. In the filling phase, there was sustained high urethral pressure, which increased above already high base points in five patients. In the prevoiding phase, nine patients had a delayed sphincter relaxation; and in the voiding phase, five had dysfunctional dyscoordinated voiding, three incomplete relaxation, one precipitous relaxation, and two were unable to void. There are also reports of abnormal EMG recordings (19). Perez-Marrero et al. (2) found some dysfunctional voiding with detrusor–sphincter dyscoordination but considered this finding inconsistent with the diagnosis of interstitial cystitis. We have found hyperactive EMG (perianal skin electrodes) in five of 155 patients, and we attributed it to lack of full relaxation of the activity of the sphincter as suggested by Schmidt and Vapnek (18). We also found decreased mean MFR (16.7 ml/sec) on Uroflow, with mean voided volume of 263 ml. Because MFR is volume dependent, we used Liverpool nomograms (20) to assess flow in relation to volume. We found that Uroflow results of female patients with interstitial cystitis fell into the 12th percentile of the normal population. Also, 11 of 142 women had low MFR (<15 ml/sec), MUCP > 150 cm H_2O, no residual volume, and, on cystoscopic examination, a well-suspended bladder neck and no cystocele, which by our criteria may indirectly indicate notably increased urethral resistance. Uroflow was described as normal by Perez-Marrero et al. (2) in all patients with interstitial cystitis. A pressure–flow study would be an apprioprate test for evaluation of the bladder outlet, but the data are lacking.

It is difficult to comment on how important these findings are in relation to symptomatology and treatment results. However, they stress the importance of investigating not only the detrusor but the urethral function as well in interstitial cystitis patients. We consider the presence of dyscoordinated voiding to be worth documenting because it may be a part of the pathophysiology or cause of treatment failure in some cases.

SUMMARY

In conclusion, we believe that urodynamic studies play an important role in the diagnosis of patients with IC but, more significantly, may lead to a better understanding of the lower tract dysfunction associated with this disease. In addition, they may have therapeutic and prognostic implications.

REFERENCES

1. Bade JJ, Rijcken B, Mensink HJA. Interstitial cystitis in The Netherlands: Prevalence, diagnostic criteria and therapeutic preferences. *J Urol* 1995;154:2035–2038.
2. Perez-Marrero R, Emerson L, Juma S. Urodynamic studies in interstitial cystitis. *Urology* 1987;29:27–30.
3. Awad SA, MacDiarmid S, Gajewski JB, Gupta R. Idiopathic reduced bladder storage versus interstitial cystitis. *J Urol* 1992;148:1409–1412.

4. Parsons CL. Interstial cystitis: Clinical manifestations and diagnostic criteria in over 200 cases. *Neurourol Urodyn* 1990;9:241–250.
5. Zeidman EJ, Helfrick B, Pollard C, Thompson IM. Bacillus Calmette-Guerin immunotherapy for refractory interstitial cystitis. *Urology* 1994;43:121–124.
6. Kontturi MJ, Hellstrom PA, Tammela TL, Lukkarinen OA. Colocystoplasty for the treatment of severe interstitial cystitis. *Urol Int* 1991; 46:50–54.
7. Webster GD, Maggio MI. The management of chronic interstitial cystitis by substitution cystoplasty. *J Urol* 1989;141:287–291.
8. Alloussi S, Loew F, Mast GJ, Jung P, Schwertfeger K, Steffens J, Ziegler M. Value of the selective reversible sacral nerve blockade in the diagnosis and treatment of the urge syndrome. *Eur Urol* 1990;17: 30–34.
9. Feltis JT, Perez-Marrero R, Emerson LE. Increased mast cells of the bladder in suspected cases of interstitial cystitis: A possible disease marker. *J Urol* 1987;138:42–43.
10. Awad SA, Gajewski JB, Katz NO, Acker-Roy K. Final diagnosis and therapeutic implications of mixed symptoms of urinary incontinence in women. *Urology* 1992;39:352–357.
11. Hald T, Holm-Bentzen M. Clinical symptoms complex. In: George NJ, Gosling JA, eds. *Sensory Disorders of the Bladder and Urethra.* New York: Spring-Verlag, 1986;49–62.
12. Gillenwater JY, Wein AJ. Summary of the National Institute of Arthritis, Diabetes, Digestive and Kidney Disease Workshop on Interstitial Cystitis, National Institutes of Health, Bethesda, MD, August 28–29, 1987. *J Urol* 1988;140:203–206.
13. Perez-Marrero R, Emerson LE, Feltis JT. A controlled study of dimethylsulfoxide in interstitial cystitis. *J Urol* 1988;140:36–39.
14. Moore KH, Nickson P, Richmond DH, Sutherst JR, Manasse PR, Heilliwell TR. Detrusor mast cells in refractory idiopathic instability. *Br J Urol* 1992;70:17–21.
15. Holm-Bentzen M, Larsen S, Hainau B, Hald T. Nonobstructive detrusor myopathy in a group of patients with chronic abacterial cystitis. *Scand J Urol Nephrol* 1985;19:21–26.
16. Fleischmann JD, Huntley HN, Shingleton WB, Wentworth DB. Clinical and immunological responses to nifedipine for the treatment of interstitial cystitis. *J Urol* 1991;146:1235–1239.
17. Hohenfellner M, Nunes L, Schmidt RA, Lampel A, Thuroff JW, Tanago EA. Interstitial cystitis: Increased sympathetic innervation and related neuropeptide synthesis. *J Urol* 1992;147:587–591.
18. Schmidt RA, Vapnek JM. Pelvic floor behavior and interstitial cystitis. *Semin Urol* 1991;9:154–159.
19. Schmidt RA. The urethral syndrome. *Urol Clin North Am* 1985;12: 349–353.
20. Haylen BT, Ashby D, Sutherst JR, Frazer MI, West CR. Maximum and average urine flow rates in normal male and female populations—Liverpool nomograms. *Br J Urol* 1989;64:330–338.

Interstitial Cystitis, edited by Grannum R. Sant.
Lippincott–Raven Publishers, Philadelphia ©1997.

CHAPTER 22

Oral Therapies for Interstitial Cystitis

Michel A. Pontari and Philip M. Hanno

Because the factors causing interstitial cystitis (IC) have yet to be identified, any therapy is necessarily empiric or symptomatic. The advantages of oral therapy over other routes such as intravesical are that it is noninvasive, painless, and simple to administer. Many oral therapies have been used for IC, with mixed results.

ANTIHISTAMINES

Histamine is one of the substances released by mast cells and can induce pain, vasodilation, and hyperemia. Elevated histamine levels have been found in bladder biopsies of IC patients (1–3) as well as in bladder washings (4). Elevated levels of histamine metabolites have been found in the urine of IC patients (5,6). Therefore, blockade of the actions of histamine may be expected to relieve some of the symptoms of IC. This idea was first tried by Simmons (7,8), who postulated that the local release of histamine may be responsible for or accompany the development of IC. He reported on six patients treated with pyribenzamine, with half showing some response. Theoharides has used the piperazine H_1 receptor antagonist hydroxyzine (Atarax, Vistaril), which can block the neuronal activation of mast cells (9,10). In a series of 40 patients treated with 25 mg in the morning and 25 mg up to 50 mg at bedtime, a 30% improvement in almost all symptoms was achieved. Only three patients did not respond at all. The main side effects of this drug are sedation and weakness. These studies were not blinded or placebo-controlled. The other recognized subtype of histamine receptors is H_2. Cimetidine, an H_2 blocker commonly used for treating ulcer disease, was used in nine patients with IC (11). A 66% response rate was observed when a dose of 300 mg twice daily was used for 1 month. Further placebo-controlled studies are needed to fully assess the efficacy of antihistamines in interstitial cystitis (see Chapter 30).

AMITRIPTYLINE

Amitriptyline, one of the tricyclic antidepressants, blocks the H_1 histaminergic receptor (12) and has become widely used in the oral treatment of interstitial cystitis. Tricyclic antidepressant medications have at least three other pharmacologic actions, however. These include (a) central and peripheral anticholinergic actions at some but not all sites, (b) blockade of the active transport system in the presynaptic nerve ending that is responsible for the reuptake of the released amine neurotransmitters serotonin and norepinephrine, and (c) sedation, presumably by a centrally acting mechanism but possibly related to the antihistamine properties. Other effects ascribed to this class of drugs is desensitization of α_2 receptors on central noradrenergic neurons and blockade of α-adrenergic and serotonin receptors. Theoretically, tricyclic agents have properties that would lead to predominantly β-adrenergic stimulation, which in the bladder would facilitate storage by detrusor relaxation and decreasing the excitability of smooth muscle in that area (13). Nighttime sedation may also be one of the beneficial effects.

Hanno and Wein (14) first reported a therapeutic response in interstitial cystitis after noting a response to amitriptyline in one of their IC patients concurrently being treated for depression. Renshaw (15) noted a similar response to desipramine hydrochloride. Because of these observations, the theoretically favorable pharmacologic profile of the tricyclic antidepressants for the treatment of IC, and their use in other chronic pain syndromes (16), a trial was undertaken. Hanno et al. (17) reported a statistically significant improvement in pain and daytime frequency with a dose of 75 mg orally at bedtime. Nocturia did not improve significantly. Urinary urgency and dyspareunia improved. A follow-up study (18) reported on the use of amitriptyline in patients who had failed

M. A. Pontari and P. M. Hanno: Department of Urology, Temple University School of Medicine, Philadelphia, Pennsylvania 19140.

hydrodistention and intravesical dimethylsulfoxide (DMSO) therapy. In 28 of 43 patients who could tolerate therapy for at least 3 weeks, with an initial dose of 25 mg at bedtime increasing to 75 mg over a 2-week period, 18 had a total remission of symptoms with a mean follow-up of 14.4 months. Five patients dropped out because of side effects, with sedation being the main side effect. Five patients derived no clinical benefit. This study was not randomized or placebo-controlled.

Kirkemo (19) treated 30 patients with amitriptyline and reported that 90% of patients experienced symptomatic improvement after 8 weeks of therapy. Frequency of urination improved more in patients with bladder capacity greater than 450 cc under anesthesia. This finding is also consistent with those of Hanno and Wein (20), who reported that patients with a bladder capacity greater than 600 cc under anesthesia seemed to respond the best. In a study of 11 patients with urinary frequency and pelvic pain (21), nine experienced symptomatic improvement. Five reported complete resolution of symptoms, and four had significant relief. Two did not tolerate the medication.

NIFEDIPINE

Nifedipine has also been reported to be useful in treating IC. Fleischmann et al. (22) performed an open trial of nifedipine therapy in ten IC patients. Eight of nine patients had a substantial clinical response based on the reduction of symptom score with a duration of at least 4 months, and three became asymptomatic. Changes in IL-2 inhibitor activity did not correlate with changes in symptom scores, arguing against an immune-mediated effect of nifedipine. Because calcium channel blockers cause vasodilation, Fleischmann has speculated as to whether nifedipine is acting to increase bladder blood flow. Nifedipine also has been reported to inhibit detrusor contractions (23) and to depress cell-mediated immune function (24). Similar results using nifedipine were noted in patients treated for the urethral syndrome. Hypotension is a possible side effect and must be checked at the beginning of therapy. Other side effects include headache, dizziness, and constipation.

PENTOSANPOLYSULFATE

Parsons has suggested that a defect in the epithelial permeability barrier, the glycosaminoglycan (GAG) layer, contributes to the pathogenesis of IC. In an attempt to correct such a defect, a synthetic sulfated polysaccharide in oral form that is excreted in the urine has been used in clinical trials. Sodium pentosanpolysulfate (PPS, Elmiron, Pharmacia, Piscataway, NJ) consists of a negatively charged polysaccharide ester (a polyanion) with properties of sulfated glycosaminoglycans and an affinity for mucosal membranes. As of 1996, Elmiron is available in the United States only on a compassionate use basis from the manufacturer.

In 1983 Parsons et al. (25) reported on 24 patients who received 150 mg orally twice daily for 6 to 24 months. Twenty patients (83%) experienced at least an 80% decrease in pain within 4 to 8 weeks. Three patients who initially responded experienced a recurrence of symptoms after reducing the dose of the medication and responded to increasing the dose. In an open-controlled trial, Fritjofsson et al. (26) reported total relief of bladder pain in 35% of 87 patients and partial relief in 24% after 400 mg twice a day for 6 months. In patients without bladder ulcer, there was a significant decrease in frequency of micturition from 16.5 to 13 voids per day. Nocturia improved from 4.5 to 3.5, also a statistically significant but clinically small change. An increase in the mean volume of micturition was also demonstrated. These changes were not seen in the group with ulcers.

Holm-Bentzen et al. (27), in a double-blind clinically controlled study, reported that no statistically or clinically significant effect of PPS was found compared to placebo. This study included two populations: group A, with clinically and pathologically verified interstitial cystitis (>28 mast cells/mm^2 in the detrusor on bladder biopsy); and group B, with painful bladder and fewer than 28 mast cells/mm^2 in the detrusor. In group A, pain and dysuria decreased more in the PPS group than with placebo, but no p value was given. Mean capacity under anesthesia also increased in the treatment group but not with placebo. In group B, no differences between the two were observed.

In a double-blind placebo-controlled trial of pentosanpolysulfate, subjective improvements in pain, urgency, frequency, and nocturia were observed with drug relative to placebo (28). In this study, objective improvement in average voided volume was demonstrated, but no difference in number of average daily voids between drug and placebo was observed. In a larger double-blind placebo-controlled study, Mulholland et al. (29) reported an improvement greater than 25% in 28 of the patients on PPS and 13% of placebo patients ($p = 0.03$). Improvement in pain and pressure to urinate was greater in the PPS patients, although the difference was not statistically significant. There was no significant difference in the increase in average voided volume between the two groups. Of note is that the patients involved in this study were those who had failed conventional treatment with hydrodistention, DMSO, and chlorpactin. Also, 44% of patients continued to use PPS for 6 to 18 months after the 3-month study period, indicating duration of the effect. The results of a 3-month randomized, prospective, double-blind, placebo-controlled multicenter study have been published (30). Of the patients on the drug, 32% showed a greater than 50% improvement in symptoms compared to 16% of those on placebo ($p = 0.01$). Minor adverse effects, mostly gastrointestinal, were seen in seven patients in the drug group and ten patients receiving placebo.

The long-term results of Elmiron have recently been summarized (manufacturer's letter to Food and Drug Administration, 1995).

Clinically significant improvement in pain, urgency, and overall status was reported by 74% to 88% of patients. Responses as measured by pain, urgency, frequency, and nocturia were consistently demonstrated over at least 3 years. There appears to be no tachyphylaxis with the use of the medication. Patients with more severe urgency, frequency, nocturia, and pain had higher response rates than those patients with less severe baseline symptoms. These results demonstrate that Elmiron can be a useful alternative in those patients who have failed first-line therapies.

OTHER ORAL THERAPIES

Several oral therapies for IC have been tried and essentially discarded. Deep (31) reported temporary improvement with steroids, and Badenoch (32) reported improvement in 19 of 25 IC patients treated with prednisone starting at 15 mg per day and eventually tapered to 5 mg per day. Other studies have not found steroids to be as helpful (33). The risks of chronic steroid administration are considerable and include fluid retention, osteoporosis, and aseptic necrosis of joints. Hormones have been used but not found to be successful (32,34). Antispasmodics and anticholinergics are generally not effective. The NIDDK criteria for IC specify that patients have not had symptoms relieved by these medications.

Oravisto and Alfthan tried immunosuppression and chloroquine derivatives (35). Approximately 50% of patients responded to some extent, but potential complications are significant, and neither drug has become widely used. Benzydamine, a potent antiinflammatory drug with strong analgesic effects, was initially reported to have an excellent response rate in IC (36), but a controlled follow-up trial demonstrated no responses in the first 12 patients, and the trial was discontinued (37).

PAIN MEDICATION

With the etiology and pathogenesis of this syndrome unknown, rational therapy is necessarily based on theories and unproven hypotheses. Therefore, treatments directed at symptomatic relief are an important part of oral therapy. Pain is a major feature of interstitial cystitis. The long-term, appropriate use of pain medications can and should form an integral part of the treatment of a chronic pain condition such as IC. Many nonopioid analgesics such as acetaminophen, nonsteroidal antiinflammatory drugs, and antispasmodic agents have a place in therapy (38).

The origin of pain in IC is unclear. Bladder inflammation is one likely source. With stimulation of endogenous opiate receptors, mast cells degranulate and release histamine and other pedtides. In IC, this theoretically could occur because of chronic endorphin release stimulated by pain. By blocking the patient's own endogenous stimulation of mast cell release, it may be possible to break a cycle of bladder pain and a response that may in turn make the pain worse by increasing bladder inflammation. The opiate antagonist nalmefene was tried in an uncontrolled trial with improvement in pain, frequency, and nocturia reported (39). Unfortunately, an unpublished, placebo-controlled trial failed to demonstrate the efficacy seen in the previous study.

The use of long-term opioid therapy in rare patients who have failed all forms of conservative therapy over many years should be considered. This is especially true because the results of surgery are anything but certain, and there have been reports of residual pelvic pain even after cystectomy (40,41). Opioids are effective for most forms of moderate and severe pain and have no ceiling effect other than that imposed by adverse effects. The common side effects include sedation, nausea, mild confusion, and pruritis. Respiratory depression is uncommon and rare if prescribed doses are used. Constipation can occur and is usually correctable by the use of a gentle laxative. The major reason for not using this class of drugs is the fear of addiction. Studies suggest that this risk is low when opiates are used in chronic pain patients with nonmalignant conditions (42). Chronic pain patients often receive inadequate doses of short-acting pain medications; this can start a cycle of short-term relief, anxiety, and pain, which can lead to visits to several physicians and to drug-seeking behavior that may be mistaken for true addiction. Although physical dependence on opioids is unavoidable, physical addiction, defined as a chronic disorder characterized by the compulsive use of a substance resulting in physical, psychological, or social harm to the user and continued use despite that harm, is rare. The long-acting narcotic formulations that result in steady levels of drug over many hours are preferable to shorter-acting analgesics. Chronic opioid therapy can be considered as a last resort in selected patients with IC. It is best administered in a pain clinic setting and requires frequent assessment by both patient and physician (43). Pain management in IC is fully reviewed in Chapter 23.

ASSESSMENT OF STUDIES ON IC TREATMENT

Interstitial cystitis is not only a difficult condition to diagnose but a difficult condition in which to assess therapeutic impact. It has long been recognized in protocols that use subjective criteria for assessment that improvement may be expected in up to 35% of placebo-treated patients (44). Because of the spontaneous remission rate (though temporary) for IC of 11% (35) to 50% (45), combined with the placebo improvement, it can be difficult to prove efficacy. Unfortunately, few IC treatments have been subjected to a placebo-controlled trial. This is not to say that what seems effective is not, but rather that a high index of skepticism is healthy, even in treatments tested by controlled trials (46). In many diseases an argument can be made against using a true placebo control as opposed to an orthodox treatment of approved or accepted value (47), but a good case for true placebo can readily be made for interstitial cystitis. The vagaries of the natural history, the general lack of progression of symptom severity over time, and the fact that IC is not life threatening mean that there is little to lose and much to gain by subjecting new treatments to the vigorous scrutiny of placebo control.

REFERENCES

1. Lynes WL, Flynn SD, Shortliffe L, et al. Mast cell involvement in interstitial cystitis. *J Urol* 1987;138:746–752.
2. Kastrup J, Hald J, Larsen L. Histamine content and mast cell count of detrusor muscle in patients with interstitial cystitis and other types of chronic cystitis. *Br J Urol* 1983;55:495–500.
3. Enerback L, Fall M, Alddenborg F. Histamine and mucosal mast cells in interstitial cystitis. *Agents Actions* 1989;27:113–116.
4. Lundberg T, Liedberg H, Nordling L, Theodorsson E, Owzarski A, Ekman P. Interstitial cystitis: Correlation with nerve fibres, mast cells and histamine. *Br J Urol* 1993;71:427–429.
5. Holm-Bentzen M, Sondergaard I, Hald T. Urinary excretion of a metabolite of histamine (1,4-methyl-imidazole-acetic acid) in painful bladder disease. *Br J Urol* 1987;59:230–233.
6. El-Mansoury M, Boucher W, Sant GR, Theoharides TC. Increased urine histamine and methylhistmine in interstitial cystitis. *J Urol* 1994; 152:350–353.
7. Simmons JL, Bunce PL. On the use of an antihistamine in the treatment of interstitial cystitis. *Am Surg* 1958;24:664–667.
8. Simmons JL. Interstitial cystitis: an explanation for the beneficial effect of an antihistamine. *J Urol* 1961;85:149–155.
9. Theoharides TC. Hydroxyzine in the treatment of interstitial cystitis. *Urol Clin North Am* 1994;21:113–119.
10. Ting S, Rauls DO, Reimann BE. Inhibitory effect of hydroxyzine on antigen induced histamine release *in vivo. J Allergy Clin Imunol* 1985; 75:63–66.
11. Seshadri P, Emerson L, Morales A. Cimetidine in the treatment of interstitial cystitis. *Urology* 1994;44:614–616.
12. Baldessarini RJ. Drugs and the treatment of psychiatric disorders. In: Gilman AG, Gooman LS, Rall TW, et al, eds. *The Pharmacological Basis of Therapeutics,* 7th ed. New York: Macmillan, 1985;387–445.
13. Wein AJ, Levin RM, Barrett DM. Voiding function and dysfunction. In: Gillenwater JY, Grayhack JT, Howards S, Duckett JW, eds. *Adult and Pediatric Urology.* St. Louis: Mosby Year Book, 1991;933–1100.
14. Hanno PM, Wein AJ. Editorial: intersititial cystitis. *J Urol* 1987; 138:595–596.
15. Renshaw DC. Desipramine for interstitial cystitis. *JAMA* 1988;260:341.
16. Clarke IM. Amitriptyline and perphenazine (Triptafen DA) in chronic pain. *Anesthesia* 1981;36:210–212.
17. Hanno PM, Buehler J, Wein AJ. Use of amitriptyline in the treatment of interstitial cystitis. *J Urol* 1989;141:846–848.
18. Hanno PM. Amitriptyline in the treatment of interstitial cystitis. *Urol Clin North Am* 1994;21:89–92.
19. Kirkemo AK, Miles BJ, Peters JM. Use of amitriptyline in interstitial cystitis. *J Urol* 1990;143:279A.
20. Hanno PM, Wein AJ. Conservative therapy of interstitial cystitis. *Semin Urol* 1991;4:143–147.
21. Pranikoff K. *Amitriptyline therapy for patients with urinary frequency and pelvic pain.* Paper presented at the 1995 Interstitial Cystitis Symposium, National Institutes of Health, Bethesda, MD, January 9–11, 1995, p 67.
22. Fleischmann JD, Huntley HN, Shingleton WB, Wentworth DB. Clinical and immunological response to nifedipine for the treatment of interstitial cystitis. *J Urol* 1991;146:1235–1239.
23. Zar MA, Irivani MM, Luheshi GN. Effect of nifedipine on the contractile responses of the isolated rat bladder. *J Urol* 1990;143:835–839.
24. Corteza Q, Shen S, Revie D, et al. Effects of calcium channel blockers on *in vivo* cellular immunity in mice. *Transplantation* 1989;47: 339–342.
25. Parsons CL, Schmidt JD, Pollen JJ. Successful treatment of interstitial cystitis with sodium pentosanpolysulfate. *J Urol* 1983;130:51–53.
26. Fritjofsson A, Fall M, Juhlin R, Persson BE, Ruutu M. Treatment of ulcer and nonulcer interstitial cystitis with sodium pentosanpolysulfate: a multicenter trial. *J Urol* 1987;138:508–512.
27. Holm-Bentzen M, Jacobsen F, Nerstrom B, Lose G, Kristensen JK, Pedersen RH, Krarup T, Feggetter J, Bates P, Barnard R, Larsen S, Hald T. A prospective double-blind clinically controlled multicenter trial of sodium pentosanpolysulfate in the treatment of interstitial cystitis and related painful bladder disease. *J Urol* 1987;138: 503–507.
28. Parsons CL, Mulholland SG. Successful therapy of interstitial cystitis with pentosanpolysulfate. *J Urol* 1987;138:513–516.
29. Mulholand SG, Hanno P, Parsons CL, Sant GR, Staskin DR. Pentosan polysulfate sodium for therapy of interstitial cystitis. *Urology* 1990; 35:552–558.
30. Parsons CL, Benson G, Childs SJ, Hanno P, Sant G, Webster G. A quantitatively controlled method to study prospectively interstitial cystitis and demonstrate the efficacy of pentosanpolysulfate. *J Urol* 1993; 150:845–848.
31. Dees JE. The use of cortisone in interstitial cystitis: a preliminary report. *J Urol* 1953;69:496–502.
32. Badenoch AW. Chronic interstitial cystitis. *Br J Urol* 1971;43:718–721.
33. Pool TL. Interstitial cystitis: clinical considerations and treatment. *Clin Obstet Gynecol* 1967;10:185–191.
34. Burford EH, Burford CE. Hunner ulcer of the bladder: a report of 187 cases. *J Urol* 1958;79:952–955.
35. Oravisto KJ, Alfthan OS. Treatment of interstitial cystitis with immunosuppression and chloroquine derivatives. *Eur Urol* 1976;2:82–84.
36. Walsh A. Benzydamine: a new weapon in the treatment of interstitial cystitis. *J Urol* 1977;68:43–44.
37. Walsh A. Interstitial cystitis: observations on diagnosis and treament with anti-inflammatory drugs, particularly benzydamine. *Eur Urol* 1977;3:216–217.
38. Rummans TA. Nonopioid agents for treatment of acute and subacute pain. *Mayo Clin Proc* 1994;69:481–490.
39. Stone NN. Nalmefene in the treatment of interstitial cystitis. *Urol Clin North Am* 1994;21:101–106.
40. Baskin LS, Tanagho EA. Pelvic pain without pelvic organs. *J Urol* 1992;147:683–686.
41. Irwin PP, Galloway NTM. Surgical management of interstitial cystitis. *Urol Clin North Am* 1994;21:145–151.
42. Gourlay GK. Long-term use of opiods in chronic pain patients with nonterminal disease states. *Pain Rev* 1994;1:62–76.
43. Portenoy RK, Foley KM. Chronic use of opioid analgesics in nonmalignant pain: report of 38 cases. *Pain* 1986;25:171–186.
44. Benson H, Epstein MD. The placebo effect. *JAMA* 1976; 232:1225.
45. Held PJ, Hanno PM, Wein AJ, Pauly MV, Cahn MA. Epidemiology of interstitial cystitis: 2. In: Hanno PM, Staskin DR, Krane RJ, Wein AJ, eds. *Interstitial Cystitis*. London: Springer-Verlag, 1990;29–48.
46. Schulz KF, Chalmers I, Hayes RJ, et al. Empirical evidence of bias; dimensions of methodological quality associated with estimates of treatment effects in controlled trials. *JAMA* 1995;273:408–412.
47. Rothman KJ, Michels KB. The continuing unethical use of placebo controls. *N Engl J Med* 1994;331:394–398.

Interstitial Cystitis, edited by Grannum R. Sant.
Lippincott–Raven Publishers, Philadelphia ©1997.

CHAPTER 23

The Causes and Treatment of Pain in Interstitial Cystitis

Daniel Brookoff

"Pain is a more terrible lord of mankind than even death itself."

Albert Schweitzer (1)

For many patients with chronic interstitial cystitis (IC), pain is the prominent feature of their disease. For some, pain is the prominent feature of their lives. Although the pain of IC can be comparable to that of advanced cancer, interstitial cystitis has not yet attracted much attention from physicians specializing in pain treatment. Textbooks on pain management barely mention IC and give no recommendations for treatment (2,3). In the first half of this chapter, the pathophysiological basis for severe chronic pain in IC is reviewed. This should allow us to see severe pain of interstitial cystitis as a medical problem that is worthy of treatment. An approach to the medical treatment of interstitial cystitis pain is then described.

THE PATHOPHYSIOLOGY OF PAIN IN INTERSTITIAL CYSTITIS

Normal Pain and Abnormal Pain

The ability to sense pain is a vital bodily function. Normal pain is the perception of a potentially harmful stimulus. Normally, pain is an important alarm that can warn a person of threatened or ongoing tissue damage and bring an illness to medical attention. The sensation of pain in IC is not normal pain and provides no useful information. Because patients with chronic pain from IC differ from patients with normal pain (Table 1), they often do not get appropriate treatment for their pain.

Chronic pain can slow healing (4), subvert therapies for medical problems (5), and even endanger life. Among cancer patients, uncontrolled pain has long been recognized as an important contributing factor to suicides (6). Untreated pain may also be an important contributor to the high rate of suicides and suicide attempts among patients with IC (7).

Processes of Abnormal Pain: Hypersensitization, Hyperalgesia, and Allodynia

Though the exact cause of IC is not known, there is a growing understanding of the processes that give rise to chronic visceral pain. Bladder inflammation in IC can cause hypersensitization of the chemosensitive afferent bladder nerves, causing *hyperalgesia,* the perception of high-intensity pain in response to a low-intensity pain stimulus. With continued inflammation, mechanoreceptive nerves in the bladder wall generate pain signals in response to small increases in intravesicular pressure. This perception of pain in response to an innocuous stimulus (such as mild distention) is called *allodynia.*

Over time, if there is no analgesic treatment, persistent pain signals transmitted from the bladder to the central nervous system cause changes in the cells of the dorsal horn of the spinal cord, which can acquire the ability to transmit pain signals to the brain with little or no peripheral stimulation. This process has been termed *central hypersensitization.* With persistent pain over years, the pain signal can become embedded in the central nervous system, and the patient no longer needs a bladder to experience pain. This explains why, in some patients with long-standing IC, treatment aimed at the bladder can stop working, and the patients become incurable.

D. Brookoff: Department of Medical Education, Methodist Hospital, Memphis, Tennessee 38104.

TABLE 1. *The difference between acute ("normal") pain and pain of chronic interstitial cystitis*[a]

Normal pain	Interstitial cystitis pain
Meaningful, linear, reversible	Meaningless, irreversible
Well-defined, recent onset	Persistent over time
Clear proximal cause	Cause obscure
Autonomic activation	Autonomic adaptation and vegetative signs

[a]Adapted from Payne (170), with permission.

Chronic Pain Treatment: Healing the Incurable

Medical training, with its strong emphasis on cure, may sometimes reduce our attention to patients who cannot be cured. This certainly applies to many patients with long-standing IC, for whom traditional therapy is often unsatisfactory (8). Patients with severe pain caused by IC may not be cured, but their pain can be healed (9). When there is no good treatment for a patient's interstitial cystitis, there will almost always be an effective treatment for pain (10). To leave a patient to suffer with treatable pain is a show of disrespect for that patient and a breach of our ethics as caregivers (11). When confronted with a patient with severe pain of IC, physicians often ask themselves whether the patient should receive treatment for pain. Perhaps the question should be "Why should this person be left in pain?"(9).

The Scope of Pain in Interstitial Cystitis

"Interstitial cystitis is a disease of extremes."

Campbell's Urology (12)

Many patients with interstitial cystitis have been left in pain. A large epidemiologic study found that 55% of patients with IC reported constant or daily pain, and 57% characterized their pain as severe or excrutiating (13). A separate study of 50 patients with pain from interstitial cystitis at Duke University reported an average duration of pain of over 7 years (14). Acccording to a standard measurement tool, the McGill Pain Inventory, the pain of interstitial cystitis was found to be more severe than the pain of advanced cancer. In large part because of undertreated pain, patients with chronic IC have a lower measured quality of life than comparable patients with end-stage kidney disease on dialysis (15).

Types of Pain

There are at least three distinct types of clinical pain (16). *Somatic pain,* the model for "normal" pain, originates in skin, muscle, and bone and is usually well localized and described in nonemotional terms (e.g., "sharp"). Somatic pain related to incision or disruption of tissues (such as a burn or other destructive injury) is usually worst at the time of injury and rapidly tapers off. Doctors feel comfortable treating somatic pain because it is usually an indicator of a remediable injury.

Much of the pain of IC is *visceral pain.* The viscera generate pain in response to inflammation, distention, or increased pressure (17). Visceral pain is not necessarily linked to visceral injury. The pain is not well localized, is often referred (18), and produces stronger autonomic and affective responses than somatic pain (19). The increased emotional content in visceral pain is physiological and not characterologic.

A third type of pain, *neuropathic pain,* can be a component of the pain of IC. Neuropathic pain is usually related to disruption of nerves and is typically experienced by patients with herpes zoster, diabetic neuropathy, and "phantom limb" syndrome. This type of pain can be caused by the formation of neuromas, the development of hypersensitivity of nerves following injury, abnormal nerve regeneration, or the formation of *ephapses*—abnormal electric connections formed between remodeling or regenerating nerves that give rise to abnormal nerve pathways wherein a stimulus that should give rise to a nonpainful sensation causes pain (20). Neuropathic pain can be agonizing and require high doses of analgesics for relief. Patients with neuropathic pain often report a shooting, burning, or electric component to the pain.

Normal Bladder Sensation

The normal bladder does not have a broad repertoire of sensation. Most sensory messages in the healthy bladder relate to distention and contraction. The first sensation of bladder fullness occurs between 100 and 200 ml of urine. It brings with it no sense of urgency and can be easily overcome (21). Between 300 and 500 ml, the sensation of fullness becomes constant, and urgency develops. If the volume increases to more than 600 ml, the individual will begin to experience discomfort and eventually pain, which is often described as deep and gnawing. Micturition is usually associated with relief, not discomfort.

Sensation in the Inflamed Bladder

Important changes occur in sensory function when the bladder is inflamed. Bladder capacity is decreased, and there is an exaggerated sense of urgency, even at small volumes. Micturition is associated with pain and discomfort. The pain sensed from an inflamed bladder has a different quality from the pain felt in a noninflamed bladder, with the former being described as "burning" and having an especially disagreeable character, whereas the latter is a deep dull sensation that does not evoke as much emotion and can often be overcome. These differences suggest that sensations from healthy and inflamed bladders are carried along different pathways (22).

In chronic IC, bladder inflammation may cause hypersensitization of chemosensitive bladder afferent nerves. Hypersensitization may occur by any one or a combination of the processes thought to give rise to IC—exposure of the bladder wall to urinary toxins, persistent infection, or other processes that cause the release of vasoactive substances by activated inflammatory cells such as mast cells. Substances implicated in the hypersensitization process include histamine, platelet-activating factor, serotonin (all of which are released by mast cells), catecholamines, prostaglandins, hydrogen and potassium ions, bradykinin, adenosine, substance P, and nerve growth factors (23). Bradykinin has been implicated as an important mediator of pain in visceral organs (24) and can cause hypersensitization of peripheral nerves, resulting in the generation of a pain signal from a nonpainful stimulus (25).

Animal Models of Persistent Bladder Inflammation

In animal models of chemically induced cystitis, nondestructive concentrations of chemical irritants cause an inflammatory reaction with release of vasoactive substances from chemosensitive afferent fibers in the bladder wall (26). These animals show sensory changes that are similar to those seen with cystitis in humans (26), including an increase in bladder motility. These changes may persist for some time after the irritant has been removed. These sensory changes are related to the way sensory information from the bladder is processed by nerves in the epithelial and adventitial layers of the bladder and are not a result of dysmotility or of changes in the muscles in the bladder wall (22). With repeated exposures to chemical irritants, the bladder can become more sensitized to chemical irritation, and these animals exhibit hyperalgesia and allodynia.

In animal models, nerve growth factor (NGF) is an important mediator of peripheral hyperalgesia. Nerve growth factor also causes central hyperalgesia through its trophic effect on nerve cells in the dorsal horn of the spinal cord. In experimental models, nerve growth factor is a mediator that can turn an acute injury into a persistent pain problem. Antagonists to nerve growth factor can block the development of chronic visceral pain syndromes that resemble interstitial cystitis (22,27) (see Chapter 8).

Nociceptors and Interstitial Cystitis Pain

Inflammatory mediators in the bladder wall stimulate afferent pain nerves (nociceptors), which synapse with dorsal horn cells in the spinal cord. The main chemical transmitters of the pain signal across the synapse are glutamate and aspartate. Stimulation of opioid receptors on peripheral neurons or at the presynaptic terminal in the spinal cord can slow or stop synaptic transmission. This is one of the methods by which high-dose systemic or intraspinal opioids block pain (28). The spinal cord cells that process the input of pain signals have several different types of glutamate receptors (29). AMPA receptors are always exposed and may mediate signals for both acute and chronic pain (30). With persistent stimulation, the receiving cells in the spinal cord reveal a different type of glutamate receptor, the NMDA receptor (31) (Fig. 1).

NMDA Receptors and Chronic Pain

With persistent NMDA receptor activation, spinal cord cells undergo trophic changes, and the pain resulting from subsequent stimulation becomes exaggerated and prolonged (32). This is an important mechanism for the generation of a "pain memory" in the spinal cord that can cause IC patients to become refractory to intravesical therapies (33). NMDA-receptor-driven formation of new connections in the spinal cord provides a physiological basis for the expansion of the affected field in chronic visceral pain (Fig. 2). Patients with IC can experience pain in the vulva, lower extremities, back, and previously unaffected areas of the abdomen. NMDA receptor activation is critical to the development and maintenance of

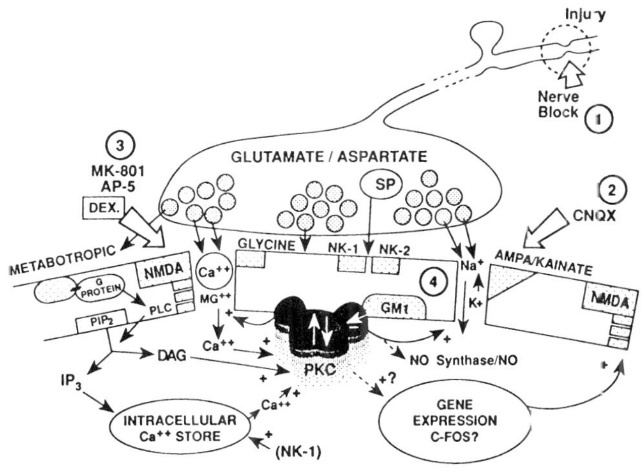

FIG. 1. Schematic diagram of possible excitatory synaptic mechanisms initiated by glutamate/aspartate release from nociceptive afferents and the intracellular cascade of molecular events triggered by NMDA/non-NMDA receptor activation. Potential pharmacologic interventions for postinjury neuropathic pain are indicated by circled numbers and include (1) peripheral nerve anesthetic blockade, (2) blockade of non-NMDA glutamate receptors, (3) blockade of NMDA receptors, and (4) blockade of translocation of protein kinase C by G_{M1} ganglioside. (From Price et al., ref. 31, with permission.)

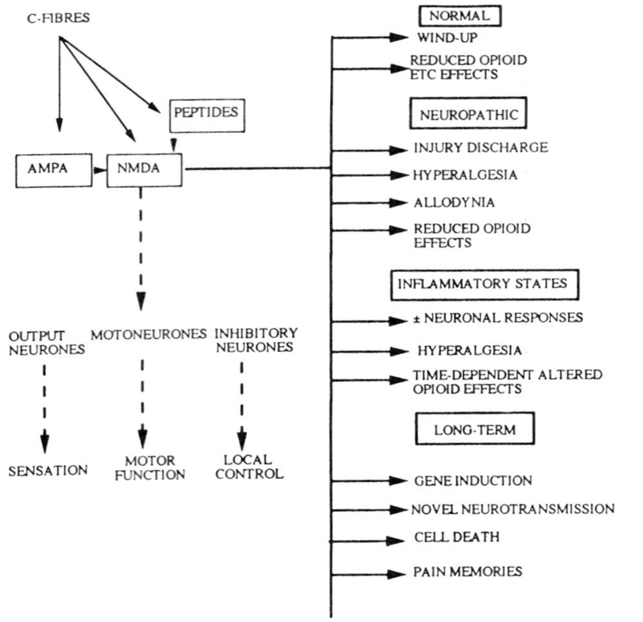

FIG. 2. The consequences of NMDA receptor activation for pain. (Adapted from Price et al., ref. 31, with permission.)

hyperalgesia and allodynia and to the development of narcotic tolerance and dependence (34). In addition, nitric oxide synthesis in the spinal cord may contribute to the establishment of hyperalgesia and mediate the ability of spinal cord cells to respond to NMDA agonists and to other pain mediators, such as substance P, released from nociceptor terminals (35).

Stimulation of NMDA receptors accelerates the production of mRNA for the c-*fos* oncogene protein in spinal cord cells (Fig. 1). In some respects, c-*fos* production can be regarded as a biochemical marker of chronic pain. With persistent visceral inflammation, an increase in c-*fos* production can be detected up the spinal cord and eventually into the thalamus (36). In certain IC patients with chronic bladder pain, the pain can persist despite complete anesthetic blocks in the low thoracic cord (S. DuPen, Swedish Hospital, Seattle WA, *personal communication*) or after cystectomy. The concept of central sensitization rationalizes the utility of trying a differential spinal anesthetic block before considering cystectomy. If the patient continues to perceive bladder pain after a spinal anesthetic at the T_{10} level, it can be taken as an indicator that the pain signal is being generated at a higher level in the spinal cord and that surgery on the bladder will not result in pain relief.

Silent Afferents and Interstitial Cystitis

The urinary bladder has a dual system of afferent innervation. Most of the sensations of distention and the pain of acute cystitis are carried by fibers of the pelvic nerve (37), as well as the hypogastric and lumbar splanchnic nerves. In the healthy bladder, these latter two pathways are usually inactive and are called *silent afferents* (22).

Persistent chemical irritation causes activation of the bladder's silent afferents. Persistent inflammation can also lead to recruitment of initially unresponsive nerve fibers with terminals in the epithelial or adventitial layers of the bladder that are sensitive to mechanical stimulation. Inputs from these nerves into the central nervous system can lead to central changes that result in centrally mediated hypersensitivity (22). This can also lead to a change in the type of stimulus needed to trigger a pain signal, from chemical irritation to mild distention.

Thus, IC pain can evolve from an early stage when it is dependent on irritative chemical stimuli (and thus amenable to intravesical treatments) to a stage at which it can be sustained by distention by small volumes of urine. In animals subjected to persistent chemical irritation, the silent mechanosensitive nerve endings in the mucosa become awakened by the irritative process and begin to transmit a message of pain with minor stimuli (38). In the chronically irritated bowel, normal mechanoreceptors in the muscle layer that are sensitive to tension respond to distention and contraction of the gut while novel mechanoreceptors in the mucosal layer transmit pain signals in response to stroking and light touch (23). This provides a plausible physiological explanation of how stimuli that normally cause no discomfort can elicit severe pain in a patient with interstitial cystitis. Similar mechanisms have been invoked for severe pain in certain cases of severe noncardiac chest pain, chronic arthritis, and chronic headache (23).

Neurogenic Edema as a Contributor to Interstitial Cystitis

There is growing evidence that peripheral inflammation can lead to the generation of nerve impulses from the spinal cord that can promote and maintain inflammation in the end organ. This is called *neurogenic inflammation.* If the pain signal is too intense or too prolonged, a pathologic response (called a *dorsal root reflex*) can occur in which dorsal horn cells release mediators that cause action potentials to fire antidromically back down afferent nerves to the periphery, releasing inflammatory mediators (39). Dorsal root reflexes are abnormal and occur only after there has been persistent inflammation. This model of central nervous system control over peripheral inflammation has been invoked to explain some of the chronic pain states that do not respond well to standard treatments, such as certain forms of chronic headaches and intractable arthritis (40). The sympathetic nervous system may also transmit impulses that cause peripheral inflammation. These nerve fibers do not come into play until after the initial inflammatory reaction has been established (41). This may be an important part of the mechanism of chronic pain and tissue damage in post-traumatic conditions such as reflex sympathetic dystrophy that are similar in many ways to interstitial cystitis (42) (see Chapter 16).

Pain and the Brain

Descending pathways from the brain via the bulbospinal tracts can modify the function of the pain receptors in the spinal cord. These influences can be either excitatory or inhibitory. Inputs into the brain can influence all of the following: the generation of pain signals from the spinal tract, the magnitude of pain threshholds, the referral areas for pain, and the receptive field for pain (43). The primary neurotransmitters in the inhibitory tracts are endogenous opioids and α_2-adrenergic agonists, the former mediating pain inhibition originating from the periaqueductal gray area in the midbrain and the latter from the locus ceruleus (44). The ability of descending pathways to facilitate pain was demonstrated in experiments in which the dorsal horn activity in monkeys increased when the monkey was led to expect that a noxious stimulus was about to be applied (45). The facilitatory pathways are probably mediated, in part, by the sympathetic nervous system and norepinephrine.

Our understanding of the pathways of pain in the brain and bulbospinal tract explains how the brain's response to pain messages can be magnified by acute emotional reactions such as anxiety, fear, depression and helplessness (46). Neurohumoral changes associated with the stress response, grieving, anxiety, or depression can influence the expression of visceral hyperalgesia at supraspinal, spinal, and peripheral sites.

Pain signals from the spinal cord are processed at different sites in the brain, e.g., the limbic system, the thalamus, and the cortex. Limbic system involvement may explain why there may be a great deal of arousal and emotion associated with visceral pain. It provides a physiological explanation why certain types of visceral pain cause patients to "lose control" while the same patient with severe somatic pain (e.g., from an incision or a fracture) can feel a lot of pain but can "grin and bear it." This also provides a neurochemical explanation of why therapies aimed at reducing anxiety and relieving depression are useful components of pain treatment. Unfortunately, when these treatments work, some physicians may be prone to think that the pain circuit is entirely "psychological" and that the patient is neurotic or imagining the symptoms. Worse yet, physicians may interpret the complaints of unimaginable or "nonphysiological" pain as a ruse designed to get intoxicating drugs. Understanding the neuronal pathways of pain allows us to develop a neuropharmacologic explanation for the success of analgesics, antidepressants, anxiolytics, relaxation training, and hypnosis in decreasing pain in IC (47).

Experimental Pharmacology and Visceral Pain

New pharmacologic therapies for chronic visceral pain are being developed based on recent findings regarding the physiology of pain (Fig. 2). For example, substances that increase the sensory threshholds of visceral nociceptors such as somatostatin (48) or the 5-HT_3 antagonists ondansetron and granisetron (49) may eventually prove useful in dampening the pain signal. NMDA-receptor antagonists have also been used in clinical research and have been found to have analgesic effects (50). Unfortunately, the currently available NMDA-receptor-blocking drugs, such as phencyclidine, ketamine, and high-dose dextromethorphan, have side effects that currently prevent their use for chronic pain (51). Another pharmacologic strategy that may prove useful is the use of adenosine to down-regulate NMDA receptors (52). There is increasing interest in using drugs that block or deplete substance P, such as capsaicin, lidocaine, and mexiletine, in the treatment of chronic visceral pain. Another promising approach to chronic bladder pain may be to use inhibitors of nerve growth factor (53).

THE MANAGEMENT OF PAIN IN INTERSTITIAL CYSTITIS

Assessing Pain in the Patient with Interstitial Cystitis

> "Every physician must be rich in knowledge and not only of that which is written in books. His patients must be his books; they will never mislead him, and by them he will never be deceived."
>
> *Paracelsus* (54)

One of the most frustrating features of treating pain is the lack of objective measures to gauge pain and assess the outcome of our treatments. Although there are measures of pain that are precise, such as survey instruments and visual analog scales (55), these are rarely used in routine clinical practice, where pain is usually assessed indirectly (56).

The most important part of assessing pain is listening to and believing our patients. Nearly all the patients I have seen for chronic pain of interstitial cystitis have been told by a caregiver at some point that their pain was not real and were invariably labeled "drug seeking" by their frustrated physicians. This group includes several patients who had undergone cystectomy and whose pain has persisted. In treating interstitial cystitis, the following definition of pain (taken from a textbook of nursing) is the most useful: *"Pain is whatever the experiencing person says it is, existing whenever she or he says it does" (57).*

Confounding Factors in Pain Assessment

Many physicians have difficulty believing reports of severe pain, even in cancer patients (58). Even physicians in practices where there are expected to be many patients in severe pain, such as medical oncology, often do not have an organized approach to the assessment of pain (59). The evaluation of chronic pain may be time consuming, and pain may be obscured by other problems (e.g., altered relationships with family members, issues related to disability). There may be no realistic hope of cure for chronic pain—only treatment. It must be recognized that treatment will probably have to continue for a prolonged time. Factors such as insomnia, fatigue, anxiety, fear, and anger (60) may affect the perception of pain.

Functional Assessment of Pain

The evaluation of chronic pain can be framed in an operational format using criteria by which progress can be measured (61). These measures of pain are related to:

1. *The patient's report of the sensation of pain.* A pain diary can help objectify pain, and numerical pain scales can be worked into the diary. If it is understood that the caregiver will review the diary carefully, then the patient often will not feel the need to "act out" a month's worth of pain at every doctor's appointment. The diary can identify exacerbating and ameliorating factors. For example, many patients with interstitial cystitis will have flares of pain after long car rides. The patient and physician can use the diary to develop effective preventive stragies, such as preemptive use of analgesic medications (62).
2. *Functional status at work.* Most patients with interstitial cystitis are of working age (13). The patient's ability to work, the number of days of work that were missed because of pain, and the specific types of activities undertaken at work can be a used as functional indices of pain.
3. *Functional status at home.* The first thing that patients in pain stop doing are the important activities that are carried on outside of work, such as going to church, spending time in family activities, and taking part in sports or hobbies. In some cases of successful treatment, the patient will continue to report pain or discomfort, but the level of activity will rise. Keeping track of activities is a useful measure of treatment progress.
4. *Emotional state of the patient during office visits.*
5. *Somatic preoccupation.* This relates to the degree to which the patient remains focused on bodily symptoms to the exclusion of other issues. It may be useful to maintain contact with a close family member in order to assess this.
6. *Use of analgesic medications.* If the patient is given an adequate supply of effective short-acting "as-needed" pain medications and told to use them whenever there is pain, then the number of pills consumed becomes a measure of pain. This also provides a useful way to assess the utility of other treatment maneuvers.

Setting Goals

It is important to develop a set of goals in collaboration with the patient to guide treatment and assess progress. At first, these may be very simple, such as being able to spend an afternoon out with the family or being able to sleep through the night. With time, the goals may get more complicated, such as a return to work or recreational activities. This approach involves taking time with patients and finding out about their lives. It also involves finding out what is missing from life because of the pain and what needs to be restored. Another factor to evaluate is pain intensity. This indicates the urgency with which relief is needed, and it influences the selection of medication, the route of administration, and the rate of dose titration (63).

The evaluation must be comprehensive enough to yield effective strategies for dealing with all sources of the pain. This certainly includes a thorough medical evaluation but may often include psychological, functional, and social evaluations.

A complete assessment of chronic pain means developing an appreciation for how pain has invaded the patient's life and contributed to changes in behavior, attitudes, and relationships. The goal of pain treatment is to enable the patient to reclaim that life.

Medical Treatment of Pain Caused by Interstitial Cystitis

> "Pain is now recognized as a fundamental cause of morbidity and mortality and should thus be treated as aggressively as any pathogen."
>
> *Benedetti and Butler* (64)

Increased understanding of the physiological basis of chronic pain has led to the development of safe and effective treatments for chronic cancer pain (65). In many cases, these treatments are also safe and effective for patients with chronic noncancerous pain (66). Chronic pain, in and of itself, is now recognized as a legitimate complaint that is worthy of specific medical treatment (67). In nearly all cases of severe pain from interstitial cystitis, we should be able to offer treatment that will result in quick, effective, and safe pain relief. This does not obviate the need to pursue other specific treatments. Indeed, when severe pain is controlled, other "specific" treatments for interstitial cystitis work better.

An Approach to the Treatment of Severe Pain

The therapeutic strategies that are generally used for chronic pain of cancer form a useful approach to the treatment of chronic pain in selected patients with painful nonmalignant diseases (68). This is a useful approach with patients with long-standing severe nociceptive or neuropathic pain, such as patients with long-standing IC (69). The approach outlined below is based on a standard approach to severe cancer pain (63).

Opioid Medications

Analgesic medications are the primary mode of treatment for pain. For mild to moderate pain, acetaminophen, aspirin, or other nonsteroidal antiinflammatory agents are suitable. For severe pain, opioid medications are the mainstays of treatment. All patients with chronic pain of moderate or greater severity should have a trial of an opiate medication, irrespective of the pathophysiological mechanism underlying the pain (70). A single practitioner has to take responsibility for pain treatment and write all prescriptions for pain medications. Patients with moderate pain are usually treated with a weak opioid such as codeine, hydrocodone, or oxycodone. These are usually formulated in combination with acetaminophen or aspirin.

Opioids customarily used to treat severe pain are morphine, hydromorphone, levorphanol, methadone, and fentanyl. The latter is formulated as a long-acting transdermal patch. Because they have recently been reformulated in higher-dose preparations, oxycodone and hydrocodone have become useful for the treatment of severe pain. Oxycodone is becoming increasingly recognized for its utility as a strong opioid with a very tolerable side-effect profile (71). Until recently, its use was limited by the fact that it was manufactured in combination with aspirin or acetaminophen, but new single-agent formulations allow for its use in higher doses. In oral form, morphine and oxycodone are equipotent (72), but oxycodone appears to cause fewer side effects (73).

Many patients with interstitial cystitis will have had previous exposure to opioids. Unfortunately, the usual strategy used to treat interstitial cystitis pain with opioid analgesics calls for intermittent dosing on an "as-needed" basis (5). In this approach, analgesics are used only when the pain recurs. The pain medications used are often short-acting and given with insufficient frequency. This discontinuous provision of analgesia subjects patients with continuous pain to periods of pain, anticipation, and anxiety. This can generate pain-avoidance behaviors that physicians erroneously characterize as "manipulative" or "drug seeking" (74).

For the patient who is opiate-naive, treatment is usually started with a short-half-life drug (such as oxycodone, hydromorphone, or morphine). When using these short-half-life opioids, most patients will require dosing every 3 to 4 hr (63). Sample drugs and starting doses for severe pain include oxycodone 10 to 15 mg, codeine 30 to 60 mg, morphine 15 to 30 mg, hydromorphone 2 to 4 mg, and levorphanol 2 to 4 mg (63). If the starting dose is not enough to produce comfort, it can be doubled. Tramadol has recently been introduced into the American market as a medication with opioid-like analgesic effects (75). I have tried it in more than ten patients with interstitial cystitis pain, but without success.

Long-Acting Opioids

For patients with continuous or frequently recurring pain, a controlled-release opioid preparation can be started once there has been a good response to the short-half-life opioid. These preparations include long-acting morphine and oxycodone, which allow dosing intervals from 8 to 12 hr. The daily dose should be roughly equivalent to the daily consumption of the short-acting medication. The long-half-life drugs, such as levorphanol and methadone, and the fentanyl patch can be very useful for the treatment of severe chronic pain in interstitial cystitis, but they are usually reserved as second-line drugs because they are more difficult to titrate and can have delayed-onset side effects. For most patients, in order to control pain with methadone, the drug must be administered at intervals (three to four times per day) that are shorter than the drug's half-life. The physician must be aware of the possibility of delayed toxicity (primarily sedation) (76).

Titration of Opioids

All patients who receive long-acting opioids such as controlled-release morphine, oxycodone, the fentanyl patch, or methadone should be supplied with a fast-acting "rescue drug" given on an as-needed basis to treat pain that breaks through the regular medication schedule. The general dose of the rescue drug is between 5% and 15% of the 24-hr base-line dose (63). The daily consumption in milligrams of the rescue drug can be used an indicator of how much the controlled-release drug is falling short of providing adequate relief and can guide upward adjustment of the dose of the controlled-release drug. By titrating the drug dose to the pain, the patient can quickly find a dose of controlled-release medication that provides good relief.

In selecting the best opioid for the patient, it is important to carefully review the patient's history of medication use and side effects. In a study of cancer patients requiring opioid analgesics, 44% required two or more drug trials, and 20% required three or more trials before achieving satisfactory pain relief with tolerable side effects (77). Certain medical considerations will also guide the choice of opioid drug; for example, morphine, meperidine, and propoxyphene should not be used in patients with renal failure (78). Meperidine is not an appropriate drug to use in the management of chronic pain because it has a long-lived metabolite that will accumulate with sustained dosing and can cause central nervous system excitability, multifocal myoclonus, and seizures (79).

Patients may do very well at the beginning of treatment with opioids and find within a few weeks that they are beginning to encounter more pain. This is especially true for patients who had severely limited their activities while they were in pain. This is not a sign of tolerance to the medications (80). This usually occurs in association with an increase in activity and is a call for retitration of the medications.

Side Effects of Opioid Medications

Many of the side effects of opioids are transient and include nausea and vomiting, itching, and somnolence. Between 10% and 40% of patients suffer opioid-induced nausea (81), which can be treated with an antiemetic such as promethazine or prochlorperazine (pills or suppositories). If patients are getting good pain relief with an opioid but having a problem with the nausea, they can take their antiemetic on a scheduled basis (e.g., four times a day) for a few days until the nausea resolves. If the nausea is primarily postprandial or related to bloating and early satiety, metoclopramide can be an effective antiemetic in doses of 10 to 20 mg three times per day. For some patients, antihistamines such as hydroxyzine may be useful as antiemetics. Because many patients with interstitial cystitis have had experience with this medication (82), it may be an easier medication to start. Tolerance to opioid-induced nausea usually develops within a week.

Some patients develop itching and hives with opioids as the result of a direct nonallergic effect on mast cells. It is more common with the naturally occurring opioids (e.g., codeine, morphine) than with the synthetic medications. This problem is easily relieved with antihistamines.

Initiation or escalation of opioid medications can produce sedation or somnolence, though patients with severe pain may feel more alert or more "normal" while using opioid analgesics (83). Tolerance to this effect usually develops within days or weeks. If the sedation is not tolerable but the analgesia is satisfactory, the opioid dose can be reduced by 25% until the sedation lifts. If sedation persists, it may be useful to reduce or eliminate other sedating medications, e.g., antihistamines and antiemetics, that are used to counteract opioid side effects. Many patients with interstitial cystitis are also taking benzodiazepines or other sedative-hypnotics, and these can be reduced or eliminated. Myoclonus is sometimes seen as a side effect of opioid use, and if this is discomforting, it can be treated with a benzodiazepine. Clonazepam is a good choice for this problem because it is relatively less sedating than other benzodiazepines (84).

One of the side effects of opioids to which patients do not develop tolerance is constipation. This can be especially problematic for patients with interstitial cystitis because many of them also suffer from irritable bowel syndrome (13) and can have exacerbations of bladder pain when their bowel function becomes disordered. It is important to get patients on a good bowel regimen. Many patients start out with a stool softener (e.g., docusate) and a mild fiber-based cathartic (e.g., senna), but most will need to use osmotic diuretics such as milk of magnesia, magnesium citrate, or lactulose, and these may as well be started early. These laxative agents are safe and not "habit-forming" like the stimulant laxatives. Some patients with interstitial cystitis notice a decrease in their bladder symptoms with the successful establishment of a bowel-training regimen.

The most feared side effect of opioids is respiratory depression. If the patient is carefully titrated on opioid medications, respiratory depression does not occur (63). Suppression of different brain centers by opioids progresses in an orderly fashion, with cortical suppression preceding effects on the brainstem. Respiratory depression occurs gradually and is signaled by a declining respiratory rate. This means that a patient who is awake and complaining of pain is not in imminent danger of suffering an overdose. If the source of pain is abruptly removed, then a dose of opioid that was well tolerated can suddenly become sedating. This becomes clinically important when a patient on opioids requires an anesthetic or neurolytic procedure (85). Otherwise, respiratory depression is generally not encountered among patients on long-term oral opioids for chronic pain (86).

Another opioid side effect is stimulation of the release of antidiuretic hormone (64). This may cause dependent edema and may also be related to the urinary retention and increase in bladder capacity in some patients on opioids. Part of this effect may be related to an increase in tone of the sphincter vesicae that can be caused by opioids (87). There is no evidence that long-term opioid administration in a medical setting causes organ toxicity (88).

Tolerance to Opioids

Some patients will develop tolerance to opioid medications. This is true for many of the unwanted side effects of opioids, such as nausea. Other factors can confer tolerance; for example, severe pain allows patients to tolerate the sedative side effects of opioids (89). There is controversy over whether tolerance develops to the pain-relieving effects of opioids. Studies of patients on long-term opioids indicate that once pain relief is established, the dose stabilizes for a prolonged period of time unless there is an acceleration of the underlying disease process (66). There have been some concerns generated from animal studies that long-term opioid use and tolerance might actually worsen hyperalgesia (34). This has not been my experience in treating the pain of interstitial cystitis, where the large majority of patients reach a stable dose and are able to decrease their analgesic medications once they have obtained sustained relief. Most of the data on opioid tolerance and physical dependence in humans involve subjects who were not in pain (90)!

Physical Dependence and Opioids

Physical dependence can become a feature of opioid use. Physical dependence is defined as the condition in which, after continued use, abrupt withdrawal or reversal of a medication will cause physical symptoms (i.e., withdrawal symptoms). Physical dependence is a medical issue, not a psychological or a spiritual problem (91). It can easily be managed by gradually tapering the medication as an outpatient if it is no longer indicated. Often, if a urologic treatment or adjunctive therapy begins to work for an interstitial cystitis patient who has been on opioids, that patient will begin to report some new sedation on what had been a tolerable opioid dose or will stop using "as-needed" pain medications. This is the time to consider slowly tapering the long-acting pain medications. The ease with which patients who are being treated for pain can be detoxified shows that physical dependence is not a problem for patients who are using their medications appropriately (92).

Appropriate Use Versus Abuse

The fear of drug abuse and drug addiction is the major reason physicians are reluctant to prescribe opioid medications for patients with severe pain. Drug abuse is the inappropriate use of a medication for a nonmedical problem. The appropriate role of medicine is to prolong and maintain life, promote function, and provide comfort from symptoms. If a patient who has been precluded from living life fully by a medical problem (e.g., physical pain) is using a medication to get back into life, then he or she is using that medication appropriately (72). If that patient is using medications to escape existential problems (such as family, social, or financial problems), then that patient is abusing drugs. If there is a question of abuse, it is up to the physician to determine whether the medications are being used to participate in life or to escape life. The patient's mood and activities and the reports of family members can be helpful indicators. It is important that the patient knows about these parameters and is helped to discriminate between these two types of use.

Drug Addiction and Pseudoaddiction

Drug abuse can become the driving force in a person's life, leading to a compulsive pattern of drug abuse and socially inappropriate or dangerous behaviors. This is the

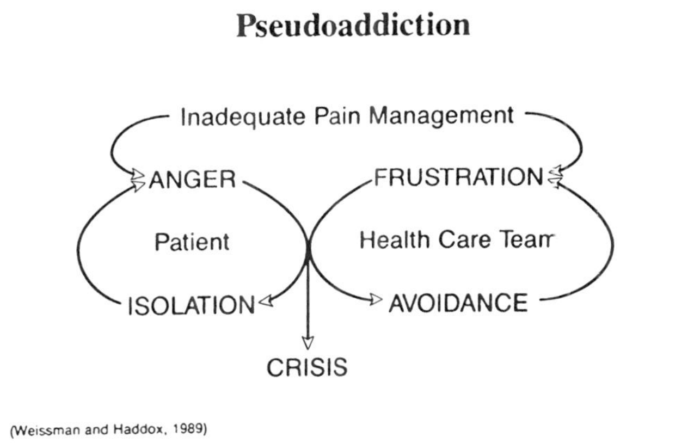

FIG. 3. Pseudoaddiction has been defined as "an iatrogenic syndrome of abnormal behavior developing as a direct consequence of inadequate pain management." (From Weissman and Haddox, ref. 97, with permission.)

definition of drug addiction (93). Drug addiction arises out of drug abuse. The medical use of opioids is not associated with the development of addiction (94–96). If a physican prescribes a pain medication in good faith for the treatment of pain, anyone who leaves the practice an addict was already an addict before the treatment. If a caring physician sincerely suspects that this may be part of the patient's problem, then that patient should be referred for evaluation by a psychologist or psychiatrist who has experience working with patients with chronic pain.

The inappropriate labeling of a patient as an addict can alienate the patient from caregivers and family and deepen isolation and prolong suffering. Most of the interstitial cystitis patients who have been referred to me have been accused by caregivers of being drug addicts and denied appropriate pain treatment, leading to isolation and anxiety. They may have behaved in ways that appeared manipulative or obsessive and that antagonized their caregivers. This constellation of behaviors has been termed *pseudoaddiction* (97). Pseudoaddiction, an iatrogenic problem related to undertreated pain, can be effectively and legitimately treated (Fig. 3).

Many of the behaviors that patients exhibit to get relief of pain are often misinterpreted as signs of drug abuse or drug addiction. Dr. Russell Portenoy (66) has classified the behaviors related to opioid use into those that are predictive of addiction and those that may be signs of pseudoaddiction (Table 2).

Nonopiate Medications for Interstitial Cystitis Pain

Opioids are a good first step in rescuing a patient in severe pain with interstitial cystitis. Once some relief is achieved, other pain managment approaches, such as adjuvant medications, nonpharmacologic treatments, and, possibly, more aggressive urologic treatments should be

TABLE 2. *Drug-related behaviors categorized by those that are indicators of abuse and addiction and those that may be related to undertreatment of pain*[a]

Probably predictive of drug abuse or addiction
Selling prescription drugs
Stealing or borrowing drugs from others
Injecting oral formulations
Obtaining prescription drugs from a nonmedical source
Concurrent abuse of alcohol or use of illicit drugs
Multiple dose escalations or other noncompliance with therapy despite warnings
Seeking prescriptions from other physicians or emergency departments without informing the prescriber or after warnings to stop
Evidence of deterioration of functioning related to drug use
Repeated resistance to changes in therapy despite adverse effects from the medication
Behaviors not necessarily predictive of abuse (may be related to undertreatment of pain)
Aggressive complaining about the need for more medicine
Drug hoarding during periods of reduced symptoms
Requesting specific medications
Unsanctioned dose escalation or noncompliance on one or two occassions
Unapproved use of the medication to treat another symptom
Reporting psychic effects not intended by the physician
Resistance to a change in treatment despite some side effects, with anxiety about return of symptoms

[a]Adapted from Portenoy (66), with permission.

used. I have found that all these treatments work better when some initial pain relief has been provided.

Antidepressants

Antidepressant medications are useful as analgesics in the treatment of chronic pain (98). They stimulate the descending nociceptive modulating pathways and thus potentiate the analgesic effects of opioid medications. The tricyclic antidepressants work better than other drugs of this class (99). Amitriptyline, imipramine, and doxepin appear to work better than nortriptyline or desipramine (100), though desipramine has been found to be useful in neuropathic pain (101). Clomipramine may be one of the most potent tricyclics in terms of analgesia, but its use has been limited by side effects, which can include convulsions and hepatotoxicity (102). The analgesic effects of the tricyclics are independent of the antidepressant effects and occur more quickly and at lower doses. The degree of pain relief *per se* is modest relative to that of the opioids (103). Tricyclics are often used in combination with opioids and augment their analgesic effects (104).

Many interstitial cystitis patients are sensitive to the tricyclics and suffer disturbing side effects at low doses (e.g., 25 mg at bedtime). Paradoxically, this appears to predict a good response, and it is worth spending the time and effort to get the patient to persevere with this drug. This may mean starting at a bedtime dose of 5 or 10 mg of amitriptyline and titrating up to bedtime doses between 50 and 100 mg (to a maximum of 200 mg). Usually, the dose can be increased every 3 to 4 days if the patient is tolerating the side effects. The anticholinergic effects of the tricyclics cause bladder retention and sedation, and this may translate into the first good night's sleep in months. Although the analgesic effects may be seen within a week of using a therapeutic dose, a reasonable trial of tricyclics should last from 8 to 12 weeks (105). Tricyclic antidepressants are safe to use in conjunction with opioids (106).

Most of the analgesic effects of antidepressants are related to their effects on norepinephrine rather than on serotonin (107). The tricyclics are therefore a better choice of antidepressants than selective serotonin reuptake inhibitors (SSRIs) for interstitial cystitis pain. If there is severe concurrent clinical depression, an SSRI may be more useful in the short term. A combination of SSRI in the morning and a small dose of a tricyclic at bedtime has been effective in depressed patients with chronic pain (108).

The side effects of the tricyclic antidepressants are related to their antihistaminic and anticholinergic effects. These include morning sedation, postural hypotension, and dry mouth, which will usually abate within 2 weeks on a stable dose. Some patients will report weight gain (as a result of appetite stimulation) or constipation (109). Several patients whom I cared for started lactating while on tricyclics, with normal serum prolactin levels and negative cranial MRIs. This resolved with withdrawal of the medication or a short course of bromocriptine. At high doses, tricyclics can cause cardiac conduction abnormalities. This can make these drugs especially dangerous for patients who are at risk for overdose.

Anticonvulsants and Antiarrhythmics

Anticonvulsant and antiarrhythmic medications may be helpful in treating neuropathic pain (110). One study suggested that the response of pain to anticonvulsants and antiarrhythmics can be predicted by the response to an intravenous infusion of lidocaine (111), though this is controversial. One technique is to administer intravenous lidocaine at a rate of 4 mg/min for 1 hr. Pain relief should be acheived when the serum lidocaine level is between 1.5 and 2.0 μg/ml (112). This has to be done in a setting where cardiac rhythm and blood pressure can be closely monitored and where there are personnel trained in cardiac resuscitation. Pain relief is usually experienced during the infusion and may last for days or weeks (113).

An empirical trial of an oral lidocaine-like drug is reasonable in patients with poorly controlled neuropathic pain (114), especially painful peripheral neuropathy. One with which I have had success in treating pain of interstitial cystitis is mexiletine. Mexiletine has been used for a variety of neurogenic pain syndromes (115–117) including radiation-induced pelvic pain with hyperalgesia and allodynia (118). In addition to stabilizing nerve cell membranes, mexiletine may also inhibit the release of substance P in the central nervous system (119). Mexiletine can be started at 150 mg at bedtime and escalated to three times per day (taken with food) as tolerated. Mexiletine usually begins to give pain relief in IC after a dose of 150 mg three times per day has been taken for more than 2 weeks. The most common side effects are hypotension and nausea, and I have had to stop the medication in nearly half of (more than 20) patients in whom I have tried it. This is consistent with the proportion of intolerable side effects rates in other studies of the use of mexiletine (120). Always make sure that the patient does not have an atrioventricular block on a base-line electrocardiogram or a history of seizures before starting this medication.

Carbemazepine has long been used for a variety of neurogenic pain syndromes, but there is a shortage of large controlled studies supporting its effectiveness in pain originating in the central nervous system (121). In tic douloureux, 70% of patients acheive good relief with carbemazepine (122). Pain relief in this condition is related to serum levels between 24 and 43 μmol/liter (123). The usual dosage is 200 mg started once in the evening and escalated over 2 weeks to three times per day. Carbemazepine may also have some antidepressant effects. This medication should be taken with food and can be escalated up to a total daily dose of 1,800 mg. Common side effects include nausea, dizziness, ataxia, and somnolence. If these side effects occur in a patient who is getting good pain relief from the medication, a useful strategy can be to discontinue the drug completely for 24 hr and then resume treatment at a daily dose that is 200 mg lower. The most serious side effect of carbemazepine is neutropenia, which usually occurs in the first 3 months of treatment. Other anticonvulsants used in the treatment of neuropathic pain include phenytoin, barbiturates, and valproate.

There have been reports of success using the newly released anticonvulsant gabapentin in the treatment of neurogenic pain caused by reflex sympathetic dystrophy and diabetic neuropathy (124). In my experience with this medication, I have seen several responses in interstitial cystitis with doses ranging from 900 to 1,800 mg per day (as either three divided doses or one nighttime dose). Some patients on gabapentin will report improved cognition and a sense of well-being in addition to pain relief (124a).

Benzodiazepines

There is considerable controversy over the use of benzodiazepines for chronic pain. Some physicians feel that they are inappropriate (125). Other investigators have found that certain benzodiazepines, such as alprazolam, have analgesic effects that are independent of their sedative effects (126). Alprazolam may be useful because it has some actions that are similar to those of the heterocyclic antidepressants, including a direct effect on β receptors in the central nervous system (127). In a recent study of patients with chronic, nonmalignant pain, 73% showed improvement after 2 weeks of low-dose (0.5 mg three times per day) alprazolam (128). Another benzodiazepine, clonazepam, has been effective in treating lancinating neuropathic pain (129). As with other benzodiazepines, tolerance and dependence can occur, but this is unusual in patients who take the medications for less than 6 months in low doses (130).

Other Drugs with Analgesic Effects

Hydroxyzine, an antihistamine that is commonly used in the treatment of interstitial cystitis, enhances the analgesic effects of opioids and has some analgesic effects of its own (131). Other medications that have been useful in central pain syndromes include clonidine (132) and propranolol (133). Neuroleptic drugs, such as phenothiazines, have not been useful as analgesic adjuvants with the exception of methotrimeprazine (which is available only as a parenteral medication) (134).

Psychostimulants such as amphetamine and methylphenidate have found limited use as adjuvant analgesics in the treatment of cancer pain (135). Their primary use is to counteract sedation in patients requiring high-dose opioids (136). Other medications that may soon become available include formulations that will block pain mediators such as bradykinin (137), excitatory amino acids (137), and cholecystokinin, which inhibits the release of enkephalins and may mediate visceral pain (138).

Local Anesthetic Procedures

Because peripheral nerves and nerves in the spinal cord are invested with opiate receptors, local application of opioids may be a useful analgesic strategy for patients with interstitial cystitis. In other painful diseases, small, systemically inactive doses of opiate medications have been shown to have significant analgesic effects when applied to inflamed tissue (140). This has certainly been useful in the treatment of pain from inflamed joints (141) and may be useful for other inflamed visceral tissues (142). There have been no reports of which I am aware of the use of intravesicular opioids in interstitial cystitis. Our expanded understanding of the neurophysiology of pain and the finding that local application of opioid drugs is especially effective in inflamed tissues may make the use of intravesicular opioids a therapy worth exploring (28).

Applying local anesthetics to the bladder or the nerves carrying pain signals to the spinal cord should also produce some pain relief in interstitial cystitis. This explains the limited utility of oral bladder anesthetics such as phenazopyridine and the intravesicular instillation of lidocaine (143). Another approach to pain management is injection of local anesthetics, opiates, or neurolytic agents into the nerves that represent the "silent afferents" that were mentioned previously using a superior hypogastric nerve block (144). This approach has been successful for severe pelvic pain caused by cancer. Another invasive anesthetic approach is percutaneous cordotomy (145), but this will usually result in severe bladder dysfunction and is associated with the risk of developing sleep apnea (146).

Intraspinal injection of opioids with or without local anesthetics can be a useful option for patients with severe intractable bladder pain (147). This may be especially useful in interstitial cystitis because intrathecal injection of epidural morphine in humans generally increases bladder capacity and relaxes the detrusor muscle (148). This could relieve urinary urgency and bladder spasm in addition to alleviating bladder pain. With the widespread use of efficient implantable drug delivery systems (149), this is an option that should be available to a growing number of patients with long-standing unremittent pain secondary to interstitial cystitis.

Intrathecal infusions of opioids with or without local anesthetics have been found to be appropriate and effective for selected patients with nonmalignant visceral pain (150) and with neuropathic pain (151). Although there are no studies of intraspinal opioids in the treatment of interstitial cystitis of which I am aware, I have referred several patients for placement of an indwelling pump and intrathecal catheter. All of them had previously experienced a good response to an intrathecal injection of morphine (12 to 24 hr of reduced pain). Five of these patients, who had been in crippling pain on high doses of opioid medications, have obtained excellent relief and have been able to discontinue their oral medications. With an increased understanding of the spinal receptors that can modulate processing of the pain signal, we can expect to see many new medications that will be applied intraspinally (such as α_2 agonists) that will relieve severe pain and "undo" the hyperalgesia and allodynia that make severe interstitial cystitis so agonizing (152).

Nonpharmacologic Treatments for Pain

Another way to interrupt the pain signal in interstitial cystitis is through the use of neurostimulators or TENS units. This modality has met with some success in patients with small-capacity ulcerated bladders (153). In addition to being anesthesized or mechanically stimulated, the nerve fibers carrying the pain signal from the bladder to the spinal cord can be interrupted by photoradiation with a neodymium:YAG laser (154) or surgical disruption (155).

Psychological approaches to pain management can decrease the perception of pain, decrease psychological distress related to pain (156), and decrease the use of medical resources (157). Psychological treatments should be incorporated into a comprehensive approach to pain management. These approaches include relaxation training, hypnosis (158) and cognitive therapy (159). Group therapy or membership in a support group can be very useful in providing psychological support, validation of the pain, and encouragement for patients with chronic pain (160). It is also useful to encourage patients to seek spiritual support (161) and to refer them to resource materials about pain management. One book that has proven especially useful for my patients with severe pain is *Managing Pain Before It Manages You* by Margaret Caudill, M.D., Ph.D., who has successfully treated patients with severe pain from interstitial cystitis (10).

OBSTACLES TO TREATING PAIN

An important consideration in pain management is that there are historical and cultural obstacles to using available treatments that must be recognized and overcome by the patient and by the caregiver. Some health professionals still label patients with chronic pain as "just complainers" or withhold appropriate pain treatment because they "do not want their patients to become addicted" (9). Actually, the concern of physicians for pain relief is relatively new in our history. For most of the history of Western medicine, physicians did not have the technical means to provide pain relief. Though ancient Greek, Hebrew, and Arabian physicians knew about the analgesic effects of opium, morphine was not extracted until 1803, and the early salicylate compounds 20 years later; the hypodermic syringe did not come into use until the 1840s.

Coincident with the rise of anesthesia and analgesic technology, an ethos evolved in American medicine in the mid-19th century that the primary role of medicine was to save lives and that the relief of suffering was, at most, only a secondary concern for physicians (162). The same time period saw the development of social Darwinism and the rise of an ethic in 19th-century America that has been called the "cult of toughness and callousness" (163). This involved a glorification of insensitivity, manifested as a reaffirmation of the "manly ability to endure pain," and brought with it an insensivity to the suffering of others (164). In fact, until recently, many cancer patients with terrible pain were abandoned by their physicians and left to die in pain and intense loneliness (165).

In the past 40 years, this has been accompanied by an increasing and exaggerated fear among health care professionals of causing addiction. Patients in pain have been labeled "drug seeking" when they should have been seen as "relief seeking." To call someone "drug seeking" is to make a judgement about his or her psychological makeup that is profound and dangerous if misapplied. Most patients with severe chronic pain are undertreated, and many report considering suicide because of feelings of hopelessness associated with their pain (166). Studies show that the overwhelming majority of patients in pain are not drug seekers. Even though some practitioners will have an *a priori* distrust of patients for whom they prescribe pain-relieving medications, 95% of patients with intense long-standing pain will either take the medications exactly as prescribed or take less than the prescribed amount (167).

Another obstacle to relieving the pain of interstitial cystitis is the fact that most of the sufferers are women (13). Since Victorian times, women have been seen as hypersensitive to pain, and pain was seen as part of the normal female experience (163). Dr. Oliver Wendell Holmes marveled at how women "are so much more fertile in their capacities of suffering than men" (168). Unfortunately, this attitude persists among some physicians, and it can be an important obstacle to the effective treatment of chronic pain in interstitial cystitis. This may explain why almost no mention is made of pain in chapters on interstitial cystitis in textbooks of general urology. In some cases, the only analgesic treatments that are recommended for intractable bladder pain are surgical (8). It is worth considering the possibility that, for many patients who have suffered with severe pain from interstitial cystitis for years, it isn't the pain that has been intractable, it is the physician (169)!

Acknowledgments

This work was supported by a grant from the Methodist Hospitals Foundation and inspired by my patients, who continue to live with interstitial cystitis and continue to teach me. This chapter is dedicated to Dr. W. Jerry Deaton and Dr. H. Michael McSwain, two urologists who have unceasingly given the kindest care to patients with interstitial cystitis.

REFERENCES

1. Schweitzer A. *On the Edge of the Forest Primeval.* New York: Macmillan, 1931;62.
2. Bonica JJ, ed. *The Management of Pain.* Philadelphia: Lea & Febiger, 1990.
3. Wall PD, Melzack R, eds. *Textbook of Pain.* New York: Churchill Livingstone, 1994.
4. Portenoy RK. Pain and quality of life: clinical issues and implications for research. *Oncology* 1990;4:172–178.
5. Melzack R. The tragedy of needless pain. *Sci Am* 1990;262:27–33
6. Breitbart W. Cancer pain and suicide. In: Foley K, Bonica JJ, Ventafridda V, eds. *Advances in Pain Research and Therapy.* New York: Raven Press, 1990;399–412.
7. Ratner V, Slade D, Greene G. Interstitial cystitis: a patient's perspective. *Urol Clin North Am* 1994;21 1-5.
8. Messing EM. Interstitial cystitis and related syndromes. In: Walsh PC, Retik AB, Stamey TA, Vaughan ED Jr, eds. *Campbell's Urology.* Philadelphia: WB Saunders, 1992 982–997.
9. Somerville MA. Death of pain: pain, suffering and ethics. In: Gebhart GF, Hammond DL, Jensen TS, eds. *Progress in Pain Research and Management.* Seattle: IASP Press, 1994:41–58.
10. Caudill MA. *Managing Pain Before It Manages You.* New York: Guilford Press, 1995.
11. Cain JM, Hammes BJ. Ethics and pain management: respecting patient wishes. *J Pain Symptom Manage* 1994;9:160–165.
12. Walsh A. Interstitial cystitis. In: Harrison JH, ed. *Campbell's Urology* Philadelphia: WB Saunders, 1978:1070–1082.
13. Koziol JA. Epidemiology of interstitial cystitis. *Urol Clin North Am* 1994;21:7–20.
14. Berwick L. Interstitial cystitis patients may require specialized team care. *Urol Times* 1991;March:1.
15. Held PJ, Hanno PA, Wein AJ, Pauly MV, Cahn MA. Epidemiology of interstitial cystitis. In: Hanno PM, Staskin DR, Krane RJ, Wein AJ, eds. *Interstitial Cystitis.* London: Springer-Verlag, 1990:7–15.
16. Payne R. Pathophysiology of cancer pain. In: Foley KM, Bonica JJ, Ventafridda V, eds. *Advances In Pain Research and Therapy.* New York: Raven Press, 1990;13–26.
17. Bonica JJ. History of pain concepts and pain therapy. *Mt Sinai J Med* 1991;58:191–202.
18. Cervero F. Sensory innervation of the viscera: a peripheral basis of visceral pain. *Physiol Rev* 1994;74:95–138.
19. Ness T. Historical and clinical perspectives of visceral pain. In: Gebhart GF, ed. *Visceral Pain.* Seattle: IASP Press, 1995:3–24.
20. Bennett GJ. Evidence from animal models on the pathogenesis of painful peripheral neuropathy and its relevance for pharmacotherapy. In: Basbaum AI, Besson JM, eds. *Towards a New Pharmacotherapy.* New York: John Wiley & Sons, 1991:68–82.
21. Morrison JFB. Sensations from the lower urinary tract. In: Torrens M, Morrison JFB, eds. *The Physiology of the Lower Urinary Tract.* London: Springer Verlag, 1987;89–131.
22. McMahon SB, Koltzenburg M. Silent afferents and visceral pain. In: Fields HL, Liebeskind JC, eds. *Progress in Pain Research and Management,* Vol 1. Seattle: IASP Press, 1994;11–30.
23. Mayer E. Clinical implications of visceral hyperalgesia. *Contemp Intern Med* 1994;6:42–54.
24. Manning DC, Raja SN, Meyer RA, Campbell JN. Pain and hyperalgesia after injection of bradykinin in humans. *Clin Pharmacol Ther* 1991;50:721–729.
25. Koltzenburg M, Kress M, Reeh PW. The nociceptor sensitization by bradykinin does not depend on sympathetic neurons. *Neuroscience* 1992;46:465–473.
26. McMahon SB, Abel C. A model for the study of visceral pain states: chronic inflammation of the chronic decerebrate rat urinary bladder by irritant chemicals. *Pain* 1987;28:109–127.
27. Woolf CJ, Safich-Garabedian B, Ma Q-P, Crilly P. Nerve growth factor contribution to the generation of inflammatory sensory hypersensitivity. *Neuroscience* 1994;62:327–331.
28. Stein C. The control of pain in peripheral tissue by opioids. *N Engl J Med* 1995;332:1685–1690.
29. Sommer B, Seeburg PH. Glutamate receptor channels: novel properties and new clones. *Trends Pharmacol Sci* 1992;13:291–296.
30. Mao J, Mayer DJ, Hayes RL, Lu J, Price DD. Differential roles of NMDA and non-NMDA receptor activation in induction and maintenance of thermal hyperalgesia in rats with painful peripheral mononeuropathy. *Brain Res* 1992;598:271–278.
31. Price DD, Mao J, Mayer DJ. Central neural mechanisms of normal and abnormal pain states. In: Fields HL, Liebeskind JC, eds. *Progress in Pain Research and Management,* Vol 1. Seattle: IASP Press, 1994:61–84.
32. Woolf CJ, Thompson SW. The induction and maintenance of central sensitization is dependent on N-methyl-D-aspartic acid receptor activation; implications for the treatment of postinjury pain hypersensitivity states. *Pain* 1991;44:293–307.
33. Mayer EA, Gebhart GF. Functional bowel disorders and the visceral hyperalgesia hypothesis. In: Mayer EA, Raybould HE, eds. *Basic and Clinical Aspects of Chronic Abdominal Pain.* New York: Elsevier, 1993;3–14.
34. Mao J, Price DD, Mayer DJ. Mechanisms of hyperalgesia and morphine tolerance: a current view of their possible interactions. *Pain* 1995;62:259–274.
35. Meller ST. The role of nitric oxide in the development and maintenance of the hyperalgesia produced by intraplantar injection of carrageenan in the rat. *Neuroscience* 1994;60:367–374.

36. Lima D, Esteves F, Coimbra A. c-*fos* activation by noxious input of spinal neurons projecting to the nucleus of the tractus solitarius in the rat. In: Gebhart GF, Hammond DL, Jensen TS, eds. *Proceedings of the Seventh World Congress on Pain.* Seattle: IASP Press, 1994:423–436.
37. Bors E, Ma KT, Parker RB. Observations on some modalities of bladder sensation. *J Urol* 1956;76:566–575.
38. McMahon SB. Neuronal and behavioral consequences of chemical inflammation of the rat urinary bladder. *Agents Actions* 1988;25: 231–233.
39. Sluka KA, Willis WD, Westlund KN. The role of dorsal root reflexes in neurogenic inflammation. *Pain Forum* 1995;4:141–149.
40. Rees H, Sluka KA, Westlund KA. The role of glutamate and NMDA receptors in the generation of dorsal root reflexes by acute arthritis in the anesthetized rat. *J Physiol* 1995;484:437–444.
41. Levine JD, Moskowitz MA, Basbaum AI. The contribution of neurogenic inflammation in experimental arthritis. *J Immunol* 1985;135: 843–847.
42. Galloway NTM, Gabale DR, Irwin PP. Intersitial cystitis or reflex sympathetic dystophy of the bladder? *Semin Urol* 1991;9:148–153.
43. Fields HL, Basbaum AI. Brain stem control of spinal pain transmission neurons. *Annu Rev Physiol* 1978;40:217–248.
44. Basbaum AI, Fields HL. Endogenous pain control systems: brainstem pathways and endorphin circuitry. *Annu Rev Neurosci* 1984;7:309–338.
45. Dubner R, Hoffman DS, Hayes RL. Neuronal activity in medullary dorsal horn of awake monkeys trained in a thermal discrimination task: task related responses and their functional role. *J Neurophysiol* 1981;46:444–453.
46. Price D, Harkins SW. The affective–motivational dimension of pain. *Am Pain Soc J* 1992;1:229.
47. Whorwell PJ, Prior A, Faragher EB. Controlled trial of hypnotherapy in the treatment of severe refractory irritable-bowel syndrome. *Lancet* 1984;2:1232–1236.
48. Plourde V, Mertz H, Sytnik B. Effects of somatostatin analogue on sensory perception to rectal balloon distension. *Dig Dis Sci* 1992;37: 976–982.
49. Steadman CJ, Talley NJ, Phillips SF. Selective 5-hydroxytryptamine type 3 receptor antagonism with ondansetron as treatment for diarrhea-predominant irritable bowel syndrome: a pilot study. *Mayo Clin Proc* 1992;67:732–737.
50. Mathisen LC, Skjelbred P, Skoglund LA, Oye I. Effect of ketamine, an NMDA receptor inhibitor, in acute and chronic orofacial pain. *Pain* 1995;61:215–220.
51. Church J, Lodge D. N-Methyl-D-aspartate antagonism is central to the actions of ketamine and other phencyclidine receptor ligands. In: Domino EF, ed. *Status of Ketamine in Anesthesiology.* Ann Arbor, MI: NPP Books, 1990;501–519.
52. Gungor T. Adenosine related compounds as potential antinociceptive agents. *Abstr Am Chem Soc* 1993;206:219.
53. McMahon SB, Bennett DLH, Priestly JV, Shelton D. The biological effects of endogenous nerve growth factor on adult sensory neurons revealed by a trkA-IgG fusion molecule. *Nature Med* 1995;1:774–780.
54. Jacobi J. *Paracelsus: Selected Writings.* Princeton, NJ: Princeton University Press, 1951.
55. McGuire DB. Measuring pain. In: Frank-Stromberg M, ed. *Instruments for Clinical Nursing Research.* Norwalk, CT: Appleton & Lange, 1988;333–356.
56. Turk DC, Melzack R. The measurement of pain and the assessment of people experiencing pain. In: Turk DC, Melzack R, eds. *Handbook of Pain Assessment.* New York: Guilford Press, 1992:3–14.
57. McCaffery M. *Nursing Management of the Patient with Pain.* Philadelphia: JB Lippincott, 1979;11.
58. Grossman SA, Sheidler VR, Swedeen K. Correlation of patient and caregiver ratings of cancer pain. *J Pain Symptom Manage* 1991;6: 53–57.
59. Von Roenn JH, Cleeland CS, Gonin R. Physicians' attitudes and practice in cancer pain management: A survey from the Eastern Cooperative Oncology Group. *Ann Intern Med* 1993;119:121–126.
60. Rowlingson JC. Classification and assessment of chronic pain. In: Raj PP, ed. *Current Review of Pain.* Philadelphia: Current Medicine Publishing, 1994:37–46.
61. Feuerstein M. Definitions of pain. In: Tollison CD, ed. *Handbook of Chronic Pain Management.* Baltimore: Williams & Wilkins, 1989;2–5.
62. McQuay HJ. Do preemptive treatments provide better pain control? In: Gebhart GF, Hammond DL, Jensen TS, eds. *Proceedings of the Seventh World Congress on Pain.* Seattle: IASP Press, 1994709–724.
63. Cherny NI, Portenoy RK. The management of cancer pain. *CA* 1994; 44:262–303.
64. Benedetti C, Butler SH. Methods, procedures and techniques for the symptomatic control of pain. In: Bonica JJ, ed. *The Management of Pain.* Philadelphia: Lea & Febiger, 1990:1637–1639.
65. Chapman CR, Foley KM, eds. *Current and Emerging Issues in Cancer Pain.* New York: Raven Press, 1992.
66. Portenoy RK. Opioid therapy for chronic nonmalignant pain: current status. In: Fields HL, Liebeskind JC, eds. *Progress in Pain Research and Management.* Seattle: IASP Press, 1994:595–620.
67. Loeser JD, Egan KJ. *Managing the Chronic Pain Patient.* New York: Raven Press, 1989.
68. Brookoff D, Polomano R. Treating sickle cell pain like cancer pain. *Ann Intern Med* 1992;116:364–368.
69. Schofferman J. Long-term use of opioid analgesics for the treatment of chronic pain of non-malignant origin. *J Pain Symptom Manage* 1993;8:279–288.
70. Jadad AR, Carroll D, Glynn CJ, Moore RA, McQuay HJ. Morphine responsiveness of chronic pain: double blind randomised crossover study with patient-controlled analgesia. *Lancet* 1992;339:1367–1371.
71. Poyhia R, Seppala T, Olkkola KT, Kelso E. The pharmacokinetics and metabolism of oxycodone after oral and intramuscular administration. *Br J Clin Pharmacol* 1992;33:617–621.
72. Twycross RG. Opioids. In: Wall PD, Melzack R, eds. *Textbook of Pain.* New York: Churchill Livingstone, 1994:943–962.
73. Kantor TG, Hopper M, Laska E. Adverse effects of commonly ordered narcotics. *J Clin Pharmacol* 1981;21:1–8.
74. Portenoy RK, Foley KM. Chronic use of opioid analgesics in nonmalignant pain. *Pain* 1986;25:171–186.
75. Lee CR, McTavish D, Sorkin EM. Tramadol, a preliminary review of its pharmacodynamic and pharmacokinetic properties and therapeutic potential in acute and chronic pain states. *Drugs* 1993;46:313–340.
76. Fainsinger R, Schoeller T, Bruera E. Methadone in the treatment of cancer pain: a review. *Pain.* 1993;52:137–147.
77. MacDonald N, Der L, Allan S, Champion P. Opioid hyperexcitability: the application of alternate opioid therapy. *Pain* 1993;72:2266–2272.
78. Chan GL, Matzke GR. Effects of renal insufficiency on the pharmacokinetics and pharmacodynamics of of opioid analgesics. *Drug Intell Clin Pharmacol* 1987;21:773–783.
79. Kaiko RF, Foley KM, Grabinski P. Central nervous system excitatory effects of meperidine in cancer patients. *Ann Neurol* 1983;13: 180–185.
80. Kanner RM, Foley KM. Patterns of narcotic drug use in a cancer pain clinic. *Ann NY Acad Sci* 1981;362:161–172.
81. Campora E, Merlini L, Pace M. The incidence of narcotic-induced emesis. *J Pain Symptom Manage* 1991;6:428–430.
82. Theoharides TC. Hydroxyzine in the treatment of interstitial cystitis. *Urol Clin North Am* 1994;21:113–119.
83. Bruera E, Macmillan K, Hanson J, MacDonald RN. The cognitive effects of the administration of narcotic analgesics in patients with cancer pain. *Pain* 1989;39:13–16.
84. Eisele JH, Grigsby EJ, Dea G. Clonazepam treatment of myoclonic contractions associated with high-dose opioids. *Pain* 1992;49:231–232.
85. Foley KM. Clinical tolerance to opioids. In: Basbaum AI, Bessom J, eds. *Towards a New Pharmacotherapy of Pain.* New York: John Wiley & Sons, 1991;181–204.
86. Zenz M, Strumpf M, Tryba M. Long-term oral opioid therapy in patients with chronic nonmalignant pain. *J Pain Symptom Manage* 1992;7:69–77.
87. Benedetti C. Intraspinal analgesia: an historical overview. *Acta Anaesthesiol Scand* 1987;31:17–32.
88. Kreek MJ. Medical complications in methadone patients. *Ann NY Acad Sci* 1978;311:110–134.
89. Coyle N, Adelhardt J, Foley KM, Portenoy RK. Character of terminal illness in the advanced cancer patient: pain and other symptoms in the last four weeks of life. *J Symptom Pain Manage* 1990;5:83–93.
90. Portenoy RK. Opioid tolerance and responsiveness: research findings and clinical observations. In: Gebhart GF, Hammond DL, Jensen TS, eds. *Proceedings of the Seventh World Congress on Pain.* Seattle: IASP Press, 1994:247–288.
91. Foley KM. The decriminalization of cancer pain. In: Hill CS, Fields WS, eds. *Advances in Pain Research and Therapy, Vol 11. Drug*

Treatment of Cancer Pain in a Drug-Oriented Society. New York: Raven Press, 1989;5–18.
92. Buckley FP, Sizemore WA, Charlton JE. Medication management in patients with chronic non-malignant pain. A review of the use of a drug withdrawal protocol. *Pain* 1986;26:153–166.
93. World Health Organization. Expert Committee on Drug Dependence 16th report. *WHO Tech Rep Ser* 1969;407:23–43.
94. Perry S, Heidrich G. Management of pain during debridement: a survey of U.S. burn units. *Pain* 1982;13:267–280.
95. Medina JL, Diamond S. Drug dependency in patients with chronic headache. *Headache* 1977;17:12–14.
96. Porter J, Jick H. Addiction rare in patients treated with narcotics. *N Engl J Med* 1980;302:123–126.
97. Weissman DE, Haddox JD. Opioid pseudoaddiction—an iatrogenic syndrome. *Pain* 1989;36:363–366.
98. Magni G. The use of antidepressants in the treatment of chronic pain. *Drugs* 1991;42:720–748.
99. Tura B, Tura SM. The analgesic effect of tricyclic antidepressants. *Brain Res* 1990;518:19–22.
100. Siddal PJ, Mather LE. Systemic approaches to the treatment of acute and chronic pain. In: Raj PP, ed. *Current Review of Pain.* Philadelphia: Current Medicine Publishers, 1994:79–92.
101. Max MB, Kishore-Kumar R, Schafer SC, Meister B, Gracely RH, Smoller B, Dubner R. Efficacy of desipramine in painful diabetic neuropathy: a placebo-controlled trial. *Pain* 1991;45:3–9.
102. Peters MD, Davis SK, Austin LS. Clomipramine: an anti-obsessional tricyclic antidepressant. *Clin Pharmacol* 1990;9:165–178.
103. Max MB. Antidepressants as analgesics. In: Fields HL, Liebeskind JC, eds. *Progress in Pain Research and Management.* Seattle: IASP Press, 1994:229–246.
104. Botney M, Fields HL. Amitriptyline potentiates morphine analgesia by a direct action on the central nervous system. *Ann Neurol* 1983;13:160–164.
105. Hanno PM. Amitriptyline in the treatment of interstitial cystitis. *Urol Clin North Am* 1994;21:89–91.
106. Rummans TA. Nonopioid agents for the treatment of acute and subacute pain. *Mayo Clin Proc* 1994;69:481–490.
107. Max MB, Lynch SA, Muir J. Effects of desipramine, amitriptyline and fluoxetine on pain in diabetic neuropathy. *N Engl J Med* 1992;326:1250–1256.
108. Smith GR. The epidemiology and treatment of depression when it coexists with somatoform disorder, somatization or pain. *Gen Hosp Psych* 1992;14:265–272.
109. Watson CPN. Antidepressants as adjuvant analgesics. *J Pain Symptom Manage* 1994;9:392–405.
110. Tanelian DL, Victory RA. Sodium channel blocking agents and their use in neuropathic pain conditions. *Pain Forum* 1995;4:75–80.
111. Rowbotham MC, Reisner LM, Fields HL. Both intravenous lidocaine and morphine reduce the pain of post-herpetic neuralgia. *Neurology* 1991;41:1024–1028.
112. Boas RA. Covino BG, Shahwarian A. Analgesic response to IV lignocaine. *Br J Anesth* 1982;54:501–505.
113. Bonica JJ, Buckley FP. Regional analgesia with local anesthetics. In: Bonica JJ, ed. *The Management of Pain.* Philadelphia: Lea & Febiger, 1990:1883–1966.
114. Glazer S, Portenoy RK. Systemic local anesthetics in pain control. *J Pain Symptom Manage* 1991;6:30–39.
115. Dejgard A, Petersen P, Kastrup J. Mexiletine for treatment of chronic painful diabetic neuropathy. *Lancet* 1988;1:9–11.
116. Awrbuch G. Treatment of thalamic pain syndrome with mexiletine. *Ann Neurol* 1990;28:233–235.
117. Chabal C, Jacobson L, Mariano A, Chaney E, Britell CW. The use of mexiletine for the treatment of pain after peripheral nerve injury. *Anesthesiology* 1992;76:513–517.
118. Colclough G, Carter A, Ackermann WE. Mexiletine for chronic pain. *Lancet* 1993;342:1484–1485.
119. Kamei J, Hitosugi H, Kawashima N, Aoki T, Ohhashi Y, Kauya Y. Antinociceptive effect of mexiletine in diabetic mice. *Res Commun Chem Pathol Pharmacol* 1992;77:245–248.
120. Campbell RWF. Mexiletine. *N Engl J Med* 1987;316:29–34.
121. Boivie J. Central pain. In: Wall PD, Melzack R, eds. *Textbook of Pain.* New York: Churchill Livingstone, 1994:871–902.
122. Loesser J. Tic doloreux and atypical facial pain. In: Wall PD, Melzack R, eds. *Textbook of Pain.* New York: Churchill Livingstone, 1994:669–710.
123. Tomson T, Tybring G, Bertilsson L, Ekbom K, Rane A. Carbemazepine in trigeminal neuralgia. *Uppsala J Med Sci* 1980;31:45–46.
124. Mellick GA, Seng ML. The use of the newly-introduced anticonvulsant gabapentin in the treatment of reflex sympathetic dystrophy and a phobic disorder. *Am J Pain Manage* 1995;5:7–9.
124a. Handforth A, Treiman DM. Efficacy and tolerance of long-term, high-dose gabapentin: additional observations. *Epilepsia* 1994;35:1032–1037.
125. Butler SH, Murphy TM. Use and abuse of drugs in chronic noncancerous pain states. In: Loesser JD, Egan KJ, eds. *Managing the Chronic Pain Patient.* New York: Raven Press, 1989:129–142.
126. Fernandez F, Adams F, Holmes V. Analgesic effects of alprazolam in patients with chronic organic pain of malignant origin. *J Clin Pharmacol* 1987;7:167–169.
127. Sethey VH, Hodges DH. Role of beta-adrenergic receptors in the antidepressant activity of alprazolam. *Res Commun Chem Pathol Pharmacol* 1982;36:329–332.
128. Westbrook L, Cicala RS, Wright H. Effectiveness of alprazolam in the treatment of chronic pain: results of a preliminary study. *Clin J Pain* 1990;6:32–36.
129. Swerdlow M, Cundill JG. Anticonvulsant drugs used in the treatment of lancinating pain. *Anesthesiology* 1981:36:1129–1133.
130. Uhlenhuth EH, DeWitt H, Balter MB, Johanson CE, Mellinger GD. Risks and benefits of long-term benzodiazepine use. *J Clin Pyschopharmacol* 1988;8:161–166.
131. Beaver WJ, Freise G. Comparison of the analgesic effects of morphine, hydroxyzine and their combination on patients with postoperative pain. *Adv Pain Res Ther* 1976;1:553–557.
132. Glynn C, Dawson D. Sanders R. A double-blind comparison between epidural morphine and epidural clonidine in patients with chronic non-cancer pain. *Pain* 1988;34:123–128.
133. Scadding JW, Wall PD, Parry CBW, Brooks DM. Clinical trial of propranolol in post-traumatic neuralgia. *Pain* 1982;14:283–292.
134. Patt RB, Proper G, Reddy S. The neuroleptics as adjuvant analgesics. *J Pain Symptom Manage* 1994;9:446–453.
135. Bruera E, Watanbe S. Psychostimulants as adjuvant agents. *J Pain Symptom Manage* 1994;9:412–415.
136. Bruera E, Fainsinger R, MacEachern T, Hanson J. The use of methylphenidate in patients with incident cancer pain receiving regular opiates: a preliminary study. *Pain* 1992;50:75–77.
137. Cheronis JC. Kinin antagonists. *Lancet* 1991;338:1011–1020.
138. Klamt JG. Intrathecal administration of lamotrigine induces analgesia in acute and chronic pain models in rats. *Br J Pharmacol.* 1994;112:340–343.
139. Maletinska L. Pharmacological characterization of new cholecystokinin analogues. *Eur J Pharmacol* 1992;222:233–240.
140. Stein C. Peripheral analgesic actions of opioids. *J Pain Symptom Manage* 1991;6:119–124.
141. Stein C, Comisel K, Yassouridis A, Herz A, Peter K. Intraarticular morphine produces analgesia following arthroscopic knee surgery. *Anesthesiology* 1990;73:766.
142. Schulte-Steinberg H, Weninger E, Jokisch D. Intraperitoneal versus intrapleural morphine or bupivacaine for pain after laparoscopic cholecystectomy. *Anesthesiology* 1995;82:634–640.
143. Asklin B, Cassuto J. Intravesical lidocaine in severe interstitial cystitis: case report. *Scand J Urol Nephrol* 1989;23:311–312.
144. Plancarte R, Amescua C, Patt RB, Aldrete JA. Superior hypogastric plexus block for pelvic cancer pain. *Anesthiology* 1990;73:236–243.
145. Patt R. Pain therapy. In: Frost EAM, ed. *Clinical Anesthesia in Neurosurgery.* Boston: Butterworth, 1990:259–280.
146. Patt RB. Superior hypogastric plexus block: a new therapeutic approach for pelvic pain. *Am Pain Soc Bull* 1995;5:7–10.
147. Wang JK. Intrathecal morphine for intractable pain secondary to cancer of the pelvic organs. *Pain* 1985;21:99–102.
148. Rawal N, Mollefors K, Axellson K, Lindgardh G, Widman B. An experimental study of urodynamic effects of epidural morphine and of naloxone reversal. *Anesth Analg* 1983;62:641–648.
149. Waldman SD. Implantable drug delivery systems: practical considerations. *J Pain Symptom Manage* 1990;5:169–174.
150. Krames ES, Lanning RM. Intrathecal infusional analgesia for nonmalignant pain: analgesic efficacy of intrathecal opioid with or without bupivacaine. *J Pain Symptom Manage* 1993;8:539–548.
151. Hassenbusch SJ, Stanton-Hicks M, Covington EC, Walsh JG, Guthrey

DS. Long-term intraspinal infusions of opioids in the treatment of neuropathic pain. *J Pain Symptom Manage* 1995;10:527–543.
152. Sosnowski M, Yaksh TL. Spinal administration of receptor-selective drugs as analgesics: new horizons. *J Pain Symptom Manage* 1990;5: 204–213.
153. Fall M. Use of transcutaneous electrical nerve stimulation in the management of chronic interstitial cystitis. In: Hanno P, Staskin DR, Krane RJ, Wein AJ, eds. *Interstitial Cystitis.* New York: Springer-Verlag, 1990;169–173.
154. Malloy TR, Shanberg AM. Laser therapy for interstitial cystitis. *Urol Clin North Am* 1994;21:141–144.
155. Irwin PP, Galloway NTM. Surgical management of interstitial cystitis. *Urol Clin North Am* 1994;21:145–151.
156. Kelly JF. Psychological approaches to the management of chronic pain. In: Raj PP, ed. *Current Review of Pain.* Philadelphia: Current Medicine Press, 1994:117–128.
157. Caudill M, Schnable R, Zuttermeister P, Benson H, Friedman R. Decreased clinic use by chronic pain patients: response to behavioral medicine intervention. *Clin J Pain* 1991;7:305–310.
158. Hilgard ER. The alleviation of pain by hypnosis. *Pain* 1975;1:213–231.
159. Turk DC, Meichenbaum D, Genest M, eds. *Pain and Behavioral Medicine: A Cognitive–Behavioral Perspective.* New York: Guilford Press, 1983.
160. Umlauf RL. Psychological interventions for chronic pain following spinal cord injury. *Clin J Pain* 1992;8:111–118.
161. Doyle D. Have we looked beyond the physical and the psychosocial? *J Pain Symptom Manage* 1992;7:302–311.
162. Somerville MA. Pain and suffering at the interfaces of medicine and law. *Univ Toronto Law J* 1986;26:286–317.
163. Pernick MS. *The Calculus of Suffering: Pain, Professionalism and Anesthesia in Nineteenth Century America.* New York: Columbia University Press, 1985;98–99.
164. Pernick MS. The calculus of suffering in nineteenth century surgery. *Hastings Cent Rep* 1983;13:26.
165. Katz J. *Silent World of Doctor and Patient.* New York: Free Press, 1984.
166. Livengood JM, Parris WCV. Early detection of measures and triage procedures for suicide ideation in chronic pain patients. *Clin J Pain* 1989;8:164–169.
167. Hitchcock LS, Ferrell BR, McCaffery M. The experience of chronic nonmalignant pain. *J Pain Symptom Manage* 1994;9:312–318.
168. Holmes OW. *Currents and Countercurrents in Medical Science.* Boston: Ticknor and Fields, 1861.
169. Wall PD. Introduction. In: Wall PD, Melzack R, eds. *Textbook of Pain.* New York: Churchill Livingstone, 1994:1–8.
170. Payne R. Cancer pain: anatomy, physiology and pharmacology. *Cancer* 1989;63:2266–2274.

Interstitial Cystitis, edited by Grannum R. Sant
Lippincott–Raven Publishers, Philadelphia ©1997.

CHAPTER 24

Psychological Aspects of Interstitial Cystitis

Naomi B. McCormick

Little has been written about interstitial cystitis (IC) until recently. However, even less has been written about the psychological aspects of this painful bladder disease. A *Medline* data-base search of all English articles on interstitial cystitis published between 1985 and 1995 produced 295 records, only seven (2%) of which concerned the psychosocial adjustment of IC patients. The *Nursing and Allied Health Data Base* yielded 11 articles on IC published between 1991 and 1994. Fortunately, six (55%) of these addressed psychosocial as well as medical aspects of the disease. To date, psychologists have published an embarrassing total of three articles on interstitial cystitis in English-language scientific or clinical journals (1–3). Not a single article about interstitial cystitis was listed in the *PsyLIT* (psychology) *Data Base* between January 1990 and June 1995! In fact, nurses, not psychologists, and Denise Webster in particular, another contributor to this book, published most of the research on IC patient psychological adjustment (4–11).

How then shall I describe the psychological aspects of a disease described so poignantly by Jennefer Richmond, an IC patient and nurse?

> The tell-tale signs were there again—frequency, urgency and pain on passing urine—I did not know...that the next four years were to be the most miserable I have ever experienced....I could not go more than 15 to 20 minutes without having to empty my bladder. (12, p. 72)

The unfortunate tendency to attribute psychopathology to the chronically ill is well demonstrated in the following passage from an article by Finnish psychologists who made an unfavorable comparison between women with interstitial cystitis and a normal control group treated for acute bacterial cystitis:

> Patients with interstitial cystitis had less effective coping strategies; in other words, they react to frustration by giving up. They also had a lower level of internal locus of control...; they do not believe that they had control over their lives, believing that chance or fate plays a dominant role. They had a low self-regulation score. This means that they are indecisive, tend to ask the opinions of other people, and do not stand up for their rights. Their scores on...interest in sexual matters were significantly lower than were the scores of patients in the control group....[They] said they were extremely sensitive to sensory stimuli. In other words, they cannot endure pain. (1, p. 71)

This description is flawed. The pathologic portrait of the supposedly typical IC patient is painted by experts who have no personal experience with the disease. To the outsider who has never had severe chronic pain, who sleeps well at night and finds sexual excitement and activity pleasurable, not agonizing, patients who seem tense, irritable, mildly depressed, and out of control of their lives appear on the surface to be poorly adjusted indeed. From the standpoint of chronically ill persons, however, it is amazing how well we cope.

Recall again Richmond's IC narrative. I empathize not so much as a psychologist but as an IC patient. Interstitial cystitis plays a major role in structuring daily activities and reducing patient energy. When one suffers from painful, chronic illness, there is no denying that disease limits choices and life experiences. No, it does not surprise me that the painful bladder patients studied by Keltikangas-Jarvinen and her colleagues appeared somewhat passive and indecisive. Given my own fatigue and sleep deprivation, I sometimes find even simple tasks at work or driving decisions a bit challenging. And I am not shocked that these IC patients are somewhat disinterested in sex.

In contemplating the psychological aspects of chronic diseases such as interstitial cystitis, one should remember the "chicken and egg" problem. Which came first—the chicken or the egg; the psychological symptoms or the

N. B. McCormick: Department of Family Studies and Psychology, University of Northern Iowa, Cedar Falls, Iowa 50614-0332.

disease? The question is unanswerable. The crisis of illness is managed with whatever developmental, emotional, and family resources the patient has available, good or poor. Simultaneously, illness itself takes its toll on personality and the social support system. The psychological problems exhibited by an IC patient may predate, be caused by, or interact with the physical illness. Whatever the case may be, it is unjust to deny the medical reality of the patient's illness as demonstrated in these unintentionally cruel conclusions drawn by Keltikangas-Jarvinen, Auvinen, and Lehtonen:

> The [IC] patients in our study associated the onset of the disease with some stressful events in their lives. Life changes recorded have, however, been the events of ordinary life...This supports the hypothesis concerning the psychic helplessness of patients. A number of drastic events did not predispose the individual to interstitial cystitis; it was triggered off by an incapacity to cope with ordinary life. The high discomfort experienced by these patients may be related to their personality, that is, to their exceptionally high sensitivity to pain rather than to the real pain caused by the disease. (1, pp. 71–72)

From a scientific point of view, a correlational study comparing the interview, questionnaire, and projective technique responses of interstitial cystitis patients with those of a control group does not justify making inferences about the causes of IC. It is human to be somewhat superstitious and try to connect a negative outcome with a particular event or situation. I have heard many IC patients offer equally fanciful hypotheses about the origins of their disease. Speculation, even wild and false speculation, gives us a sense of personal control over our involuntary illness experience.

I hope I have been persuasive and have laid to rest, once and for all, the harmful idea that interstitial cystitis patients are psychologically disturbed by definition, somehow unconsciously willing painful bladder illness on themselves. The mental health of IC patients is just as varied as that of the rest of the population. Some of us are immature and self-centered; others are well adjusted and socially sensitive. Our numbers probably include the statistically expected numbers of psychotic, neurotic, "average," and even extraordinarily well functioning individuals. What makes us different, then, is how IC affects our personalities and intimate relationships and how, in turn, we draw on our own psychological resources to face IC.

Because of the paucity of psychological research on interstitial cystitis patients, this chapter includes studies and clinical descriptions of a wide variety of chronically ill patients, especially those who suffer from other painful medical conditions. Five key issues for health care practitioners and IC patients alike are addressed: illness as a stressor; the psychological adjustment of chronically ill persons; the physician–patient relationship; a description of high-functioning or psychologically self-actualizing patients who have chronic illness; and philosophic issues relevant to coping with chronic illness.

ILLNESS AS A STRESSOR

Ambiguity and Delayed Diagnosis

One of the most stressful aspects of interstitial cystitis has been the ambiguous meaning of symptoms and the difficulty patients face getting a correct diagnosis. After several years of being misdiagnosed and receiving numerous uncomfortable and unnecessary treatments for the incorrect urological disorder, I was almost relieved to learn that I had IC. My experience was not unusual in the 1980s. It took a very hearty individual indeed to manage this situation psychologically. As leaders of the Interstitial Cystitis Association recollected:

> Some [patients]...simply went to the library and diagnosed themselves, returning to the doctor armed with medical literature. They had to convince the doctor that their pain was real—no easy task....Sometimes it took years to find a doctor willing to treat them...; they often had to educate their doctors about the available treatments. (13, p. 2)

Research suggests that the typical IC sufferer of the 1980s visited between two and five physicians and was in medical limbo up to about 5 years before being diagnosed correctly (14). Minority women were especially likely to endure painful bladder symptoms a long time before being diagnosed with interstitial cystitis (15). As long as IC was underdiagnosed, there was a strong risk that physicians would erroneously attribute the patient's voiding and bladder pain to psychiatric problems (5). More than 45% of the women with IC studied by Webster had been misdiagnosed with a gynecologic disorder (5). An additional 43% had been falsely labeled as having a psychiatric disorder.

Individuals with complaints that do not appear to have a readily known physiological basis tend to be labeled as "somaticizers, hypochondriacs, or overutilizers" (16, p. 191). But, as Draucker points out so well, many such individuals may suffer from "rare, difficult-to-diagnose, or typically underdiagnosed illnesses" (16, p. 191). Having an underdiagnosed disease such as interstitial cystitis, which responds suboptimally to treatment, interferes with effective coping in four ways. First, the ambiguity or uncertainty of one's medical condition makes it difficult for the patient to plan how to avoid harm; there is no obvious strategy for managing symptoms. Second, self-blame is inevitable if health care providers tell the patient that symptoms are caused by psychological problems. Self-blame contributes to lowered self-esteem, helplessness, and a sense that the patient has lost control over life. Third, if a medical disorder is misdiagnosed as psychiatric in nature, patients are unable to obtain the medical information that would help them regain not only their health but feelings of efficacy and autonomy. Misdiagnosis interferes with cognitive mastery and patient self-care. Fourth, people constantly engage in social comparisons. If they are falsely diagnosed as having a psychiatric problem, medical patients cannot help but make negative social comparisons regarding their strength and competence. Patients don't just suffer from interstitial cystitis. Historically, many have suffered as much or more from being told that their bladder problems were all in their heads.

Symptoms

The primary IC symptoms, frequent voiding and chronic pain, distress patients and their loved ones (14,17,18). Some patients live lives of "intractable pain," requiring "as many as 60 trips to the bathroom daily, making travel impossible and leaving many patients homebound...[with] chronic sleep deprivation and depression" (19, p. 63). According to the 1987 Urban Institute study, more than three of four female interstitial cystitis patients suffer from pain in the bladder, vagina, and urethra, urgency and frequent voiding, and sleep deprivation as a result of waking up repeatedly to void at night (20). Half or more of these same patients complained that it was difficult to work full time or ride in a car, that they had difficulty emptying their bladder, that pain was relieved only briefly when voiding, and that sexual intercourse was painful. Those who had milder cases of IC described unpredictable and disturbing flare-ups. Patients who had severe IC noted that they experienced continuous sensations of pressure, burning, and stabbing in the pelvic area.

Many women with IC report that their symptoms are worse from midcycle until menstruation (10,20). Often, patients are not sure what precipitates acute IC symptoms, although a number think that increased stress, changes in diet, and overwork play their part. Worse still, IC patients often suffer from other inflammatory diseases such as lupus, arthritis, and irritable bowel syndrome, which in themselves can be disabling conditions. Finally, the unpredictability of interstitial cystitis makes it difficult for patients to plan ahead (11). Eagerly anticipated work and social activities might have to be canceled on a last-minute basis.

Sexuality

Interstitial cystitis has a devastating impact on sexuality (1,7,9,14,19–22). Most patients complain of decreased interest in sexual interactions, and between 60% and 90% of heterosexual women with IC report that sexual intercourse is sometimes or always painful.

There is no systematic research on the sexual problems faced by men with IC, but Evans suggests that these men also experience painful intercourse (23). Adding to the sexual concerns of men with IC, a number have undergone prostate surgery as a result of prior misdiagnosis. Unfortunately, this type of surgery increases their risk for erection difficulties (24).

One-third of women with IC complain that having their genitals touched and, most of all, experiencing orgasms exacerbates pain (7,21). Because they fear additional pain and often live with constant, excruciating pain, many IC patients reduce the frequency of their sexual activities dramatically, especially that of sexual intercourse (9,21). Decreased sexual contact and enjoyment of sexual interactions can be very depressing to those who previously took great pleasure and pride in sexual expression.

It is not unusual for partners to report that they have developed sexual dysfunctions out of sympathy for their loved one who suffers from IC. Specifically, arousal or erection difficulties may be precipitated by anxiety about harming a partner during sexual activity; these difficulties, in turn, may interfere with sexual enjoyment during the all too few times that IC patients desire or initiate lovemaking (2,21).

Interstitial cystitis can destroy the romantic ambiance (2,21). Frequent trips to the toilet during lovemaking interfere with a couple's sexual mood. The sensation of pain may cloud patients' awareness of sexual excitement. Equally problematic, IC patients occasionally report having sex with partners regularly, even though it is painful, because of guilt, fear of rejection, or a sense of duty.

Sexual activity is particularly painful for younger, premenopausal women (9). To make matters worse, a number of medications used by patients to control pain or reduce urgency may interfere with lubrication, arousal, and orgasm (25–30). Antidepressants, used by IC patients to reduce urgency and pain, inhibit lubrication, make genital contact uncomfortable, and even delay or prevent orgasm and ejaculation.

PSYCHOLOGICAL ADJUSTMENT

Mental Health

Patients with symptoms of interstitial cystitis may be misdiagnosed as having a somaticization disorder (5). As Denise Webster explains, medical conditions that are difficult to diagnose, that respond poorly to treatment, and that afflict women more than men are often suspected by physicians to be symptomatic of psychiatric disturbance. Forty-three percent of the women with IC who participated in Webster's research had been told previously that they had a psychiatric, not a urologic, disorder.

Today, the debate about the psychiatric status of IC patients has taken a new turn. A growing number of mental health professionals have associated IC patients' symptoms of genital pain and pain during intercourse with a possible history of sexual abuse (6). I agree that sexual abuse and assault are all too common female experiences (31). However, this is no excuse to again blame women for their urologic symptoms. Many women who have experienced sexual abuse or coercion never develop interstitial cystitis. Even if a patient recalls having been sexually abused, this is not evidence that her suprapubic pain and discomfort during intercourse are caused by psychopathology rather than bladder disease. I believe "that to pathologize another's behavior and redefine her life history for her is violence of the highest order" (6, p. 83).

Although there is no empirical evidence that IC is caused by psychopathology, the disease can have serious psychological consequences (1,20). Those who are seriously ill do not necessarily become depressed (32). However, depression becomes increasingly likely the longer an individual has been ill and the more demands illness makes, psychologically and physically. Indeed, research on women with a variety of illnesses suggests that disabling conditions, physical inactivity, and chronic, severe pain intensify the risk for depression, especially among older women (33,34). A patient's prolonged physical illness can also lead to depression in the spouse and other family members as well as to increased family tension (35).

Preliminary research suggests that women with moderate to severe IC may be more susceptible to depression than both average women and those who suffer from nonpainful serious medical conditions. Interstitial cystitis patients are significantly more likely to admit being depressed and having suicidal thoughts than both the general population and kidney dialysis patients (14,20). Research on pain patients who do not have IC is worth considering. One such study suggested that chronic pain patients who did not have cancer seemed to suffer even more than cancer patients, some of whom also lived with pain (36). All of the patients were judged to be free of major psychiatric problems; none were severely depressed. Nonetheless, in this study, the chronic pain patients felt less control over their lives, engaged in more social avoidance as a result of their pain, and were less capable of identifying and expressing their feelings than the cancer patients, some of whom also experienced pain. Pain patients with and without cancer were more anxious than both chronically ill patients who were free of pain and a control group of physically healthy individuals. Pain often pushes individuals into social withdrawal.

The excruciating daily pain associated with IC may be harder on patients than life-threatening but less painful conditions. Health care providers should use supportive psychotherapy and antianxiety or antidepressant medications to treat the emotional distress that sometimes results from relentless pain (37). Physicians and nurses can also help patients strategize ways that they can be productive and enjoy life as much as possible despite IC. Researchers have noted that seriously ill people can and often do lead self-reliant and independent lives (38).

Researchers have identified two types of chronically ill persons who suffer from such painful conditions as IC, which respond suboptimally to conventional medical care: *problem solvers* and *avoiders and self-blamers* (39,40). Problem solvers actively seek information about their illness, make full use of available social support, and engage in self-care with enthusiasm. Avoiders and self-blamers, in contrast, futilely wish for a miracle cure, deny the reality of their chronic illness, and/or blame themselves for getting sick. Not surprisingly, problem solvers are significantly less physically disabled and freer of depression than the equally ill patients who engage in avoidance and self-blame. "Functioning may be significantly affected by psychological factors, including how patients appraise and cope with the stress of their illness" (39, p. 297). If they are able to make the best of a bad situation, IC patients can and do lead happy productive lives.

Coping with Chronic Pain and Urgency

Most IC patients are aware of their pain on a daily basis; one-third of the women in one study regarded their pain as intolerable (1). Interstitial cystitis also hurts patients economically and recreationally (20). Living with pain and urgency, the IC patients often structure their lives around access to public toilets. The demands of illness and often frequent treatments may interfere with patients' productivity at work. Some patients can no longer work outside their homes or full time. Others are afraid to seek new, better jobs, terrified that their IC symptoms would not be understood or accepted by a new employer. As a result of severe IC symptoms, patients may have to forgo leisure and social activities that were once highly gratifying and seek help with childcare and housework.

Psychological adjustment to IC and other diseases is determined in part by the patient's ability to accept illness (41). A German study of chronically ill individuals with a variety of diagnoses indicated that those who saw illness as a positive challenge were less anxious, less depressed, and more emotionally stable than patients who regarded their illness as either an enemy, punishment, or sign that they were damaged human beings. Adjustment to chronic illness and medical gains were especially good if patients had an *internal locus of control* (thought that they could control their outcomes) and engaged in *moderate denial* (refused to allow illness to threaten their self-image).

Self-efficacy is the extent to which an individual feels competent to manage a task, including coping with illness. Cognitive–behavioral psychotherapists report that chronic pain patients who are higher in self-efficacy function better psychologically than equally disabled individuals who lack confidence in their own abilities (42). This has important implications for clinicians:

> A person's self-statements and appraisal of events mediate feelings and behavior. Thus, therapeutic instruction to modify self-defeating, pain-related cognitions and the limitation created by avoidant pain behavior may bring about an amelioration of the pain experience. (42, p. 165)

How can these insights into affirming cognitions be put to use? Let me use myself as an example. When I am in pain, I try to reframe the sensations so as to give myself maximum control over the experience. Instead of telling myself that "I cannot stand the pain," I remind myself that "the pain is difficult to tolerate but is not dangerous or permanent." I remind myself that medications and various self-help procedures will help me control the pain sooner or later. Also, I remind myself that I have excellent bladder capacity when dilated in my urologist's office so that my sensations of urgency do not necessarily represent a need to void every 5 min. I also tell myself that my situation will become more tolerable if I try to ignore my urgency and suprapubic pain or put them into the background. I usually do this by involving myself in an interesting activity (such as reading, listening to music, light exercise, or writing). If none of these strategies are sufficient, I give myself permission to be emotionally upset and do not view this as a sign that I am psychologically imbalanced.

One of my mentors, Albert Ellis, the founder of Rational–Emotive Behavior Therapy, taught me this. I use cognitive–behavior techniques daily, not only on myself but in my work with psychotherapy clients and college students. At age 82, with poor eyesight, hearing loss, a serious case of diabetes, and associated urinary problems, Albert Ellis works harder and with more pleasure than many individuals half his age. Accepting his illness as an unalterable reality, Ellis disputes self-pity and anger by saying to himself:

> Too damned bad!..It's hard doing so many things to keep myself in a relatively healthy condition—but it's much harder, and in the long run much more painful and deadly, if I don't keep doing this! (43, p. 47)

Sometimes IC patients respond to pain and urgency by worrying, smoking, and crying (4). But other, more adaptive strategies are also employed. Many IC patients acquire strategies for managing pain and illness completely on their own or by learning from other IC patients. As Kristene Whitmore comments: "Patients who cope best...are those who take an active role in managing their lives" (37, p. 121).

Patients who are high in self-efficacy manage their diets by avoiding foods that exacerbate IC symptoms such as spicy, highly acidic foods, alcohol, and caffeine (3,8,10). A variety of activities for minimizing the distress of IC symptoms have been reported and include keeping busy or engaging in engrossing activities, seeking emotional support from family and friends, experimenting with various postures and sleeping positions, wearing comfortable, loose clothing, using cold or heat to reduce sensations of pain, avoiding jolting exercise or travel, and being conscientious of hygiene to reduce the chances of bladder infection (3,4,8,10).

To cope with chronic pain and urgency, interstitial cystitis patients have a wide variety of cognitive strategies. In my own interview study of a small group of IC patients, most women said that they coped with the disease by reminding themselves that they had no choice but "to accept the disease," that the disease needed to be "put into perspective" and should not be allowed to "take over their lives," and, finally, that they should give themselves credit for doing their best to function despite IC (3). In Denise Webster and Tim Brennan's (10) research with a larger sample of women, the two most popular psychological strategies for coping with acute IC symptoms were praying and a self-reminder that the patient will feel better eventually.

Interstitial cystitis patients need not manage their symptoms without professional help. Behaviorally oriented clinicians report good outcomes in helping patients reduce pain sensations while increasing bladder capacity and decreasing daily voids (44,45). The problem is that the same patients who do well with behavioral bladder training are those who would do well on their own, individuals who are motivated to work hard despite having chronic illness. The challenge to urologists, nurses, and psychotherapists is how best to help IC patients who are low in self-efficacy and regard their illness as an enemy or punishment for past misdeeds and personal inadequacy. For better or worse, a patient's best ally in coping with IC is high frustration tolerance.

Adjusting to Sexual Difficulties

Most IC patients report that their symptoms interfere with sexual responsiveness and enjoyment, although a few indicate that interstitial cystitis has had no effect on their sexuality or has challenged them to be sexually more creative and energetic (2,3,21,24). Some remarkable IC patients have retained or even enhanced sexual pleasure by initiating erotic activity and choreography to reassure partners that they truly desire sex, catheterizing themselves to anesthetize their bladders before sexual intercourse, and keeping a plastic-lined garbage can at bedside for voiding so they do not have to interrupt lovemaking with frequent visits to the toilet (24).

One of the most popular sexual self-care strategies is to avoid sexual activity, especially intercourse, when IC symptoms are troubling (9,22). Interstitial cystitis patients also report emptying their bladders before and after sexual activity, avoiding prolonged intercourse, experimenting with sexual positions and activities that minimize pressure on the urethra, minimizing postcoital irritation by cleansing sexual secretions and spermicides, and taking pain-controlling or antispasmodic medications before sexual activity (9,21,22). Some IC patients report that oral sex is more pleasurable and less likely to bring about discomfort than intercourse (24).

In order to make a satisfactory sexual adjustment to IC, patients may find it helpful to give up our culture's incredible obsession with intercourse and orgasms. Sex is more or should be much more than genital juxtapositions or the insertion of tab A into slot B accompanied by orgasms (31,46). Sex ideally includes all aspects of intimacy, sharing the "feeling of merged boundaries, physical and emotional, in a very special way" (46, pp. 2–3 of transcript).

Traditional sexual scripts need to be replaced by doing such things as holding a partner who masturbates to orgasm or sharing a sensual massage (21). Regardless of how often patients feel up to sex or how varied (or not) their sexual activities have become, they need to remind themselves that they are lovable, sexual persons who do not have to engage in frequent genital gymnastics in order to prove they are adequate human beings or good lovers (24). Unflinching self-acceptance and a solid, open relationship with a loving partner are prerequisites to satisfactory sexual adjustment despite IC.

Family Issues

Research suggests that happily married persons enjoy better health than those who have unsatisfactory marriages (47). Related to this, chronically ill persons who have supportive partners and families cope better with pain and other symptoms than their less fortunate counterparts (33). Interstitial cystitis generally is not associated with marital or family disruption (20). In fact, IC patients frequently turn to their partner or spouse for emotional support (4,10).

In workshops, I have talked to numerous partners of IC patients about their experiences (17). A number complain of a worsened quality of life. Specifically, healthy partners say that their partner's IC has contributed to disturbed sleep, increased household and childcare responsibilities, financial hardships, increased social isolation, and numerous hours wasted in physicians' waiting rooms. Their biggest complaint, however, comes from their empathy for their spouse's suffering. Partners despair that there is nothing they could do to relieve their loved one's pain.

On the positive side, some couples have told me that the challenge of IC has actually improved their relationship (17,24). These individuals note that communication and trust have increased, that both the patient and spouse have greater self-acceptance, and that they appreciate more than ever "the little things" they were still able to do together. Some couples report enhanced teamwork and intimacy and the eroticization of nongenital sex in response to the challenge of interstitial cystitis.

Clinical observations and research suggest that chronic illness is most likely to have a negative impact on families when the patient can no longer engage in self-care, when the family or the patient cannot stop grieving over the loss, and when constant pain interferes with the patient's emotional availability to other family members (48). Because sex-role socialization prepares men for the caretaker role less than women, some have suggested that men are not as good at taking care of a physically ill spouse as are women. In contrast with this assumption, men make up the majority of caretakers of IC patients, and I have rarely heard complaints about their sensitivity or competence.

A study of the husbands of women who had rheumatoid arthritis supports my hypothesis that men can be excellent caretakers for chronically ill family members (49). A spouse's personality problems and conflict in the relationship, not medical impairment, predicted poor psychological adjustment. Specifically, unsupportive, negative, argumentative interactions with a spouse were associated with decreased mental health for both chronically ill women and their healthy husbands.

Despite a woman's chronic illness, some families are well adjusted, even if the woman is depressed (32). Depressed, chronically ill women who had solid marriages described their families as coping with the wife's or mother's illness by becoming introspective or psychologically minded, by talking about feelings more, by negotiating the process of daily family interactions, by planning for the future, and by interpreting family dynamics to solve problems. As Woods and Lewis explain:

> A strong relationship with an adult partner may buffer the effects of [a chronically ill mother's] depressed mood, with emotional support from the partner and more active paternal involvement attenuating the consequences of maternal depression for children. (32, p. 145)

A chronically ill patient's physical distress alone does not predict poor family adjustment (50). According to an intensive case study of 11 families in which the mother had a chronic (and sometimes life-threatening) illness, well-adjusted families faced fewer stresses outside the mother's illness than poorly adjusted families (which were bombarded by multiple stressors such as unemployment, poverty, death of a significant person, and alcoholism). Well-functioning families were able to "view the illness experience in a positive light as a family....These positive effects ranged from having a greater awareness of the relationship between diet and illness to making changes in one's basic orientation towards life" (50, pp. 586–587). In the well-functioning families, chronically ill women discussed positive things with their spouses and children such as "a greater appreciation of life, of living in the here and now and achieving a better balance between work and other aspects of one's life" (50, p. 587).

Chronic illness may stimulate psychological growth in individuals and families. This takes place when families take pride in coping well with adversity and enhancing their social support network (50). In these situations, children are proud of their new duties and competencies. Indeed, the primary support figure for a chronically ill woman is her spouse or life partner. Often, the rest of her support system is organized around this relationship.

Social Support

Not everyone is fortunate enough to have a supportive life partner, and the availability of socially supportive relationships greatly reduces pain-precipitated depression (34).

Interstitial cystitis support groups play an important role in the patient's sense of self-efficacy and well-being by providing information about the disease, group support, and validation through shared experiences (4). When faced with an acute attack of bladder pain, IC patients turn first to their spouses or romantic partners (10). Other IC patients are their second most important source of social support, followed by friends and other family members. Few IC patients regard their physicians and nurses as a major source of support when they experience acute symptom "flares."

Social support is desirable, although almost half of the IC patients studied by Webster and Brennan (10) said that they preferred to withdraw from others when their symptoms were worse. This should not be construed as a sign of poor psychological adjustment. Sometimes, the best source of support during an IC attack is the patient her- or himself.

THE PHYSICIAN–PATIENT RELATIONSHIP

Frustration and Anger

Interstitial cystitis is a recipe for frustration; the experience of most interstitial cystitis patients and their physicians is far from ideal. Years go by before many IC sufferers are diagnosed correctly (14,15). There is no completely satisfactory medical therapy for this disease (51). One in four patients reports that no treatments alleviate the symptoms (14). Because of these factors and the chronic pain of many patients, it is not surprising that some IC patients present themselves to physicians as angry and uncooperative (37).

Unfortunately, anger is contagious. Observational studies of outpatient interviews provide strong evidence of a positive correlation between patients' and their physicians' tones of voice and emotional expressions (52, p. 85). Angry interactions beget dislike, and physician dislike for a patient is one of the best predictors of patient dissatisfaction with medical care. Dissatisfied patients are less likely to comply with recommended treatments, return to a physician, trust the health care system, or expect improvement. Debra Roter and Judith Hall give us insight into this problem:

> the prevailing fact of routine medical practice is that many serious medical conditions are chronic...and therefore do not offer the rewards of a cure nor the variety and excitement of an acute condition. Patients with chronic conditions may also cease acting very appreciative since they are not getting cured and indeed may be on a downward slide. Finally, patients who do not feel good are likely to be grumpy [and] unresponsive...; patients whose distress is of an emotional nature may be particularly erratic or unrewarding in interpersonal interaction. Thus, it is not too surprising if physicians have more feelings of liking for their patients in better condition (52, p. 52).

Research suggests that physicians like male patients more than female ones and healthier patients more than less healthy ones (52,53). What does this imply for the typical interstitial cystitis patient who is likely to be a woman who complains of chronic symptoms that respond poorly to treatment? Vicki Ratner, the founder and President of the Interstitial Cystitis Association, reminds us that "although a disease may not be life threatening, its impact on one's life may be devastating....[especially with an illness like] IC...that involves severe pain" (54, p. 25). Empathy, not just medication, has healing properties.

Restructuring the Physician–Patient Relationship

Until there is a cure for IC, the most important thing a physician can do is to provide IC patients with an emotionally supportive relationship. The doctor–patient relationship needs to be structured so that there is more time to listen to patients' stories:

> Patients need to feel that their doctor takes a personal interest in them as individuals, likes them, is concerned and committed to their welfare....The fulfillment of the basic need to feel known and understood begins with the telling of the patient's story. Telling one's story can also be therapeutic in its own right in providing a cathartic release and the opportunity for insight and perspective. For physicians, the patient story provides the context for clinical insight necessary for understanding and interpreting the many symptoms and clues the patient provides. (52, p. 6)

How can physicians establish or rebuild rapport with an angry, complaining patient? First, they should not personalize the patient's anger. A simple *reflection of feelings,* mirroring a patient's feelings back, sometimes helps defuse an angry patient. The physician could say something like this: "I can hear how angry you are at this disease and how frustrated you are that up until now, none of the treatments seemed to have worked very well." Most patients are grateful when they are heard and appreciate physicians who are honest about the limitations of prevailing treatments.

Patients who hold on to their anger may benefit from other interactive approaches. If anger gets in the way of effective medical care, it may be helpful to comment on the relationship process (what has gone wrong in the interaction). As a psychotherapist, when my attempts at empathy backfire and it is clear that a patient is purposefully ignoring helpful advice, I say something like this as calmly and firmly as possible: "I feel like you are contradicting every suggestion I have made. I appreciate that you are very angry, but right now, your anger is a real barrier to my ability to help you." Another helpful technique is exploring the cognitive (intellectual) source of a patient's anger. Here, the physician explores and helps patients dispute or argue with the beliefs that contribute to their hostility (55). I might ask a patient: "Yes, I hear your anger. What are you saying to yourself about this disease that is making you so angry?" Expected responses might be: "It's not fair that I'm this sick" or "I can't stand this much pain." Responses like this are an opportunity to explore the basic unfairness of life and help them reframe their illness experience to one that encourages greater hopefulness, increased flexibility, and more appreciation for their own psychological and social resources. Sometimes, all a patient needs is to have his or her strength and courage acknowledged.

With a physician's or nurse's help, patients can reframe their illness experience from viewing IC as a catastrophe that is beyond their control to perceiving painful bladder disease as a difficult life experience that they can somehow do their best to manage. The physicians and nurses who have helped me the most have been those who recognized that my occasional expression of anxiety or tearfulness during an office visit is a legitimate reaction to the difficulties of living with IC. It is not wise to refer a patient for psychiatric care solely because she or he was tearful when describing symptoms or loss experienced as a result of interstitial cystitis. There is nothing inherently adaptive about being emotionally inexpressive. In fact, some psychologists suggest that the opposite may be true (56). Emotional expression aside, if a patient is able to function well at home and or at work within the limits imposed by bladder disease, it is reasonable to conclude that she or he is coping well. Acknowledging this can be enormously helpful.

HIGH-FUNCTIONING PATIENTS

High-functioning patients can be an inspiration both to other IC sufferers and to their health care providers. Psychologists, nurse scientists, and medical sociologists have contributed much to our understanding of high-functioning patients with chronic illness.

Healthful Beliefs

There is a large and growing research literature on the relationship between beliefs about illness and the psychological adjustment of chronically ill persons. Generally, chronically ill individuals who feel in control of their lives, who are willing to put up with discomfort in order to resume normal activities, and who are high in self-efficacy function better and are happier than their passive counterparts (42,47). It is beneficial to teach patients cognitive methods and behavior strategies for controlling pain and maximizing their activity level.

Illness may be viewed as an enemy, as a sign of being a damaged or flawed person, or as a positive challenge. Chronically ill persons who accept their illness as a positive challenge have significantly better mental health than those who blame themselves for being ill or are bitterly resentful (41). A chronically ill person's beliefs about illness have direct bearing on family well-being too. In one study, the severity of a woman's chronic illness had no impact on her husband's mental health (49).

Denise Webster, Tim Brennan, and I have researched healthful beliefs employed by IC patients and their spouses (4,11,17). Responses from workshop participants suggest that the best-adjusted patients are those who accept that they have a right to be chronically ill and who make peace with IC by resolving that the disease is difficult but not impossible to live with. The most widely used cognitive strategies for managing IC are: seeking information or learning as much as possible about the illness, self-validation or accepting the legitimacy of the illness experience, taking responsibility for one's own health, and engaging in downward social comparisons (or realizing that other people may have worse problems than oneself) (11). The most popular stress-reduction techniques among IC patients are a combination of spiritual and practical strategies: refusing to let the disease take over one's life, putting the illness in perspective, having faith that one can adapt to life with this illness, keeping needed medications on hand, carefully considering all possible self-care and medical options, and spending quiet time alone when IC symptoms are especially troubling.

Many women rely on faith to cope with their IC; this can be faith in themselves, faith in their physicians or nurses, or faith in God or religious principles. As Webster and Brennan explain, "it may be that having faith in anything or anyone is more important than the focus of the faith" (11, p. 18). A 20-year German study revealed that many chronically ill individuals go through a positive developmental process, passing from depression and inactivity when first diagnosed with chronic illness to eventual "openness and an affirmative life attitude" (38, p. 77). Many chronically ill persons are "able to cope very actively and effectively with the illness and its consequences" after initial adjustment problems (38, p. 78). Which chronically ill persons function best over time? The answer is those who "are actively involved in shaping their lives and in mastering the challenges of life....in a responsible way" (38, p. 78). When compared with physically healthy adults their age, the chronically ill participants in this longitudinal study made more plans and had more realistic plans for the future, reported greater social satisfaction, and were more active within their families and the surrounding community.

A qualitative study of 40 adults who either had a chronic illness or cared for a family member who did indicates that those who thrive psychologically despite physical disability are those who construct *normalizing* stories about themselves, reframing illness as a "normal" or customary human experience. As one patient said:

> It's just treating things that occur in your life as things that occur in your life and not as...major determinants of who you are. That they're facts of life and you deal with them....You cope...as you go along....Normal to me is psychologically healthy more than...physically....Here you got this physical illness, but let's try to deal with it just like you got brown hair and brown eyes—it's part of you....So it's keeping things in perspective—that's normalcy. (57, p. 10)

By reframing physical illness to something that is normal and even inspirational, the patient can replace fear with competence, saying to her- or himself: "I've been through this, and I can manage" (57, p. 13).

Compassion for others is characteristic of patients who normalize illness. Compassionate patients acknowledge that their lives are difficult but probably not so difficult as those of many others. Being a normal person is transformed into an acceptance of physical abnormality—reconstructing chronic illness into an ordinary or expected state of events.

The dominant view in our culture is that life with an incurable chronic illness is, by definition, problematic and miserable. This point of view is inevitably linked to a health care model that focuses on "servicing" sickness more than helping patients "get on with life" (57, p. 20). Chronically ill individuals who normalize their illness challenge physicians and nurses to develop new ways to think about patient, nurse, and doctor roles.

Self-Care

Patients who cope best with interstitial cystitis are those who take responsibility for learning as much as possible about their disease and symptom management (37,58). Physicians, nurses, and psychotherapists can help IC patients by instructing them in bladder retraining, diet, stress reduction, and pain control. But, patients can also become self-care experts in their own right by seeking information from ICA support groups and engaging in independent research. Increasing numbers of chronically ill persons research their own diseases (59). Taking advantage of on-line data bases, interactive computer programs, electronic mail lists for disabled persons, telephone hotlines, educational videos, health magazines, and public libraries, well informed patients make the best health care choices possible. Furthermore, well informed patients increase the mutuality of the doctor-patient relationship, exchanging information freely and regarding their physicians as colleagues, not authority figures (52).

Self-care generates self-efficacy. Describing the hidden benefits of learning to manage her bladder disease, an IC patient from one of my couples' workshops exclaimed: "Now I take better care of the rest of me!" (17). At this same workshop, a number of IC patients and their spouses indicated that the illness experience had inspired them to reassert control over their lives by making self-care a family activity. Spouses and other family members, not just IC patients, reported improving their diet, establishing and maintaining a regular exercise program, and engaging in more stress-reducing and pleasurable activities together.

There is empirical support for the stress-reduction benefits of capable self-care. In one study, the psychosocial adjustment of women with diabetes mellitus was negatively related to the presence of outside stressors (60). Women who faced few stressors were well adjusted to chronic illness; those who experienced multiple stressors were more poorly adjusted. Not surprisingly, diabetic women favored *problem-focused coping* (managing their illness by trying to eliminate stress or improve their environment) over *palliative coping* (engaging in wishful thinking or avoidance).

Intimate Relationships

There are no systematic studies of how intimate partners and children influence the psychological adjustment of IC patients or how an IC patient's disease affects the family. Studies with other chronic diseases suggest that partners and children can be enormously beneficial. In a 3-year study of women with nonmetastatic breast cancer, fibrocystic disease, and diabetes, researchers reported that marital adjustment was inversely related to the severity of a woman's illness and to the length of time she had been ill (32). In contrast, an intensive case study of 11 families in which the mother suffered from a chronic and, in some cases, life-threatening illness found that the demands of a woman's illness alone did not predict impaired individual or family psychological adjustment (50).

Research suggests that chronically ill women function best when they have an emotionally supportive partner and children who willingly assume responsibilities that patients are too disabled to perform without assistance (32,50). Well-functioning, chronically ill women and their loved ones have been described as unusually introspective or psychologically minded, doing their best to understand family process and appreciate the here and now.

In some of my workshops at meetings of the Interstitial Cystitis Association, spouses and family members have talked about how IC inspired them to improve communication and increase their trust in one another and self-acceptance (17,24). Several couples adjust to IC by focusing on their relationship, not the disease, and increasing their intimacy in multiple ways.

Activism

The Interstitial Cystitis Association (ICA) was founded in 1984 to bring IC patients together and educate the general public and medical community about the disease (13,19,54). Then and now, the ICA seems to play a key role in patient adjustment. Thanks to ICA support groups, patients feel less alone with their illness. Because of ICA efforts to fund research, more patients have hope that their symptoms can be relieved and that a cure eventually will be found. Thanks to ICA-sponsored education, fewer patients are misdiagnosed, and increasing numbers of physicians have learned how better to help IC patients.

To date, nobody has compared the psychological adjustment of IC patients who are activists with those who are isolated from the ICA and similar grass-roots organizations for physically disabled persons. From what I have seen from the ICA leaders I have met, I hypothesize that ICA activism is positively associated with being a well-functioning individual for two reasons. First, very depressed persons usually do not have the energy to become activists. Second, given the disease's suboptimal response to medical treatment, IC activism may be the only kind of control many of us exercise over our disease. Efforts to take control of our lives, however undertaken, generally make human beings feel better.

PHILOSOPHICAL ISSUES

In our culture, which worships physical strength and perfection, a disabling medical condition like interstitial cystitis is likely to be regarded with denial and shame (61). Susan Wendell uses her own experience with physical disability to address the marginalization of chronically ill persons:

> I realized after a year that waiting to get well, hoping to recover my healthy body, was a dangerous strategy. I began slowly to identify with my new disabled body and to learn to work with it....I also began to experience the world as structured for people who have no weaknesses....Coming into the public world with illness, pain, or a devalued body, we encounter resistance....Much of our experience goes underground because there is no socially acceptable way of expressing it....A few close friends may share it, but there is a strong impulse to protect them for it too, because it seems so private, so unacceptable. I found...even answering the question, "How are you?" becomes...conflict-ridden....I don't want to risk...discomfort and rejection by telling [people]...what they don't want to know. (62, pp. 381; 389)

Interstitial cystitis, like other painful and disabling conditions, has philosophical (not just psychological) implications. To cope with IC, patients have to dispute Western culture's insistence that health and physical vigor are virtues and that chronically ill persons are inadequate and blameworthy for "allowing themselves" to become disabled (62). To help patients with IC, physicians need to broaden their self-image beyond the heroic idea of caring for the acutely ill (who respond rapidly to their treatments) to the more frustrating but nurturing task of caring for the chronically ill (who may remain unimproved or become worse over time despite their best efforts). To live with IC, perhaps even to thrive psychologically despite IC, patients need to "come out of our collective water closets" (61). Interstitial cystitis patients and others benefit when patients acknowledge publically, without shame, that we have painful bladder disease and that we do our best to both live with IC and fight for a cure.

REFERENCES

1. Keltikangas-Jarvinen L, Auvinen L, Lehtonen T. Psychological factors related to interstitial cystitis. *Eur Urol (ENM)* 1988;15:69–72.
2. McCormick NB, Vinson RK. Sexual difficulties experienced by women with interstitial cystitis. *Women Ther* 1988;7(2–3):109–119.
3. McCormick NB, Vinson RK. Interstitial cystitis: How women cope. *Urol Nurs* 1989;9(4):11,14–17.
4. Webster D. Comparing patients' and nurses' views of interstitial cystitis: A pilot study. *Urol Nurs* 1990;10(3):10–15.
5. Webster D. Interstitial cystitis: Women at risk for psychiatric misdiagnosis. *Clin Issues Perinat Women Health Nurs* 1993;4(2):236–243.
6. Webster D. Reframing women's health: Tension and paradox in framing interstitial cystitis. *J Women Health* 1993;2(1):81–84.
7. Webster DC. Sex and interstitial cystitis: Explaining the pain and planning self-care. *Urol Nurs* 1993;13(1):4–11.
8. Webster D, Brennan T. Use and effectiveness of physical self-care strategies for interstitial cystitis. *Nurse Pract* 1994;19(10):55–61.
9. Webster DC, Brennan T. Use and effectiveness of sexual self-care strategies for interstitial cystitis. *Urol Nurs* 1995;15(1):14–22.
10. Webster DC, Brennan T. Self-care strategies used for acute attack of interstitial cystitis. *Urol Nurs* 1995;15(3):86–93.
11. Webster DC, Brennan T. Use and effectiveness of psychological self-care strategies for interstitial cystitis. *Health Care Women Int* 1995; 16(5):463–475.
12. Richmond J. The tyranny of interstitial cystitis. *Nurs Times* 1994;90 (October 26–November 1):72.
13. Ratner V, Slade D, Greene G. Interstitial cystitis: A patient's perspective. *Urol Clin North Am* 1994;21(1):1–6.
14. Slade DKA. Interstitial cystitis: A challenge to urology. *Urol Nurs* 1989;9(3):5–7.
15. Sant G. Interstitial cystitis in minority women. *J Assoc Acad Minor Physicians* 1993;4(3):89–92.
16. Draucker CB. Coping with a difficult-to-diagnose illness: The example of interstitial cystitis. *Health Care Women Int* 1991;12:191–198.
17. McCormick NB. *When your spouse has interstitial cystitis.* Paper presented at the Interstitial Cystitis Association fifth national meeting, New Orleans, ICA, May 1990.
18. Women and health. *New Directions for Women* 1987;16(November–December):6.
19. Ratner V, Slade D, Whitmore KE. Interstitial cystitis: A bladder disease finds legitimacy. *J Women Health* 1992;1(1):63–68.
20. Chalker R, Whitmore K. *Overcoming Bladder Disorders*. New York: Harper & Row, 1990.
21. McCormick NB. Is there sex after IC? *ICA Update* 1990;5(3):4–5.
22. Webster D. Survey on sexual problems and IC. *ICA Update* 1993;8 (4):4.
23. Evans R. *Men with IC.* Paper presented at the Interstitial Cystitis Association seventh national meeting, Orlando FL, ICA, October, 1993.
24. McCormick NB. *Sex despite interstitial cystitis.* Paper presented at the Interstitial Cystitis Association eighth national meeting, San Diego, ICA, October, 1995.

25. Angier N. Drug works, but questions remain. *The New York Times* 1993; 143(December 13):B8.
26. Linn A. Drugs that can ruin your sex life. *Ladies Home Journal* 1994; September:92,98,100–101.
27. Masters WH, Johnson VE, Kolodny RC. *Human Sexuality*, 5th ed. Philadelphia: JB Lippincott, 1993.
28. McCormick NB. Undesirable sexual side-effects of medications. *ICA Update* 1995;10(2):5–6.
29. Riley AJ, Peet M, Wilson C. eds. *Sexual Pharmacology.* Oxford: Clarendon Press, 1993.
30. Schover LR, Jensen SB. *Sexuality and Chronic Illness: A Comprehensive Approach.* New York: Guilford Press, 1988.
31. McCormick NB. *Sexual Salvation: Affirming Women's Sexual Rights and Pleasures.* Westport, CT: Prager, 1994.
32. Woods NF, Lewis FM. Women with chronic illness: Their views of their families' adaptation. *Health Care Women Int* 1995;16:135–148.
33. Roberto KA. The study of chronic pain in later life: Where are the women? *J Women Aging* 1994;6(4):1–7.
34. Turk DC, Okifuji A, Scharff L. Assessment of older women with chronic pain. *J Women Aging* 1994;6(4):25–42.
35. Roy R. Influence of chronic pain on the family relations of older women. *J Women Aging* 1994;6(4):73–88.
36. Dalton JA, Feurestein M. Fear, alexithymia and cancer pain. *Pain* 1989; 38(2):159–170.
37. Whitmore KE. Self-care regimens for patients with interstitial cystitis. *Urol Clin North Am* 1994;21(1):121–130.
38. Kruse A, Lehr U. Longitudinal analysis of the developmental process in chronically ill and healthy persons—Empirical findings from the Bonn longitudinal study of aging (BOLSA). *Int Psychogeriatr* 1989;1(1): 73–85.
39. Bombardier CH, D'Amico C, Jordan JS. The relationship of appraisal and coping to chronic illness adjustment. *Behav Res Ther* 1990;28: 297–304.
40. McCormick NB. Positive side-effects of chronic illness. *ICA Update* 1995;10(3):3.
41. Schussler G. Coping strategies and individual meanings of illness. *Soc Sci Med* 1992;34:427–432.
42. Kores RC, Murphy WD, Rosenthal TL, Elias DB, North WC. Predicting outcome of chronic pain treatment via a modified self-efficacy scale. *Behav Res Ther* 1990;28:165–169.
43. Sleek C. Coping with disabilities the Albert Ellis way. *Am Psychol Assoc Monit* 1995;26(10):47.
44. Chaiken DC, Blaivas JG, Blaivas ST. Behavioral therapy for the treatment of refractory interstitial cystitis. *J Urol* 1993;149:1445–1448.
45. Frye, K. Understanding interstitial cystitis. *J Urol Nurs* 1993;12(1): 367–371.
46. Webster D. *Sexuality and IC.* Paper presented at the Interstitial Cystitis Association seventh national meeting, Orlando, ICA, October, 1993.
47. Bullers S. Women's roles and health: The mediating effect of perceived control. *Women Health* 1994;22(2):11–30.
48. Chronic illness: How a serious illness affects the family. *Univ Texas Lifetime Health Lett* 1993;5(9):3,8
49. Manne SL, Zautra AJ. Couples coping with chronic illness: Women with rheumatoid arthritis and their healthy husbands. *J Behav Med* 1990;13:327–342.
50. Hough EH, Lewis ML, Woods NF. Family response to mother's chronic illness: Case studies of well and poorly adjusted families. *West J Nurs Res* 1991;13:568–596.
51. Gillenwater JY. The role of the urologist in urinary tract infection. *Med Clin North Am* 1991;75:471–480.
52. Roter DL, Hall JA. *Doctors Talking with Patients, Patients Talking with Doctors: Improving Communication in Medical Visits.* Westport, CT and London: Auburn House, 1993.
53. Hall JA, Epstein AM, DeCiantis ML, McNeil BJ. Physicians' liking for their patients: More evidence for the role of affect in medical care. *Health Psychol* 1993;12:140–146.
54. Ratner, V. Lighting strikes twice: Perils of the patient as woman. *J Women Health* 1992;1(4):249–251.
55. Ellis A, Abrahms E. *Brief Psychotherapy in Medical and Health Practice.* New York: Springer, 1978.
56. Jourard SM. *The Transparent Self,* rev ed. New York: Van Nostrand Reinhold, 1971.
57. Robinson CA. Managing life with a chronic condition: The story of normalization. *Qual Health Res* 1993;3(1):6–28.
58. Taking charge of interstitial cystitis. *Harvard Women Health Watch* 1994;2(3):2–3.
59. Licht J. Research your own illness: Libraries, computer databases and other resources can open a patient's eyes. *Washington Post Health* January 25, 1994;10(4):7.
60. White NE, Richter JM, Fry C. Coping, social support, and adaptation to chronic illness. *West J Nurs Res* 1992;14:211–224.
61. McCormick NB. *Coming out of our water closet: Attacking shame associated with interstitial cystitis.* Paper presented at the Interstitial Cystitis Association gala 10th anniversary luncheon and benefit, New York, ICA, September 15, 1994.
62. Wendell S. Toward a feminist theory of disability. In: Holmes HB, Purdey L, eds. *Feminist Perspectives in Medical Ethics.* Bloomington: Indiana University Press, 1992;63–81.

Interstitial Cystitis, edited by Grannum R. Sant.
Lippincott–Raven Publishers, Philadelphia ©1997.

CHAPTER 25

A Nursing Paradigm for Interstitial Cystitis

Denise C. Webster, Carol Dalton, and Rita M. Martel

NURSING ROLES

Nursing approaches to helping patients with interstitial cystitis (IC) reflect the great diversity of patient presentations and needs as well as the broad range of nursing roles. The latter depend on educational preparation, legal definitions of the scope of nursing, and the setting in which the nurse provides care. In the setting of a team approach, in which each profession contributes specialized knowledge and skills to treatment of the client's health concerns, the nurse's role involves a combination of delegated and independent activities, including prescriptive privilege. Outpatient practices may reflect role requirements related to differing rural and urban needs and/or the nurse's experience with managing particular conditions.

We represent different nursing roles: a women's health nurse practitioner in private practice (C.D.), a nurse practitioner specializing in gerontology, bladder retraining, and pelvic floor rehabilitation in a major medical center hospital (R.M.), and a nurse educator/researcher/clinical specialist in psychiatric nursing (D.W.). Although there are considerable differences in our roles in relation to IC patients, we share a set of core values and beliefs.

THEORIES OF NURSING AND NURSING'S METAPARADIGM

Many health professionals are surprised to learn that nurses do not necessarily accept a single biomedical model of health and illness (1). There are now more than 25 recognized theories of nursing, each of which provides its own form of guidance for working with patients. There are, however, areas of agreement about the focus of the discipline of nursing. All nursing theories implicitly or explicitly address or define health, the importance of environment, the centrality of the patient/client, and the importance of the therapeutic relationship between nurse and patient (2). Each nursing theory may have its distinct definitions for these concepts and the relationships among them. Because nurses operate from a variety of different paradigms, including a wide range of nursing theories, we approach chronic illness and IC differently. In addition to theoretical concepts regarding the person, health, and environment, our nursing practice embodies the assumptions, values, and beliefs of the individual practitioner. Among these are the beliefs that helping a client with a chronic illness requires a holistic perspective of the person and health and a commitment to empowering the client to direct and monitor her own care. The following sections describe a nursing paradigm for IC, incorporating theory, research, and clinical practice.

The person with IC, usually a woman, is seen as manifesting an underlying unity of body, mind, and spirit. Furthermore, the person is seen as having the inherent capacity and resources to heal when placed in the best position for nature to act on her (3). A holistic perspective, then, requires an individualized approach to care that recognizes the uniqueness of each person; uniqueness may be traced to biological and sex differences as well as to developmental and cultural aspects. This individual uniqueness means we cannot treat people with standard protocols or programs of care designed to treat a hypothetically average patient. In this model, the client's perspective becomes central, and her experience is seen as a valid and valued source of information about what is likely to be helpful. One example of this view is a nurse's definition of pain as being "whatever the experiencing person says it is" (4).

A holistic definition of health refers to a harmony or integrity of body, mind, and spirit rather than the health of

D. C. Webster: School of Nursing, University of Colorado Health Sciences Center, Denver, Colorado 80262.
C. Dalton: Wellspring for Women, Boulder, Colorado 80302.
R. M. Martel: Department of Obstetrics and Gynecology, University of Colorado Health Sciences Center, Denver, Colorado 80262.

an isolated body system (5). Consequently, some treatments undertaken from a nursing perspective may deal with a symptom with an appreciation for its representativeness of the whole person. Physical, psychological, emotional, and spiritual health are equally important dimensions in a holistic understanding of the client's condition. The medical diagnosis is usually confined to the physical dimension, which is used as only part of the overall nursing diagnosis. For example, clients with interstitial cystitis may have other medical diagnoses, such as vulvodynia, fibromyalgia, or irritable bowel syndrome (6). Many nurses are comfortable working with clients who wish to use complementary as well as allopathic approaches for healing. A women's health nurse practitioner with specialized knowledge of herbs and dietary supplements might suggest, as part of a healing program of care, dietary and herbal approaches to reducing general inflammatory responses. Patients receiving biofeedback and electrical stimulation often have dramatic improvements in their ability to reduce symptoms of urinary frequency and pain, whether the source of the pain has been identified as IC, dyspareunia, vulvodynia, or pelvic pain of unknown origin. Clients referred for hypnosis for pain management often identify multiple sources of stress that exacerbate their pain or keep them in a state of psychological and physiological hyperarousal. Adequate pain management involves developing skills for reducing these stressors and accessing resources for healing.

A holistic perspective also envisions the individual as embedded in a larger system, which often includes family and other loved ones, community, and vocational, recreational, and spiritual/religious resources. Many women find support groups an invaluable resource for giving and getting information, advice, support, and assistance (7). For other women, having a large network of friends and family can be as much a source of stress as a support (8). Helping patients decide how best to care for themselves may involve making some conscious decisions about how to maintain a balanced sense of responsibility for themselves and others. Often patients want their loved ones to be actively involved in helping them manage their illness. In cases in which spouses/partners are willing and able to be part of the process, their contributions may be invaluable. If the client identifies spiritual resources as important to her, these resources should be honored and incorporated in whatever ways the client finds meaningful.

NURSING–CARING

Some nurse theorists have described nursing as synonymous with caring and/or caring as synonymous with healing (3,5,9–11). Not all nurses would subscribe to such a definition, but it has much in common with the traditional view of women as healers and with the concepts of caring/healing described by Florence Nightingale (12). Historically, women healers have attributed holistic understandings of persons and health to the relationship between the individual and the community and to the "virtues of nature" as healing resources. Sickness is often seen as a passage toward wholeness that benefits from having a companion or caretaker on the journey. This romanticized version of the therapeutic relationship obviously bears little resemblance to the reality of the current health care experience. Among the requirements placed on this kind of relationship are the creation of cooperative, egalitarian interactions and commitment to pooling resources and knowledge. A process that empowers the client usually involves demystifying health care, validating their experiences, and maintaining the client's dignity during often impersonal and dehumanizing procedures (13,14). Too often we focus only on problems, deficits, and sickness to the exclusion of also recognizing a person's inherent resources, strengths, and health. Although time constraints often dictate the focus of an interaction, exclusive attention to problems can reinforce the patient's sense of diminishment and subtly foster a dependent relationship in which the patient's role is to be "compliant" (15).

ASSESSMENT AS INTERVENTION

Language and Labels

Because the predominant model of illness in Western medicine has been rooted in a belief in the separateness of body and mind, patients with any illness that eludes medical intervention may have been confronted with pronouncements of their illness as being "just in your mind" or "psychosomatic." In this context, body–mind relationships are often seen by clients and health professionals alike as pathologic (16). Because such interpretations may convey pejorative meaning, it is important to listen carefully to the client's perspective of what brought on her illness. It is equally important to provide any feedback to clients cautiously, to avoid unintentionally psychopathologizing the very normal experiences of body–mind phenomena. For example, nurses may label patients with IC as being "type A," which can reflect an observation that they often appear to be in a state of hyperarousal (17). This can be construed by patients to mean they are being held responsible for having created their own illness, a classic example of "blaming the victim." A state of hyperarousal may be very understandable for clients who have ongoing pain of unexplained origin and/or are experiencing an acute flare of their symptoms of pain, urgency, and frequency. Because nurses tend to seek pragmatic solutions that are acceptable to the client, the questions the nurse asks and the language the nurse uses can constitute healing interventions in themselves. In response to the question "What makes it worse?" does the client indicate that stress (among other things) seems to make symptoms worse? If so, does the ability to reduce arousal relieve or reduce the symptoms? What strategies has she used to try to manage the symptoms, and how have these worked?

Developing Trust

Development of a trusting relationship may require an openness to hearing and validating what the patient has been through, her physical suffering and, often, her frustrations in trying to obtain care. Some have had multiple unsuccessful surgeries. Often patients find their illness has changed their self-concept as a woman, mother, daughter, sister, or wife, and they may wish to discuss these concerns with someone who is able to hear their feelings. Many patients come to us with the added burden of feeling discounted and/or humiliated. Nurses can help normalize these experiences by letting the client know that other people would have similar feelings under the circumstances. For example, one woman was told after her hysterectomy to think of her vagina as "her husband's sock," a metaphor that made her feel both depersonalized and dirty. Another woman had been told to manage her pain by "getting drunk," and yet another was told her pain was probably caused by guilt about having sexual intercourse. Many have been told they are "overinterpreting" their experiences or that there is "nothing more that can be done." In our experience, respectful listening to the story of the illness is an important source of information about the ways the client has come to view the illness and how the nurse might be most helpful.

In some cases, unless the client has come from a long distance for the appointment, the first session may be entirely devoted to the development of trust in a climate of safety and hopefulness, through hearing and validating the client's experience. If the client is in active pain, has dyspareunia, or has fear of instrumentation, any potentially intrusive procedures should be avoided during the first visit. Agreed-on "homework," to be carried out before the next session, may include tracking voiding patterns or identifying current self-care practices and their effectiveness in preventing or managing symptoms.

Identifying Goals

Perhaps the most important question we ask a client is, "What are your hopes for coming here?" Unless we know a client's goals, hopes, and expectations, we may flounder in all the details that constitute a holistic assessment or create an idealized plan of care that bears little resemblance to what the client is seeking. However, it may be equally important to help clients identify small, identifiable, and manageable steps toward a goal. Success in these small steps can build confidence and competence, whereas the uncompromising demand for complete recovery carries a high probability of failure. Sometimes it is necessary to ask, "What level of pain relief would be acceptable to you?" In many cases, just providing clients with the tools to determine their progress can have a healing effect. Keeping logs on the use and effectiveness of many self-care strategies can be empowering for some clients, as they identify a broader repertoire of strategies or measure progress in manageable increments. Are there some self-care strategies that she uses to prevent symptoms that may differ from those she uses to manage mild to moderate symptoms? How are flares similar to or different from the lower levels of symptoms, and what seems to help manage these acute exacerbations? For others, keeping logs seems to increase the experience of discomfort, and they may need to distract themselves from symptoms or focus primarily on identifying periods of comfort and activities that increase comfort.

Symptoms

Patients with IC are usually seen by nurses because they are experiencing urinary urgency, frequency, and/or suprapubic pain, which may or may not be relieved by voiding. Many also have had bladder hyperdistention and a bladder biopsy. To obtain accurate base-line data about patients' current bladder capacity and interval between voids, they are often given a 24-hr voiding diary (urolog) to complete. The urolog is for 2 to 3 days in the week. Patients may be unfamiliar with terms such as "void" or "leaking point," so it is important to use their own terms or avoid using medical jargon. Ask the patient to note fluids drunk, what times, and how many ounces. A "bladder bonnet" can be used under the toilet seat to measure each voiding. It may be best if they do not change their usual patterns during this time. In giving instructions, it is important to determine the amount of hydration that is desirable. Many clients are actually overhydrated because they have been told to "force fluids." Some interpret this to mean "as much as possible" and drink more than 4 liters of fluid a day. We recommend eight (8-oz) glasses of fluid per day, stopping at 8 p.m. except for sips of water or ice chips. When we determine clients' preferred choice of fluids, we may discover, without showing disapproval or surprise, that many IC patients find caffeinated and acidic fluids aggravate their symptoms. Clients may also use the urolog to become more familiar with their bodies in relation to thoughts, feelings, and sensations before and after voiding.

Assessment of the IC patient should include not only her experiences of urgency and frequency (daytime and at night) but different types and sites of pain, possibly related to other medical diagnoses. Are there changes in symptoms that accompany menstrual cycles? Did her symptoms first arise during the perimenopause, posthysterectomy, or associated with a developmental change?

What other kinds of symptoms has she had, and what does she make of these? Does she have any ideas about why she might be having these symptoms at this point in her life? The purpose of these questions is not to "pigeonhole" patients into preconceived categories that "explain" IC but to obtain, from the clients' perspective, how the illness fits into their lives, relationships, and responsibilities. Information about losses associated with having IC may help client and nurse make connections between changes in severity of illness and the stresses associated with the illness itself. Job loss and/or relationship difficulties may contribute to the depression and anxiety of having any chronic illness. Does the client need a referral to seek disability support?

Occasionally, a client will connect her pain with a history of physical and/or sexual abuse or other traumatic experiences (18). It is not uncommon for the experience of pain and a prevailing sense of helplessness to revive memories of earlier pain and helplessness (19,20). Because of the range of life experiences that could be construed as potentially traumatic, it seems important to ascertain if the patient feels there is any connection between these experiences and her current experience. If so, what does she believe will be helpful to her in dealing with the situation now? If the client believes she would benefit from counseling, and the nurse is not prepared to provide such counseling, a referral may be appropriate. In such a case, the referral would be in response to a client's expressed needs and desires rather than to a preconceived belief that "all pelvic pain patients" have some shared history and/or need a particular type of treatment.

Resources

Ascertaining the client's current resources is at least as important as ascertaining the signs and symptoms of illness. A recent study of 138 women with interstitial cystitis revealed that most had an astonishing repertoire of self-care and coping strategies that they used to manage living with IC (7,21–23). Taken as a whole, these ways of thinking about having IC and activities avoided or undertaken to manage having IC demand nothing less than the need to redefine oneself to manage living with a chronic illness. This redefinition often involves clarifying priorities and refining energy expenditures as well as learning new ways of eating, moving, relating, and resting. On whom or what can they depend? For what kinds of information, advice, support, or assistance? In the midst of these changes, many feel compelled to learn everything they can about the illness and the range of possible treatments for it. Some will feel overwhelmed if they are provided with huge amounts of material written for professionals. Others will want all the information they can obtain. Some will want information about the availability of support groups for them and/or their partners. Others would prefer to choose the type, timing, and source of the information they desire. Because of this variation, it may be best to simply ask clients what needs they have for information and what kind of contact, if any, they would like to have with others who have IC. When ascertaining their current coping and self-care strategies, it is important to ask which they actually find helpful rather than to suggest that there are "good" and "bad" ways to manage having IC.

Biofeedback is a good example of an assessment that is an intervention in itself and of an approach that also can become a self-care strategy (24–27). Many clients experience vaginal/vulvar pain intermittently or constantly and often react by tightening the pelvic floor muscles. This can activate a pain loop that leads to more pain. In most cases, there is a markedly elevated level of muscular electrical activity when clients are asked to relax the pelvic floor muscle. The treatment goal is to educate the muscles to relax at will. The client can then learn to relax at will during pain and can reduce or eliminate the pain. Many are able to reduce the amount of medications needed (e.g., narcotics, antiinflammatory, tranquilizers, antidepressants). By providing clients with graphic information about their ability to voluntarily relax or contract selected muscles, we teach clients a skill that can modify their pain. Many women with dyspareunia and pelvic pain have increased urethral pressures. The effect of a spasm in the pelvic floor can be demonstrated by having the client maintain a clenched fist for a period long enough for her to experience discomfort and fatigue in the entire arm. Not all IC patients will have this pelvic floor problem or be able to trace their dyspareunia to this source. However, those who do can benefit from assessment/intervention using vaginal or rectal electromyography (EMG) biofeedback, which is a computerized program projected on a monitor for nurse and patient to observe. A base line can be determined during an office visit. Sessions of up to 15 min may be tolerated, using either a vaginal or rectal probe or an EMG-sensing garment without probe insertion. Sometimes a patient has both spasm and inability to contract muscles voluntarily. Most can be taught in the office to isolate the pelvic floor muscles and voluntarily relax and contract them, followed by practice at home, with or without portable home units. The procedure involves determining the ability to relax or contract the pelvic floor muscle on command, followed by evaluating the level of pelvic floor muscle relaxation. Many women perform pelvic floor exercises (Kegel exercises) improperly and will benefit from learning how to avoid using buttocks, abdomen, thighs, and doing a Valsalva while attempting to meet their contraction goals. First, determine the desired number of seconds contracting based on base line, increasing incrementally over time. Clients initially should relax 8 to 10 sec between contractions.

A similar process, using surface electromyography, evaluates the level of abdominal (Valsalva) or thigh contractions. These contractions can be demonstrated on the computer monitor to help the client alter behaviors that may have become habitual in response to pain (28,29). Surface patches can be placed anywhere on body where there seems to be tension to further teach and demonstrate how it looks on monitor and how it feels to relax particular muscle groups. Sessions with the nurse may be done weekly. Most clients require a total of four to six 15- to 30-min sessions. Although home units are recommended, clients can practice these techniques without the use of external monitors. For clients who are able to relax but have a weak pelvic floor, the nurse might suggest use of graduated vaginal weights.

SELF-CARE FOR INTERSTITIAL CYSTITIS

Many of the suggestions that follow were derived from the above study of the use and effectiveness of self-care (7,21–23). The structure of the sections reflects the different types of self-care that women said they used. In most cases, only four or five examples of the strategies found to be most effective in each category are described.

Hygiene

Frequently, the instructions nurses provide for patients with IC are measures actually more useful for patients with bladder infections (17). Consequently, they encourage women to wipe from front to back, wear cotton underpants, avoid tight clothing, use white toilet paper, and avoid scented soaps. It should be noted that some recycled white toilet papers may be irritating because of chemicals used in recycling. Because most IC patients are not able to trace their symptoms to an infection, they may feel misunderstood if these are the only helpful ideas the nurse can offer. Nevertheless, most IC patients are scrupulous in carrying out these practices, if only to avoid a concomitant infection. What patients actually find most effective, however, is avoiding tight clothing, emptying the bladder at regular intervals, resting during the day, drinking only water, and avoiding constipation (21).

Many IC patients have either been told to increase their voiding frequency or done so on their own to "keep the bladder empty," in an attempt to reduce the pain associated with a full bladder. In addition to helping them determine their average voiding interval and volumes, it may be helpful to let women know that they will never totally empty their bladder unless they self-catheterize. Once they learn this, they are sometimes less prone to void as frequently. If they void at intervals of 15 min or less, it may be important to work with them to use a bladder-holding protocol, i.e., to suppress urges to void and increase the interval to 30 min. After 1 week, if this is tolerated with no increase in the level of pain, we recommend they increase the voiding interval 15 min per week until they void at 3-hr intervals, as tolerated.

Often patients find that the combination of medications to manage pain, relative physical inactivity, diminished fluid intake, and avoiding fruits and vegetables places them at risk for having chronic constipation. Maintaining a regular bowel-emptying schedule involves having adequate roughage in the diet. For those who find they cannot meet these requirements with fruits and vegetables, daily psyllium seed powder (Metamucil) may be helpful. If constipation/flatus is a problem acidophilus in pill form or α-galactosidase (Beano) may be helpful. Clients should avoid laxatives, as these lead to bowel dependence. Clients may also need to limit chocolates and nuts, which can cause bloating and trigger increased pelvic discomfort. Many patients find bananas, dairy products, and white flour contribute to constipation. Adequate water intake and regular exercise, as tolerated, are also important to maintaining bowel regularity.

Diet

Most diet-related self-care strategies for IC patients involve avoiding foods associated with an increase in symptoms of frequency and/or pain. These include alcohol, citrus (including tomatoes), coffee, spices, citric acid, and carbonated beverages (21). However, eliminating all potentially offending foods can provide an additional stress. Sometimes patients are afraid to eat anything, for fear of having a flare. Because having a chronic illness usually means having to deprive oneself of many former pleasures, it is important to keep additional deprivations to a minimum. Most can handle bland foods and starches unless they have a specific grain or milk allergy. We usually suggest that people eliminate foods that clearly cause symptoms and then experiment with other foods to find as many as possible that can be enjoyed.

Medications

In the self-care study, several medications were reported to be effective for preventing symptoms of IC (21,22). These included two prescription medications—antidepressants and antibiotics—and two over-the-counter medications—calcium carbonate (Tums) and sodium bicarbonate. For managing mild to moderate symptoms, sodium bicarbonate and Tums were still on the list, whereas treatment for symptoms of acute attack included bladder analgesics, antispasmodics, antidepressants, and narcotics. The rationale for using these medications appears in other chapters in this book.

Obviously, if one serves as a primary practitioner, it is necessary to rule out urinary tract infection and to treat any infection with the appropriate antibiotic. Bladder spasms may be reduced by taking a small dose of anticholinergic medication such as oxybutynin (Ditropan), 2.5 mg (a half tablet) once daily, in the morning if most of the pain is associated with voiding during the day or at bedtime if nocturia of at least twice a night is present. The ability to sleep uninterruptedly and regularly is vital to the reparative process. Occasionally medications to facilitate sleep may be of benefit.

Diet and Food Supplements to Reduce Inflammatory Responses

One common factor in interstitial cystitis is inflammation. Prostaglandins are a group of hormones the body produces that play a primary role in both the onset and the relief of inflammation. Paradoxically, one set of prostaglandins and other biochemicals increase inflammation whereas another set of prostaglandins and biochemicals suppress or moderate inflammation (29). Balancing prostaglandins is one of the keys to controlling inflammation. Two basic foods are essential to balance prostaglandins: fiber and fatty acids. Fatty acids play a role in properly balancing prostaglandins, and fiber helps bind excess prostaglandins and other metabolic by-products, inactivating them and flushing them from the body. If these are absorbed rather than excreted, they tend to cause more inflammation.

Prostaglandins that increase inflammation consist primarily of arachidonic acid, which is obtained from animal products, corn oil, and soybean oil. Arachidonic acid is made from linolenic acid and is essential in small quantities for good health. The problem is that most of us eat too many foods that contain large quantities of linolenic acid. Beneficial prostaglandins are made from another fatty acid, eicosapentaenoic acid (EPA). This last is one of the ω-3 fatty acids that are part of a larger group, polyunsaturated fatty acids. These are primarily found in marine plants (e.g., seaweed) and cold-water fish. Wild animals, such as deer, rabbit, and elk, also have some EPA in their tissues, although not nearly as much as fish. Three other fatty acids are important: docosahexaenoic acid (DHA), α-linolenic acid (ALA), and γ-linoleic acid (GLA). The ALA is converted into EPA, and DHA is made from EPA in the body. Therefore, it is important to ingest adequate amounts of ALA and DHA (through diet and supplements) so that all of the EPA is available to be converted into prostaglandins.

Fiber reduces inflammation. Both a high-fiber diet and fiber supplements are helpful. It is somewhat difficult to eat the recommended amount of fiber without increasing calories far beyond the body's needs, so it may be necessary to recommend a fiber supplement that contains a mixture of soluble and insoluble fiber. If this increases flatulence and bloating, the patient can reduce the supplement amount and gradually increase it as the body adjusts. Beano is a digestive enzyme product that can help reduce gas caused by extra fiber. When increasing fiber, be sure to increase water intake as well. Fiber without water tends to act as a dry sponge and create constipation.

In addition to these dietary supplements, patients generally choose one or two of the following fatty acid supplements: evening primrose oil, borage oil (GLA), mackerel oil (EPA), blackcurrant seed oil, or flaxseed oil. Other nutrients are necessary for the positive action of the fatty acids in the body. Patients may use a multivitamin mineral as a base foundation for supplementation. Other vitamins and minerals that are helpful in manufacturing prostaglandins are calcium and magnesium, vitamin E, and B-complex vitamins. Cold-processed food-based supplements seem to provide faster and more effective relief of symptoms than synthetic varieties.

Another source of inflammation can be a histamine reaction. To see if this seems to be a likely possibility, look for other symptoms of allergies, such as itchy eyes and ears, scratchy throat, sneezing, and head congestion. If some or all of these symptoms are present, then high histamine levels may be part of the IC puzzle. To treat this, the patient should first lower her exposure to potential allergens. If seasonal pollens are suspected, close the bedroom window, wash hair at night, change pillow cases frequently, and keep animals out of the bedroom and off the bed. If certain foods such as dairy products seem to increase the symptoms, then avoid those. Natural supplements that often help to relieve histamine reactions are garlic, alfalfa tablets, vitamin C with bioflavonoids (or perhaps just the bioflavonoids if the C seems to be a bladder irritant). Some patients find that sustained-release vitamin C is less irritating. Over-the-counter or prescription antihistamines can also prove to be helpful.

An adrenal hormone, dehydroepiandrosterone (DHEA), is one of the natural hormones used to treat a variety of health problems associated with inflammation. It is helpful, however, only if the DHEA level is low or low normal to begin with. A simple blood test for DHEA sulfate can give you this information (30).

A variety of herbal remedies may be helpful for IC patients. One cornsilk blend (Cornsilk/Pipsissawa Compound by Wind River Herbs) seems to be very soothing to the urinary tract. Be careful of using herbal formulas or individual herbs used to treat cystitis, as these may be too harsh and actually increase symptoms.

Hormonal conditions such as premenstrual syndrome (PMS) and low-estrogen conditions associated with amenorrhea and menopause can often increase symptoms of IC. Two types of PMS seem to aggravate IC. The first PMS type is caused by prostaglandin imbalance and includes symptoms of joint and muscle pains, headaches, acne, nausea, and irritability along with increased IC symptoms. Symptoms may be relieved with the program described previously for managing inflammation and prostaglandins. The second type of PMS is caused by low progesterone. This PMS type includes symptoms of mood swings, tearfulness, depression, fatigue, breast tenderness, and bloating along with increased IC symptoms. Menstruating IC patients may benefit from using micronized oral progesterone tablets from ovulation until menstruation to reduce the symptoms, along with diet and supplements. The supplements include vitamin E, B complex, zinc, and a soy-based protein powder used in a drink.

Low estrogen affects the integrity of the cells lining the vagina, bladder, and urethra. Low estrogen also can affect the muscle tone of the pelvic floor, causing a decrease in bladder control. Many women who do not have IC develop problems with frequency of urination, pressure, and decreased bladder control when their estrogen levels are too low. Estrogen replacement therapy (ERT) can often reduce these symptoms, although it is often necessary to use a vaginal estrogen cream as well as oral therapy. For women who cannot or who choose not to use traditional ERT, a variety of phytoestrogens such as estriol tablets and vaginal creams are available. There are also triestrogen tablets and creams, which contain 80% estriol, 10% estrone, and 10% estradiol.

Herbal preparations can help the body to produce more of its own hormones. Preparations include licorice root, vitex, black cohosh, motherwort, and ginseng. Women who have a tendency to high blood pressure should be careful when using ginseng or licorice root, as it can increase blood pressure. One popular formula is Women's Tonic 2 by Wind River Herbs, which contains dong quai, chaste tree berry, wild yam root, motherwort, black cohosh, American ginseng, and St. John's wort.

Body Comfort

Body comfort strategies reported to be most effective for managing symptoms include wearing loose clothing, getting a massage, putting a heating pad on the pubis or pubis and lower back, as well as taking warm baths and using meditation. Additional strategies for managing acute attacks include slow breathing, imagery/relaxation tapes, and meditation (22).

Many visualization/imagery/relaxation/self-hypnosis tapes are commercially available. Through experimentation, patients usually find one or more that they are able to use. For best results, however, regular daily practice of meditation or one of the above methods will make the strategy more effective when needed to manage an acute attack. These strategies also can be useful to help manage the straining and discomfort many have during acute attacks. The same visualization/relaxation technique can be used to help relax the pelvic floor if they find they are straining at other times.

Women with any type of pelvic congestion or pelvic and bladder pain may benefit from increased circulation and relaxation. Two types of hot compresses may be helpful. Castor oil packs are made from castor oil (preferably cold pressed) and four pieces of wool or cotton flannel cut large enough to fit over the bladder/pelvic area. Layer the flannel and pour castor oil into the center until saturated. Lay this directly onto the skin so that it covers the bladder area. Cover the cloth with a plastic bag and then with a heat source, such as a heating pad. Leave on as long as desired but at least 30 min. These compresses should not be used during heavy menses. After removing the pack, wash the skin with a solution of 1 tsp baking soda to 1 pint water to wash off the oil. The flannel pack can be stored in a plastic bag in the refrigerator and reused up to 20 to 30 times (31).

Ginger compresses can be made by grating a two-inch piece of ginger root or 1 teaspoon of ginger power (not as potent). Add ginger to 1 quart of boiled water. Remove from the heat and cover and steep for 15 to 20 minutes before straining out the ginger. Dip cloth or cotton towel into the ginger water and apply to the bladder area. Cover with plastic and a heat source. Leave on as long as desired at a comfortable temperature. Ginger water can be refrigerated and warmed up for additional treatments.

Psychological Self-Care

Among the most effective self-care strategies for managing IC are stress-reduction and cognitive techniques. The most effective stress-reduction strategy for women in the self-care study was attending an IC support group (7). Not surprisingly, then, helping others with IC was also seen as an effective self-care strategy. Among the most effective cognitive coping strategies are educating oneself about IC, accepting the experience as real (i.e., rejecting views that IC is "just in the head"), and taking responsibility for one's own health, e.g., by developing an individualized self-care program. In addition, perhaps because it raises endorphin levels or DHEA, patients say that seeking activities and people that make them laugh is very helpful. Another important thing patients do to take care of themselves is refusing specific treatments. For the patient who has taken the time to know her body and respect her experience, refusing a treatment can be an empowering and wise decision.

Managing an acute attack requires slightly different cognitive and stress-reduction approaches (22). Among the most effective of these are praying, using positive self-talk, and remembering that it will get better, as well as having faith in self, health professionals, or a spiritual source. Practical approaches to managing symptoms include spending time alone, not being embarrassed about the need to urinate anywhere, and keeping needed medications on hand. In helping patients develop their self-care plans, it is important to explore their past coping—what has and has not been helpful. Because attacks are often unexpected, it may be helpful to have a list of "things to do" to manage an attack and to keep a personal "first aid" kit stocked for these times, rather than having to gather things together under duress.

Distraction strategies are among the most effective ways to manage moderate or flare symptoms. The self-care study found that doing crafts and hobbies, keeping busy, throwing oneself into work, listening to or playing music, distracting oneself with memories, or reading for pleasure were very effective. To manage an attack, in addition to these strategies, many distracted themselves by watching TV. Fewer were able to "relocate" the pain, but those who did found it effective. Relocating pain to a smaller or less disturbing area of the body, or focusing one's attention on areas of comfort, are among the more effective hypnotic approaches for managing any type of acute or chronic pain (32–35).

As noted above, the single most effective self-care strategy was attending an IC support group. Although not all patients are inclined to join such groups, many find them a rich source of information, advice, assistance, and support. Most patients seek information and advice from physicians; however, the most effective information and advice was seen to come from other patients and books. Sometimes nurses have lists of other IC patients who have agreed to have their phone numbers given to new IC patients. Advice from a significant other was also seen as more effective than advice from a nurse or physician. Understandably, those who are closest to patients have more specialized knowledge about their unique needs and resources. Nurses should be able to direct clients to available support groups and books and determine, with the client, if it would be helpful to include the partner and family when identifying resources for managing the multiple needs associated with having a chronic illness.

Effective sexual self-care involves an active involvement by clients and their sexual partners (36). The most effective sexual self-care strategies include avoiding intercourse when having symptoms, avoiding unlubricated intercourse, avoiding sexual positions that put pressure on the urethra, and avoiding direct clitoral stimulation. The nurse may also discuss ways to be intimate that do not necessarily include intercourse if it is painful (23,37–39). If dyspareunia is present, some patients experience promising results with vaginal electrical stimulation. It appears that the electrical stimulation, delivered by an inserted rectal or vaginal probe, acts to block afferent pain impulses (26,40). Electrical stimulation can be used in combination with exercises to help clients learn what a proper contraction feels like (by matching the image in the monitor with their sensations). A home unit with settings at 10 to 20 Hz can be used initially for 15 min daily, increasing to 30 min daily.

Couples often benefit from stress reduction and relaxation exercises. In one family, several of the children joined their mother every evening in listening to a soothing relaxation tape with subliminal messages for healing. As with any chronic illness, those who provide support also have needs. The caretaker/support role can be draining, and relationships may be strained. Even the most loving, supportive spouse often feels guilty, unable to vent feelings of anger or depression. In some areas, spouses, partners, family, or friends have either been included in IC support groups or developed groups to meet their special needs. Nurses who have specialized skills in counseling couples and families and/or in facilitating support groups may have a special role in developing these resources.

Clearly, managing a chronic illness/chronic pain condition such as IC can be time consuming and exhausting for patients who already have limited energy. The nurse who can work with the client to identify priorities for self-care and develop a step-by-step program for healing will find the time and energy well spent. Although rapid resolution of any long-term illness is unlikely, nurses can provide a caring relationship and a sense of hopefulness that in IC, as in life, "slow and steady" will eventually be rewarded.

RESOURCES

- Interstitial Cystitis Association, P.O. Box 1553, Madison Square Station, New York, NY 10159-1553. (212) 979-6057.
- Instant protein powder. Available from Shaklee Corporation, San Francisco, CA 94111. (714) 670-3818.
- Triestrogen tablets and creams. Available from Belmar Pharmacy, Lakewood, CO. (303) 763-5533; and Bezweken Women's Health Care Products, Beaverton, OR. (800) 743-2256.
- Wind River Herbs. Jackson Hole, WY. (800) 903-4372.

REFERENCES

1. Webster D. A nurse looks at medical students looking at nursing. *Nurs Outlook* 1988;36:130–135.
2. Fawcett J. *Conceptual Models of Nursing Practice.* Philadelphia: FA Davis, 1989.
3. Erickson H, Tomlin E, Swain M. *Modeling and Role-Modeling: A Theory and Paradigm for Nursing.* Englewood Cliffs, NJ: Prentice-Hall, 1983.
4. McCaffery M, Beebe A. *Pain: Clinical Manual for Nursing Practice.* St Louis: CV Mosby, 1989.
5. Watson J. *Nursing: Human Science and Human Care.* Norwalk, CT: Appleton-Century-Crofts, 1985.
6. ICA Research Update. Connections between IC, vulvodynia, and fibromyalgia to be investigated. *ICA Update* 1994;9:7.
7. Webster D, Brennan T. Use and effectiveness of women's psychologic self-care strategies for IC. *Health Women Int* 1995;16:463–475.
8. Belle D, ed. *Lives in Stress: Women and Depression.* Beverly Hills, CA: Sage Publications, 1982.
9. Newman M, Sime M, Corcoran-Perry S. The focus of the discipline of nursing. *Adv Nurs Sci* 1991;14(1):1–6.
10. Benner P, Wrubel J. *The Primacy of Care: Stress and Coping in Health and Illness.* Menlo Park, CA: Addison-Wesley, 1989.
11. Montgomery C. *Healing Through Communication: The Practice of Caring.* Newbury Park, CA: Sage, 1993.
12. Achterberg J. *Woman as Healer.* Boston: Shambhala, 1991.
13. Webster D, Lipetz M. Changing definitions, changing times. *Nurs Clin North Am* 1986;2:87–97.
14. Webster D. Solution-focused approaches in psychiatric-mental health nursing. *Perspect Psychiatr Care* 1990;26:17–24.

15. Montgomery C, Webster D. Caring, curing, and brief therapy: a model for nurse psychotherapy. *Arch Psychiatr Nurs* 1994;8:291–297.
16. Webster D. Interstitial cystitis: Women at risk for psychiatric misdiagnosis. *Clin Issues Perinat Women's Health Nurs* 1993;2:236–243.
17. Webster D. Comparing patient and nurse views of interstitial cystitis: a pilot study. *Urol Nurs* 1990;10:10–15.
18. McCormick N. Sexual Abuse and IC: When bladder disease isn't the worst thing that ever happened. *ICA Update* 1991;6:6–7.
19. Rossi EL. *The Psychobiology of Mind–Body Healing*, rev ed. New York: WW Norton, 1993.
20. Webster D. Interstitial cystitis: Paradigms and paradox. *J Women's Health [Suppl]* 1993;2:81–84.
21. Webster D, Brennan T. Use and effectiveness of physical self-care strategies for IC. *Nurse Pract* 1994;19:55–61.
22. Webster D, Brennan T. Women's physical and psychological self-care for acute attack states of interstitial cystitis. *Urol Nurs* 1995;15:86–93.
23. Webster D, Brennan T. Use and effectiveness of sexual self-care strategies for interstitial cystitis. *Urol Nurs* 1995;15:14–22.
24. Fall M, Carlson C, Erlandson B. Electrical stimulation in interstitial cystitis. *J Urol* 1980;123:192–195.
25. Dijkema HE, Weil WH, Mijs PT, Janknegt. Neuromodulation of sacral nerves for incontinence and voiding dysfunctions. *Eur Urol* 1993;24(1):22–26.
26. Schmidt RA, Wapnek JM. Pelvic floor behavior and interstitial cystitis. *Semin Urol* 1991;9:154–159.
27. Whitmore KE. Self-care regimens for patients with interstitial cystitis. *Urol Clin North Am* 1994;21:121–130.
28. Chaiken DC, Blaivas JG, Blaivas ST. Behavioral therapy for the treatment of refractory interstitial cystitis. *J Urol* 1993;149:1445–1448.
29. Scala J. *The Arthritis Relief Diet.* New York: Penguin Books, 1989.
30. Gaby A. *Preventing and Reversing Osteoporosis.* Rocklin, CA: Prima Publishing, 1995.
31. Northrup C. *Women's Bodies, Women's Wisdom.* New York: Bantam Books, 1994.
32. Caudill M. *Managing Pain Before It Manages You.* New York: Guilford Press, 1995.
33. Catalano, E. *The Chronic Pain Control Workbook.* Oakland, CA: New Harbinger Press, 1987.
34. Davis M, Eshelman E, McKay M. *Relaxation and Stress Reduction Workbook*, 3rd ed. Oakland, CA: New Harbinger Press, 1988.
35. Zahourek R, ed. *Clinical Hypnosis and Suggestion in Patient Care.* New York: Brunner/Mazel, 1990.
36. Webster D. Sex and IC: Explaining the pain and planning self-care. *Urol Nurs* 1993;13:4–11.
37. McCormick NB, Vinson RK. Sexual difficulties experienced by women with interstitial cystitis. *Women Ther* 1988;7:109–119.
38. McCormick NB, Vinson RK. Interstitial cystitis: How women cope. *Urol Nurs* 1990;19:10–15.
39. McCormick NB. Is there sex after IC? *ICA Update* 1990;5:4–5.
40. Glazer H. Biofeedback shows promising results for IC and vulvar pain. *ICA Update* 1994;9:2.

Interstitial Cystitis, edited by Grannum R. Sant.
Lippincott–Raven Publishers, Philadelphia ©1997.

CHAPTER 26

Use of Lasers in Interstitial Cystitis

Allan M. Shanberg and Terrence Malloy

Interstitial cystitis, as demonstrated in many other chapters in this book, is a perplexing and difficult disease for both patient and urologist. It definitely has a spectrum of presenting complaints and a multitude of treatment options. Patient complaints range from severe frequency of urination to marked pain on urination or pelvic pain. The etiology of this disease remains unknown but may be related to some dormant microbes (1), although others claim an autoimmune phenomenon (2).

The overwhelming majority of patients seen with this disorder are female. Because of the initial difficulty in establishing a diagnosis, it is not unusual for many of our patients to have already undergone several pelvic surgical procedures, including hysterectomy. Objectively, in our hands, the diagnosis of interstitial cystitis is made by exclusion of the other bladder disorders that can present with the same symptoms, e.g., carcinoma *in situ,* tuberculosis, malakoplakia, chemical or bacterial cystitis, yeast cystitis, and referred pain from upper tract disease (3).

The majority of patients referred to both of us and to a tertiary care hospital have already had an extensive workup. Our recommendation, at a minimum, includes an intravenous pyelogram (IVP), cystometric studies, and cystoscopy under anesthesia with bladder biopsy. The recent introduction of the potassium leak test as described by Parsons is helpful, and we are currently using this as well (4). Cystoscopy under anesthesia is generally the most reliable objective study because frequently, when the bladder is distended and then collapsed, the typical petechial hemorrhages of interstitial cystitis become visible (Fig. 1). Bladder biopsy has been controversial for ascertaining the presence, absence, or increased numbers of mast cells. We have suggested for many years that reviewing the biopsy is important in making this diagnosis, not only to exclude other disease but also in noting the marked inflammatory reaction present in both the lamina propria and the muscularis layer of the bladder (Fig. 2) (4–7).

In 1985, we reported our first experience in the use of the Nd:YAG laser in this disease (8). Since that time we have been able to define those patients whom we think could benefit from laser therapy and also, more importantly, to reduce the major and serious complication of small bowel perforation associated with laser therapy by modifying our various techniques (9).

PATIENT CRITERIA FOR ND:YAG LASER THERAPY OF IC

All of our patients have failed conventional means of therapy such as DMSO, bladder stretching, heparin instillations as recently reported by Parsons, cortisone instillations, and various oral medications such as antihistamines and amitriptyline (10–14).

All patients with only frequency of urination and not pain were excluded from our current treatment protocol; as we have recently reported (9), painful bladder and, most specifically, the patient with Hunner's ulcer disease associated with interstitial cystitis have the best results from laser photoirradiation. Unfortunately, the spectrum of this disease allows many patients to have frequency alone as a primary component of their symptoms, but we have found that these patients have a poor response to laser photoirradiation.

TECHNIQUE OF LASER PHOTOIRRADIATION

We currently recommend that all patients be simultaneously laparoscoped at the time of laser therapy. The IC patients have an extremely thin bladder, and loops of small and large intestine have been reported to perforate after laser therapy. The laparoscopy allows the surgeon to

A. M. Shanberg: Department of Urology, University of California, Irvine, Orange, California 92868.
T. Malloy: Department of Urology, University of Pennsylvania, Philadelphia, Pennsylvania 19104.

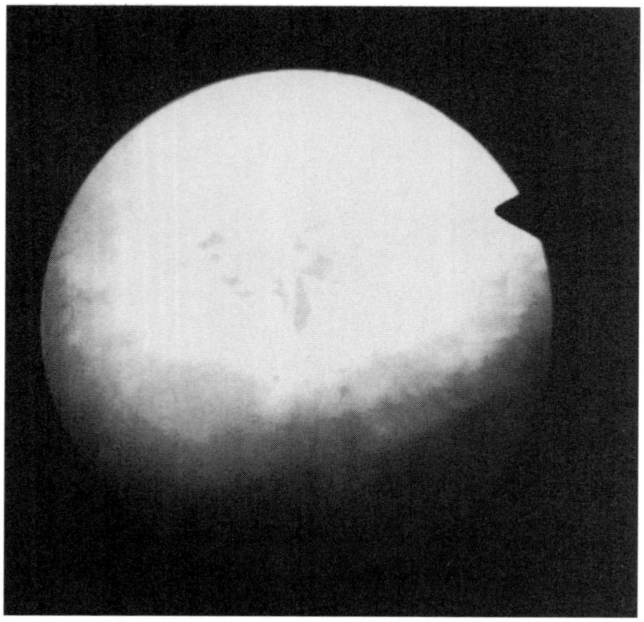

FIG. 1. Petechial hemorrhage in a bladder with interstitial cystitis.

free small bowel adhesions from the bladder and push the bowel away while a second surgeon is performing the laser photoirradiation. The laparoscopic surgeon can also watch the bladder being treated from an intraperitoneal view, enabling him to see the serosa of the bladder blanch and turn chalk white, an indication that therapy should be discontinued in an area.

The bladder needs to be treated in a constantly collapsed state. Minimal irrigation should be used; frequent emptying produces better results than using a continuous-flow cystoscope. If the bladder is distended, this will thin the bladder wall and increase the risk of forward scatter, which can result in small bowel perforation. We use the Nd:YAG laser with either a right-angle fiber or a straight 5° deflecting fiber at a power of 20 to 25 W and 2-sec pulse duration. We are careful to keep the fiber 1 to 3 mm from the bladder wall and to move the fiber continuously to avoid accumulation of laser energy in one area; we also are careful not to touch the bladder with the fiber during treatment. Total laser dosage is also limited to 25,000 J at any one treatment to prevent pelvic visceral damage.

If a Hunner's ulcer is present, this is treated until it visually turns chalk white. Then the petechial hemorrhagic areas, as well as the most severely inflamed areas, are also treated until they turn chalk white, using the same criteria. If the patient has a good response with pain relief, and multiple areas remain untreated during the first treatment, we may bring the patient back and retreat the remaining inflamed areas 6 weeks later. All patients are admitted to the hospital overnight for observation and sometimes pain control. A Foley catheter is left in place overnight, and an epidural anesthetic is frequently used for 12 to 24 hr.

COMPLICATIONS

Pelvic pain for 24 to 48 hr posttreatment is frequent, but in patients with Hunner's ulcer disease, it is often impressive how soon they notice the absence of bladder pain and decrease of frequency of urination. We have not seen small or large bowel perforation with the combina-

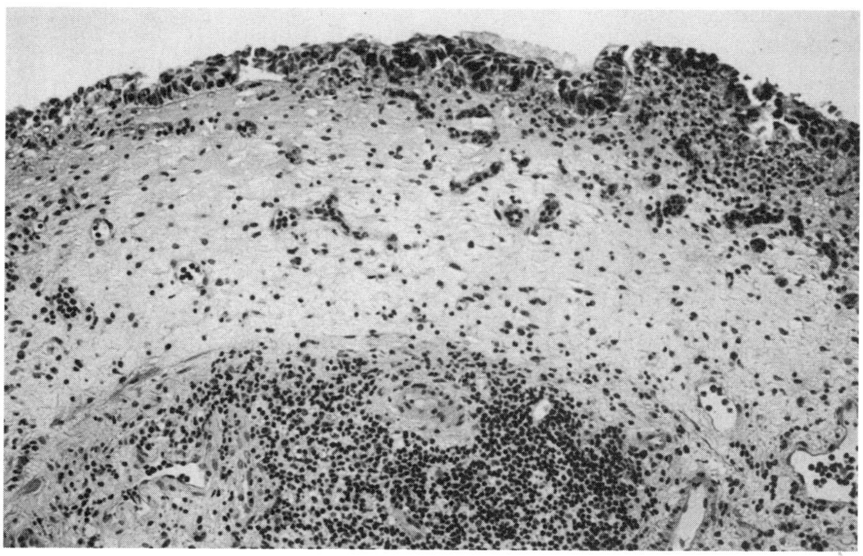

FIG. 2. Biopsy demonstrating inflammatory changes.

tion of decreased dosage, treating a collapsed bladder, and adjunctive laparoscopy, but all patients should be warned of this significant risk from laser photoirradiation of interstitial cystitis.

RESULTS

In the 10 years since our original report (8), we have accumulated experience in 59 patients treated in both institutions. In the last several years we have declined to treat patients with severe frequency alone as the component of their interstitial cystitis syndrome because the patients we treated in the earliest group with frequency alone and no pain had the poorest results from laser therapy. In the group of patients presenting with Hunner's ulcer disease, there were 28 patients. Twenty of these patients exhibited significant pain relief, decreased frequency, and improvement of their bladder capacity. This group of patients with Hunner's ulcer disease frequently exhibits the most dramatic response with rapid relief of symptoms following laser therapy.

The next group of 20 patients presented with severe pain but no evidence of Hunner's ulcer. These patients did have biopsy evidence quite consistent with IC as manifested by severe inflammatory changed described previously. Ten of these patients (50%) exhibited significant improvement in their symptom complex, again measured by decreased pain, improved bladder capacity, and general improvement in well-being. The remaining ten patients showed no significant improvement in their symptom complex.

In the last group of patients, originally treated with frequency alone as the major component of their disease (11 patients) at the beginning of our experience there was very little improvement and we have abandoned laser therapy in this sub-group of patients.

SUMMARY AND CONCLUSIONS

Laser photoirradiation of interstitial cystitis is not a cure of this disease. Many of these patients will return 1 to 2 years later with a recurrence of their symptoms of pain, and endoscopy will reveal new disease or new Hunner's ulcer in areas of the bladder not previously treated. Frequently these patients continue to obtain palliation of their symptoms from repeat laser therapy, and we have several patients who have been treated intermittently over the last 10 years and have been able to save their bladders without undergoing cystectomy. In data recently published by Gillespie (15), she has recently used a KTP laser (wavelength 532 nm) to attempt to denervate the pain fibers of the bladder by cutting these fibers alongside the ureterovesicle junction. Her results in this preliminary paper are interesting and exciting and may also shed some knowledge on the reasons our patients have had significant pain relief from our laser photoirradiation, i.e. denervation of the bladder. This observation is purely speculative at this time but may explain some of our findings.

REFERENCES

1. Domingue GJ, Ghoniem GM, Bost KL, Fermin C, Human LG. Dormant microbes in interstitial cystitis. *J Urol* 1995;153(4):1321–1326.
2. Ratliff TL, Klutke CG, Hofmeister M, He F, Russell JH, Becich J. Role of the immune response in interstitial cystitis. *Clin Immunol Immunopathol* 1995;74(3):209–216.
3. Hanno PM. Diagnosis of interstitial cystitis. *Urol Clin North Am* 1994;21(1):63–66.
4. Parsons CL, Stein PC, Bidair M, Lebow D. Abnormal sensitivity to intravesical potassium in interstitial cystitis and radiation cystitis. *Neurol Urodyn* 1994;13(5):515–520.
5. Johansson SI, Fall M. Pathology of interstitial cystitis. *Urol Clin North Am* 1994;21(1):55–62.
6. Pang XK, Cotreau-Bibbo MM, Sant GR, Theoharides TC. Bladder mast cell expression of high affinity oestrogen receptors in patients with interstitial cystitis. *Br J Urol* 1995;75(2):154–161.
7. Sant GR, Theoharides TC. The role of the mast cell in interstitial cystitis. *Urol Clin North Am* 1994;21(1):41–53.
8. Shanberg AM, Chalfin SA, Tansey LA. Treatment of interstitial cystitis with the neodymium-YAG laser. *J Urol* 1985;134:885.
9. Malloy TR, Shanberg AM. Laser therapy for interstitial cystitis. *Urol Clin North Am* 1994:21(1):141.
10. Theoharides TC: Anti-depressants, antihistamines, interstitial cystitis and cancer. *J Urol* 1995;154(4):1481.
11. Parsons CL, Housley T, Schmidt JD, Lebow D. Treatment of interstitial cystitis with intra-vesical heparin. *Br J Urol* 1994;73(5):504–507.
12. Hanno PM. Amitriptyline in the treatment of interstitial cystitis. *Urol Clin North Am* 1994;21(1):7–20.
13. Childs SJ. Dimethyl sulfone ($DMSO_2$) in the treatment of interstitial cystitis. *Urol Clin North Am* 1994;21(1):85–88.
14. Sant GR, Larock DRKL. Standard intra-vesical therapies for interstitial cystitis. *Urol Clin North Am* 1994;21(1):73–83.
15. Gillespie L. Destruction of the vesicoureteric plexus for the treatment of hypersensitive bladder disorder. *Br J Urol* 1994;74:40–43.

Interstitial Cystitis, edited by Grannum R. Sant.
Lippincott–Raven Publishers, Philadelphia ©1997.

CHAPTER 27

Electric Stimulation in the Management of Interstitial Cystitis

Philip E. V. Van Kerrebroeck

Various forms of electric stimulation have been used to treat interstitial cystitis (IC) (1). Recent studies on the effect of electric stimulation on the behavior of the bladder, urethra, and pelvic floor in various forms of lower urinary tract dysfunction have sparked new interest in the treatment possibilities of electric stimulation in IC (2). Moreover, the increasing evidence of a neurogenic origin of entities such as detrusor instability, urgency–frequency syndromes, urethral syndrome, and the pelvic pain syndrome make it logical to suspect a role for neurogenic dysfunction in the genesis of classical interstitial cystitis (3–6).

In the past, several treatment modalities for IC have been proposed that resulted in an interruption or destruction of the afferent innervation of the bladder or blockade of the sensory nerve ends of the bladder mucosa. Endoresection of ulcers (7), cystolysis (8), and deafferentation at the level of the sacral roots (9) or at the level of the spinal cord (10) all produced immediate relief of symptoms as a consequence of inhibition of sensory information. Moreover, anterolateral chordotomy resulted in relief not only of the symptoms but also of the pathologic aspect of the disease (10).

Bladder distention (11) and dimethylsulfoxide instillations (12) as well as topical application of local anaesthetics similarly exert their action by changing sensory nerve endings (13).

Application of transcutaneous electric nerve stimulation (TENS) is another form of treatment that aims at relieving pain in conditions of various etiologies by influencing sensory signals. Experience with two different applications, intravaginal and suprapubic stimulation, has existed for several years, although the number of well-conducted studies is limited. A newer form of therapy is the application of current directly in the neighborhood of the sacral nerves (neuromodulation).

INTRAVAGINAL ELECTRIC STIMULATION

Intravaginal electric stimulation (IVS) has been widely used to inhibit the hyperactive bladder with good results (14). Therefore, empirically, several patients with other forms of functional problems of the lower urinary tract, including interstitial cystitis, have been treated with intravaginal electric stimulation. However, the number of well-controlled studies on the use of intravaginal electric stimulation in classic interstitial cystitis is very limited. Moreover, the results of these studies were rather disappointing in terms of the subjective effect of the treatment as well as tolerance for the method itself.

With acute stimulation under anaesthesia, bladder capacity could be increased in patients with interstitial cystitis. Because of these initial results, chronic stimulation has been applied. A flexible electrode carrier mounted on an inflatable device was used with alternating pulses of 10 Hz and a pulse width of 2 ms. The voltage was adjusted by the patients to a level at which stimulation was perceived. The appliance was used continuously during daytime and stopped at night. Only a limited number of patients, generally with the combination of interstitial cystitis and detrusor instability, continued the treatment on a chronic basis (15). The major drawback of IVS was pain and hypersensitivity to pressure during the treatment. Because several months of treatment is necessary to obtain an effect, the majority of patients gave up this treatment.

A trial with randomization between intravaginal electric stimulation and transcutaneous electric stimulation

P. E. V. Van Kerrebroeck: Department of Urology, University Hospital Maastricht, NI 6202 AZ Maastricht, The Netherlands.

revealed several advantages of this latter method, and therefore, IVS is now rarely used in patients with interstitial cystitis.

TRANSCUTANEOUS ELECTRIC STIMULATION IN INTERSTITIAL CYSTITIS

Transcutaneous electric stimulation (TENS) is used extensively in a number of pain conditions. It is a cheap and noninvasive method that can influence the sensory signals from a painful area.

The primary intention with the use of peripheral electric stimulation is to relieve pain by stimulation of myelinated afferents in order to activate segmental inhibitory circuits (16). The probable mechanism of action of TENS is through the so-called "gate-control" system (17). Because of its reported effects on motoric dysfunction of the lower urinary tract, TENS may be suspected to have a direct effect on reflexes controlling autonomic functions (18).

Generally, a device is used consisting of a pulse generator with amplifier and two electrodes. The pulses may be delivered continuously or as trains of stimulation. Continuous stimulation seems to be preferable for treating pain conditions. Biphasic pulses are preferable because of the resulting zero net charge flow with this pulse type. This results in reduction of electrochemical reactions at the contact site between electrodes and tissue. However, because of their technical simplicity, many devices use unipolar rectangular pulses, and there have been no reports of serious complications. Frequencies used for TENS vary from 1 to 100 Hz. No systematic evaluation of the optimal frequency has been performed, and 50 Hz seems to be most commonly used. Short pulses (0.1 to 0.2 msec) are most effective in terms of charge transfer for a threshold effect to activate a peripheral nerve.

Two carbon-rubber electrodes are used, which permits excitation of afferent fibers without significant side effects. Because the size of the electrodes has an influence on the current density obtained, a minimum of 4 cm^2 has been advised (19).

The stimulus intensity required to elicit sensation of stimulation and the threshold for pain sensation varies between individuals. In general, the maximum tolerable intensity is used. Although other sites, perineal and even tibial, have been successfully explored, the electrodes are most commonly placed in the suprapubic region 10 to 15 cm apart, immediately above the symphysis pubis (20–22).

Perhaps one of the most important factors for successful treatment of interstitial cystitis with TENS is the counseling of the patient. Specially trained nurses or therapists are best able to instruct the patient and to take the time necessary in the initial phase as well as during the follow-up. The time necessary for TENS to produce a significant effect on the bladder symptoms varies widely. The effect, however, is cumulative but rather slow to appear in interstitial cystitis. The standard recommendation is to start with 0.5 to 2 hr of treatment twice daily, but the duration of a treatment session will depend on the severity of the pain.

Results with suprapubic TENS in well-controlled studies are scarce. One study mentions 60 patients, 33 of whom were classified as having classic interstitial cystitis (with Hunner's ulcer at cystoscopy), and 27 with nonulcer cystitis (23). High- or low-frequency TENS (2 to 50 Hz) was used, with the patients advised to start with the high frequency. If there was no effect within 1 month, low-frequency stimulation was to be used instead. Some patients reported a faster effect with low-frequency stimulation, but the muscle twitches were experienced as unpleasant by some. The majority of patients continued with the high-frequency TENS treatment. Follow-up is present from 9 months to 17 years. Overall, the effect of TENS was more marked on the bladder pain than on the micturition frequency. In nine patients there was a remission of symptoms after treatment for more than 1 year. However, the majority of the patients had to use the stimulator intermittently to remain free of symptoms. Some patients underwent cystoscopy several years after treatment and relief of their symptoms. Interestingly, disappearance of the local lesions or of the bleeding after dilation was found (20).

MAXIMAL PELVIC FLOOR STIMULATION

Maximal pelvic floor stimulation by means of vaginal and anal electrodes has yielded good results in a preliminary study (22). These series mainly comprised women with the nonulcer type of interstitial cystitis. Further experience and well-controlled studies are required to confirm these results. At present, no such studies are available, and current information is mainly predicated on case presentations.

DIRECT SACRAL NERVE STIMULATION

Based on the suspected role for neurogenic dysfunction in the genesis of classical interstitial cystitis (3–6), direct sacral nerve stimulation has recently been explored in the treatment of interstitial cystitis. The actual form of this type of electric stimulation with surgically implanted devices is defined as neuromodulation (2). Neuromodulation, however, is a general name indicating an invasive technique of electric stimulation with physiological mechanisms in common with TENS. Neural stimulation with implanted electrodes is explored in various forms of dysfunction of the lower urinary tract because these syndromes are associated with labile sacral reflex behavior, and the dampening of sacral nerve excitability is associated with a therapeutic benefit.

The advantage of the method is that, before implantation of a permanent electrode, trial stimulation can be performed with a temporary percutaneous electrode. During this 3- to 4-day period of temporary stimulation, information can be collected on the subjective effect of the stimulation. The objective effect can be judged based on the voiding diaries. Such a test or trial period of stimulation has proven to be an effective way to assess the therapeutic potential of chronic sacral nerve stimulation. The S_3 nerve is most frequently used. A wire electrode (3-0 flexon pacer wire) or a thin temporary electrode is inserted into the foramen via an angiocath guide or a special needle and connected to an external pulse generator (Medtronic Inc., Minneapolis, MN). The stimulation is continued for 3 to 4 days with a fixed pulse width of 200 μsec and a frequency setting of 15 Hz. If the trial is successful, then the patient can be considered for implantation of a permanent neural prosthesis. A permanent electrode with four contact points is then placed in the foramen that corresponds to the sacral nerve tested and connected to a pulse generator (Itrell-II, Medtronics Interstim, Maastricht, The Netherlands). The parameters of stimulation can be programmed with an external programmer. The amplitude is set at a comfortable level with a frequency of 10 Hz and a pulse width of 200 μsec. The method seems to be safe over the years, and the clinical effect persistent.

Various disease entities have been treated with this type of stimulation, including a limited number of patients with interstitial cystitis. In a review chapter on this method of stimulation, patients with interstitial cystitis are classified among the female dysfunctional voiding syndromes (24). Of a total of 71 patients with voiding dysfunction, 50 (70.4%) showed a very significant symptom improvement. However, 21 (29.6%) were unaffected by the stimulation. The author states that this form of stimulation is more efective in managing symptoms associated with identifiable muscle function than symptoms that are mostly sensory in nature. The results so far support the view that the therapeutic benefit is a result of modulation of neural reflex excitability.

The (limited) experience with neuroprosthetic implants has shown that electric stimulation can be used on a long-term basis to treat problems of voiding dysfunction. The exact place of this treatment modality in interstitial cystitis, however, still has to be determined with further clinical experience.

CONCLUSIONS

The experience with the use of electric stimulation in patients with interstitial cystitis is based on open, non-controlled studies with small numbers of patients. Because of the lack of reported benefits in a significant percentage of patients, few centers have adopted these techniques as part of their standard treatment algorithms. It is common experience that electric stimulation for pain treatment involves a significant placebo effect. Therefore, controlled studies in this field are difficult to design. Another problem is the lack of adequate and objective tools to measure pain reduction. A strong argument in favor of electric stimulation is the fact that the beneficial effect of electric stimulation exceeds the reported placebo effect in placebo-controlled drug studies (25,26).

This finding is in agreement with the general experience that the magnitude of placebo effect in interstitial cystitis is rather low. The finding of objective cystoscopic amelioration after TENS treatment suggests that the effects are based on organic changes, at least in some patients.

The reported effects of TENS, along with a long-term follow-up and the parallel disappearance of objective signs and symptoms, are a sufficient basis for further research and clinical application of this technique. For patients resistant to all forms of conservative treatment and who are at the point of accepting invasive and often mutilating surgery, neuromodulation offers an attractive alternative.

REFERENCES

1. Fall M, Erlandson B, Sundin T. Intravaginal electrical stimulation: clinical experiments on bladder inhibition. *Scand J Urol Nephrol* 1978; 44(Suppl):41–47.
2. Tanagho EA, Schmidt RA. Electrical stimulation in the management of the neurogenic bladder. *J Urol* 1988;140:1331–1335.
3. Pariver F, Bradbook RA. Interstitial cystitis. *Br J Urol* 1986;58:239–244.
4. Christmas TJ, Rode J, Chapple CR. Nerve fibre proliferation in interstitial cystitis. *Virchows Arch* 1990;416:447–451.
5. Hanno P, Levin RM, Monson FC. Diagnosis of interstitial cystitis. *J Urol* 1990;143:278–281.
6. Hohenfellner M, Nunes L, Schmidt RA. Interstitial cystitis: increased sympathetic innervation and related neuropeptide synthesis. *J Urol* 1992;147:587–591.
7. Greenberg E, Barnes R, Stewart S. Transurethral resection of Hunner's ulcer. *J Urol* 1974;111:764–766.
8. Worth PHL, Turner-Warwick RT. The treatment of interstitial cystitis by cystolysis with observations on cystoplasty. *Br J Urol* 1973;45:65–71.
9. Meirowsky AM. The management of chronic interstitial cystitis by differential sacral neurotomy. *J Neurosurg* 1969;30:604–607.
10. Nesbit RM. Anterolateral chordotomy for refractory interstitial cystitis with intractable pain. *J Urol* 1947;57:741–744.
11. Dunn M, Ramsden PD, Roberts JBM. Interstitial cystitis treated by prolonged bladder distention. *Br J Urol* 1977;49:641–654.
12. Sant GS. Intravesical 50% dimethyl sulfoxide (RIMS-50) in treatment of interstitial cystitis. *Urology* 1987;29(Suppl):17–21.
13. Aldenborg F, Fall M, Enerback L. Proliferation and transepithelial migration of mucosal mast cells in interstitial cystitis. *Immunology* 1986;58:411–416.
14. Fall M, Erlandson BE, Sundin T, Waagstien F. Intravaginal electrical stimulation. Clinical experiments on bladder inhibition. *Scand J Urol Nephrol* 1977;44(Suppl):41–47.
15. Fall M. Use of transcutaneous electrical nerve stimulation in the management of chronic interstitial cystitis. In: Hanno PM, Staskin DR, Krane RJ, Wein AJ, eds. *Interstitial Cystitis.* London: Springer Verlag, 1990;169–173.
16. Fall M. Transcutaneous electrical nerve stimulation in interstitial cystitis: up-date on clinical experience. *Urology* 1987;24(suppl):40–42.
17. Melzack R, Wall PD. Pain mechanisms: a new theory. *Science* 1965; 150:971–979.
18. de Groat WC. Excitation and inhibition of sacral parasympathetic neurons by visceral and cutaneous stimuli in the cat. *Brain Res* 1971;18: 499–503.

19. Woolf CJ. Segmental afferent fibre-induced analgesia: transcutaneous electrical nerve stimulation and vibration. In: Melzack R, Wall PD, eds. *Textbook of Pain,* 2nd ed. London: Churchill Livingstone, 1989; 884–896.
20. Fall M, Carlsson CA, Erlandson BE. Electrical stimulation in interstitial cystitis. *J Urol* 1980;123:192–195.
21. McGuire EJ, Shi-Chun Z, Horwinski ER, Lytton B. Treatment of motor sensory detrusor instability by electrical stimulation. *J Urol* 1983;129: 78–79.
22. Eriksen BC. Painful bladder disease in woman: effect of maximal electric pelvic floor stimulation. *Neurourol Urodyn* 1989;8:362–363.
23. Fall M, Lindström S. Transcutaneous electrical nerve stimulation in classic and nonulcer interstitial cystitis. *Urol Clin North Am* 1994; 21:131–139.
24. Schmidt RA. Neurostimulation of bladder and urethra. In: Webster G, Kirby R, King L, Goldwasser B, eds. *Reconstructive Urology.* Boston: Blackwell Scientific Publications, 1993;591–601.
25. Holm-Bentzen M, Jacobsen F, Nerström B. A prospective double-blind clinically controlled multicenter trial of sodium pentosanpolysulfate in the treatment of interstitial cystitis and related painful bladder disease. *J Urol* 1987;138:503–507.
26. Mulholland SG, Sant GR, Hanno P. Pentosan polysulphate sodium for therapy of interstitial cystitis: a double-blind placebo-controlled clinical study. *Urology* 1990;35:552–556.

Interstitial Cystitis, edited by Grannum R. Sant.
Lippincott–Raven Publishers, Philadelphia ©1997.

CHAPTER 28

Surgical Treatment of Interstitial Cystitis

Markus Hohenfellner, Jürgen Linn, Christian Hampel, Joachim W. Thüroff

At the turn of the century, when interstitial cystitis was first gaining recognition as a clinical entity (1–4), only limited possibilities for conservative treatment existed. As a result, the decades immediately following witnessed the development of a variety of surgical therapies. Then, as now, it was generally agreed that conservative treatments should be exhausted before surgery was considered. This requirement became progressively more complicated as investigations into the cause and pathophysiology of interstitial cystitis (both still largely undetermined) resulted in many hypotheses, some highly controversial. Nevertheless, many of these hypotheses provoked new forms of conservative treatment.

Not all patients assigned the diagnosis of interstitial cystitis have the same disease (5). Patients with pelvic pain and sensory urgency and frequency despite a large anatomic bladder capacity are included along with those with small, contracted bladders. Second, many patients exhibit significant interaction between their somatic disease and their personality, leaving doctors undecided whether the patient's psychological status is the origin or the result of the condition (6–8). Third, tragic outcomes of highly invasive surgical approaches to interstitial cystitis have been observed (9,10). Thus, it seems crucial to exhaust all conservative means beforehand. However, in the face of a growing number of available but often ineffective forms of conservative treatment, patients understandably are reluctant to await relief of the irritating and painful symptoms that restrict their lives (8). This may explain why these patients have a tendency to change physicians, a phenomenon observed over 40 years ago (8,11). Each start with a new physician brings the possibility that the patient will be exposed anew to a full cycle of conservative treatment. Actually, to many patients, the possibility of a surgical solution is never even mentioned (8), even though 10% to 28% (12,13) may be eligible for operative intervention. Although we do not advocate the surgical approach as an early form of treatment, we believe that the initial outlining of a step-by-step approach to interstitial cystitis should raise the possibility of surgery in the event of failure of conservative therapy. This helps patients keep faith with the variety of conservative options. Additionally, the patient's ordeal may be shortened significantly by diagnostic measurements that make clear where conservative therapy is likely to fail.

M. Hohenfellner, J. Linn, C. Hampel, J. W. Thüroff: Department of Urology, University of Mainz, 55101 Mainz, Germany.

DIAGNOSTIC EVALUATION

The diagnostic workup should be extensive and include psychological and pathophysiological aspects (14). Even in these cost-conscious times, the patient with interstitial cystitis should not be operated on in haste. It is essential to obtain a thorough history, including such factors as family and professional environments, nutritional habits, and any previous conservative efforts, to get a feeling for the patients and their wishes. Few things are worse than the outcome of unsuccessful surgery for pelvic pain and/or bladder discomfort when the pelvic organs in actuality are not the origin but rather the target of pathologic sensations (9).

The clinical workup must be complete as well. Entities that mimic the symptoms of interstitial cystitis, such as bacterial urinary tract infections, urinary stones, tumors in the small pelvis, neurologic disorders, and particularly carcinoma *in situ* of the bladder (especially in men) must be excluded (7,15–18). Thus, cystoscopy under anesthesia is an integral part of the workup, not only to measure anatomic bladder capacity but also to biopsy the bladder for related histopathology and to exclude carcinoma *in situ* (19,20). The initial finding of a small, contracted bladder with only a low anatomic capacity may forestall long and erratic trials of conservative treatment that will never be able to restore the compliance of the chronically inflamed and consequently disintegrated bladder wall. Anatomic bladder capacity may not only be used as a prognostic tool for the value of conservative treatment; it may also help to decide the type of surgical approach (20). In patients in whom bladder capacity is normal, surgical approaches aimed at restoring bladder function may be considered. In contrast, in patients in whom anatomic bladder capacity has been lost, reconstructive surgery is needed (19–23).

TRANSURETHRAL SURGERY

Hunner explored various kinds of transurethral treatments such as bladder overdistention (the "Young method") and chemical or electric ulcer fulguration in 1918 (2). None of these procedures proved to give satisfactory results, so he concluded, "We are not surprised that excision (of the ulcers) is the only method of cure" (2). Nevertheless, transurethral treatments continued (7,15,24–30), even though various authors agreed that in most cases they provided only temporary relief. Badenoch went one step further when he deliberately distended the bladder until it perforated—without success, as the symptoms recurred (24). He also speculated that the effects of cystodiathermy may result from the accompanying bladder dilation (24).

NEUROUROLOGIC PROCEDURES

The clinical symptoms of urgency and pain in interstitial cystitis correlate with histopathologic findings of altered bladder innervation (7,31–34). Surgical procedures to manipulate the innervation to reduce the bladder's hypersensitivity and reconstruct its storage function have been implemented at different neural levels.

Peripheral Denervation

One of the first to report surgical treatment of interstitial cystitis was Hunner in 1918 (2). Having at that time only a few conservative or transurethral techniques at hand, he opted for open surgical control of the elusive bladder ulcers. Although the rationale for this approach was the assumption that the main causative factor was a focal infection (7,26,30,35,36), one may speculate that in fact the surgical technique resulted—at least to some extent—in a peripheral denervation of the bladder. To gain the appropriate surgical access, Hunner freed the bladder from its surrounding tissues, and, if an ulcer was located at the posterior wall or the bottom, he detached the peritoneum completely as well (2). Over an 18-year period Hunner reported on 19 patients who underwent open surgery; of these, one died postoperatively, four experienced recurrence of symptoms after a mean interval of 13.5 months, and 14 (73.6%) were cured (follow-up unspecified). The late results, however, have been unsatisfactory, with symptoms recurring within 3 years, bringing this type of operation into general disrepute (11,30,37). Both Counseller and Badenoch, who repeated this procedure unsuccessfully in two patients, confirmed these findings (21,24).

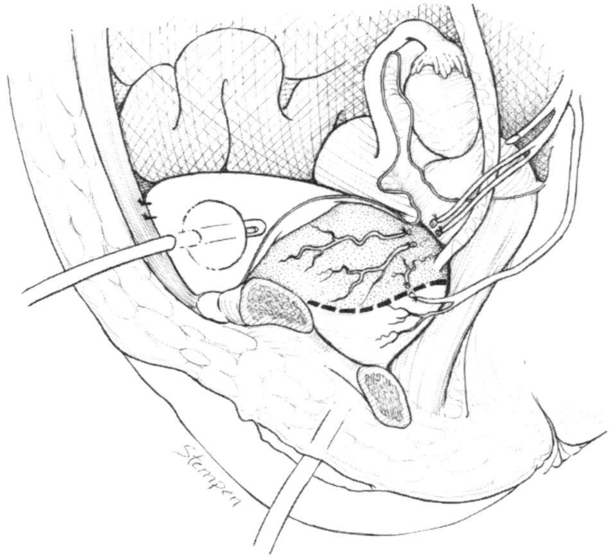

FIG. 1. Technique of cystolysis (20). Division of the superior vesical vessels and of the ascending branches of the inferior vessels via a posterior dissection down to the trigone (*dashed line* marks limit of dissection). A patch of peritoneum covering the bladder dome is sutured to the M. rectus to prevent bladder contraction during catheter drainage.

At the start of the 1970s, a similar surgical maneuver, cystolysis, was developed by Worth and Turner-Warwick to denervate the bladder peripherally (20) (Fig. 1). In their initial report, all ten patients found relief from their bladder pain, with the technique called a complete success in three and an improvement in four. A follow-up report 7 years later continued to advocate this technique (38).

Because it is impossible for a surgeon to distinguish sensory from motor fibers at this peripheral level, this procedure must affect the lower motor neuron of the bladder as well. Although Worth and Turner-Warwick did not detail the postoperative mode of bladder evacuation, Freiha and Stamey, who repeated the procedure, observed the need for Valsalva to empty the bladder in all six of their patients (39). Over a follow-up of 1.6 years, they observed a success rate of 50%. Their publication was followed by an editorial comment by Bruce H. Stewart, who wrote: "Unfortunately, most previously described bladder denervation procedures have fallen into disrepute because of high late recurrence rates. Because of the relatively short follow-up in the present series, the ultimate

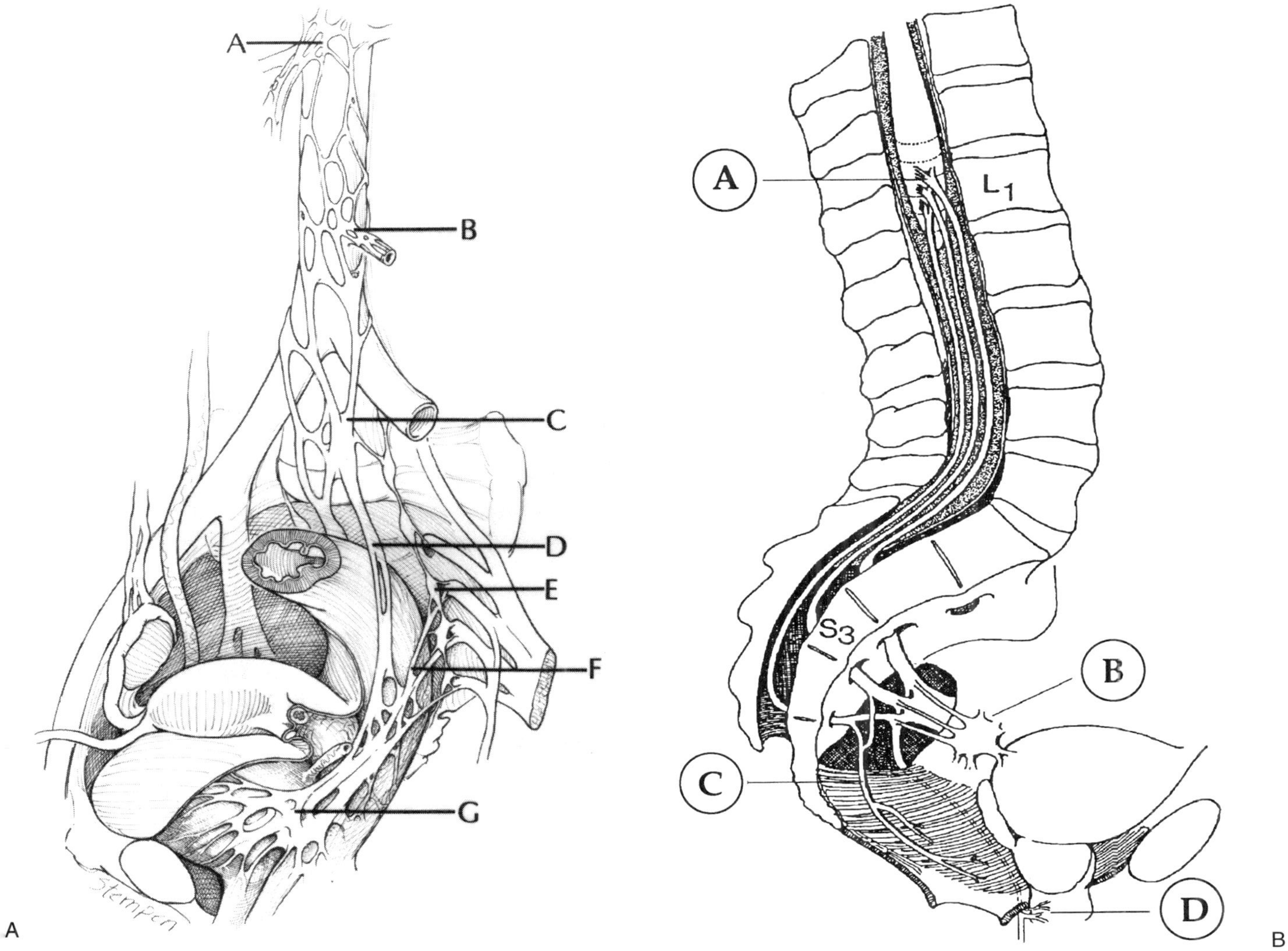

FIG. 2. Topographic anatomy of the bladder innervation. **(A)** Sympathetic and parasympathetic pathways. A, Plexus mesentericus superior; B, Arteria mesenterica inferior; C, Plexus hypogastricus superior (presacral nerve); D, Nervus hypogastricus sinister; E, Truncus sympathicus sinister; F, Nervus splanchnicus pelvicus; G, Plexus hypogastricus inferior (plexus pelvicus). **(B)** Parasympathetic and somatomotoric pathways. A, Parasympathetic sacral micturition center and somatomotoric Nucleus onuf (S_2–$S_{4/5}$); B, Plexus pelvicus; C, Nn. musculus levatori ani; D, N. pudendus.

value of this procedure will not become apparent for some time to come"(40). This skeptical judgment was confirmed by Albers and Geyer, who reported a mean 5.3-year follow-up after cystolysis (41). Seven of their 11 patients experienced recurrence of all preoperative symptoms within 4 years, three patients showed an intermediate subjective response without complete relief, and one patient had a good subjective response over 7.5 years.

Sympathetic Surgery

At the end of the last century, Jaboulay reasoned that visceral perception of pain may be transmitted to the central nervous system via nerve fibers running with the sympathetic nerves (42) (Fig. 2A). This hypothesis was used as the basis for the rationalization of the following early indications for sympathetic surgery: perineal and pelvic neuralgia (42,43), microvascular pathology (44), vaginismus, sexual hyperexcitability, and masturbation (45). Subsequently, its application was validated for management of various states of vascular disease and pain (46–51).

These therapeutic principles were first applied to the lower urinary tract by Gino Pieri in 1926. He believed that histologic evidence of malnutrition of the bladder wall suggested that periarterial nerve fibers were involved in the sclerotic thickening of the local blood vessels (52). As a consequence, he resected the superior hypogastric plexus (presacral nerve), both paravertebral sympathetic chains at the level of the sacral promontory, and the gray rami from the first, second, and third sacral ganglia to the corresponding sacral nerves (53). Learmonth then clinically confirmed Jaboulay's theory of sympathetic pain perception (54,55), evidence that is increasingly solid today (56,57). In 1931, Learmonth reported four patients with interstitial cystitis in whom he had performed a neurectomy of the superior mesenteric plexus. He considered the procedure a success in two, an improvement in one, and a failure in the fourth but pointed out his extremely short follow-up of a maximum of 4 months (54). Meticulous recording of micturition diaries revealed a marked but only transitory increase in frequency and a decrease of functional bladder capacity between the third and fifth postoperative days, a phenomenon also observed by Douglass (37). Learmonth speculated that this might be attributable to the inhibitory function of the sympathetics on smooth muscle contractility, and thus, he contributed one of the few clinical observations on a subject that has still not been explored experimentally. Douglass noted in three of five patients a significant relief of pain after excision of the superior mesenteric plexus (37). As in Learmonth's patients, none of his experienced complete recovery, although it was enough that they felt the operation was justified. He attributed the residual hypersensitivity to the preserved sensory fibers running in the dorsal sacral roots. The complete failures he considered to result from anatomic variations that might divert the sympathetic innervation through pathways other than the presacral nerve (37). Similar favorable results were reported by Nesbit after presacral neurectomy without division of the lateral sympathetics in six cases with a maximum follow-up of 11 months (58) and by Scott and Schroeder, who resected the superior mesenteric plexus and the upper part of the sacral sympathetic chain (including the first and second sacral ganglia) in three patients and considered two significantly improved (59).

The late results of sympathectomy were disappointing as it became clear that what Ormond had stated in 1935 was true: "The immediate results in most instances are good: there is relief from pain, and the frequency is lessened. But recurrence or gradual relapse is the rule." Correspondingly, Nesbit wrote 8 years after his initial publication, "The benefits that follow sympathectomy are of temporary nature only" (60). The same applied to the series of Learmonth. Jacobson et al., in 1944, reviewed all the Mayo Clinic patients in whom presacral neurectomy had been performed, among them 33 patients with interstitial cystitis who had been operated on by Learmonth (61) during the preceding 13 years. Long-term relief of pain was complete in three patients, partial in nine, and absent in 21, while frequency remained unaffected in most.

Parasympathetic Surgery

In the late 1940s, Heimburger et al. in clinical trials showed the S_2 to S_4 segment to supply the predominant innervation to the human bladder, the third sacral nerve being the most important (62) (Fig. 2B). In light of these findings and the long-term results of sympathetic surgery for interstitial cystitis, the value of parasympathetic surgery began to be investigated by several groups in the early 1950s. Moulder and Meirowsky, a urologist and a neurosurgeon at Vanderbilt University, had already contributed extensive work on the innervation of the neurogenic bladder and its surgical modification (63,64). To gain a predictive assessment on the possible effects of sacral rhizotomy in interstitial cystitis, they subjected their patients first to a bilateral S_3 sacral block with procaine. If symptoms were relieved and bladder capacity increased, a bilateral S_3 neurectomy was performed. This procedure was performed on two patients in 1954 (23) and on another in 1967. A follow-up report on all three was published in 1969 (22). At that time they were free of symptoms and had an average bladder capacity of 275 to 500 ml. Based on these observations, Milner and Garlick (65) and Mason et al. (66) repeated the Moulder–Meirowsky procedure on a total of ten patients with a follow-up of 15 months (6 to 18 months). The six patients in the first group showed an increase of functional bladder capacity from 108 to 311 ml; five were completely free of symptoms, and ulcerations (evident preoperatively) were healed. One patient had persistent pain and bleeding as a result of mucosal cracking and ulceration, although her frequency was relieved; she was the only patient in the series who had undergone an earlier surgical attempt in the form of partial cystectomy (65). In the second group, Mason et al. judged the outcome to be successful in three of four patients. In a third report, one patient with a left-sided S_2 and a bilateral S_3 sacral rhizotomy continued to enjoy a good result after 5 years (67).

In contrast to these investigators, who had sectioned the whole S_3 spinal nerve, including its ventral and dorsal roots, Bohm and Franksson modified this procedure (68). Previously, they had defined the spinal segments carrying the sensory afferents of the bladder (69) and conducted clinical investigations that led them to the conclusion that the phenomenon of pain in the small pelvis may arise from pathologic changes of the sacral nerve roots (70). Combining these findings with the observation that the symptoms of interstitial cystitis appear to constitute a condition of hypersensitivity and pain, they sectioned only the dorsal sacral roots in seven patients. This was done uni- or bilaterally on one to three segments. The side and number of segments on which the deafferentation was performed were decided on the basis of symptoms and endoscopic findings. One additional patient underwent unilateral sectioning of the dorsal and ventral sacral S_3 spinal nerve. The outcome was inconclusive. Pain was abolished in only one patient and nearly abolished in a second, while the others continued to experience considerable pain. Frequency was normalized in one patient, five patients had postoperative voiding intervals from 2 to 4 hr, and two patients had no relief. The bladder volume remained unchanged, and cystoscopically detectable lesions persisted, in all patients, although in two they healed on the side of the rhizotomy. The overall degree of success was unrelated to the unilateral or bilateral nature of the dorsal rhizotomies.

In this total of 22 patients who underwent sacral rhizotomy, the following complications and side effects were encountered: a postoperative wound infection in one, an atonic bladder of 1 month's duration in one (66), temporary hypalgesia in two, perineal numbness in one, and absent Achilles reflex in one (65).

Other Neurourologic Procedures

The most central type of denervation ever performed for interstitial cystitis has been anterolateral chordotomy. Probably the first case, performed in 1923 by Frazier and associates, was a 33-year-old woman with "intense vaginal and bladder pain extending down to sole of left foot...probably due to ulcers in bladder" (71). She was free of pain for almost 1 year after right unilateral chordotomy of the fifth thoracic segment. Subsequently, right-sided recurrence of pain was treated by a second chordotomy of the left third thoracic segment, after which she remained free of symptoms for the remaining follow-up (8 years). Side effects were transitory urinary retention and weakness of her lower limbs for about 3 weeks; complete loss of pain persisted, although so did her loss of temperature sense up to 2 inches above the umbilicus (71). Four further patients were subjected to anterolateral chordotomy by Nesbit, and all results were reported as successful after a mean follow-up of 11 months (3 to 24 months) (60). Although no significant complications and side effects have been reported and the procedure has been favorably rated by others (7,11,72), no further reports are extant.

Although temporary electrostimulation showed long-term success rates that were regarded as excellent in 20% of patients with ulcerous interstitial cystitis (73), similar results could not be obtained by chronic electrostimulation in the form of sacral neuromodulation. In our own series, 11 patients underwent percutaneous test stimulation (acute and subchronic sacral neuromodulation) that was judged successful in three. Despite the encouraging initial performance in these three patients, the system subsequently implanted for chronic sacral neuromodulation failed to achieve a reliable beneficial effect. This observation is consistent with others' (R.A. Schmidt, *personal communication*).

A totally different approach to interstitial cystitis was described by Gillespie et al. (74), based on their evaluation of ten patients in whom urgency, frequency, and pelvic pain led to the diagnosis of interstitial cystitis. The symptoms were attributed to a lateral compression of the L_5 nerve root, which was relieved by decompressive surgery. This procedure resulted in immediate relief of pain in nine of their ten patients who were followed for 6 months. However, in an MRI-based study of our own group that included 22 patients, the findings of Gillespie et al. could not be confirmed (75). Only one of the 22 had an intervertebral disk prolapse, and this patient had experienced ischialgia on the ipsilateral side for the previous 30 years. The differences in these two studies may derive from different criteria employed to confirm the diagnosis of interstitial cystitis. Additionally, it remains unclear in which way an L_5 compression could affect the function of the urinary bladder from a neurophysiological point of view.

FUNCTIONAL RECONSTRUCTION OF THE LOWER URINARY TRACT WITH INTESTINAL SEGMENTS

Bladder Augmentation: Orthotopic Bladder Substitution

Because interstitial cystitis is a benign disease that does not require radical surgery in the small pelvis, orthotopic reconstruction of the lower urinary tract is the prevailing therapeutic choice. Functional as well as aesthetic reasons make it the most widely used technique. However, it is also the technique that has produced the most controversial results, with success rates varying between 25% (10) and 100% (6,25,76) (Table 1). Any critical analysis that attempts to clarify these discrepancies must focus on three issues: indications, technique of the surgical approach to the detrusor, and technique of bladder augmentation/substitution.

To start with the last, the literature reveals that, although many different techniques of bladder augmentation have been used over the past decades, the outcome with regard to symptoms has not varied: neither the type of intestinal segment used nor the shape formed seems to play a significant role. Today there is, of course, widespread consensus that, for functional urodynamic reasons, any type of intestinal segment used for urinary storage should be detubularized (77,78). Actually, the first patient subjected to ileocystoplasty by Goodwin was a woman with a 10-year history of intractable interstitial cystitis. Her outcome as well as that of a second woman with interstitial cystitis was rated as excellent—in fact the only two excellent results among the first 14 patients with

TABLE 1. *Results of supra- or subtrigonal bladder resection and augmentation*

First author	Cystectomy (supra-/subtrigonal)	Number of patients	Success rate (%)	Follow-up (months)
Bejany (76)	Sub	5	100	52
Badenoch (24)	Supra	9	55	?
Bruce (25)	Supra	8	100[a]	36
Freiha (13)	Supra	6	67	23
Goodwin (6)	Supra	2 (3)[b]	100	18
Guillonneau (80)	Supra	8	88/75[c]	23
Hohenfellner (89)	Sub	17	82/71[d]	73
Hohenfellner (89)	Supra	6	100	26
Holm-Bentzen (84)	Supra	6	83	60
Kontturi (83)	Supra	12	83	56
Nielsen (10)	Supra	8	25	10
Nurse (29)[e]	Supra	24	70	?
Nurse (29)[f]	Supra	12	83	?
von Garrelts (79)	Supra	13	93	40
Webster (81)	Supra	19	63	38

[a]One patient required reoperation because of insufficient bladder resection.
[b]One of three patients died on the tenth postoperative day from acute coronary thrombosis.
[c]Seven patients are free of symptoms; one of these has stress incontinence grade III.
[d]Fourteen patients are free of symptoms; of these, two require conversion (one from stress incontinence grade III and one from chronic pyelonephritis).
[e]Without preoperative trigonal biopsies.
[f]With preoperative trigonal biopsies.

that type of bladder augmentation. Good to excellent results were also reported by others with ileum (24,25, 79–81), ileocecum (10,15,17,81–83), cecum (79,84), right colon (24,81), and sigmoid colon (25,79,80,82,83), independent of whether these segments were detubularized (10,25,80,81,83) or not (15,17,18,79,80,82–84). Conversely, failures were reported with the same techniques (10,24,79–81,83).

For the surgical approach to the detrusor, there is a silent but nearly general agreement that at least the supratrigonal part of the bladder should be resected. In only a few reports was the detrusor not resected, and in these the outcome was universally unfavorable (83,85). Bruce et al. (25) and Webster and Maggio (81) reported one case each in which bladder had been removed insufficiently at the first operation with resultant recurrence of symptoms; a second operation with excision of the bladder remnant down to the trigone in the first report and the bladder neck in the second solved the problem. In our own experience, three patients in whom ileum bladder augmentation had been performed at other institutions without previous detrusor resection came to us because the procedure had failed to improve their condition. They then underwent secondary supravesical diversion.

Most authors perform supratrigonal resection of the bladder (10,24,25,39,79–86); only a few perform subtrigonal resection in some (29,84) or all (76,87) of their patients (Figs. 3 and 4). The advantage of trigone preservation is that the ureteral orifices are left *in situ,* obviating ureteral reimplantation with its associated pitfalls; the disadvantage is that the trigone may be the source of symptom persistence or recurrence. Aiding the decision may be the histopathologic findings and clinical results. Hunner described the lesions as located in the free portion of the bladder (the trigone represents the fixed portion) in all of his 18 patients (2). Hand found that, in 223 patients, about half the minimal lesions were in the trigone–base area, whereas the greatest number of the advanced lesions either involved the whole of the bladder or were confined to the dome (7). Smith and Dehner reported trigone involvement in two of 28 cases (88), Nurse et al. in 13 of 25 (29), and Nielsen et al. in one of seven patients (10). However, only a few investigators (29,85) attributed failure to the retained trigone. Actually, the abovementioned success rates between 25% and 100% (Table 1) were all achieved with supratrigonal detrusor resection; therefore, the resection line seems not to be the exclusive critical issue. This was confirmed in our study of 23 patients, 17 of whom underwent subtrigonal and six supratrigonal cystectomy. After a mean follow-up of 73.1 months, 12 of the patients with subtrigonal cystectomy had results rated as excellent, one as fair, and four as failure (two patients were asymptomatic but suffered from complications). In the supratrigonal group, all six patients had excellent results after a mean follow-up of 25.5 months (89). As a basis for the decision regarding trigone preservation, Nurse et al. suggest taking biopsy samples of the trigone preoperatively (29); Whitmore and Gittes state that "the trigone is saved if it is not too diseased" (18).

This leaves as the last important point to be investigated the indication for orthotopic bladder substitution. It is impossible to compare the different reports of surgical therapy for interstitial cystitis because most of the criteria that characterize the disease are only rarely outlined in detail. However, anatomic bladder capacity is one parameter that is supplied by several authors as part of the preoperative diagnostic workup. Nielsen et al. were the first to recognize that results of orthotopic bladder substitution varied in relation to anatomic bladder capacity (10). Two of their eight patients had a bladder capacity of 200 ml on cystoscopy, and in both the outcome was successful; in the other six, with a mean anatomic bladder capacity of 524 ml (400 to 675 ml), the procedure failed. The same pattern applies to the reports of other researchers (79,81,83) (Table 2) but seems not to apply to subtrigonal cystectomy (our own unpublished observation in 17 patients).

Because the morbidity and mortality of augmentation enterocystoplasty in interstitial cystitis seem not to be different from those with other indications (90), the reader is referred to the relevant literature. Interestingly, Folsom et al. achieved comparable (or even better) results when supratrigonal bladder resection was performed without subsequent augmentation enterocystoplasty (91). They described their first case, done in 1923, as a surgical accident in which the bladder was inadvertently resected down to the trigone; then the bladder remnant was closed over an 18 French soft rubber catheter. To their surprise, the patient was entirely cured from her symptoms with no day frequency, no nocturia, and relief of pain. Seven more cases were done until 1940. Postoperatively, the patients recovered normal bladder capacity, and all were entirely relieved of their bladder distress with a follow-up of a few months to 17 years. Two patients developed vesicoureteral reflux as a sequela of the operation, one requiring bilateral surface ureterostomy.

TABLE 2. *Preoperative anatomic bladder capacity and postoperative results*

First author	Mean preoperative anatomic bladder capacity (ml): Successful outcome	Failure
Goodwin (6)	50	0
Kontturi (83)	186	300
Nielsen (10)	200	524
von Garrelts (79)	"all contracted"/93% success	
Webster (81)	192	362

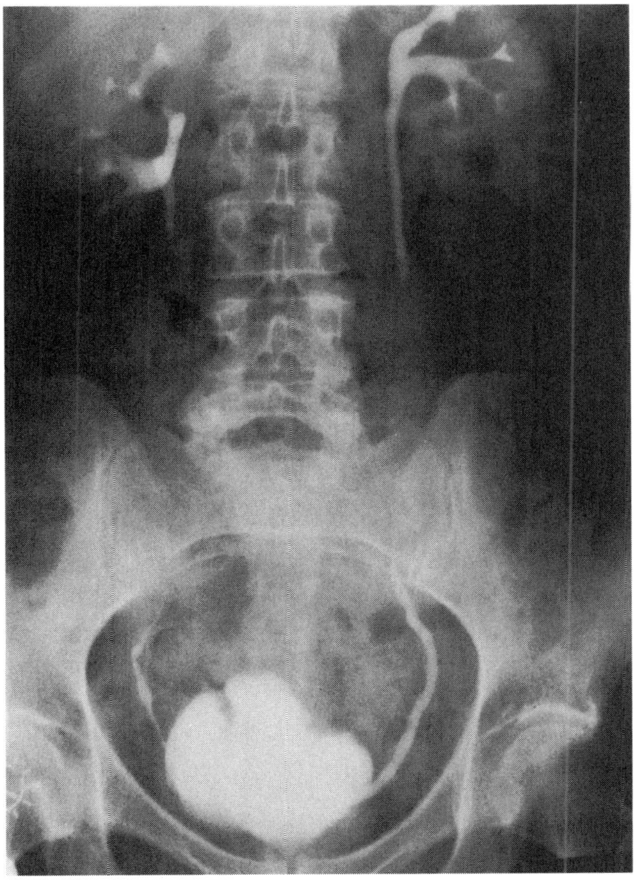

FIG. 3. Intravenous pyelogram after supratrigonal bladder resection and bladder augmentation with Mainz pouch 1.

Ureterocolic Implantation

In 1935, Ormond mentioned that this procedure had "been done [by others] in exceptionally severe and stubborn cases" without specifying data or references (30). Two years later, Counseller reported five patients, all of whom had a year-long history of interstitial cystitis with numerous forms of conservative and surgical treatment. Four had a minimum follow-up of 1 year (1 to 8 years), and the outcome in all was rated as excellent. In this preantibiotic era, Counseller endorsed preoperative intraperitoneal vaccination and implantation of one ureter at a time according to the technique of Coffey. Subsequently, other investigators confirmed the efficacy of this procedure (7,24,39,92,93). One reported a severe complication rate in that two of six patients were lost to chronic renal failure (24). However, this complication rate does not concur with that of other large series of ureterosigmoidostomy (94–98). One may speculate that the modification of this technique—detubularizing the sigma–rectum junction (Mainz pouch II) (99)—which started a renaissance of ureterosigmoidostomy in reconstructive and oncologic urology, may also be applicable in selected cases of interstitial cystitis.

Urinary Diversion

Urinary diversion with intestinal segments is the most invasive, and therefore the last, option in the therapeutic regimen of otherwise intractable interstitial cystitis. It is

A

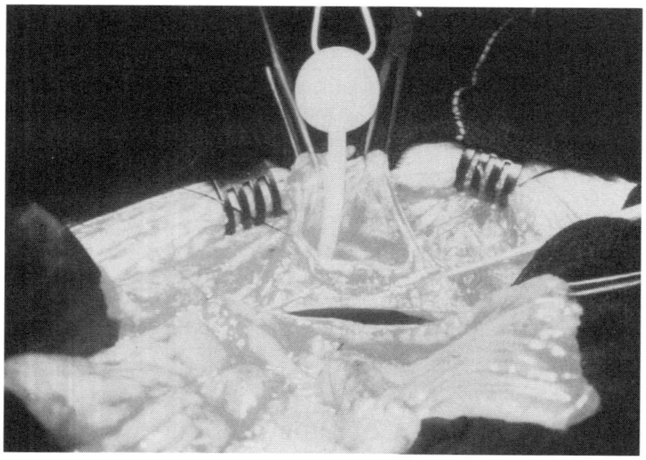

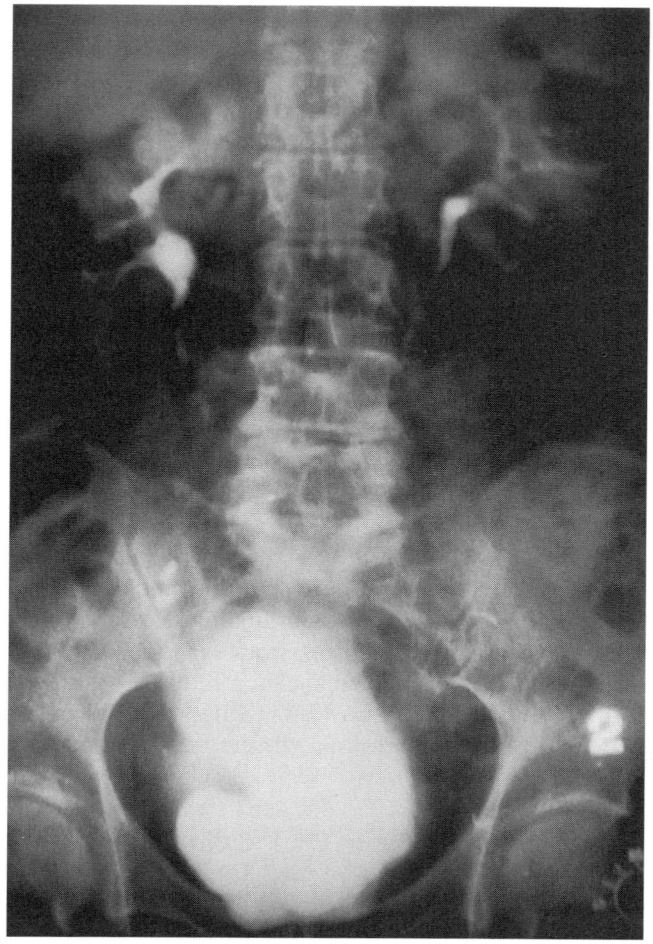

B

FIG. 4. Subtrigonal bladder resection. **(A)** Intraoperative situation preserving just a bladder neck cuff. **(B)** IVP after bladder augmentation with Mainz pouch 1.

indicated when previous bladder augmentation or substitution has failed. It may also be a primary approach *per se* (14) or when orthotopic substitution is not indicated [e.g., severe stress incontinence, inability to catheterize via the urethra, or evidence of interstitial cystitis in the trigone and urethra with the risk of urethral symptom persistence after cystectomy (7,29,88)]. However, reports of patients with persistent symptoms after cystectomy and urethrectomy (14) or with severe persistent projection of pain in the small pelvis after complete pelvic evisceration in combination with urinary and fecal diversion (9) highlight the necessity of an extremely thorough preoperative psychological and pathophysiological evaluation before any surgical treatment is undertaken.

Several essential considerations should precede urinary diversion: whether it is necessary to combine it with a cystectomy if the bladder is still *in situ;* whether it is a valid backup procedure for an unsuccessful orthotopic bladder augmentation/substitution; which type of urinary diversion to undertake.

Notably, a recent report states that the success rate of urinary diversion as a primary approach to interstitial cystitis shows a similar correlation to anatomic bladder capacity as orthotopic bladder substitution (14). Lotenfoe et al., who approached conservative refractory interstitial cystitis by urethrectomy, cystectomy, and creation of a continent colonic urinary reservoir (Florida pouch), observed a 20% success rate in five patients with a large bladder capacity (>400 cc) and 88% success in 17 patients with small bladder capacity (<400 cc) (14).

On the other hand, symptoms of interstitial cystitis cease when the storage function of the bladder is suspended. Observations of this phenomenon date back to the last century, when Simpson and Tait (100) created a temporary vesicovaginal fistula in three patients "to put the bladder in a state of complete physiological rest." They then noted immediate relief of pain (100). Also, Hunner reported a patient who was free of symptoms as long as she had a cystostomy (2). Later, different types of permanent incontinent and continent types of urinary diversion without concomitant cystectomy were performed; all led to relief of symptoms (7,13,21,24,101) except for one case reported by Wishard et al. (102). However, two of the three patients who were treated by Freiha et al. had to undergo secondary cystectomy for pyocystis (13). Therefore, in patients in whom urinary diversion is indicated as an initial surgical approach to interstitial cystitis, cystectomy is not necessary for relief of symptoms; however, colpocystotomy or secondary cystectomy may become necessary for management of pyocystis.

Several groups report urinary diversion as an ultimate procedure after failed orthotopic bladder augmentation/substitution (10,19,24,39). Except for one report (39) that noted two successes in two patients, the results are not explicitly outlined, but one may assume that they were satisfactory. At our own institution, three patients came to us from other hospitals in which an ileum bladder augmentation had been performed without previous detrusor resection. In all, the procedure had failed to improve their condition. After conversion to a continent urinary diversion with a Mainz pouch 1, two were fine. The third patient had extensive pain when catheterizing her continence mechanism such that she had to undergo conversion to incontinent urinary diversion. Her problems derived from recurrent inflammation of the bowel segment used to create the continence mechanism. Light microscopy showed changes similar to those of interstitial cystitis. Such observations had led to the assumption that interstitial cystitis may recur in transposed bowel segments (24,101,103,104). However, it has been found that this type of tissue reaction may affect all bowel segments that are exposed to urine to varying degrees (105).

Different techniques of incontinent urinary diversion have been successfully used in the treatment of interstitial cystitis. Probably the first report (mentioned above) is that of Tait, who described three patients in whom a temporary vesicovaginal fistula was created to relieve the patients of pain and allow healing of bladder ulcerations (100). Several groups have successfully used ileal conduits in the past (13,24,106). However, today we should offer the patient continent urinary diversion whenever indicated to avoid impairment of body image as far as possible.

CONCLUSION

The phenomenon of interstitial cystitis has been known now for a century, and extensive work has been done in the past. Indeed, some of the contemporary hypotheses regarding its pathophysiology were formulated more than 50 years ago. If they are not clinically helpful, as the precise nature of the disease remains undefined, the descriptions of the therapeutic challenge and past attempts at meeting it certainly are. We can benefit especially from the case reports of surgical therapy with meticulous long-term follow-up. Together with techniques available today, the consideration of older methods may help achieve a more differentiated surgical approach to those cases intractable to conservative treatment. This implies the appreciation that interstitial cystitis probably is a conglomerate of different diseases with similar symptoms but with different pathophysiological and anatomic bases. A successful strategy for treatment relies not only on the precise knowledge of symptoms, clinical findings, and histology in each patient, but also on the patient's individual personality, while choosing the least invasive means possible.

This review of the literature uncovers a variety of potentially effective surgical treatments. One important consideration is the anatomic bladder capacity (capacity under anesthesia). A large capacity permits an attempt at restitution of the storage function by bilateral neurectomy of the S_3 spinal nerve or anterolateral chordotomy; conversely, a large capacity is a negative prognostic indicator for supratrigonal bladder resection and augmentation as well as for urinary diversion. Patients with a small anatomic bladder capacity have been shown to do well after bladder resection that preserves just the trigone combined with bladder augmentation. Alternative procedures are ureterocolic implantation and continent urinary diversion. Under these circumstances incontinent urinary diversion as a primary choice seems to be outdated.

REFERENCES

1. Hunner GL. A rare type of bladder ulcer in women; report of cases. *Boston Med Surg J* 1915;172(18):660–664.
2. Hunner GL. Elusive ulcer of the bladder. Further notes on a rare type of bladder ulcer, with a report of twenty-five cases. *Am J Obstet* 1918; 78:374–395.
3. Nitze M. *Lehrbuch der Kystoskopie.* Wiesbaden: Verlag von JF Bergmann, 1907;272–274.
4. Skene AJ. *Diseases of the Bladder and Urethra in Women.* New York: William Wood & Co, 1887 (quoted in 7).
5. Fall M, Johansson SL, Aldenborg F. Chronic interstitial cystitis: a heterogeneous syndrome. *J Urol* 1987;137:35–38.
6. Goodwin WE, Turner RD, Winter CC. Results of ileocystoplasty. *J Urol* 1958;80:461–466.
7. Hand JR. Interstitial cystitis: report of 223 cases (204 women and 19 men). *J Urol* 1949;61:291–310.
8. Ratner V, Slade D, Greene G. Interstitial cystitis. A patient's perspective. *Urol Clin North Am* 1994;21:1–5.
9. Baskin LS, Tanagho EA. Pelvic pain without pelvic organs. *J Urol* 1992;147:683–686.
10. Nielsen KK, Kromann-Andersen B, Steven K, Hald T. Failure of combined supratrigonal cystectomy and Mainz ileocecocystoplasty in intractable interstitial cystitis: is histology and mast cell count a reliable predictor for the outcome of surgery? *J Urol* 1990;144:255–259.
11. Smith GG. Interstitial cystitis. *J Urol* 1952;67:903–915.
12. Oravisto KJ. Epidemiology of interstitial cystitis. *Ann Chir Gynaecol Fenn* 1975;64:75.
13. Freiha FS, Faysal MD, Stamey TA. The surgical treatment of intractable interstitial cystitis. *J Urol* 1980;123:632–634.
14. Lotenfoe RR, Christie J, Parsons A, Burkett P, Helal M, Lockhart JL Absence of neuropathic pelvic pain and favorable psychological profile in the surgical selection of patients with disabling interstitial cystitis. *J Urol* 1995;154:2039–2042.
15. deJuana CP, Everett JC. Interstitial cystitis. *Urology* 1977;10:325–329.
16. Smith JC, Badenoch AC. Carcinoma of the bladder simulating chronic cystitis. *Br J Urol* 1965;37:93–99.
17. Utz DC, Zincke H. The masquerade of bladder cancer *in situ* as interstitial cystitis. *J Urol* 1974;111:160–161.
18. Whitmore WF, Gittes RF. Reconstruction of the urinary tract by cecal and ileocecal cystoplasty: Review of a 15-year experience. *J Urol* 1983;129:494–498.
19. Webster GD, Galloway N. Surgical treatment of interstitial cystitis.

Indications, techniques, and results. *Urology [Suppl]* 1987;29(4):34–39.
20. Worth PL, Turner-Warwick R. The treatment of interstitial cystitis by cystolysis with observations on cystoplasty. *Br J Urol* 1973;45:65–71.
21. Counseller VS. Bilateral transplantation of the ureters of the female. *Am J Obstet Gynecol* 1937;33:234–248.
22. Meirowsky AM. The management of chronic interstitial cystitis by differential sacral neurotomy. *J Neurosurg* 1969;30:604–607.
23. Moulder MK, Meirowsky AM. The management of Hunner's ulcer by differential sacral neurotomy: preliminary report. *J Urol* 1956;75:261–262.
24. Badenoch AW. Chronic interstitial cystitis. *Br J Urol* 1971;43:718–721.
25. Bruce PT, Buckham GJ, Carden ABG, Salvaris M. The surgical treatment of chronic interstitial cystitis. *Med J Aust* 1977;1:581–582.
26. Bumpus HCJ. Interstitial cystitis: its treatment by overdistension of the bladder. *Med Clin North Am* 1930;13:1495–1498.
27. Greenberg E, Barnes R, Stewart S, Furnish T. Transurethral resection of Hunner's ulcer. *J Urol* 1974;111:764–766.
28. Hanno P, Ruggieri M, Wein AJ. Current status of interstitial cystitis. *World J Urol* 1990;8:212–217.
29. Nurse ED, Parry JRW, Mundy R. Problems in the surgical treatment of interstitial cystitis. *Br J Urol* 1991;68:153–154.
30. Ormond JK. Interstitial cystitis. *J Urol* 1935;33:576–582.
31. Christmas TJ, Rode J, Chapple CR, Milroy EJG, Turner-Warwick RT. Nerve fibre proliferation in interstial cystitis. *Virchows Arch [A] Pathol Anat* 1990;416:447–451.
32. Galloway NTM, Devdatta RG, Irvin PP. Interstitial cystitis or reflex sympathetic dystrophy of the bladder? *Semin Urol* 1991;9:148–153.
33. Hohenfellner M, Nunes L, Schmidt RA, Lampel A, Thüroff JW, Tanagho EA. Interstitial cystitis: increased sympathetic innervation and related neuropeptide synthesis. *J Urol* 1992;147:587–591.
34. Shickley TJ, Luthin GR, Ruggieri MR. Immunhistochemical examination of neuropeptides and m-2 muscarinic receptors in normal and interstitial cystitis (ic) bladders. *J Urol* 1992;147:462A.
35. Bumpus HCJ, Meisser JG. Focal infection and selective localization of streptococci in pyelonephritis. *Arch Intern Med* 1921;27:326–337.
36. Meisser JG, Bumpus HC. Focal infections in relation to submucous ulcer of the bladder and to cystitis. *J Urol* 1921;6:285–298.
37. Douglass HL. Excision of the superior hypogastric plexus in the treatment of intractable interstitial cystitis. *Am J Surg* 1934;25:249–257.
38. Worth PHL. The treatment of interstitial cystitis by cystolysis with observations on cystoplasty. A review after 7 years. *Br J Urol* 1980;52:232.
39. Freiha FS, Stamey TA. Cystolysis: a procedure for the selective denervation of the bladder. *J Urol* 1980;123:360–363.
40. Stewart BH. Editorial comment. *J Urol* 1980;123:363.
41. Albers DD, Geyer JR. Long-term results of cystolysis (supratrigonal denervation) of the bladder for intractable interstitial cystitis. *J Urol* 1988;139:1205–1206.
42. Jaboulay M. Le traitement de la neuralgie pelvienne par la paralysie du sympathique sacré. *Lyon Med* 1899;90:102–104 (quoted in Jacobson CF, Nesbit RM, Schroeder CF. *N Engl J Med* 1939;220:274–278).
43. Rochet V, Latarjet A. Étude sur les voies d'abord chirurgical du plexus hypogastrique et de son ganglion. *Lyon Chir* 1913;10:425–433.
44. Greenwood B. The origins of sympathectomy. *Med Hist* 1967;11:165–169.
45. van Duzen RE. Effect of resection of presacral nerve on vesical function. *South Med J* 1932;25:964–967.
46. Adson AW, Brown GE. The treatment of Raynaud's disease by resection of the upper thoracic and lumbar sympathetic ganglia and trunks. *Surg Gynecol Obstet* 1929;48:577–603.
47. Smithwick RH. The rationale and technic of sympathectomy for the relief of vascular spasm of the extremities. *N Engl J Med* 1940;222:699–703.
48. Spurling RG. Causalgia of the upper extremity: Treatment by dorsal sympathetic ganglionectomy. *Arch Neurol Psychiatry* 1930;23:784–788.
49. White JC, Bland EF. The surgical relief of severe angina pectoris. *Medicine* 1948;27:1–42.
50. de Takats G, Walter LE, Lasner J. Splanchnic nerve section for pancreatic pain. *Ann Surg* 1950;131:44–57.
51. Sadar ES, Cooperman AM. Bilateral thoracic sympathectomy-splanchnicectomy in the treatment of intractable pain due to pancreatic carcinoma. *Cleve Clin Q* 1974;41:185–188.
52. Viannay C. Du tratement chirurgical des cystites douloureuses arrivées au stade de "cystalgie," par les interventions sur le sympathique pelvien, et, en particulier, par la resection du nerf pré-sacré. *Arch Fr-Belg Chir* 1927;30:229–236.
53. Pieri G. Énervation ou ramisection? *Presse Méd* 1926;34:1141–1142.
54. Learmonth JR. Neurosurgery in the treatment of diseases of the urinary bladder II. Treatment of vesical pain. *J Urol* 1931;26:13–24.
55. Learmonth JR. Neurosurgery in diseases of the urinary bladder. *Am J Surg* 1932;16:270–274.
56. Glynn CJ, Jamous MA, Teddy PJ, Moore RA, Lloyd JW. Role of spinal noradrenergic system in transmission of pain in patients with spinal cord injury. *Lancet* 1986;2:1249–1250.
57. Levine JD, Goetzl EJ, Basbaum AI. Contribution of the nervous system to the pathophysiology of rheumatoid arthritis and other polyarthritides. *Rheum Dis Clin North Am* 1987;13:369–383.
58. Nesbit RM, McLellan FC. Sympathectomy for the relief of vesical spasm and pain resulting from intractable bladder infection. *Surg Gynecol Obstet* 1939;68:540–546.
59. Scott WJM, Schroeder CF. Denervation of the bladder for relief of intractable pain. *Ann Surg* 1938;108:730–740.
60. Nesbit RM. Anterolateral chordotomy for refractory interstitial cystitis with intractable pain. *J Urol* 1947;57:741–745.
61. Jacobson CE, Braasch WF, Love JG. Presacral neurectomy for intractable vesical pain and neurogenic vesical dysfunction. *Surg Gynecol Obstet* 1944;79:21–26.
62. Heimburger RF, Freeman LW, Wilde NJ. Sacral nerve innervation of the human bladder. *J Neurosurg* 1948;5:154–164.
63. Meirowsky AM, Scheibert CD, Hinchey TR. Studies on the sacral reflex arc in paraplegia. I. Response of the bladder to surgical elimination of sacral nerve impulses by rhizotomy. *J Neurosurg* 1950;7:33–38.
64. Meirowsky AM, Scheibert CD, Hinchey TR. Studies on the sacral reflex arc in paraplegia. II. Differential sacral neurotomy. An operative method. *J Neurosurg* 1950;7:39–43.
65. Milner WA, Garlick WB. Selective sacral neurectomy in interstitial cystitis. *J Urol* 1957;78:600–604.
66. Mason TH, Haines GL, Leversee BW. Selective sacral neurotomy for Hunner's ulcer. *J Neurosurg* 1960;17:22–26.
67. Saris SC, Silver JM, Vieira JFS, Nashold BS. Sacrococcygeal rhizotomy for perineal pain. *Neurosurgery* 1986;19:789–793.
68. Bohm E, Franksson C. Interstitial cystitis and sacral rhizotomy. *Acta Chir Scand* 1957;113:63–67.
69. Petersén I, Franksson C. The sensory innervation of the urinary bladder. *Urol Int* 1955;2:108–119.
70. Bohm E, Franksson C, Petersén I. Sacral rhizopathies and sacral root syndromes (SII–SV). *Acta Chir Scand [Suppl]* 1956;216:2–49.
71. Grant FC. Chordotomy for relief of pain in the genitourinary tract. *J Urol* 1931;25:551–558.
72. Band D. *Trans Eighth Cong Soc Int d'Urol* 1949;2:224–256.
73. Fall M. Transcutaneous electrical nerve stimulation in interstitial cystitis. *Urology [Suppl]* 1987;29:40–42.
74. Gillespie L, Levin N, Delamarter R. Lumbar nerve root compression and interstitial cystitis—response to decompressive surgery. *Br J Urol* 1991;68:361–364.
75. Brinkmann O, Lütkemeyer B, Bongartz G, Hohenfellner M, Roth S, Hertle L. *Lumbar nerve root compression causing interstitial cystitis: a magnetic resonance study in 22 patients.* Paper presented at European Association of Urology 1994, Berlin, 13–16 July.
76. Bejany DE, Politano VA. Ileocolic neobladder in the woman with interstitial cystitis and a small contracted bladder. *J Urol* 1995;153:42–43.
77. Goldwasser B, Webster GD. Augmentation and substitution enterocystoplasty. *J Urol* 1986;135:215–224.
78. Hinman FJ. Selection of intestinal segments for bladder substitution: physical and physiological characteristics. *J Urol* 1988;139:519–523.
79. von Garrelts B. Interstitial cystitis: Thirteen patients treated operatively with intestinal bladder substitutes. *Acta Chir Scand* 1966;132:436–443.
80. Guillonneau B, Toussaint B, Bouchot O, Buzelin JM. Traitement de la cystite interstitielle par cystectomie sus-trigonale et entérocystoplastie. *Prog Urol* 1993;3:27–31.
81. Webster GD, Maggio MI. The management of chronic interstitial cystitis by substitution cystoplasty. *J Urol* 1989;141:287–291.
82. Hradec H. Bladder substitution: Indications and results in 114 operations. *J Urol* 1965;94:406–417.
83. Kontturi MJ, Hellström PA, Tammela TLJ, Lukkarinen OA. Colo-

cystoplasty for the treatment of severe interstitial cystitis. *Urol Int* 1991;46:50–54.
84. Holm-Bentzen M, Klarskov P, Opsomer R, Hald T. Coecocystoplasty: an evaluation of operative results. *Urol Int* 1986;41:21–25.
85. Hanley H. Ileocystoplasty. A clinical review. *J Urol* 1959;82:317.
86. Turner-Warwick R, Ashken HM. The functional results of partial, subtotal, and total cystoplasty with special reference to ureterocystoplasty, selective sphincterotomy, and cystocystoplasty. *Br J Urol* 1967;39:3–12.
87. Linn JF, Hohenfellner M, Roth S, et al. Comparison of subtrigonal and supratrigonal cystectomy combined with orthotopic bladder substitution with Mainz-pouch I for treatment of interstitial cystitis. Submitted for publication.
88. Smith BH, Dehner LP. Chronic ulcerating interstitial cystitis. *Arch Pathol* 1972;93:76–81.
89. Hohenfellner M, Linn J, Roth S, et al. *Orthotopic bladder substitution with the Mainz pouch I in interstitial cystitis.* Paper presented to Continent Urinary Reconstruction. 2nd International Meeting, 1995, Mainz.
90. Smith RB, Van Cangh P, Skinner DG, Kaufmann JJ, Goodwin WE. Augmentation enterocystoplasty: a critical review. *J Urol* 1977;118:35–39.
91. Folsom AI, O'Brien HA, Caldwell GT. Subtotal cystectomy in the treatment of Hunner ulcer. *J Urol* 1940;44:650–666.
92. Higgins CC. *Am Intern Med* 1941;15:708–715.
93. Lower WE, Schlumberger FC. Bilateral simultaneous ureterosigmoidostomy for chronic interstitial cystitis. *Cleve Clin Q* 1939;6:181–184.
94. Allen TD. Editorial comment (Ureterosigmoidostomy: is it a viable procedure in the age of continent urinary diversion and bladder substitution?). *J Urol* 1995;153:1431.
95. Bissada NK, Morcos RR, Morgan WM, Hanash KA. Ureterosigmoidostomy: is it a viable procedure in the age of continent urinary diversion and bladder substitution? *J Urol* 1995;153:1429–1431.
96. Goodwin WE, Scardino PT. Ureterosigmoidostomy. *J Urol* 1977;118:169–174.
97. Kälble T, Tricker AR, Friedl P, et al. Ureterosigmoidostomy: long-term results, risk of carcinoma and etiological factors for carcinogenesis. *J Urol* 1990;144:1110–1114.
98. Stöckle M, Becht E, Voges G, Riedmiller H, Hohenfellner R. Ureterosigmoidostomy: an outdated approach to bladder exstrophy? *J Urol* 1990;143:770–775.
99. Fisch M, Wammack R, Müller SC, Hohenfellner R. The Mainz pouch II (sigma rectum pouch). *J Urol* 1993;149:258–263.
100. Tait, L. On the cure of the chronic perforating ulcer of the bladder by the formation of an artificial vesico-vaginal fistula. *Lancet* 1870;54:738.
101. Messing EM, Stamey TA. Interstitial cystitis. Early diagnosis, pathology, and treatment. *Urology* 1978;12:381–392.
102. Wishard WN, Nourse MH, Mertz JHO. Use of Clorpactin WCS-90 for relief of symptoms due to interstitial cystitis. *J Urol* 1957;77:420.
103. Kisman OK, Lycklama à Nijeholt AAB, v. Krieken JHJM. Mast cell infiltration in intestine used for bladder augmentation in interstitial cystitis. *J Urol* 1991;146:1113–1114.
104. McGuire EJ, Lytton B, Cornog JL. Interstitial cystitis following colocystoplasty. *Urology* 1973;2:28–29.
105. MacDermott JP, Charpied GL, Tesluk H, Stone AR. Recurrent interstitial cystitis following cystoplasty: Fact or fiction? *J Urol* 1990;144:37–40.
106. Jacobo E, Stamler FW, Culp DA. Interstitial cystitis followed by total cystectomy. *Urology* 1974;3:481–485.

Interstitial Cystitis, edited by Grannum R. Sant.
Lippincott–Raven Publishers, Philadelphia ©1997.

CHAPTER 29

Complementary Approaches in the Management of Interstitial Cystitis

Francine Mendelowitz and Robert Moldwin

Despite a dramatic increase in research efforts dedicated to promote an understanding of interstitial cystitis (IC), this disabling urologic disorder remains an idiopathic symptom complex with no known cure. Traditional allopathic treatments have been successful in providing some relief to most patients; however, no single treatment reliably controls patients' symptoms (1). This suboptimal response to traditional pain management is not exclusive to IC. It has been estimated that only 50% of patients with chronic pain syndromes achieve relief from standard medical treatments (2). Because of the limited effectiveness of traditional treatment strategies, patients with interstitial cystitis and other pain syndromes have recently sought out complementary or "alternative" approaches to their care. According to the World Health Organization, more than 70% of the world's population depend on nonallopathic methods of healing (3). More than 96% of the 22 million Americans searching for alternative therapies in 1990 were also under the medical care of a "conventional" physician (4). Americans' fascination with complementary therapy has developed alongside the wellness movement that burgeoned in the 1960s. As a result, patients have begun to take greater control of their physical health and more responsibility for managing illness. Patients with interstitial cystitis often experience a loss of control over their physical and emotional health. Discovering alternative methods of treatment and symptom management has restored hope for many of these patients. This chapter highlights the complementary approaches available to patients with interstitial cystitis.

F. Mendelowitz and R. Moldwin: Interstitial Cystitis Center, Department of Urology, Albert Einstein College of Medicine, Long Island Jewish Medical Center, New Hyde Park, New York 11040-1496.

ACUPUNCTURE

Acupuncture use dates back over 5,000 years. Although it is one of the oldest forms of medical therapy, it is among the more recent strategies employed in the treatment of interstitial cystitis. Its basic tenets correspond to the individual's state of health and a balanced flow of energy throughout the body (*yin* and *yang*), which are determined by 12 channels known as meridians and approximately 1,000 acupoints. Acupuncture involves the placement of needles into specific acupoints in order to rebalance the individual's flow of energy and to block pain. Some studies suggest that acupuncture elicits an increase in cerebrospinal fluid levels of the endogenous opiates β-endorphin and met-enkephalin. Furthermore, the effects of acupuncture can be reversed if patients receive prior administration of the morphine antagonist naloxone (5). Acupuncture is theorized to provide pain relief by stimulating large-diameter myelinated afferent nerves (Aα fibers), thereby inhibiting spinal transmission of pain via thin, unmyelinated nerves (C fibers) (pain-gate theory). Acupuncture's effect may also be related to C-fiber activation in a scenario of "counterirritation" (6).

Chang (7) reviewed acupuncture's effectiveness in patients with idiopathic urinary urgency, frequency, and dysuria. Acupuncture needles were applied to the Sp 6 point of 26 patients; 22 (84.6%) of the patients reported symptomatic improvement. Of these patients, 17 (65.4%) were asymptomatic; the remaining five experienced relief from urinary urgency and dysuria, but urinary frequency persisted. The rise in mean cystometric capacity with treatment was not clinically significant (from 222 to 258 cc).

Philip et al. (8) treated 16 patients with acupuncture for idiopathic detrusor instability. Eleven patients (69%) experienced symptomatic relief; however, few objective changes were noted on urodynamic evaluation. The small number of patients who were treated for urinary sensory/urgency syndrome showed no symptomatic changes.

Reports of acupuncture's efficacy in the treatment of IC and pelvic pain syndromes have varied. Geirsson et al. (9) investigated acupuncture and transcutaneous electric nerve stimulation (TENS) in the treatment of IC. Neither TENS nor acupuncture, when applied to the posterior tibial nerve, elicited any change in urinary frequency, mean or maximum voided volume, or pain level (recorded on visual analog scales). Only one patient presented with short-term symptom improvement after acupuncture.

Rapkin and Kames (10) studied 14 patients with pelvic pain who received 6 to 8 weeks of acupuncture therapy twice weekly. Eleven patients had at least a 50% decrease in pain, with an average 71% reduction. Two patients had less than a 50% pain reduction, and one patient experienced an increase in pain. Our clinical experience has demonstrated that multiple acupuncture sessions are generally necessary to achieve significant symptomatic relief, and therapeutic effectiveness is often related to the physician or acupuncturist who performs the treatment. Evaluation of acupuncture's effectiveness in treating IC has been hampered by these variables and the inability to conduct double-blinded studies. At the present time, acupuncture appears to be a useful, relatively noninvasive complement to traditional medical care.

DIAPHRAGMATIC BREATHING

The pain experienced by individuals with IC has been compared to the severity of pain encountered with cancer or chronic back pain (11). Most individuals react to pain by bracing and increasing the pace of breathing. Slow, diaphragmatic breathing can be an effective method of disrupting the pain cycle (12). The sympathetic nervous system is dramatically influenced by the way in which individuals breathe. During thoracic breathing, sympathetic activity increases, as does muscle tension (13). Slow diaphragmatic breathing, on the other hand, tends to decrease sympathetic tone, thereby encouraging a state of generalized relaxation. We have found the technique of diaphragmatic breathing to be particularly useful for patients who have IC associated with pelvic floor dysfunction (PFD). Pelvic floor dysfunction, or "nonneurogenic" striated sphincteric dyssynergia, is often characterized by pelvic pain, urinary frequency, urgency, hesitancy, and decreased urine flow rates. Schmidt (14) noted three patterns of abnormal pelvic floor behavior with voiding: (a) the inability of the sphincter and levator musculature to relax; (b) the inability to maintain sphincter and pelvic floor relaxation; and (c) unstable, spastic relaxation behavior in the sphincter with a postponed detrusor contraction. We have demonstrated PFD to be present in as many as 70% of IC patients meeting NIDDK criteria (15). We retrospectively evaluated 19 patients with IC meeting NIDDK criteria and associated pelvic floor dysfunction. Patients were treated with 3 months of conservative therapy including sitz baths, diazepam (2 mg three times daily), and "relaxation therapy." Relaxation therapy was accomplished with combined techniques of diaphragmatic breathing and progressive muscle relaxation. Mean urgency and pain scores decreased by 4 (0 to 10 visual analog score) and 3.5, respectively. Mean nocturia decreased by 3.4 ($p < 0.005$). These data suggest that diaphragmatic breathing and progressive muscle relaxation in conjunction with other conservative modalities can result in profound improvements in patients' symptoms. Diaphragmatic breathing is a quick and simple method to break the tension–pain–tension cycle. Continued practice of this technique has helped patients by enhancing muscle relaxation, relieving stress and pain while rehabilitating pelvic floor musculature.

PROGRESSIVE MUSCLE RELAXATION

Koziol et al. (16) demonstrated the substantial influence that stress has on pain perception by evaluating 374 IC patients and noting that stress increased pain in 61% of patients. Progressive muscle relaxation is a stress-reducing technique that was introduced in 1970 by Edmund Jacobson. Deep muscle relaxation and decreased sympathetic activity are achieved by voluntarily tightening and then relaxing specific muscle groups. It is well known that the anticipation of recurrent pain in a chronic pain syndrome can induce muscle contraction, leading to further pain and perpetuating a pain–tension–pain cycle. A reduction in muscle tension for a limited period of time can disrupt this cycle (12,17), as seen with diaphragmatic breathing.

Linton reported that patients with back and joint pain have successfully utilized relaxation techniques to manage and cope (12,18,19). Relaxation training was also found to be an effective approach for pain relief among ulcerative colitis patients (19). Twenty patients with chronic pain related to ulcerative colitis received six weekly progressive relaxation training sessions, and 20 patients were placed in a control group (untreated). Immediately after treatment and at 6-week follow-up, experimental subjects had more pain relief and rated pain as less intense on visual analog scales. Of the 20 patients who received treatment, the average intensity of pain rating decreased from 7.9 to 4.5 ($p < 0.003$). Relaxation training was taught to IC patients in our treatment center by a clinical social worker (F.M.) trained in lower urinary tract disorders. The goal of the training was to provide muscle relaxation, stress reduction, and pain management. This was achieved through face-to-face sessions and individually designed audiotapes. Twelve weeks after their initial consultation for relaxation training, patients were asked to complete a brief, anonymous survey Of those responding to the survey who received relaxation training, 14 (86%) stated that they used the techniques regularly. Of patients who received training, 76% felt that it helped their urologic condition. Forty-three percent of respondents felt that the training helped them to manage other medical and/or psychological problems, and 93% would recommend relaxation training to other patients.

HYPNOSIS

Hypnosis is one of the oldest cognitive approaches used in pain management. It involves establishing an alliance with the patient, teaching her to relax through suggestion, and then shifting her focus away from the sensation of pain (20). Melzack and Wall's gate-control theory of pain regulation supports the effectiveness of hypnosis in controlling pain (21). The gate theory suggests that presynaptic interference with efferent fibers from the cerebral cortex to the spinal cord (which can be achieved through hypnosis) modulates peripheral nociceptive input in the dorsal horn of the spinal cord (22). Success of this therapeutic tool is dependent on patient motivation, imagination, and trust in the therapist (23).

Though hypnosis cannot completely alleviate pain, it can help to modify the patient's perception of pain (24). Harding (25) studied the effects of hypnosis on 90 patients with intractable migraines. An average session lasted 30 min, and the number of sessions varied from four to seven. Follow-up studies done 6 months to 8 years after treatment found that 38% of patients had no migraines, 32% showed moderate symptom relief, and 30% experienced no relief or were lost to follow-up. Hilgard (26) investigated the use of hypnosis in patients with ischemic pain. Those patients who were highly responsive to hypnosis did not feel ischemic pain for 18 to 45 min. Our clinical experience in utilizing hypnosis to treat IC patients has not been as encouraging as the studies cited above. Patients with IC have found hypnosis to be a useful tool in managing daily stress and reducing muscle tension. Many patients have experienced temporary pain relief after receiving hypnotic intervention. Hypnosis as a complementary therapy in treating interstitial cystitis is recommended, as it has no side effects and helps to promote the patient's sense of control (27). Enhancement of patient self-control may further reduce secondary anxiety and depression (28).

BEHAVIORAL MODIFICATION

Behavioral modification strategies have been particularly effective with interstitial cystitis patients. Chaikin et al. (29) conducted research involving 42 women with refractory symptoms of IC (urgency, frequency, pain for a minimum of 2 years' duration). Therapy was directed at teaching patients to modify certain behaviors such as frequent voiding. An average of 12 weekly behavioral therapy sessions helped patients increase intervals between voids an average of 93 min ($p < 0.01$). Additionally, 98% of patients studied had a decrease in the number of daily voids by a mean of nine ($p < 0.01$), from an average of 17 voids per day to an average of eight voids per day. Functional bladder capacity increased in 38 of the 42 patients studied by an average of 73 ml ($p < 0.01$). Koprowski and Parsons (30) found that bladder retraining decreased urinary urgency, frequency, and nocturia in 15 (71%) of 21 IC patients. An increase in voided volume was noted in all patients, from a mean of 92 cc before therapy to a mean of 179 cc after treatment. We reviewed 15 IC patients with a bladder-retraining (holding) protocol. Our results paralleled previous studies with a mean increase in voided volume of 65 cc within 1 month. Unfortunately, 11 patients (73%) had a persistent sense of bladder fullness at pretherapy volumes.

Severe pain associated with bladder filling has been the only major impediment to successful implementation of such strategies. Behavior modification techniques using individualized bladder holding protocols have provided for a reduction in IC symptomatology and an increase in self-control among patients.

BIOFEEDBACK

Biofeedback assists patients to gain awareness and greater control over physiological processes through bioelectric instrumentation. An EMG facilitated biofeedback helps teach patients to relax muscles that are causing pain. Electromyographic biofeedback was initially used to treat muscle contraction (tension) headaches. Chapman (31) reported that patients receiving frontalis muscle EMG biofeedback therapy responded better than those receiving placebo medication or no treatment at all. Interestingly, the decrease in headache pain was not affected by changes in EMG activity, and the exact cause(s) for improvement were not clarified. This suggests that medical-electronic devices carry a strong clinically useful placebo effect (32).

Electromyographic biofeedback therapy has proven efficacious for patients with chronic rheumatic back pain (33). Twenty-two patients were followed in a treatment outcome study $2^1/_2$ years after either EMG paravertebral biofeedback, pseudofeedback (feedback that is not contingent on the response of the subject), or conventional medical treatment alone. Patients receiving paravertebral biofeedback reported 68.3% improvement in pain versus 13.8% improvement reported by those in the other two groups ($p < 0.001$). This study also found that biofeedback effected positive changes in attitude among patients in that they were pleased to be able to do something to manage their pain problem themselves. Our clinical experience has shown EMG biofeedback to be useful in the management of patients with IC and pelvic floor dysfunction. A retrospective study of 16 female patients aged 20 to 73 years receiving EMG biofeedback and electric stimulation was conducted. Patients received an average of six weekly sessions using an Incare Perineal Reeducation System 8900 with transvaginal probes and surface abdominal electrodes. Patients were taught to identify pelvic floor muscles and to isolate them from abdominal muscles. Mean muscle identification (pelvic contraction minus abdominal contraction) rose from 2.2 mV before biofeedback to 4.0 mV afterwards ($p = 0.025$). Eleven of 16 patients (69%) reported symptomatic improvement after treatment. As was seen with the treatment of tension headache, the treatment response did not correlate to changes in muscle identification.

Electromyographic biofeedback has been found to be useful adjunctive therapy in the treatment of IC and pelvic floor dysfunction; however, long-term follow-up studies and the role of the placebo effect should be considered for further research.

PHYSICIAN–PATIENT RELATIONSHIP

Establishment of a sound relationship between physician and patient is the most important foundation for successful treatment in chronic disorders such as interstitial cystitis (34). Patients with IC often present to physicians with exaggerated amounts of stress because of the extended length of time in which they have been forced to cope with an undiagnosed illness or an illness that has been categorized as psychological (35). When patients develop greater ease in working with physicians, they achieve a greater sense of control, and their physical symptoms and ability to tolerate pain change (36). The physician may play a unique role in influencing patients' perceptions of their health status and their ability to change that status. As reported by Kaplan et al. (37), who evaluated the effects of physician–patient interactions on the outcomes of chronic disease, physician behaviors that encourage patients' self-confidence, motivation, and positive perspective on health status can indirectly change patients' health outcomes. The placebo effect of the physician–patient relationship and the need for supportive intervention cannot be overestimated in the treatment of patients with interstitial cystitis.

CONCLUSION

Interstitial cystitis remains a chronic idiopathic inflammatory syndrome of the bladder with no uniformly successful therapy (38). Its diagnostic challenge and resistance to most conventional medical treatments have created a high economic cost (an average of $170 million per year is spent for medical care) (39) and a devastating psychosocial cost for patients. A multidimensional and multidisciplinary approach to treatment is the preferential course to take in working with interstitial cystitis. The role of complementary therapies in the management of IC has flourished in the past several years. These therapies offer renewed hope to patients and a greater sense of involvement and control in managing their disease. Continued research on the efficacy of complementary approaches in interstitial cystitis is essential to determine the long- and short-term effects of these promising treatments.

REFERENCES

1. Chalker R, Whitmore KE. The painful bladder syndrome: Interstitial cystitis and urethral syndrome. In: *Overcoming Bladder Disorders*. New York: Harper Collins, 1990;133–179.
2. Toomey TC, Ghia JN, Mao W, Gregg JM. Acupuncture and chronic pain mechanisms: the moderating effects of affect, personality, and stress on response to treatment. *Pain* 1977;3:137–145.
3. Krippner S. A cross-cultural comparison of four healing models. *Altern Ther* 1995;1:21–29.
4. Beinfield H, Korngold E. Chinese traditional medicine: an introductory overview. *Altern Ther* 1995;1:44–52.
5. Lewith GT, Kenyon JN. Physiological and psychological explanations for the mechanisms of acupuncture as a treatment for chronic pain. *Soc Sci Med* 1984;19:1367–1378.
6. Fields HL. Nondrug method for pain control. In: *Pain*. New York: McGraw-Hill, 1987;307–343.
7. Chang PL. Urodynamic studies in acupuncture for women with frequency, urgency and dysuria. *J Urol* 1988;140:563–566.
8. Philip T, Shah PJR, Worth PHL. Acupuncture in the treatment of bladder instability. *Br J Urol* 1988;61:490–493.
9. Geirsson G, Wang Y, Lindstrom S, Fall M. Traditional acupuncture and electrical stimulation of the posterior tibial nerve. *Scand J Urol Nephrol* 1993;27:67–70.
10. Rapkin AJ, Kames LD. The pain management approach to chronic pelvic pain. *J Reprod Med* 1987;32:323–327.
11. Held PJ, Hanno PM, Wein AJ, et al. Epidemiology of interstitial cystitis. In: Hanno PM, Staskin DR, Krane RJ, et al, eds. *Interstitial Cystitis*. London: Springer Verlag, 1990;27–35.
12. Schuman M. Biofeedback in the management of pain. In: Barber J, Adrian C, eds. *Psychological Approaches to the Management of Pain*. New York: Brunner/Mazel, 1982;150–167.
13. Peper E, Holt CF. *Creating Wholeness*. New York: Plenum Press, 1993; 33–103.
14. Schmidt RA, Vapnek JM. Pelvic floor behavior and interstitial cystitis. *Semin Urol* 1991;IX(2):154–159.
15. Moldwin RM, Fried-Siegel J, Mendelowitz F. Pelvic floor dysfunction and interstitial cystitis. *J Urol* 1994;151:285A.
16. Koziol JA, Clark DC, Gittes RF, Tan EM. The natural history of interstitial cystitis: A survey of 374 patients. *J Urol* 1993;149:465–469.
17. Linton SJ. Behavioral remediation of chronic pain: A status report. *Pain* 1986;24:125–141.
18. Linton SJ, Gote S, Tam KG. A controlled study of the effects of applied relaxation plus operant procedures in the regulation of chronic pain. *Br J Clin Psychol* 1984;23:291–299.
19. Shaw L, Ehrich A. Relaxation training as a treatment for chronic pain caused by ulcerative colitis. *Pain* 1987;29:287–293.
20. Sacerdote P. Techniques of hypnotic intervention with pain patients. In: Barber J, Adrian C, eds. *Psychological Approaches to the Management of Pain*. New York: Brunner/Mazel, 1982;60–83.
21. Wall PD, Melzack R, eds. *Textbook of Pain*. New York: Churchill Livingstone, 1994.
22. Wickramasekera I. Biofeedback and behavior modification for chronic pain. In: Echternach JL, ed. *Pain*. New York: Churchill Livingstone, 1987;255–266.
23. Fields HL. Nondrug methods for pain control. In: *Pain*. New York: McGraw-Hill, 1987;307–334.

24. Barber J. Incorporating hypnosis in the management of chronic pain. In: Barber J, Adrian C, eds. *Psychological Approaches to the Management of Pain.* New York: Brunner/Mazel, 1982;40–59.
25. Harding HC. Hypnosis in the treatment of migraine. In: Lassner J, ed. *Hypnosis and Psychosomatic Medicine.* New York: Springer-Verlag, 1967;131–134.
26. Hilgard ER. Pain: its reduction and production under hypnosis *Proc Am Phil Soc* 1971;115:470–473.
27. Mutter CB, Coates ML. Hypnosis in family medicine. *Am Fam Physician* 1990;42:70s–73s.
28. Koziol JA, Clark DC, Gittes RF, Tan EM. The natural history of interstitial cystitis: A survey of 374 patients. *J Urol* 1993;149:465–469.
29. Chaikin DC, Blaivas JG, Blaivas ST. Behavioral therapy for the treatment of refractory interstitial cystitis. *J Urol* 1993;149:1445–1448.
30. Koprowski P, Parsons CL. Interstitial cystitis: successful management by a pattern of increasing urinary voiding intervals. *J Urol* 1992;147: 587–591.
31. Chapman SL. A review and clinical perspective on the use of EMG and thermal biofeedback for chronic headaches. *Pain* 1986;27:1–43.
32. Wickramasekra I. A conditioned response model of the placebo effect: predictions from the model. *Biofeedback Self Regul* 1980;5:5–18.
33. Flor H, Haag G, Turk DC. Long term efficacy of EMG biofeedback for chronic rheumatic back pain. *Pain* 1986;27:195–202.
34. Ratner V, Slade D, Whitmore KE. Interstitial cystitis: a bladder disease finds legitimacy. *J Women Health* 1992;1:63–67.
35. Draucker CB. Coping with a difficult to diagnose illness: the example of interstitial cystitis. *Health Care Women Int* 1991;12:191–198.
36. Greenfield S, Kaplan S, Ware JE. Expanding patient involvement in care. *Ann Intern Med* 1985;102:520–528.
37. Kaplan SH, Greenfield S, Ware JE. Assessing the effects of physician–patient interactions on the outcomes of chronic disease. *Med Care* 1989;27:s110–s127.
38. Koziol JA. Epidemiology of interstitial cystitis. *Urol Clin North Am* 1994;21:7–20.
39. Ratner V, Slade D, Greene G. Interstitial cystitis: a patient's perspective. *Urol Clin North Am* 1994;21:1–5.

Interstitial Cystitis, edited by Grannum R. Sant.
Lippincott–Raven Publishers, Philadelphia ©1997.

CHAPTER 30

Hydroxyzine for Symptomatic Relief of Interstitial Cystitis Symptoms

Theoharis C. Theoharides and Grannum R. Sant

Interstitial cystitis (IC) is characterized by voiding frequency, nocturia, and dysuria as well as suprapubic pressure, dyspareunia, and suprapubic pain (1,2). On distention under general or spinal anesthesia, the bladder appears edematous and friable with submucosal petechial hemorrhages (glomerulations) (1,2). A number of publications have reported the presence of increased numbers of mast cells in bladder biopsies of IC patients (3–7). However, the number of bladder mast cells in controls and in patients with the nonulcerative form of IC has been reported not to differ significantly (3,8). Mast cells in the mucosa and submucosa of IC patients, however, were definitively increased over controls, and they were distinctly activated, in contrast to those in transitional carcinoma, which were also increased but were not activated (9). In addition, bladder mast cells from IC patients were more responsive to secretory stimuli than were those from normal tissue (10).

Interstitial cystitis occurs primarily in women, well over half of whom also have a history of allergies, and about one-third also report migraines and irritable bowel syndrome (IBS), all of which appear to worsen around the menstrual cycle and under stress (1,11). The therapy of IC is variable, largely because of the lack of any definitive theory as to the etiology and pathogenesis (2), even though mast-cell activation has emerged as a significant contributing factor (9,10). Over the years, systemic treatments have included glucocorticoids, the histamine-1 (H_1) receptor antagonist tripelennamine hydrochloride (Pyribenzamine) (12), intravesical dimethylsulfoxide (DMSO) (13), heparin (14), a polysulfonate (Elmiron) (15), and tricyclic antidepressants (16).

We previously demonstrated that mast cells are activated in sterile bladder and prostate inflammation (17), that bladder mast-cell secretion may be triggered by the neurotransmitter acetylcholine, and that mast-cell activation, rather than their absolute number, is a more reliable characteristic of IC (9). The unique piperazine H_1-receptor antagonist hydroxyzine blocks mast-cell activation (18). Moreover, hydroxyzine was recently shown to also block rat basophilic leukemia (RBL) cell secretion (19). The RBLs are equivalent to mucosal mast cells (MMC) (20). This drug was considered a good candidate to reduce IC symptoms because, in addition to its antihistaminic and mast-cell inhibition properties, it also reduces secretion from neurons (21) and has anticholinergic, anxiolytic, and sedative properties (Table 1). Preliminary reports on small groups of patients have been reported (22,23). Patients with IC who were prescribed hydroxyzine had a substantial improvement of symptoms after 3 to 4 months. Our experience with a larger group of 90 patients is the basis for this chapter.

MATERIALS AND METHODS

Oral hydroxyzine was prescribed as hydroxyzine hydrochloride (Atarax) or hydroxyzine pamoate (Vistaril) by the physicians responsible for the local care of their respective patients throughout the United States. In some cases, patients were allergic to the fillers or dyes used in the pill or capsule and were prescribed hydroxyzine HCl elixir instead.

Patients started with 25 mg at bedtime (QHS) for 1 week and progressed to 50 mg QHS the second week. The dose was then increased to 75 mg (50 mg QHS and 25 mg

T. C. Theoharides: Departments of Pharmacology and Experimental Therapeutics and Internal Medicine, Tufts University School of Medicine and New England Medical Center, Boston, Massachusetts 02111.

G. R. Sant: Department of Urology and Interstitial Cystitis Clinic, New England Medical Center and Tufts University School of Medicine, Boston, Massachusetts 02111.

TABLE 1. *Characteristics of hydroxyzine relevant to IC*

Mast cell secretion inhibitor
Neuron transmitter release inhibitor
H_1-receptor antagonist
Anticholinergic
Sedative
Anxiolytic

at midday) the third week or as soon as sedation became tolerable or disappeared.

Ninety IC patients, from over 200 who fit the NIH-established diagnostic criteria and had their respective physicians prescribe hydroxyzine, reported their progress. Both patients and physicians were put on notice that hydroxyzine is not approved for IC, that it should not be taken by any patient who was pregnant or contemplating pregnancy, and that it should be taken with caution by clinically depressed patients, as it may worsen untreated depression. It was also stressed that hydroxyzine is sedating, at least temporarily, and that concurrent administration of hydroxyzine and tricyclic antidepressants could increase sedation. Patients were provided with a standardized case report form in order to score the severity of their symptoms, using 10-cm (1 = best, 10 = worst) visual scales, which they filled out and returned to one of the authors (T.C.T.). All patients were female with a 1.7-year mean duration of symptoms and 5.2-month duration of treatment to date.

RESULTS

Obviously, these are results on random patients, followed by different physicians, reporting their clinical symptoms subjectively, and on a treatment regimen that varied slightly. The results are presented as percentage response of all patients who responded by phone or by returning the case report forms.

All 90 patients had been diagnosed with IC according to the NIH-established criteria, including bladder biopsy, in 72 of which mast cells were reportedly increased. All patients complained of frequency, nocturia (some as frequently as every 15 min), and pain. Of the 90 patients (Table 2), 60 had a history of allergic problems including allergic rhinitis, food allergies, drug allergies, asthma, contact dermatitis, or eczema. Thirty-five patients reported gastrointestinal problems that had been diagnosed as IBS.

TABLE 2. *Clinical conditions associated with IC*

Condition	Approximate incidence
Allergies	60/90
IBS	35/90
Migraines	25/90
Fibromyalgia	15/90

Many patients reported frequent headaches, but 25 specifically indicated migraines. Fifteen patients were also diagnosed with fibromyalgia. Most patients (83%) reported that their symptoms worsened premenstrually or at the time of ovulation. A majority of the patients indicated that their symptoms intensified after eating spicy food, chocolate, bananas, or citrus fruits or drinking beer, wine, coffee, tea, or carbonated beverages.

As shown in Table 3, the average response of all patients who had taken hydroxyzine for more than 3 months and reported their progress was about 40%. However, when results were tabulated for those patients who had a history of allergies, the mean improvement for all symptoms was about 55% (Table 4). The patients who reported the least or no benefit turned out to be those with the longest history of symptoms and/or those who were postmenopausal.

Interestingly, those patients who did best reported considerable improvement of most other symptoms, especially migraines and tolerance of foods to which they had previously been considered intolerant. Eleven patients returned to full-time work, although they had been incapacitated for years by IC, and another felt well enough to start her own business.

Some patients felt well enough and discontinued the medication, only to experience a return of symptoms within a couple of days; however, symptoms disappeared promptly on resumption of the drug. Some patients who had been on hydroxyzine for over 1 year managed to remain in remission while reducing hydroxyzine from 75 to 25 mg QHS.

The main side effect reported was sedation, especially in the morning, which lasted anywhere from 1 to 5 days every time the amount of hydroxyzine was increased. Four patients reported increased appetite, one bloating, and two developed urinary retention when the dose exceeded 50 mg/day. Two patients reported nightmares. Twenty-three were not sedated at all. All patients reported a substantial decrease in frequency of nocturia and increase in restful sleep before any other noticeable decrease in other symptoms.

DISCUSSION

These results were evaluated subjectively, without blinding or placebo controls. However, they were consistent in the extent and duration of the clinical response, especially in the younger patients with a history of allergies.

It is not entirely clear why hydroxyzine had such a beneficial effect or whether the effect was entirely related to an action on the bladder. Hydroxyzine is a piperazine H_1-receptor antagonist with a three-ring structure. It reaches a peak serum concentration about 2 hr after oral administration and is almost entirely metabolized and cleared through the kidneys and liver with a half-life that has been reported to vary from 3 to 20 hr in adults (24). Its

TABLE 3. *Effects of hydroxyzine[a] in IC Patients*

Symptoms	Improvement (% total)[a]	Number of patients[b]
Overall response	39	90
Frequency	42	90
Nocturia	53	89
Burning	38	64
Pressure	35	78
Painful intercourse	35	52

[a]At 75 mg per day for 3 months.
[b]Those who returned questionnaires or replied by phone.

TABLE 4. *Effect of hydroxyzine in IC patients with allergies*

Symptoms	Improvement (% total)[a]	Number of patients[b]
Overall response	57	55
Frequency	62	55
Nocturia	70	55
Burning	52	51
Pressure	50	47
Painful intercourse	40	39

[a]At 75 mg per day for 3 months.
[b]Those who returned questionnaires or replied by phone.

present clinical use is mostly limited to the treatment of pruritus and urticaria (25), even though it is also effective in the treatment of allergic rhinitis and in reversing histamine-induced airway obstruction (26,27).

Parenteral hydroxyzine given together with morphine has been shown to result in enhanced analgesia in the treatment of postoperative pain (28). Even though hydroxyzine is often used with opioids to treat migraines, a prospective double-blind study did not prove that hydroxyzine augments the analgesia of the opioids for the acute treatment of severe headaches (29,30). It appears that the combination of hydroxyzine and opioids may have originated in an attempt to limit the hypotension of opioid-induced histamine release from mast cells (31). However, this antihistaminic action alone is not sufficient to explain hydroxyzine's effectiveness in IC, as other common H_1-receptor antagonists are ineffective (1,2). The effect of hydroxyzine on mast cells clearly is an important part of its clinical effectiveness in reducing symptoms associated with IC (Table 1). Hydroxyzine inhibits mast-cell secretion (18,32), which means that it essentially blocks secretion of the numerous immune, vasoactive, and nociceptive mast-cell mediators (33), all of which could participate in the pathophysiology of IC (34).

Mast-cell activation in IC may result from a variety of triggers, especially neurohormonal secretagogues (33,35). Mast-cell secretion is triggered by neuropeptides (35), whereas in the brain it is also stimulated by the neurotransmitter acetylcholine and by direct nerve stimulation (36–38). Most IC patients report a worsening of their symptoms premenstrually or around ovulation, and it is important to note that although progesterone has been shown to inhibit histamine release from mast cells (39), estradiol augments secretion (40). Patients with IC also have a history of allergic problems, migraines, and IBS (41). The ability of hydroxyzine to inhibit mast-cell activation could explain its beneficial effect in other coexisting conditions because mast cells have been implicated in the pathophysiology of migraines and IBS (35,42,43). That mast cells are central to the pathophysiology of IC is supported by the fact that bowel used for bladder augmentation in IC may develop develop mast cell infiltration (44). Terminal ileal mast cells are elevated in patients with IBS (45), a syndrome similar to IC that is also exacerbated by stress (46).

Hydroxyzine also has the unique ability to inhibit neuronal depolarization by high potassium levels (21) and thus reduce secretion of neurotransmitters and neuropeptides that could trigger mast cells or damage the bladder directly (47). Mast cells have been localized close to neuronal processes in many organs, including the bladder (48). Moreover, neuropeptide-positive nerve processes are increased in the bladders of IC patients (49,50). Stress activates bladder mast cells (51), thus directly implicating the nervous system. Neurohormonal mast-cell activation results in altered or empty granules within the domain of the cell. This process is different from the exocytotic degranulation customarily seen in anaphylaxis (52). Intragranular activation is recognizable by electron microscopy, but many such mast cells would not stain with routine histochemical techniques. This explains why some authors have reported low mast-cell counts in IC patients (8). Similar intragranular activation has also been reported in gastrointestinal mast cells, where increased numbers of mast cells associated with nerves occur in ulcerative colitis (53). In fact, mast cells with extensive intragranular activation have also been noted in scleroderma and termed "phantom" mast cells (54).

Hydroxyzine has anticholinergic properties, which help reduce frequency of urination. Moreover, hydroxyzine's sedative and anxiolytic properties reduce nocturia as well as anxiety, which is often present in IC. The use of hydroxyzine QHS is indicated not only by its long half-life but by the fact that evening dosing of hydroxyzine reduces its adverse effects, although its beneficial action is maintained during the day (55). The ability of hydroxyzine to inhibit mucosal mast-cell secretion could also explain its beneficial effect against the intolerance or allergies many IC patients appear to have to foods. Red wine exacerbates IC symptoms and migraines, and it can cause serotonin release from platelets (56). Interestingly, the major hydroxyzine metabolite cetirizine (Zyrtec) appears to lack hydroxyzine's inhibitory effect on mast cells and blocks eosinophil recruitment, instead (57).

Certain antihistamines and tricyclic antidepressants have analgesic effects (58). For instance, amitriptyline has been reported to reduce symptoms of IC in about 35% of patients (16), and unpublished observations indicate similar responses to doxepin (1,34). The beneficial action of these drugs may partially be explained by the fact that amitriptyline has been reported to inhibit mast-cell secretion (59), whereas doxepin, a potent antihistaminic drug used to reduce symptoms of systemic mastocytosis, is also an analgesic (60,61). In addition, tricyclic drugs such as amitriptyline, desipramine, and imipramine have been shown to be effective in reducing the pain of diabetic neuropathy, post-herpetic neuralgia, and migraine headaches (62,63). However, all these drugs result in prolonged sedation and hypotension, and they should not be used in patients with cardiac conditions, hyperthyroidism, or hypertension.

Recently, an article in *U.S. News and World Report* (64) discussed the results of recent studies that reported that the histamine-1 receptor antagonists loratadine (Claritin), astemizole (Hismanal), and hydroxyzine (Atarax or Vistaril) as well as the antidepressants (65) amitriptyline (Elavil) and fluoxetine (Prozac) increased the growth of melanoma cells, an aggressive type of skin cancer, in mice (66). However, although amitriptyline and fluoxetine were also associated with cutaneous lymphoid hyperplasia (67), hydroxyzine was shown (all by the same researchers) to be cytotoxic against human breast carcinoma (68). The histamine-2 receptor antagonist cimetidine (Tagamet) did not have such an effect. The effect of these drugs was biphasic, augmenting tumor growth at low concentrations but inhibiting tumor growth at high concentrations. Histamine, itself, has been linked to both augmentation and inhibition of tumor growth (69). These antihistamines and antidepressants bind to an intracellular site termed the "antiestrogen binding site" (AEBS) (70), which appears to be an intracellular histamine receptor (68).

These and other apparently confusing results were recently discussed in an editorial that concluded that there is no immediate cause of concern but should promote communication among clinicians, drug safety experts, immunologists, and pharmacologists concerning these issues (71).

A small double-blind, placebo-controlled study funded in part by the Interstitial Cystitis Association (ICA) is currently in progress to ascertain the true efficacy of hydroxyzine in the treatment of interstitial cystitis.

CONCLUSIONS

In an open-label, nonconsecutive case series, 90 patients meeting the NIDDK-established criteria for IC were prescribed by their individual physicians a total of 75 mg per day hydroxyzine (50 mg at bedtime) for a mean duration of 5 months. Symptomatic response was assessed using case report forms with IC symptoms evaluated on visual analog scales. Improvement of IC symptoms was noticeable after 3 months, but the most pronounced relief of symptoms occurred in patients with a history of allergies and evidence of increased mast cells on bladder biopsy. Ten patients have remained in full remission for over 3 years. Discontinuation of the drug resulted in return of symptoms within a few days.

Hydroxyzine reduces IC symptoms because of its unique ability to inhibit bladder neuronal stimulation and mast-cell secretion of vasoactive and nociceptive mediators as well as its antihistaminic, anticholinergic, anxiolytic, and sedative effects. Hydroxyzine is recommended as a first-line treatment for patients with mild or recent symptoms, especially those with a history of allergies or documented bladder mastocytosis.

Acknowledgments

Costs associated with this work were covered by a grant from Kos Pharmaceuticals, Miami, FL. Thanks are due to Dr. V. Ratner and Ms. D. Slade as well as many IC patients for useful discussions and Ms. Linda Tamulaites and Ms. Susan Mayo for their word-processing skills.

REFERENCES

1. Sant GR. Interstitial cystitis. *Monogr Urol* 1991;12:37–63.
2. Pontari MA, Hanno PM. Interstitial cystitis. In: Walsh PC, Retik AB, Stamey TA, Vaughan ED Jr, Wein AJ, eds. *Campbell's Urology*. Philadelphia: WB Saunders, 1995;1–19.
3. Larsen S, Thompson SA, Hald T, et al. Mast cells in interstitial cystitis. *Br J Urol* 1982;54:283–286.
4. Kastrup J, Hald J, Larsen L, Nielsen VG. Histamine content and mast cell count of detrusor muscle in patients with interstitial cystitis and other types of chronic cystitis. *Br J Urol* 1983;55:495–500.
5. Aldenborg F, Fall M, Enerbäck L. Proliferation and transepithelial migration of mucosal mast cells in interstitial cystitis. *Immunology* 1986;58:411–416.
6. Lynes WL, Flynn SD, Shortliffe LD, et al. Mast cell involvement in interstitial cystitis. *J Urol* 1987;138:746–752.
7. Christmas TJ, Rode J. Characteristics of mast cells in normal bladder, bacterial cystitis and interstitial cystitis. *Br J Urol* 1991;68:473–478.
8. Hanno PM, Levin RM, Monson FC, et al. Diagnosis of interstitial cystitis. *J Urol* 1990;143:278–281.
9. Theoharides TC, Sant GR, El-Mansoury M, Letourneau RJ, Ucci AA Jr, Meares EM Jr. Activation of bladder mast cells in interstitial cystitis: a light and electron microscopic study. *J Urol* 1995;153:629–636.
10. Frenz AM, Christmas TJ, Pearce FL. Does the mast cell have an intrinsic role in the pathogenesis of interstitial cystitis? *Agents Actions* 1994;41:C14–C15.
11. Ratner V, Slade D, Whitmore KE. Interstitial cystitis: A bladder disease finds legitimacy. *J Women Health* 1992;1:63–68.
12. Simmons JL, Bunce PL. On the use of an antihistamine in the treatment of interstitial cystitis. *Am Surg* 1958;24:664–667.
13. Sant GR. Intravesical 50% dimethyl sulfoxide (RMSO-50) in treatment of interstitial cystitis. *Urology [Suppl]* 1987;29:17–21.
14. Parsons CL, Housley T, Schmidt JD, Lebow D. Treatment of interstitial cystitis with intravesical heparin. *Br J Urol* 1994;73:504–507.
15. Mulholland SG, Hanno PM, Parsons CL, Sant GR, Staskin DR. Pentosan polysulfate sodium for therapy of interstitial cystitis. A double-blind placebo-controlled clinical study. *Urology* 1990;35:552–558.
16. Hanno PM, Buehler J, Wein AJ. Use of amitriptyline in the treatment of interstitial cystitis. *J Urol* 1989;141:846–848.
17. Theoharides TC, Flaris N, Cronin CT, Ucci A, Meares E. Mast cell activation in sterile bladder and prostate inflammation. *Int Arch Allergy Appl Immunol* 1990;92:281–286.
18. Theoharides TC, Kops SK, Bondy PK, Askenase PW. Differential

release of serotonin without comparable histamine under diverse conditions in the rat mast cell. *Biochem Pharmacol* 1985;34:1389–1398.
19. Fischer MJE, Paulussen JJC, Horbach DA, et al. Inhibition of mediator release in RBL-2H3 cells by some H_1-antagonist derived anti-allergic drugs: relation to lipophilicity and membrane effects. *Inflamm Res* 1995;44:92–97.
20. Seldin DC, Adelman S, Austen KF, et al. Homology of the rat basophilic leukemia cell and the rat mucosal mast cell. *Proc Natl Acad Sci USA* 1985;82:3871–3875.
21. Konstantinidou AD, Lambracht-Hall M, Rozniecki JJ, Sugiultzoglu M, Theoharides TC. Hydroxyzine inhibits serotonin release from thalamic mast cells and neurons. *Neuropharmacology* (in press).
22. Theoharides TC. Hydroxyzine for interstitial cystitis. *J Allergy Clin Immunol* 1993;91:686–687.
23. Theoharides TC. Hydroxyzine in the treatment of interstitial cystitis. *Urol Clin North Am* 1994;21:113–119.
24. Simons ER, Simons KJ, Frith EM. The pharmacokinetics and antihistaminic property of the H_1 receptor antagonist hydroxyzine. *J Allergy Clin Immunol* 1984;73:69–75.
25. Theoharides TC. Histamine$_2$ (H_2)-receptor antagonists in the treatment of urticaria. *Drugs* 1989;37:345–355.
26. Schaaf L, Handeles L, Weinberger M. Suppression of seasonal allergic rhinitis symptoms with hydroxyzine. *J Allergy Clin Immunol* 1979;63: 129–133.
27. Kaliner M, Sigler R, Summers R, Shelhamer JH. Effects of infused histamine: analysis of the effects of H_1 and H_2 histamine receptor antagonists on cardiovascular and pulmonary responses. *J Allergy Clin Immunol* 1981;68:365–371.
28. Hupert C, Yacoub M, Turgeon LR. Effect of hydroxyzine on morphine analgesia for the treatment of postoperative pain. *Anesth Analg* 1980; 59:690–696.
29. Duarte C, Dunaway F, Turner L, Aldag J, Frederick R. Ketorolac versus meperidine and hydroxyzine in the treatment of acute migraine headache: a randomized, prospective, double-blind trial. *Ann Emerg Med* 1992;21:1116–1121.
30. Tek D, Mellon M. The effectiveness of nalbuphine and hydroxyzine for the emergency treatment of severe headache. *Ann Emerg Med* 1987; 16:308–313.
31. Lagunoff D, Martin TW, Read G. Agents that release histamine from mast cells. *Annu Rev Pharmacol Toxicol* 1983;23:331–351.
32. Simons FER. The antiallergic effects of antihistamines (H_1-receptor antagonists). *J Allergy Clin Immunol* 1992;90:705–715.
33. Galli SJ. New concepts about the mast cell. *N Engl J Med* 1993;328: 257–265.
34. Sant GR, Theoharides TC. The role of the mast cell in interstitial cystitis. *Urol Clin North Am* 1994;21:41–53.
35. Theoharides TC. Mast cells: the immune gate to the brain. *Life Sci* 1990;46:607–617.
36. Dimitriadou V, Buzzi MG, Moskowitz MA, Theoharides TC. Trigeminal sensory fiber stimulation induces morphologic changes reflecting secretion in rat dura mast cells. *Neuroscience* 1991;44:97–112.
37. Spanos C, El-Mansoury M, Letourneau R, et al. Carbachol-induced bladder mast cell activation: augmentation by estradiol and implications for interstitial cystitis. *Urology* 1996; 48:809–816.
38. Christmas TJ, Rode J, Chapple CR, Milroy EJ, Turner-Warwick RT. Nerve fibre proliferation in interstitial cystitis. *Virchows Arch [A]* 1990; 416:447–451.
39. Vliagoftis H, Dimitriadou V, Theoharides TC. Progesterone triggers selective mast cell secretion of 5-hydroxytryptamine. *Int Arch Allergy Appl Immunol* 1990;93:113–119.
40. Vliagoftis H, Dimitriadou V, Boucher W, et al. Estradiol augments while tamoxifen inhibits rat mast cell secretion. *Int Arch Allergy Appl Immunol* 1992;98:398–409.
41. Koziol JA, Clark DC, Gittes RF, Tan EM. The natural history of interstitial cystitis: a survey of 374 patients. *J Urol* 1993;149:465–469.
42. Theoharides TC. Mast cells and migraines. *Perspect Biol Med* 1983; 26:672–675.
43. Miner PB Jr. The role of the mast cell in clinical gastrointestinal disease with special reference to systemic mastocytosis. *J Invest Dermatol* 1991;96:40–44.
44. Kisman OK, Lycklama a Nijeholt AAB, van Krieken JHJM. Mast cell infiltration in intestine used for bladder augmentation in interstitial cystitis. *J Urol* 1991;146:1113–1114.
45. Weston AP, Biddle WL, Bhatia PS, Miner PB Jr. Terminal ileal mucosal mast cells in irritable bowel syndrome. *Dig Dis Sci* 1993;38:1590–1595.
46. Farthing MJG. Irritable bowel, irritable body, or irritable brain? *Br Med J* 1995;310:171–175.
47. Payan DG, Levine JD, Goetzl EJ. Modulation of immunity and hypersensitivity by sensory neuropeptides. *J Immunol* 1984;132:1601–1604.
48. Letourneau R, Pang X, Sant GR, Theoharides TC. Intragranular activation of bladder mast cells and their association with nerve processes in interstitial cystitis. *Br J Urol* 1996;77:41–54.
49. Pang X, Marchand J, Sant GR, Kream RM, Theoharides TC. Increased number of substance P positive nerve fibers in interstitial cystitis. *Br J Urol* 1995;75:744–750.
50. Hohenfellner M, Nunes L, Schmidt RA, Lampel A, Thuroff JW, Tanagho EA. Interstitial cystitis: increased sympathetic innervation and related neuropeptide synthesis. *J Urol* 1992;147:587–591.
51. Spanos C, Letourneau R, Sant GR, Theoharides TC. Degranulation of rat bladder mast cells (MC) in a non-traumatic stress model: implications for the pathogenesis of interstitial cystitis (IC). In: *NIH Interstitial Cystitis Scientific Research Symposium.* Bethesda, MD: NIH, 1995;110.
52. Dvorak AM, McLeod RS, Onderdonk A, et al. Ultrastructural evidence for piecemeal and anaphylactic degranulation of human gut mucosal mast cells *in vivo. Int Arch Allergy Appl Immunol* 1992;99:74–83.
53. Dvorak AM, McLeod RS, Onderdonk AB, et al. Human gut mucosal mast cells: ultrastructural observations and anatomic variation in mast cell–nerve associations *in vivo. Int Arch Allergy Appl Immunol* 1992;98: 158–168.
54. Claman HN, Choi KL, Sujansky W, Vatter AE. Mast cell "disappearance" in chronic murine graft-vs-host disease (GVHD)-ultrastructural demonstration of "phantom mast cells." *J Immunol* 1986;137: 2009–2013.
55. Goetz DW, Jacobson JM, Apaliski SJ, Repperger DW, Martin ME. Objective antihistamine side effects are mitigated by evening dosing of hydroxyzine. *Ann Allergy* 1991;67:448–454.
56. Jarman J, Glover V, Sandler M. Release of [^{14}C]5-hydroxytryptamine from human platelets by red wine. *Life Sci* 1991;48:2297–2300.
57. Campoli-Richards DM, Buckley MMT, Fitton A. Cetirizine: A review of its pharmacological properties and clinical potential in allergic rhinitis, pollen-induced asthma, and chronic urticaria. *Drugs* 1990;40: 762–781.
58. Rumore MM, Schlichting DA. Analgesic effects of antihistamines. *Life Sci* 1985;36:403–416.
59. Theoharides TC, Bondy PK, Tsakalos ND, Askenase PW. Differential release of serotonin and histamine from mast cells. *Nature* 1982;297: 229–231.
60. Sullivan TJ. Pharmacologic modulation of the whealing response to histamine in human skin: identification of doxepin as a potent *in vivo* inhibitor. *J Allergy Clin Immunol* 1982;69:260–267.
61. Hameroff SR, Cork RC, Weiss JL, Crago BR, Davis TP. Doxepin effects on chronic pain and depression: a controlled study. *Clin J Pain* 1985;1:171–176.
62. Max MB, Lynch SA, Muir J, Shoaf SE, Smoller B, Dubner R. Effects of desipramine, amitriptyline and fluoxetine on pain in diabetic neuropathy. *N Engl J Med* 1992;326:1250–1256.
63. Welch KMA. Drug therapy of migraine. *N Engl J Med* 1993;329: 1476–1483.
64. Brink S. A different kind of cancer risk. *US News & World Report* 1995.
65. Brandes LJ, Arron RJ, Bogdanovic RP, et al. Stimulation of malignant growth in rodents by antidepressant drugs at clinically relevant doses. *Cancer Res* 1992;52:3796–3800.
66. Brandes LJ, Warrington RC, Arron RJ, et al. Enhanced cancer growth in mice administered daily human-equivalent doses of some H_1-antihistamines: predictive *in vitro* correlates. *J Natl Cancer Inst* 1994;86: 770–775.
67. Crowson AN, Magro CM. Antidepressant therapy: a possible cause of atypical cutaneous lymphoid hyperplasia. *Arch Dermatol* 1995;131: 925–929.
68. Brandes LJ, Macdonald LM, Bogdanovic RP. Evidence that the antiestrogen binding site is a histamine or histamine-like receptor. *Biochem Biophys Res Commun* 1985;126:905–910.
69. Theoharides TC. Neuroimmunology of tumor growth: the role of mast cells. *Int J Immunopathol Pharmacol* 1988;1:89–98.
70. Sudo K, Monsma J, Katzenellenbogen BS. Antiestrogen binding sites distinct from the estrogen receptor: subcellular localization, ligand specificity, and distribution in tissues of the rat. *Endocrinology* 1983;112:425–434.
71. Theoharides TC. Antidepressants, antihistamines, interstitial cystitis and cancer. *J Urol* 1995;154:1481–1482.

Interstitial Cystitis, edited by Grannum R. Sant.
Lippincott–Raven Publishers, Philadelphia ©1997.

CHAPTER 31

Intravesical Therapies for Interstitial Cystitis

Dennis R. La Rock and Grannum R. Sant

Interstitial cystitis (IC) continues to be an enigmatic urologic syndrome in spite of the recent upsurge of scientific inquiry into its causes and pathophysiology (1–4). Diagnosis is based on symptomatology, endoscopic evaluation under anesthesia, and exclusion of specific bladder diseases. The recognition of the "nonulcer" variety of IC in 1978 led to increasing rates of diagnosis, especially in younger, premenopausal women (5–7). Because the pathophysiology of IC is unknown, treatment is frequently empirical, and a variety of systemic, intravesical, cystoscopic, and surgical treatments have been employed in IC. Investigators and clinicians rely on subjective measures and symptom scores to determine efficacy because there are no pathognomonic or objective measures of disease activity or severity. Furthermore, the variable natural history of IC makes evaluation of therapy an imprecise undertaking.

Intravesical pharmacotherapy is one of the mainstays in the treatment of IC, and intravesical dimethylsulfoxide (DMSO) is one of only two drugs approved by the Food and Drug Administration (FDA) for IC (8,9). However, other intravesical agents are used to treat the increasing number of patients being diagnosed with IC (10). These drugs are used singly or in combination with DMSO. This chapter summarizes the current approaches to intravesical therapy of IC.

OVERVIEW

In spite of the increasing prevalence of IC, its etiology remains unknown (11,12). The lack of specific pathognomonic disease markers has led to a number of etiologic postulates including autoimmune mechanisms, bladder mastocytosis, and a dysfunctional bladder epithelium associated with alterations in surface glycosaminoglycans (GAGs) (12–14). There is a current consensus that IC is not a single "cause-specific" disease but a syndrome characterized by bladder inflammation initiated by a variety of stimuli: mechanical, allergic, inflammatory, environmental, neuroimmunoendocrine, etc. (11,14).

The treatment of IC is empirical and nonspecific (10,15). Intravesical therapies target the bladder mucosal lining and/or bladder wall inflammation, leading to symptomatic relief of pain, frequency, and urgency. Intravesical treatment includes both single and multiple drug therapy. The rationale of combined therapy, e.g., DMSO plus steroids or heparin, is based on the additive antiinflammatory effects of the individual drugs (10).

Studies of intravesical therapy are hampered by the variable natural history of IC. Chronicity is a hallmark of IC, and a patient's clinical course is frequently punctuated by flare-ups and quiescence. Spontaneous remission rates of 10% to 15% have been reported in IC, but these figures beg a somber interpretation because of the lack of a specific disease marker and the subjective nature of IC symptoms (16,17). Young, sexually active women with IC may experience a worsening of their symptoms whenever bacterial cystitis is superimposed on their chronic symptoms of IC.

The lack of objective disease measures and the unpredictable natural history of IC present problems with drug studies of IC (Table 1). Randomized, double-blind, placebo-controlled studies are ideal for the assessment of therapeutic drug benefit, but such studies are the exception rather than the rule in IC. However, recent studies of sodium pentosanpolysulfate (Elmiron) and Nalmefene (an opioid agonist mast cell inhibitor) utilized the prospective, placebo-controlled model (18,19). Blinded studies of intravesical drugs have not been performed because of study design limitations. For example, dimethylsulfoxide (DMSO) administration is associated with a garlic breath, whereas sodium oxychlorosene

D. R. La Rock and G. R. Sant: Department of Urology and Interstitial Cystitis Clinic, New England Medical Center and Tufts University School of Medicine, Boston, Massachusetts 02111.

TABLE 1. *Drug studies in interstitial cystitis: Problems*

Variable natural history of IC
Spontaneous remissions
Placebo-response rate in drug studies
Coexistent urinary tract diseases
e.g., urinary tract infections
Lack of specific disease markers
Lack of objective response criteria
Few double-blind studies performed

lavage (Clorpactin) is painful and requires the administration of general or regional anesthesia (8,17). Thus, intravesical DMSO cannot be compared to placebo instillation of saline or water because the characteristic DMSO odor would betray the patients receiving DMSO. The obvious logistic limitations of placebo-controlled studies include the difficulty of keeping the drugs from being identified (smell and taste with DMSO; pain and need for anesthesia with Clorpactin), the impossibility of doing a head-to-head comparison of DMSO and Clorpactin, and finally, the lack of accepted objective response criteria.

An alternative to the dilemma of double-blind studies in IC is the use of a symptom-scoring index similar to the AUA/WHO symptom index for benign prostatic hyperplasia. A symptom index for IC has recently been validated, and this will likely offer a methodology for elucidating the natural history of IC and prove useful in testing drug efficacy (oral and intravesical) in IC (20) (see Chapter 34).

TREATMENT GOALS IN INTERSTITIAL CYSTITIS

The subjective symptoms of pain, frequency, and urgency do not easily allow for statistical evaluation of treatment outcomes. This difficulty is further compounded by the uncertain and unpredictable natural history of the disease. Although many patients accept the chronicity of their symptoms, some gravitate from physician to physician in search of the "magic bullet" to cure their disease (7).

The goal of therapy is the elimination or neutralization of the cause of IC. Because the causative factors are unknown, treatment is necessarily empirical. The majority of patients can expect meaningful symptom relief, albeit never total or permanent, with available therapies. Realistic determination of treatment efficacy requires a better knowledge of the natural history of IC, the use of uniform diagnostic criteria, and the identification of specific histologic (e.g., mast cell) or biochemical disease markers (7,14). The placebo response rate in IC is high because of the intermittency and subjectivity of its symptoms. Clear definitions of efficacy and treatment outcomes—subjective, objective, or representing "global well-being"—are required. Treatment frequently controls symptoms without influencing the endoscopic appearance of the bladder or the microscopic features of the disease.

The physician should aim to control or ameliorate the symptoms while providing support and understanding to the patient. Patients should be educated about the natural history and treatment options of IC and be reassured that IC is not a harbinger of systemic disease or malignancy. The rationale for the various therapies should be explained, and the lack of a specific cure emphasized. This will reduce the possibility of subsequent patient disenchantment and allows the physician to change easily from one treatment modality to another as needed. Many patients also benefit from concomitant psychotherapeutic support and counseling regarding coping mechanisms, family support, pain management, etc.

INTRAVESICAL PHARMACOTHERAPY: PRINCIPLES

Oral drug efficacy in IC is affected by drug pharmacokinetics and distribution. Most oral drugs are excreted in low amounts in the urine, either unchanged or as inactive metabolites. Side effects are relatively common with antihistamines, tricyclic antidepressants, steroids, etc., because high doses and/or prolonged courses of treatment are needed to achieve therapeutic benefits. The variable success of oral agents is partially explained by the pharmacokinetic vagaries of drug absorption, metabolism, and renal excretion. The small proportion of active drug that reaches the bladder accounts for the reduced *in vivo* effectiveness of many oral drugs.

Intravesical drug administration overcomes many of the problems associated with oral therapy (Table 2). High drug concentrations are achieved in the bladder, and the relatively poor absorption from the bladder results in a low incidence of systemic side effects. The drugs exert their effect directly on the inflamed bladder wall or the dysfunctional bladder lining without being influenced by

TABLE 2. *Intravesical instillations in IC*

Advantages:
Lack of significant systemic side effects
High drug concentrations
Minimal absorption
Noninterference by renal, liver metabolism
Single-agent, multiagent therapy
Disadvantages:
Morbidity of catheterizations
Patient discomfort
Urinary tract infections
Costs: visits, catheters, trays, etc.
Need for anesthesia
Clorpactin

drug interaction, metabolism, or the effects of liver, gastrointestinal, or renal function. High drug concentrations are delivered topically (i.e., locally) to the diseased organ, i.e., the inflamed bladder, and this reduces the potential for side effects or drug interaction.

Intravesical pharmacotherapy has certain disadvantages (Table 2). The morbidity of bladder catheterization is real, although the risk of urinary tract infection with clean, intermittent catheterization is low (21,22). Most patients receive intravesical therapy in the doctor's office, and this adds to treatment costs in terms of the office visit, time away from work, the costs of catheters, lubricants, topical anesthetics (in some patients), catheter trays, etc. Some patients may develop a transient chemical cystitis with irritation and bleeding or an occasional systemic effect, e.g., with Bacillus Calmette-Guérin (BCG) (8,23).

Intravesical therapy is the mainstay of IC treatment and the standard against which other treatments are measured (Table 3). Drugs such as silver nitrate, dimethylsulfoxide, and Clorpactin exert their effects directly on the bladder wall when administered intravesically. Short "dwell times" (usually 15 to 60 min) in the bladder reduce the chance of systemic absorption while delivering high drug concentrations to the inflamed bladder. Dimethylsulfoxide (RIMSO-50) is the only approved intravesical drug for the treatment of IC. However, silver nitrate and oxychlorosene sodium (Clorpactin WCS 90) have been used for many years to treat interstitial cystitis (24–26), and they are of proven safety and acceptable morbidity. Recently, two pilot studies have shown promise for new intravesical agents, i.e., BCG and hyaluronic acid (Cystistat) (23,27).

TABLE 3. *Intravesical agents used for IC*

Drugs
Dimethylsulfoxide (RIMSO-50)
Sodium oxychlorosene (Clorpactin WCS-90)
Heparin
Steroids
Sodium bicarbonate
Silver nitrate
Hydrodilation
Simple
Helmstein
Sodium pentosanpolysulfate (Elmiron)
Cromolyn sodium
Lidocaine
Doxorubicin
Bacillus Calmette-Guerin (BCG)
Cystistat (hyaluronic acid)
Mode of therapy
Single agent
Multiagent cocktails
Sequential therapy

INTRAVESICAL THERAPIES

Bladder Hydrodilation

Bladder hydrodistention is an essential component of the diagnostic evaluation of suspected IC as well as a useful therapy. Hydrodistention has been used since 1930 to treat IC, with variable success. The two common techniques for distention are simple hydraulic filling and intravesical (Helmstein) balloon hydrodistention. Treatment regimens aimed at increasing voiding intervals are surrogates for self-dilation (28,29). Such treatment is possible only if the patient does not suffer undue pain as a result of increasing voiding intervals.

Some patients report transient symptomatic relief after initial diagnostic cystoscopy and hydrodilation. The bladder is usually filled by passive gravity filling (pressure of 60 to 80 cm H_2O) for 2 to 3 min. Because the methods and treatment response criteria for hydrodistention are not standardized, true assessment of its therapeutic efficacy is impossible. About 20% of our patients experience short-term symptomatic relief (<3 months) following cystodistention. Bladder hydrodistention probably causes transient/partial ischemia or mechanical damage to the submucosal nerve plexus and stretch receptors in the bladder and leads to reduced pain and frequency and increased bladder capacity (9,22).

A greater degree of distention is achieved using the Helmstein intravesical balloon (30). A continuous epidural anesthetic is started in the cystoscopy suite and maintained for 3 hr in the recovery room. Saline or water is periodically added to the intravesical balloon whenever the bladder pressure, as measured by a sphygmomanometer, falls below the halfway point between systolic and diastolic blood pressures. The Helmstein procedure can double the bladder capacity and is especially useful in patients with markedly reduced (<300 to 400 ml) bladder capacities. The duration of response is usually a few months, and repeat hydrodistentions are needed. This risk of bladder rupture is reduced if hydrodistention is not performed at the time of bladder biopsy. Patients with thin bladder walls are also at increased risk of perforation. Gross hematuria frequently develops following removal of the Helmstein balloon, and bladder drainage with a large foley catheter (gravity or three-way irrigation) may be necessary. Backache and flank discomfort may occur during the hydrodistention because of the obstruction of urine flow into the bladder (10).

Silver Nitrate

The caustic, antiseptic, and astringent properties of silver nitrate render it useful for the treatment of interstitial cystitis (24). The activity of the silver nitrate depends on its concentration and the duration of its "dwell time" in the bladder. Bladder penetration is negligible because the silver ion is precipitated.

Various dosage and treatment schedules of silver nitrate instillation have been recommended. Concentrations range from 1:5,000, 1:2,000, 1:1,000 to as high as 1% to 2% (1 to 2:100). Higher concentrations require local or general anesthesia for administration. Silver nitrate intravesical "dwell times," though not standardized, vary between 2 and 10 min. Silver nitrate monotherapy as well as combination therapy with bladder distention, bladder mucosal anesthesia (e.g., with cocaine hydrochloride), and bladder fulguration have been used (9,24). Treatment intervals vary but average 6 to 8 weeks. One treatment protocol employs gradually increasing concentrations on successive days.

A cystogram is required to exclude patients with vesicoureteral reflux. Biopsies should not be performed at the time of treatment because of the risk of silver nitrate extravasation into the surrounding tissues (9). Leakage into the peritoneum, pelvis, and retroperitoneum can be potentially serious and even fatal.

Because silver nitrate is frequently combined with hydrodistention and fulguration of ulcerated areas, assessment of its efficacy is difficult. The overall reported success rate with intravesical silver nitrate monotherapy is about 50% after 1 year (9,10). Intravesical silver nitrate therapy is safe and inexpensive, and dilute solutions can be administered in the office. However, the drug has not been evaluated in controlled clinical trials, and intravesical dimethylsulfoxide (DMSO) is currently the drug of choice for "first-line" intravesical therapy.

Sodium Oxychlorosene (Clorpactin WCS-90)

Oxychlorosene sodium is a mixture of hypochlorous acid and the sodium salt of dodecylbenzene sulfonic acid. Hypochlorous acid is liberated following intravesical instillation, and the sulfonic acid augments drug penetration and the germicidal action of the hypochloride. Clorpactin exerts a "detergent" action on the bladder mucosa, and a 0.2% solution can be administered with local anesthesia at weekly intervals (four to six treatments). The "bleaching" effect of the Clorpactin is difficult to reconcile with the hypothesis that a damaged bladder mucopolysaccharide layer is related to the development of the disease (9,10,17).

The initial rationale for the use of Clorpactin in the 1950s was based on the similarity between the "classic form" of interstitial cystitis with small, scarred, ulcerated bladders and tuberculosis of the bladder (26,31). Clorpactin was used to treat bladder tuberculosis, and this led to its empirical use in interstitial cystitis based on the unsubstantiated belief that IC is caused by unidentified bacteria.

A 0.4% Clorpactin solution is commonly used, but it requires a general or regional anesthetic because intravesical instillation is painful. Repeat instillations are frequently needed, as only about one-third of the patients achieve long-term remission of their symptoms. Relief of pain and discomfort can be quite dramatic, and remissions may last for up to 6 to 12 months. The risk of multiple Clorpactin instillations include the additive morbidity of multiple anesthetics and the theoretical concern of repeated insults and damage to the bladder mucosa. However, in over 80 patients treated at our Interstitial Cystitis Clinic with repeat lavage (up to eight to ten times), there has been no cumulative bladder mucosal dysplasia, reduced bladder capacity, or *de novo* initiation of vesicoureteral reflux. Furthermore, there has been no mortality or morbidity attributable to the multiple anesthetics (17).

Intravesical Clorpactin is usually reserved for patients who fail to respond to intravesical DMSO or silver nitrate therapy. Before instillation, position and configuration of the ureteral orifices should be carefully examined. If the orifices appear incompetent, a cystogram should be done to exclude vesicoureteral reflux (9,17). Reflux of Clorpactin into the ureters or renal pelvis can lead to fibrosis and later complications (31). Clorpactin can be administered to patients with reflux provided that the ureteral orifices are occluded with small, Fogarty-type embolectomy catheters and the patient is placed in a steep reversed Trendelenburg position.

The majority of patients experience troublesome urgency, frequency, dysuria, and pain for a few days following Clorpactin instillation (17). An indwelling Foley catheter left in for 24 to 48 hr postinstillation promotes patient comfort. Patients frequently require narcotic analgesics for control of pain and anticholinergics for relief of frequency and urgency. Suprapubic pain/pressure and dyspareunia seem to respond better than urinary frequency, urgency, and nocturia. However, treatment responses have not been prospectively analyzed or categorized. There is no standard protocol for Clorpactin lavage. Previous reports used varying concentrations (0.2% to 0.4%), differing frequencies of administration, and either local or general/regional anesthesia. Messing and Stamey reported a 79% success rate after six instillations, success being defined as >6 months of symptomatic improvement (5,31).

Our current technique of Clorpactin lavage is outlined in Table 4. The patient requires a general or regional anesthetic. Cystoscopy is performed, followed by a standard bladder hydrodilation for 2 to 3 min at a pressure of 60 to 80 cm H_2O. The bladder capacity is measured, and the presence and degree of glomerulations terminal hematuria, and ulcerations are assessed. A freshly prepared (within 6 hr) 0.4% solution of Clorpactin is then instilled into the bladder via a 20F 5-cc balloon foley catheter. The perineum is protected with a moist towel from the caustic effects of inadvertent spillage or pericatheter leakage of Clorpactin. The volume of Clorpactin instilled is usually 250 to 500 cc. This amount is dependent on the bladder

TABLE 4. *Technique of Clorpactin lavage*

Cystoscopy under anesthesia (general, regional)
Passive bladder hydrodilation
Measurement of bladder capacity
Shield perineum, introitus with moistened bowel
Keep foley balloon snug at bladder neck (especially in women)
Instill 0.4% Clorpactin solution via indwelling foley
Use a volume 50–60% of bladder capacity
"Dwell time" 5–7 min
Repeat instillations three or four times
Drain Clorpactin, irrigate foley with normal saline

capacity as determined at the time of the bladder hydrodilation. A volume of approximately half of the measured capacity is employed to allow adequate drug contact drug with the bladder mucosal surface. Larger volumes may spontaneously leak around the catheter and cause caustic burns to the external meatus, vaginal introitus, or perineum.

"Dwell time" is usually 5 to 7 min, after which the bladder is drained; the process is then repeated for a total of three or four times, for a cumulative "dwell time" of 15 to 25 min. At the end of the lavage, the Clorpactin is drained, and the bladder is copiously irrigated with normal saline. The perineum and vaginal introitus are also irrigated. During the filling and lavage stages of the treatment, the Foley catheter is gently extended so that the balloon is snug at the bladder neck so as to reduce the chances of pericatheter leakage. The foley catheter is left for gravity drainage overnight; the patient is discharged, and the catheter is removed 1 to 2 days later. Most patients experience a worsening of their symptoms in the immediate postoperative period, and this can last for days to weeks. Adequate preoperative counseling is important in this regard so that patients have realistic postoperative expectations.

There is no way to predict the response to Clorpactin lavage, the duration of any response, or the number of treatments required to achieve it. Comparisons with placebo are needed to confirm the effectiveness of Clorpactin lavage. Subjective assessment using symptoms scores and global assessment indicates that 50% to 60% of patients achieve meaningful symptomatic improvement (17). Clorpactin can be instilled as single treatment or as a course of treatment, e.g., six instillations at monthly or biweekly intervals. Because of the costs and the potential risks—anesthetic and surgical—of repeated lavage, our preference is for single lavage therapy.

Dimethylsulfoxide (RIMSO-50)

Dimethylsulfoxide (DMSO) has many pharmacologic properties—antiinflammatory, analgesic, muscle relaxant, mast cell stimulation, and collagen dissolution—that make it appealing for the treatment of interstitial cystitis (8,10). The initial technique of topical suprapubic application has been superseded by the intravesical instillation of an aqueous 50% solution (RIMSO-50), which was approved by the FDA in 1978 for the treatment of interstitial cystitis.

Dimethylsulfoxide is a widely used drug for the treatment of IC because of its affordability, ease of office administration, and proven safety (Table 5). RIMSO-50 is administered in the office via a small (8F or 10F) urethral catheter after the urethra is anesthetized with 2% lidocaine jelly. It is inadvisable to administer DMSO at the time of bladder biopsy. Treatment should not begin until the bladder biopsy sites are healed, usually 3 to 4 weeks postoperatively. This avoids significant absorption via the unhealed biopsy sites. A sterile urine is a prerequisite for intravesical DMSO instillation. A careful urinalysis should be done before each instillation. Patients with pyuria/bacteriuria should not receive treatment unless the urine is sterile and any urinary tract infection has been treated.

Instillations are given every 1 to 2 weeks for four to eight treatments. The frequency and duration of treatment are empirical. A small number of patients experience a temporary worsening of their symptoms initially. This is probably a result of DMSO-induced release of histamine from mast cells or of a transient chemical cystitis. Fifty milliliters of RIMSO-50 is instilled into the bladder, the catheter is removed, and the patient is instructed to hold the medication in the bladder for 15 to 20 min before voiding. Longer "dwell times" of up to 1 to 2 hr are associated with annoying bladder discomfort, which can lead to patient dissatisfaction. After the initial course of treatment, subsequent instillations are administered depend-

TABLE 5. *Intravesical dimethylsulfoxide therapy*

Monotherapy
Combination therapy
DMSO + steroids
DMSO + heparin
DMSO + steroids + bicarbonate
Treatment regimens
Nonstandardized
Once or twice weekly for four to eight treatments
Maintenance therapy (variable)
Relapses
Relapse rate 35–40%
60–80% relapsers respond to further DMSO treatment
Response
Overall response rate 50–90%
Slightly better with "nonulcer" patients
Drawbacks
Chemical cystitis in 5–10%
Initial worsening of symptoms in 10–15%
Transient garlic breath in 20–40%

ing on the severity of symptoms and the temporal response to treatment.

Many patients experience a garlic-like breath odor and a similar taste in their mouths because of the pulmonary excretion in expired air of a small percentage of the DMSO. These symptoms are self-limiting and rarely last for more than 24 to 48 hr (8,22,32). About 10% of patients experience a transient chemical cystitis manifested by bladder spasms and irritability, and they benefit from short courses of oral anticholinergics (e.g., Pro-Banthine, or oxybutynin) or belladonna and opium suppositories (10). Numerous clinical studies with DMSO have failed to demonstrate changes in the ocular refractive index or the development of lens opacities in humans. However, the manufacturer still recommends slit-lamp eye examinations before and during RIMSO-50 treatment. Dimethylsulfoxide is teratogenic in animals and should be avoided during pregnancy. (8)

Both forms ("early" and "classic") of interstitial cystitis respond to RIMSO-50 treatment (8,22,32,33). Patients with "classic" IC—ulcerated, small capacity bladders—experience a 50% to 70% symptomatic improvement (Table 5). Some authors report parallel improvements in bladder capacity and endoscopic appearance of the bladder. However, it is difficult to truly assess these parameters because DMSO responders do not routinely undergo cystoscopy. Patients with "nonulcer" disease respond to intravesical DMSO therapy with reported response rates of 50% to 90%.

The overall relapse rate after a 4- to 8-week course of treatment is between 35% and 40%, but 50% to 60% of relapsers respond to additional intravesical DMSO treatment (8,22). The timing of treatment in "relapsers" depends on their symptoms. Most patients who relapse require treatment at 1- to 2-monthly intervals. Response rates are variously defined in the reported series, and this makes comparisons difficult. One study did report objective urodynamic and cystoscopic improvement in patients receiving intravesical DMSO. Patients with the more severe symptoms may need monthly prophylactic instillations. In general, the bladder capacity and bladder mucosa remain unchanged following intravesical DMSO treatment. Although most studies of intravesical DMSO have been uncontrolled, urodynamic and symptomatic significance was demonstrated in a placebo-controlled, double-blind crossover study (32,34).

Intravesical DMSO is safe, cheap, efficacious, and free of local or systemic toxicity. Suitably motivated and trained individuals can be taught the technique of intermittent catheterization for instillation of DMSO (21). This allows self-treatment. Patients can administer treatment whenever bladder symptoms warrant, and this avoids the cost, in terms of time and money, of repeated visits to the physician's office.

RIMSO-50 therapy is frequently augmented in patients who do not respond to the initial course of treatment and in those with eosinophilic inflammation in their bladder biopsies. Hydrocortisone (100 mg) mixed with 50 ml of RIMSO-50 is usually beneficial (8,10). The antiinflammatory actions of the two drugs are additive, with the DMSO serving as a "vehicle" to enhance penetration of the hydrocortisone into the bladder wall. The intravesical instillation of steroids (e.g., hydrocortisone or Kenalog) avoids the side effects of systemic steroid therapy (Table 5). Although oral steroids have been used in the past to treat IC, and with good results, the deleterious effects of high-dose oral steroid therapy (e.g., fluid retention, osteoporosis) for a chronic disease such as IC resulted in the near abandonment of this form of therapy. In our experience, 25% to 30% of the patients who do not respond to DMSO monotherapy will get symptom improvement when steroids are added to the DMSO (10).

Heparin (5,000 units) and sodium bicarbonate (1 ampoule), which enhances steroid activity, have been recommended to increase the antiinflammatory activity of the DMSO–steroid mixture (22,34). Although a variety of intravesical "cocktails" are available, we prefer a simplified approach to intravesical therapy starting with RIMSO-50 monotherapy (16). Multiagent intravesical cocktails are useful in selected patients, but it is difficult to attribute specific therapeutic benefits to individual drugs in the mixture. Reported treatment outcomes with intravesical heparin and DMSO mixtures are not significantly better than with DMSO alone (22).

Open and controlled clinical studies have demonstrated the beneficial effects of intravesical DMSO in both types of interstitial cystitis (ulcerative and nonulcerative). Its safety is proven, and there are few side effects. Many patients with IC benefit from intravesical DMSO at some point in their clinical course.

Heparin

Intravesical heparin, in a dose of 10,000 IU monthly, reduces relapses in patients who respond to RIMSO-50, and it has been recommended for maintenance therapy. Heparin, an anionic polyelectrolyte, has antiinflammatory and "surface-protective" actions as well as inhibitory effects on fibroblast proliferation, angiogenesis, and smooth muscle proliferation. It also mimics the antiadherence characteristics of the bladder glycosaminoglycan (GAG) mucosal lining, and this property makes it a theoretically attractive drug for treatment because of the putative etiology of a GAG deficiency in interstitial cystitis (9). This is also the rationale for treatment with the oral agent—sodium pentosanpolysulfate (Elmiron) (18,35). Treatment with intravesical heparin (10,000 units in 10 ml sterile water) three times per week for 3 months resulted in clinical remission of symptoms in 27 of 48 patients (56%) (36), and the remission was maintained in 80% to 90% of patients for up to 1 year if they continued maintenance intravesical heparin therapy.

A recent report demonstrated a decrease in the relapse rate from 52% in patients treated with DMSO alone to 20% in those maintained with monthly instillations of heparin and followed for 12 months (37). This approach holds promise for future improvement in reducing treatment relapses after intravesical DMSO therapy. Heparin has also been administered by endoscopic, intralesional injections of Hunner's ulcers supplemented by intravenous therapy. More recently, subcutaneous heparin has been shown to alleviate symptoms, particularly pelvic and bladder pain, and be associated with a fall in serum and urine levels of eosinophilic cationic protein (38). Recent reports, however, suggest that it is no better than placebo.

Other Intravesical Agents

The continuing search for a satisfactory treatment of IC has led to the use of a variety of intravesical drugs (Table 3). Pilot studies of intravesical pentosanpolysulfate sodium (Elmiron) suggest a therapeutic benefit, with earlier responses compared to oral administration. However, published reports are lacking. Intravesical disodium cromoglycate (cromolyn sodium), a mast cell inhibitor, showed promise in an early study with amelioration of symptoms in six of nine patients (39). However, the responses were short-lived, and most patients required subsequent treatment with hydrodilation. Intravesical lidocaine (200 mg lidocaine in 40 ml normal saline) has been anecdotally reported to control pain and frequency in a single patient with "classic" interstitial cystitis. Twice-weekly instillations for 1 hr were used, but symptoms recurred within 3 months of stopping the treatment (40).

Intravesical doxorubicin (Adriamycin) has also been used in three patients with the ulcer type of interstitial cystitis (41). Irritative voiding symptoms resolved in all the patients accompanied by complete healing of their ulcers. Weekly treatments (50 mg doxorubicin in 50 ml normal saline) for 6 weeks followed by monthly instillations were used with bladder "dwell times" of 2 hr. Frequency, urgency, and dysuria were common side effects. Follow-up in this study was short (only 5 weeks in two of the three patients), and further documentation of the efficacy of this regimen is required before it enters the therapeutic mainstream.

Two recent pilot studies show efficacy of intravesical BCG (Bacillus Calmette-Guerin) and Cystistat. (23,27) Intravesical BCG was used in five patients with refractory IC who had failed standard treatment. Patients had 6 weekly treatments and they were evaluated pre- and post-treatment by symptoms questionnaires and water cystometry. All showed reduced medication requirement and improved symptom scores (pain, frequency, etc.) as well as increased bladder capacity. Most importantly, three patients reported complete relief of symptoms! Although the mechanism of action of BCG in IC is unknown (anti-inflammatory versus immunotherapy, etc.), these promising results suggest that a prospective, randomized, double-blind placebo-controlled study is needed to confirm these findings and determine optimal dosage and treatment schedules (23).

On the assumption that the bladder epithelial mucosal lining is defective in IC, the glycosaminoglycan hyaluronic acid (Cystistat) was instilled intravesically in a group of 25 patients with refractory disease (27). The drug dosage was 40 mg weekly for 4 weeks, followed by monthly administration. By 20 weeks, about 70% of patients had a positive response (complete or partial), but the response decreased beyond 6 months. There was no significant toxicity or morbidity associated with hyaluronic acid therapy. Double-blind, placebo-controlled studies are ongoing in Canada, and they should define the role of Cystistat in the therapeutic armamentarium.

These two new agents show obvious promise and would add greatly to the therapeutic options available to the urologist if their efficacy is confirmed by prospective, placebo-controlled trials.

SUGGESTED INTRAVESICAL TREATMENT ALGORITHM

Treatment of IC usually begins with endoscopic diagnosis and the hydrodilation done as part of the initial cystoscopy (3,7). Following diagnosis, treatment is begun with some form of oral or intravesical therapy. Intravesical therapy can be employed as "first-line" treatment or reserved for patients who fail to respond to oral therapy with anticholinergics, antiinflammatories, antihistamines, Elmiron, etc.

Dimethylsulfoxide, singly or in combination, is the first avenue of intravesical treatment. It is administered on an outpatient basis and with little morbidity. DMSO monotherapy is our preferred choice for initial intravesical therapy (7,10). Patients who fail to respond to four to six weekly instillations are empirically switched to DMSO combination therapy for two to four weekly treatments. Some patients who fail DMSO monotherapy benefit from the addition of steroids (either hydrocortisone or Kenalog). The antiinflammatory properties of steroids are particularly noticeable in IC patients in whom bladder biopsies show microscopic evidence of eosinophilic inflammation. The known antiallergic activity of steroids may add to the therapeutic benefit of DMSO in such patients.

Heparin and sodium bicarbonate are also employed for intravesical DMSO combination therapy (8,22). However, in our experience, these drugs add little to the efficacy of DMSO—-steroid instillations. Heparin maintenance, 10,000 IU administered monthly, does appear to reduce relapses in patients who respond to an initial course of DMSO or DMSO and steroids. This approach

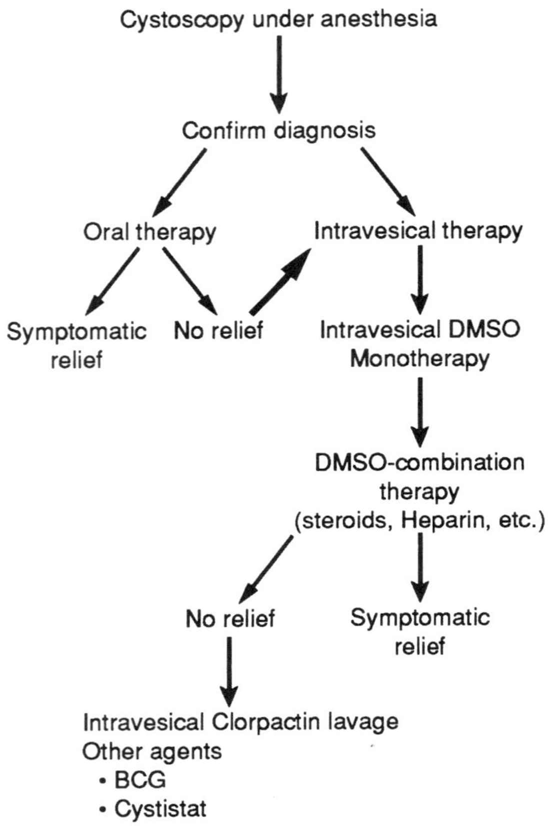

FIG. 1. Suggested treatment algorithm.

to maintenance therapy merits further study, and if its efficacy is confirmed, it should reduce the number of patients requiring alternative forms of therapy. Patients who fail to respond to DMSO—monotherapy or combination therapy—are candidates for Clorpactin lavage.

Clorpactin is reserved for DMSO nonresponders and patients with the most severe symptoms. Clorpactin is not employed as first-line intravesical treatment because its administration requires anesthesia (regional or general), and many patients are reluctant to consider Clorpactin treatment because of the potential morbidity, e.g., pain, bladder irritation. The complication rate with Clorpactin lavage is low, and we have encountered no serious complications—anesthetic or surgical—with its use. The mechanism of action of Clorpactin is uncertain, although the symptoms of pain/pressure seem to respond more than those of frequency and nocturia.

Intravesical DMSO and Clorpactin are currently the most widely used and effective intravesical agents in our therapeutic armamentarium. However, they are not panaceas, and many patients require alternative forms of treatment. Our current treatment algorithm for interstitial cystitis is outlined in Fig. 1.

CONCLUSIONS

The treatment of interstitial cystitis is difficult and frequently frustrating for the patient and physician. Treatment is hampered by the lack of a clear understanding of its pathophysiology, and this makes it difficult to objectively assess disease severity and/or progression.

Clearly, there are drawbacks to intravesical therapy. Responses to intravesical lavage are variable in duration, unpredictable, and unamenable to objective measurement. Multiple treatments are frequently needed, as with DMSO, and multiple anesthetics may be required for Clorpactin therapy. There have been no double-blind, placebo-controlled studies comparing the mainstays—Clorpactin, DMSO—of intravesical treatment.

We hope that current research into the pathogenesis and causation of interstitial cystitis will lead to an improved understanding of this disease or syndrome. The introduction of newer, more specific intravesical therapies will surely follow such advances.

REFERENCES

1. Hunner GL. Elusive ulcer of the bladder. *Am J Obstet* 1918; 78:374–377.
2. Gillenwater JY, Wein AJ. Summary of the National Institute of Arthritis, Diabetes, Digestive and Kidney Diseases Workshop on Interstitial Cystitis, National Institutes of Health, Bethesda, MD, August 28–29, 1987. *J Urol* 1988;140:203–206.
3. Hanno P, Levin RM, Monson FC, Teuscher C, Zhou ZZ, Ruggieri M, Whitmore K, Wein AJ. Diagnosis of interstitial cystitis. *J Urol* 1990; 143:278–281.
4. Sant GR. Diagnosis of interstitial cystitis—a clinical, endoscopic and pathologic approach. In: Hanno PM, Staskin DR, Krane RJ, Wein AJ, eds. *Interstitial Cystitis*. London: Springer-Verlag, 1990;107–113.
5. Messing EM, Stamey TA. Interstitial cystitis: early diagnosis, pathology and treatment. *Urology* 1978;12:381–392.
6. Meares EMM Jr. Interstitial cystitis—1987. *Urology* 1987;29(4 Suppl): 46–48.
7. Sant GR. Interstitial cystitis. *Monogr Urol* 1991;12(3):37–63.
8. Sant GR. Intravesical 50% dimethyl sulfoxide (RIMSO-50) in treatment of interstitial cystitis. *Urology* 1987;29(4 Suppl):17–21.
9. Hanno PM, Wein AJ. Medical treatment of interstitial cystitis other than Rimso-50, Elmiron. *Urology* 1987;29(4:Suppl):22–26.
10. Sant GR, La Rock DR. Standard intravesical therapies for interstitial cystitis. *Urol Clin North Am* 1994;21(1):73–83.
11. Fall M, Johansson SL, Aldenborg F. Chronic interstitial cystitis: a heterogenous syndrome. *J Urol* 1987;137:35–38.
12. Ratliff TL, Klutke CG, McDougall EM. The etiology of interstitial cystitis. *Urol Clin North* Am 1994;21(1):21–30.
13. Sant GR, Meares EM Jr. Interstitial cystitis—diagnosis, pathogenesis and treatment. *Infect Urol* 1990;3:24–30.
14. Theoharides TC, Sant GR. Bladder mast cell activation in interstitial cystitis. *Semin Urol* 1991;9:74–87.
15. Sant GR. Interstitial cystitis—pathogenesis, evaluation and treatment. *Urol Ann* 1990;3:171–196.
16. Messing EM. The diagnosis of interstitial cystitis. *Urology* 1987;29 (4 Suppl):4–7.
17. La Rock DR, Sant GR. Intravesical clorpactin lavage for refractory interstitial cystitis. *Infect Urol* 1995;8(5):151–157.
18. Mulholland SG, Hanno P, Parsons CL, Sant GR, Staskin DR. Pentosan polysulfate sodium for therapy of interstitial cystitis. A double-blind placebo-controlled clinical study. *Urology* 1990;35:552–558.
19. Stone NN, Sherman F. Pilot study of the opiate antagonist nalmefene (IVX-B-111) in patients with interstitial cystitis. *J Urol* 1990;143:280A.
20. O'Leary MP, Sant GR, Whitmore K, et al. The interstitial cystitis symptom index. *J Urol* 1996;155(Suppl):439A.

21. Biggers RD. Self administration of dimethyl sulfoxide (DMSO) for interstitial cystitis. *Urology* 1986;28:10–11.
22. Hanno PM, Wein AJ. Conservative therapy of interstitial cystitis. *Semin Urol* 1991;9:143–147.
23. Zeidman EJ, Helfrick B, Pollard C, Thompson IM. Bacillus Calmette-Guerin immunotherapy for refractory interstitial cystitis. *Urology* 1994;43:121–124.
24. Pool TL, Rives HF. Interstitial cystitis: treatment with silver nitrate. *J Urol* 1944;51:520–522.
25. O'Conor VJ. Clorpactin WCS 90 in the treatment of interstitial cystitis (abstract). *Q Bull Northwest Univ Med School* 1955;29:392–394.
26. Wishard WN, Nourse MH, Mertz JHO. Use of clorpactin wcs 90 for relief of symptoms due to interstitial cystitis. *J Urol* 1957;77:420–422.
27. Morales A, Emerson L, Nickel JC, Lundie M. Intravesical hyaluronic acid in the treatment of refractory interstitial cystitis. *J Urol* 1996; 156(1):45–48.
28. Blaivas S, Blaivas JG. Successful treatment of sensory urgency and interstitial cystitis with behaviour modification. *J Urol* 1986;135:189A.
29. Parsons CL, Kaprowski PF. IC: Successful management by increasing urinary voiding intervals. *Urology* 1991;37:207–212.
30. Dunn M, Ramsden PD, Roberts JBM, Smith JC, Smith PJB. Interstitial cystitis treated by prolonged bladder distension. *Br J Urol* 1977; 49:641–645.
31. Messing EM, Freiha FS. Complication of clorpactin wcs 90 therapy for interstitial cystitis. *Urology* 1979;13:389–392.
32. Perez-Marrero R, Emerson LE, Feltis JT. A controlled study of dimethyl sulfoxide in interstitial cystitis. *J Urol* 1988:140:36–39.
33. Barker SB, Matthews PN, Philip PF, Williams G. Prospective study of intravesical dimethyl sulfoxide in the treatment of chronic inflammatory bladder disease. *Br J Urol* 1987;59:142–144.
34. Perez-Marrero R, Emerson LE. Interstitial cystitis. *Can J Obstet Gynecol* 1990;116:4–8.
35. Fritjofsson A, Fall M, Juhlin R, Persson BE, Ruutu M. Treatment of ulcer and non-ulcer interstitial cystitis with sodium pentosanpolysulfate: multicenter trial. *J Urol* 1987;138:508–512.
36. Parsons CL, Housley T, Schmidt JD, Lebow D. Treatment of interstitial cystitis with intravesical heparin. *Br J Urol* 1994;73(5): 504–507.
37. Perez-Marrero R, Emerson LE, Maharajh DO, Juma S. Prolongation of response to DMSO by heparin maintenance. *Urology* 1993;41(1 Suppl):64–66.
38. Lose G, Jespersen J, Frandsen B, Hojensgard JC, Astrup T. Subcutaneous heparin in the treatment of interstitial cystitis. *Scand J Urol Nephrol* 1985;19:27–29.
39. Edwards L, Bucknall JE, Makin C. Interstitial cystitis: possible cause and clinical study of sodium cromoglycate. *Br J Urol* 1986;58:95–96.
40. Asklin B, Cassuto J. Intravesical lidocaine in severe interstitial cystitis. Case report. *Scand J Urol Nephrol* 1989;23:311–312.
41. Khanna OP, Loose JH. Interstitial cystitis treated with intravesical doxorubicin. *Urology* 1990;36:139–142.

Interstitial Cystitis, edited by Grannum R. Sant.
Lippincott–Raven Publishers, Philadelphia ©1997.

CHAPTER 32

Interstitial Cystitis: A Women's Health Perspective

Vicki Ratner and Debra Slade

In the past 10 years, the picture of interstitial cystitis (IC) has changed dramatically. Patients are getting diagnosed more quickly and treated more effectively. Research funding has increased significantly, and researchers are painstakingly uncovering clues about this enigmatic disease. Yet we still do not know the cause or, more likely, causes; there is no definitive diagnostic test or marker for the disease; and there are no uniformly effective treatments. There are an estimated 500,000 cases of IC, but probably many more remain undiagnosed. Although IC has 25 times the number of sufferers as hemophilia, 17 times the number of cystic fibrosis, and is more common than multiple sclerosis, it remains unrecognized by many in the medical community. We still don't know why 90% of IC sufferers are women or why it strikes so many young, healthy women. From a women's health perspective, we have many challenges to face before we conquer this disease.

THE IC PATIENT'S PERSPECTIVE

Interstitial cystitis, a chronic inflammatory condition of the bladder wall, is a devastating disorder. Unremitting pain and urinary frequency of up 70 times a day wreak havoc in patients' personal, family, and professional lives. Many people with IC find travel difficult or impossible. Some must work reduced schedules, and others are forced to go on disability. Many abstain from sex rather than risk exacerbation of their symptoms. Many give up sports and leisure activities, and others are unable to fulfill essential family obligations. A 1987 study by the Urban Institute revealed that the quality of life of IC patients is worse than that of women on dialysis for end-stage renal disease.

The personal testaments of IC patients continue to document a sad story of medical ignorance and indifference. One woman wrote to Ann Landers describing "years of nonstop pain, 40 to 60 bathroom trips a day, little sleep, lots of tests, 12 doctors, hundreds of allergy shots, diets, antibiotics, and six unnecessary operations." Another confides that she consulted ten doctors—a family physician, a gynecologist, an internist, and several urologists—for 4 agonizing years before being diagnosed with IC. "I was told that the pain was all in my head—that it was due to the stress of studying law or, at one point, to grief over my father's recent death. The pain was unbearable. It felt like a knife being turned inside of me." These are just two examples of the thousands of letters that the ICA has received.

When treatments alleviate symptoms, many patients are able to manage their disease effectively and lead near-normal, productive lives. "After being diagnosed with IC, I was an emotional and physical wreck," one patient recalls. "Numerous doctors dismissed my symptoms. At the insistence of a friend, I consulted a urologist who initiated DMSO instillations. Within a month, I was back to my normal life, and have been mostly well for four years."

In spite of new treatments and pain management techniques, far too many patients are still misdiagnosed, and many diagnosed patients are not helped by any treatment. Far too many are still told that they will just have to learn to live with their pain. Indeed, the Urban Institute study found that IC patients have suicidal thoughts four times more frequently than the general population. "Sometimes I wish I was dead because the misery and pain are unbearable," one female IC patient wrote to the ICA. "If I had cancer, I would know sooner or later that I would be either in remission or dead, but with IC, I only suffer day

V. Ratner and D. Slade: Interstitial Cystitis Association, New York, New York 10159.

after day, without any hope of getting better. So many times I have thought of killing myself to get out of the pain and mental suffering caused by this disease." The grim fact is that suicides have been reported. Recently, the ICA received this note from the widower of an IC patient. "Enclosed are three donations made in memory of my wife Joanna...who was diagnosed with IC following a hysterectomy. Like many other sufferers, Joanna was told it was in her head after tests turned up nothing. A cystoscopy revealed the disease, [but] the extreme pain and despair over chances for a cure caused her to end her life on April 8, 1995."

Creative use of standard treatments, as well as ancillary therapies, dietary changes, stress control, pain management, and information on a plethora of helpful coping techniques might have saved Joanna's life and the lives—and quality of life—of numerous IC patients. This information is available, and access to it should be provided by all practitioners who treat IC patients.

PATIENT ACTIVISM PUTS IC ON THE MAP

The Interstitial Cystitis Association was born out of patient desperation. My own story (V.R.) is well known. I was stricken with IC in medical school, and although I had access to the "best" medical care, I endured the classic syndrome of misdiagnosis and mistreatment that has all too often been the lot of IC sufferers. Determined that others should not have to endure the pain and uncertainty of protracted and sometimes fruitless medical odysseys, I searched out a few other IC patients. In the living room of my apartment in New York City in 1984, we agreed on the need for an assertive, determined patient advocacy organization. Just emerging from the isolation of having a so-called "rare" disease, we had no idea of how many IC patients there were. We began to get a clue, however, when I appeared on ABC's "Good Morning, America" in 1985. We got 10,000 letters of response within the first 2 weeks.

The ICA is a grassroots patient advocacy and educational organization established to provide a support network for IC patients and their families, to educate the public and the medical community about the realities of IC, and to insist on research to search for its cause, better treatments, and, ultimately, a cure.

Our success in these areas has greatly exceeded our early, rather modest expectations. In 1987, we prompted the National Institute of Diabetes, Digestive, and Kidney Diseases (NIDDK) to sponsor a 2-day medical conference devoted entirely to IC. The ICA had significant input into this meeting, which resulted in improved diagnostic criteria and a commitment from the NIDDK to support the establishment of a national data base of IC patients. Participating in this meeting was a core group of physicians and other researchers who came with more questions than answers but were committed to provide scientific expertise and leadership in the struggle to raise awareness and understanding of IC among their colleagues. Since then, this group of dedicated physicians has grown significantly, joined by research scientists, nurses, and other practitioners who are working with us to conquer IC.

Today, the ICA coordinates a support network of over 15,000 people in the United States and has offshoots in Canada, England, and Germany as well. In communities across the country in nearly every state in the United States, IC patients have organized support groups, medical meetings, media campaigns, political action campaigns, and very successful fundraising drives. And they have even promoted initiatives to improve access to restrooms. The ICA produces a quarterly newsletter, the *ICA Update,* bringing patients the latest information on research, information on scientific conferences, the latest in treatments, coping strategies, and provides a comprehensive resource catalog. We also sponsor a biannual national meeting that features a medical symposium reviewing current research and workshops on treatments and coping strategies for patients and their families. Over the years, ICA members have appeared on national television, and articles on IC have appeared in *Readers Digest, U.S. News and World Report, The New York Times, The Washington Post, Modern Maturity, Ms., Longevity, Ladies Home Journal, Good Housekeeping,* and other national magazines. Our media exposure has been a critical link in reaching thousands of desperate IC sufferers who would otherwise have gone undiagnosed.

Because of advocacy by the dedicated members of the ICA family, the lives of patients are significantly better. Dr. Philip Hanno, Chair of the Department of Urology at Temple University School of Medicine, paid us a supreme compliment by saying that "the ICA is a textbook example of what a strong patient advocacy group can accomplish for a little known disease." Over the years we've been privileged to work closely with Dr. Hanno and the other members of our Medical Advisory Board in our struggle to unravel the complex enigmas of this disease.

PARTNERSHIP WITH THE NATIONAL INSTITUTES OF HEALTH

Until 1987, not a single penny of federal research funds had been spent on IC. Early on, we recognized that an intensive research effort was needed to gain some insight into the disease and to move toward finding a cure. The ICA initiated a political action campaign that consisted of Congressional visits and a letter-writing campaign to Senators and Representatives. Patients told their heart-wrenching stories before Congressional committees. As a result of these successful annual campaigns, and through the support of Senator Harry Reid from Nevada, Congress has earmarked $11 mllion specifically for IC and related research, via the National Institutes of Health (NIH). Because of our continued efforts, since 1990, funding for IC has increased 145%, exceeded only by increases for breast cancer (200%) and ovarian disease (157%).

Today, the Urology Division of the NIH works in partnership with the ICA and has been extremely supportive of developing and promoting interest in IC in the research community. Without the tremendous commitment of NIH, under the direction of Dr. Lee Nyberg, Director of Urology, the range and depth of research would never have evolved. Scientific conferences on IC have been held regularly since 1987. In January 1995, the NIDDK sponsored a 3-day meeting on IC and basic bladder research that revealed new insights and promising leads toward new therapies. Another conference followed in October.

Because of intense competition with other more established diseases for research money, the ICA instituted its own fund-raising campaign to provide seed money to researchers so that they might obtain preliminary results. To date, we have funded many projects that have gone on to receive NIH funding.

SCIENTIFIC PROGRESS

Until about 1986, scientific interest in interstitial cystitis was minimal. In editions of *Campbell's Urology* before 1986, the section on psychosomatic disorders included IC, which it characterized as a disorder that "may represent the end stage of a bladder that has been made irritable by emotional disturbance...a pathway for the discharge of unconscious hatred." On this basis, thousands of desperate IC patients were told "it's all in your head," and advised to take vacations, drop out of school, get married, get unmarried, or to see a psychiatrist. Fortunately, this erroneous bit of medical dogma has been corrected.

Before 1986, it was difficult to find a urologist who believed that IC existed. Dr. Daniel Brookoff, a pain management specialist and a member of the ICA's Medical Advisory Board, has observed that "There's nothing like an effective treatment to make a doctor believe a disease and want to treat it." Unfortunately, he notes, that reasoning also occurs in reverse. "If there is no cure and there is no uniformly effective treatment, then there must be no disease." Today, these incorrect assumptions about IC have changed substantially.

Further testament to the immense progress made over the past decade in raising awareness about interstitial cystitis is its treatment in the scientific and medical press. Ten years ago, IC was barely a footnote in medical texts; now it has become the sole subject of prestigious scientific publications. A supplement to *Urology* (Vol. 29, 4) edited by Grannum R. Sant, M.D. was published in April 1987. A comprehensive volume, *Interstitial Cystitis* by Drs. Philip M. Hanno, David R. Staskin, Robert J. Krane, and Alan J. Wein, was published in 1990. The February, 1994 issue of the *Urologic Clinics of North America* was devoted entirely to IC. Most recently, a supplement to *Urology* (vol 49, 5A) edited by Drs. Alan Wein and Philip Hanno was published in May 1997. The publication of these works along with discussion on IC in a variety of other scientific journals, including this landmark text, further enhances the visibility and status of this once widely ignored disease.

The medical progress has been impressive. We now have a clearer picture of the natural history of interstitial cystitis. We now have enough information to begin separating IC patients into subgroups according to what may cause their symptoms and, consequently, which treatments may be most effective. Pain management, avoided in the past because of fears about drug dependence, is now being employed, and patients who lived—sometimes for decades in unremitting pain—are getting some relief. Surgery, formerly thought appropriate for about 10% of IC patients, is now recommended only as a last resort when all other remedies have failed. Finally, patients are learning how to be assertive about their needs and are insisting on access to a wide range of treatment options. They are also insisting on a cooperative relationship with their physicians and support staffs.

THE CHALLENGES

The progress cited above is impressive by any standards, but serious challenges remain. Perhaps foremost is to maintain the current level of federal research funding. This becomes more and more difficult in the current political climate mandating few increases and many cuts to the federal budget.

It is essential that funding levels be maintained in order for researchers to gain a better understanding of IC and to begin to examine the relationship between IC and other conditions such as irritable bowel disease, chronic fatigue syndrome, fibromyalgia, endometriosis, and vulvodynia, which are becoming increasingly common among the IC patient population. In addition, the relationship between IC and abacterial prostatitis and prostatodynia in men needs to be elucidated to determine if they are really the same disease. We need to increase our efforts to educate all doctors, especially urologists, gynecologists, internists, and family practice physicians, about IC. It is unconscionable that some patients still have to doctor-hop repeatedly before having their symptoms understood and taken seriously.

THE PROGNOSIS

From a women's health perspective, it seems fair to say that the prognosis for a cure for IC is, at best, guarded. A group of largely female patients is seeking treatment from a medical community dominated by men. The field of urology remains focused on prostate disease and male sexual dysfunction. Of the approximately 8,600 Board-certified urologists in the United States, only 85 are women. Urologists must become more responsive to female urologic problems, and gynecologists, who often fill the role of women's primary care physician, and increasingly, family physicians, must be trained in the diagnosis and treatment of urologic problems.

Dramatic and profound changes in our health care system are putting the most vulnerable, especially the poor and those who are plagued with chronic diseases like IC, at risk. Without the guarantee of universal coverage, many IC patients may ultimately be forced into bankruptcy by astronomical medical bills. Gatekeepers of health maintenance organizations (HMOs) may deny coverage for a disease that is not universally agreed on as a "disease" as well as refuse to refer the patient to a knowledgeable urologist when a diagnosis has been made.

In order not to lose what we have won, we must maintain a united front. We must not accept misdiagnosis and mistreatment silently. We must let the medical community and Congress know that the pain and disruption of IC are too severe to be ignored. From ground zero in 1985, we have come a surprising distance. With determination, talented researchers, and sufficient funding, we will find a cure.

Interstitial Cystitis, edited by Grannum R. Sant.
Lippincott–Raven Publishers, Philadelphia ©1997.

CHAPTER 33

Health-Related Quality-of-Life Issues in Interstitial Cystitis

Anita K. Wagner, Carolyn C. Shea, and Grannum R. Sant

Interstitial cystitis (IC) greatly impacts patients' lives, and its burden extends far beyond symptoms of pelvic pain and urgency into the physical, social, role, and emotional functioning and well-being of patients, leading to disability, social isolation, unemployment, depression, and even suicide (1,2). Although clinicians are well aware of the impact IC has on the daily lives of their patients, the standardized measurement of this impact in research and clinical practice has been elusive. The focus of the lengthy process of diagnosing, treating, and researching interstitial cystitis (IC) has largely been the physical aspects of the disease. The impact of the emotional and quality-of-life implications of IC has only been recently identified and evaluated.

Daily interactions with patients, their families, social supports, as well as health care providers, both directly and indirectly affected by IC, have identified and emphasized the need for further research, evaluation, and understanding of the impact of the disease and its impact on patient quality of life.

In this chapter, we describe the use of standardized patient-completed, health status measures in patients with IC. Specifically, the following issues are addressed: the concepts and methods of standardized health status measurement; the general health status of IC patients as assessed by the SF-36 Health Survey instrument; potential applications of health status measurement in IC research and patient care; and the need for future studies.

C. C. Shea, and G. R. Sant: Department of Urology and Interstitial Cystitis Clinic, New England Medical Center and Tufts University School of Medicine, Boston, Massachusetts 02111.

A.K. Wagner: Department of Neurology, Tufts University School of Medicine and The Health Institute, New England Medical Center, Boston, Massachusetts 02111.

MEASUREMENT OF HEALTH-RELATED QUALITY OF LIFE

The goal of medical care for most patients is the achievement of a more fulfilling life and the preservation of functioning and well-being (3). Since the beginning of this century, the redefinition of health, together with innovations in health-status measurement technology, have focused on standardized assessments of patients functioning and well-being in their daily lives. In 1941, Dr. Henry Sigerest introduced a positive definition of health when he wrote that "health is not simply the absence of disease; it is something positive, a joyful attitude toward life, a cheerful acceptance..., responsibilities.... the care is not complete before the patient has been readjusted socially and enabled to resume his old position or adjust... to a new one" (4). In 1947, the Constitution of the World Health Organization defined health as "a state of complete physical, mental, and social well-being and not merely the absence of disease and infirmity" (5).

The multidimensional definition of health has been nicely illustrated by Ware (6) using the analogy of a pond (Fig. 1): when a rock is thrown in a pond, the ripples go out all over the pond. Similarly, the symptoms of IC, or its treatment (e.g., intravesical dimethylsulfoxide, oral tricyclic antidepressants, antihistamines) affect multiple domains of an individual s life, his or her health status, or health-related quality of life (HQL).

Incorporating this broad definition of health in the assessment of the quality of medical care services, Lembke postulated in 1952 that "the best measure of quality is not how well or how frequently a medical service is given, but how closely the result approaches the fundamental objectives of improving life, relieving distress, restoring function and preventing disability" (7). In the 1990s, an era of health care cost containment, assessment

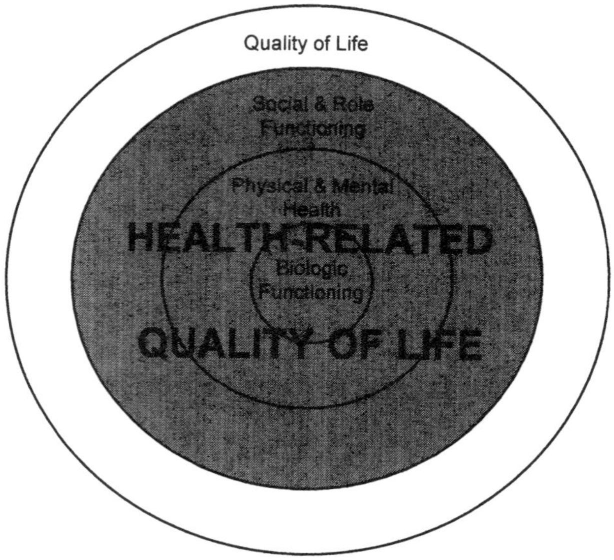

FIG. 1. Health status concepts.

of patients' functioning and well-being as a part of health care quality evaluation has become crucial (8).

Because the patient is the best source of information regarding the achievement of the goals of health care (9), his or her point of view in monitoring the quality of medical care outcomes has been increasingly recognized (8), and standardized patient questionnaires have been developed. During the past 50 years, the techniques of constructing patient-based outcomes measures and the content of such measures have been refined. Psychometric theory and methods to develop health status measures have led to the development of reliable and valid measures of functioning and well-being, i.e., patient-completed health status or HQL questionnaires (8,9).

The HQL questionnaires are broadly categorized into generic and specific questionnaires. Generic measures assess concepts that are globally relevant, including ability to function in everyday life and emotional well-being (10). They are not specific to any age, disease, or treatment group. Because generic measures are designed to be broadly applicable across populations with differing diseases and treatments, they allow for comparisons between different conditions (11). Generic measures estimate the HQL burden of a particular condition in relation to that of another, and they allow comparison of the HQL of patients with a specific disease, such as IC, to that of patients without a chronic condition. Specific measures focus on the impact of a particular disease and its treatment on specific concepts and domains (12). A modular approach, combining general and specific measures, has also been recommended (12–14).

Table 1 lists the health concepts represented in ten commonly used generic health status questionnaires (8). Although some concepts, such as sleep and cognitive function, are represented less frequently than others, there is consensus regarding the inclusion of physical, social, and role functioning, which are represented in all the measures.

A widely used general health status measurement instrument is the MOS (Medical Outcome Study) SF-36 (Short Form-36) Health Survey (15–17), which allows for comprehensive and precise measurement of general health. Broad and in-depth measurement of the general domains of HQL are achieved. With the advent of this practical and psychometrically tested and validated general instrument, comparisons of HQL across different populations are possible. With eight multiitem scales, the SF-36 measures the patient's perception of the following health concepts: physical functioning, role limitations related to physical problems, bodily pain, general health perceptions, vitality, social functioning, role limitations

TABLE 1. *Content of widely used general health surveys*[a]

Concepts	QWB	SIP	HIE	NHP	QLI	COOP	EuroQOL	Duke	MOS FWBP	MOS SF-36
Physical functioning	•	•	•	•	•	•	•	•	•	•
Social functioning	•	•	•	•	•	•	•	•	•	•
Role functioning	•	•	•	•	•	•	•	•	•	•
Psychological distress		•	•	•	•	•	•	•	•	•
Health perceptions (general)			•	•	•	•	•	•	•	•
Pain (bodily)		•	•	•	•	•	•	•	•	
Energy/fatigue	•		•	•				•	•	•
Psychological well-being			•					•	•	•
Sleep		•		•				•	•	
Cognitive functioning		•						•	•	
Quality of life			•			•			•	
Reported health transition						•			•	•

[a]Modified from Ware (8), with permission. QWB, Quality of Well-Being Scale; SIP, Sickness Impact Profile; HIE, Health Insurance Experiment Surveys; NHP, Nottingham Health Profile; QLI, Quality-of-Life Index; COOP, Dartmouth Function Charts; EuroQOL, European Quality-of-Life Index; Duke, Duke Health Profile; MOS FWBP, MOS Functioning and Well-Being Profile; MOS SF-36, MOS 36-Item Short Form Health Survey.

TABLE 2. *Information about SF-36 scales and summary measures and the interpretation of low and high scores*[a]

Scale	Label	No. of items	No. of levels	Meaning of scores: Low scores	Meaning of scores: High scores
Physical functioning	PF	10	21	Significant limitations in performing all physical activities, including bathing or dressing, because of health	Performs all types of physical activities, including the most vigorous, without limitations related to health
Role: physical	RP	4	5	Problems with work or other daily activities as a result of physical health	No problems with work or other daily activities as a result of physical health
Bodily pain	BP	2	11	Very severe and extremely limiting pain	No pain or limitations caused by pain
General health	GH	5	21	Evaluates personal health as poor and believes it is likely to get worse	Evaluates personal health as excellent
Vitality	VT	4	21	Feels tired and worn out all of the time	Feels full of pep and energy all of the time
Social functioning	SF	2	9	Extreme and frequent interference with normal social activities related to physical or emotional problems	Performs normal social activities without interference from physical and emotional problems
Role: emotional	RE	3	4	Problems with work or other daily activities as a result of emotional problems	No problems with work or other daily activities as a result of emotional problems
Mental health	MH	5	26	Feelings of nervousness and depression all of the time	Feels peaceful, happy, and calm all of the time
Physical health summary	PCS	36	567	Substantial limitations in self-care, physical, social, and role activities; severe bodily pain; frequent tiredness; health rated "poor"	No physical limitations, disabilities, or decrements in well-being; high energy level; health rated "excellent"
Mental health summary	MCS	36	493	Frequent psychological distress, substantial social and role disability caused by emotional problems; health in general rated "poor"	Frequent positive affect; absence of psychological distress and limitations in usual social/role activities from emotional problems; health rated "excellent"

[a]From Schweitzer et al. (20) and Deyo and Patrick (22), with permission.

arising from emotional problems, and general mental health. It also includes a single item that examines change in health over time.

The eight SF-36 scales can be grouped into scales that predominantly assess either physical health (the physical functioning, role-physical, and pain scales) or mental or emotional health (the mental health, role-emotional, and social functioning scales). Within physical health, the physical functioning scale measures limitations in performing daily physical activities, such as walking, carrying groceries, etc.; the role-physical scale assesses disability resulting from physical limitations; and the pain scale assesses the severity of pain and resulting limitations. Similarly, the mental health scale measures functioning, and the role-emotional scale measures disability resulting from limitations within the mental health domain. Scales that have been found to contain attributes of both the mental and the physical domain are the social functioning, general health perceptions, and vitality scales (15). Based on factor-analytic studies, two summary scores, the physical component summary (PCS) and the mental component summary (MCS), can be constructed (18). Table 2 provides information about the SF-36 health status scales and their interpretation.

THE HEALTH-RELATED QUALITY OF LIFE OF PATIENTS WITH INTERSTITIAL CYSTITIS

The SF-36 questionnaire has been completed by 172 patients with interstitial cystitis (IC). These patients were either evaluated or beginning treatment at the Interstitial Cystitis Clinic at New England Medical Center. After confirming that the SF-36 met standard criteria of data quality and psychometric requirements, patient SF-36 scale scores were compared with those of an age- and gender-matched sample from the general United States population (16,19).

The SF-36 scale scores in IC are represented in Fig. 2. SF-36 scales are ordered such that the scales on the left half of the graph are those mostly measuring physical health components, and those at the right are the scales mostly measuring mental health components (16,18). Scale scores range from 0, indicating worst health, to 100, indicating best health, in each domain. Compared to

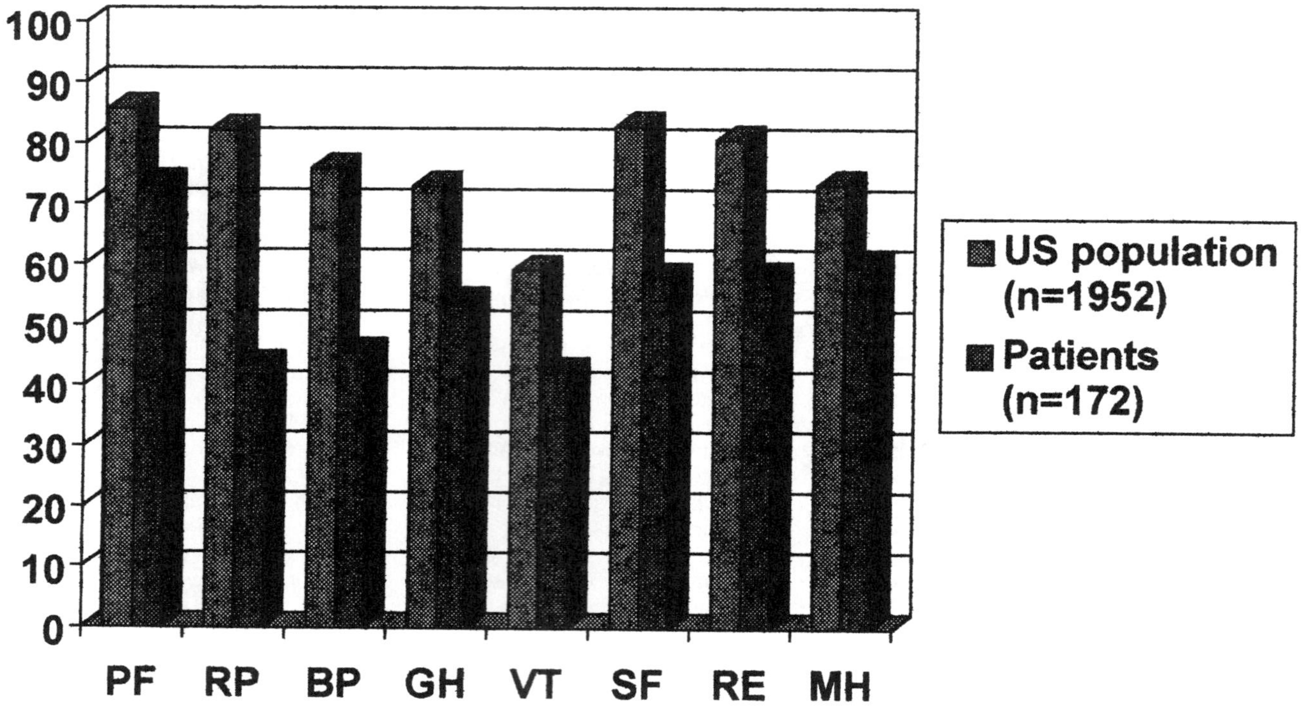

FIG. 2. Comparison of IC patient's SF-36 scale scores with those of the age- and gender-matched U.S. population.

the general population, patients with symptoms of IC scored significantly ($p < 0.001$) lower in all eight domains of health assessed by the SF-36. Knowledge gathered from the Medical Outcomes Study (19) underscores the societal relevance of IC patients' lower health status. For example, compared to the bodily pain scale score of the age- and gender-matched general population, the IC patients' lower (i.e., more pain) pain score goes hand in hand with a close to threefold increase in the likelihood of patients not being able to work because of their health (34.7% versus 12.9%) (16).

The PCS and MCS scores of IC patients were compared with those of the general population and patients with selected medical conditions. Figure 3 illustrates the PCS and MCS scores for the general U.S. population, IC patients, outpatients seen at the New England Medical Center Psychiatry Clinic, and patients with rheumatoid arthritis. Both PCS and MCS are standardized to have a mean of 50 and a standard deviation of 10 in the general U.S. population (18). To assess differences in general health as perceived by the patients, scores in this comparison are not adjusted for age and gender differences. Most of the IC patients in our sample were female (96.5%), while the gender distribution in the other samples was more even (57.2% of the general population sample, 61.1% of the psychiatric patients, and 59.1% of the arthritis patients are female). These demographic differences notwithstanding, comparisons of PCS and MCS quantify the general health burden experienced by IC patients in both the physical and mental health domains. Among the three chronic conditions, IC patients evaluate their physical health as poorer (PCS = 41.1) than the general population (PCS = 50) as well as poorer than patients from an ambulatory psychiatry clinic (PCS = 49.8). However, IC patients judge their physical health as better than arthritis patients (PCS = 35.9). These PCS scores suggest that IC patients are about six times more likely than individuals in the general population to cut down on work time because of health problems. However, they are only half as likely to do so as patients with arthritis (18).

Patients with IC (MCS = 42.0) experience more mental health impact than patients with arthritis (MCS = 53.9); however, as expected, the mental health impact of psychiatric outpatients (MCS = 32.5) is almost one standard deviation larger. The Medical Outcome Study demonstrated that scores are related to criteria such as life satisfaction, psychiatric morbidity, and utilization of health care services (18). Patients with IC score about 8 points lower on MCS than the general population, and this translates into about a 1.5-fold decrease in the probability of IC patients being satisfied with their lives, a twofold increase in the probability of screening positive on a three-item screen for depressive symptoms, and a 1.7-fold higher likelihood of receiving mental health care services within the next 6 months. These data indicate that IC patients experience a substantial impact on their

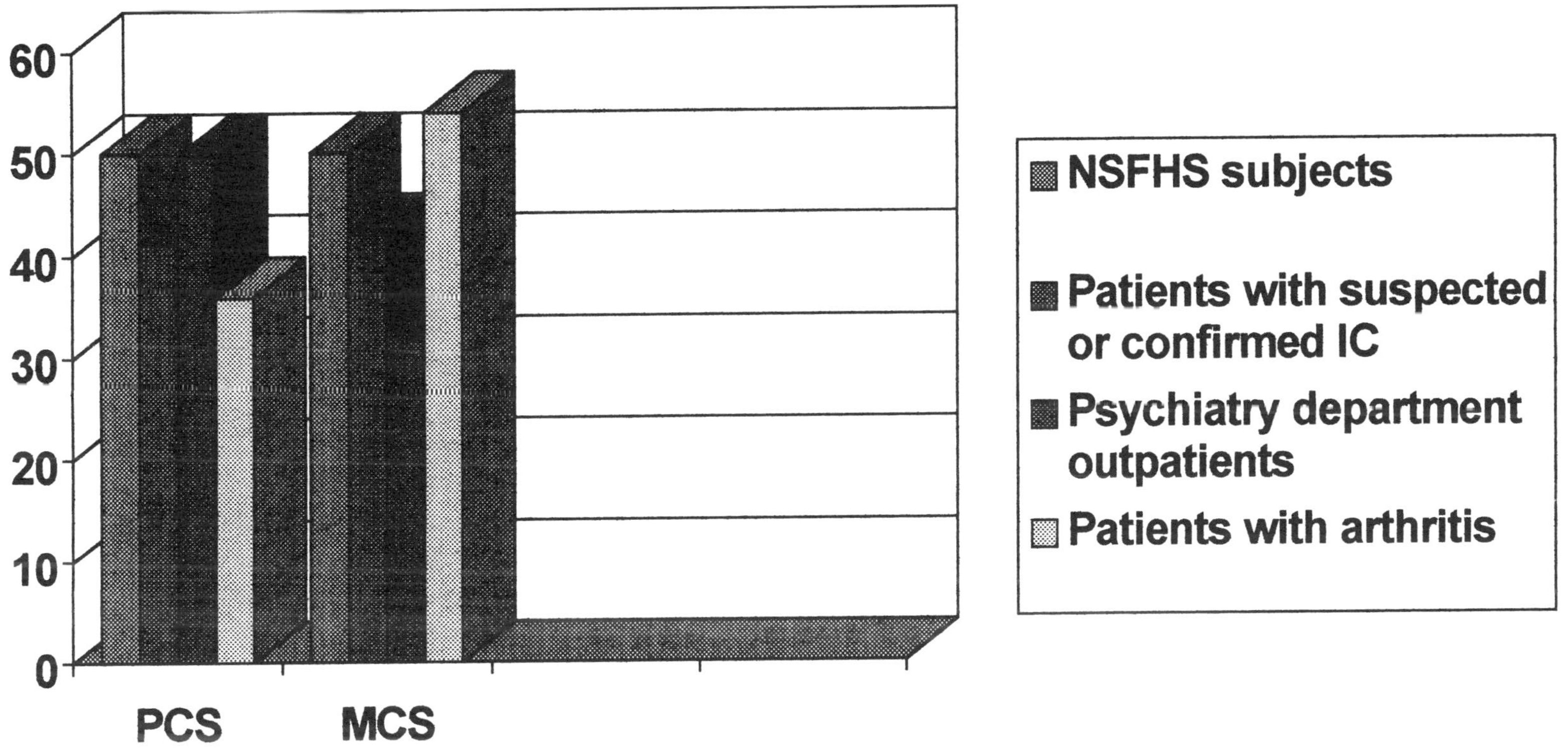

FIG. 3. Comparison of SF-36 physical and mental component scale scores for IC patients with those of the general U.S. population and those of patients with other chronic conditions.

HQL—an impact that can be quantified using a general health status measure such as the SF-36. These HQL measures may have multiple applications in a disease/syndrome such as interstitial cystitis. Our SF-36 health survey validates the many problems and concerns verbalized by patients newly diagnosed with IC and those learning to live with it.

APPLICATIONS OF HEALTH-RELATED QUALITY-OF-LIFE ASSESSMENT

General health status measures can be used to monitor the health of populations and estimate the burden of disease; evaluate health-care policy; assess benefits of treatment in clinical trials; monitor and improve health care outcomes; and support decision making in individual patient care (8). Utilization of health status measurement has many potential applications in IC research and patient care.

Population-Based Uses of HQL Measures

Estimating the Burden of Interstitial Cystitis

Standardized assessment of patients' HQL quantifies patients' experiences and contributes to a better understanding of the relative burden IC places on their lives. The characteristic profile of IC patients HQL, compared to that of other chronic conditions, could aid in the decision making of health care professionals, patients, and policy makers. Similarly to recently published data on the health status of patients with chronic fatigue syndrome (20), misconceptions about the severity or "reality" of the burden associated with IC symptoms may be alleviated when the similarities and differences between IC patients' health status profiles and those of patients with other chronic conditions are required.

The burden of illness falls primarily on the IC sufferer and directly impacts every aspect of that person's life. The physical symptoms of IC and the implications of chronic illness affect interactions with family and social supports, intricacies of personal and professional relationships, execution of job responsibilities, as well as development of coping mechanisms. Constant awareness of the chronicity of illness, especially pain, can escalate feelings of helplessness, hopelessness, and frustration. Pain lowers the quality of life as it compromises the ability to carry out normal activities of daily living. Quality-of-life issues are the impetus behind every phone call, every visit, every interaction between client and health care provider—physician and nurse.

Assessing Treatment Benefits in Clinical Trials

Increasingly, development of new pharmacologic and nonpharmacologic treatment modalities requires demonstration of their effectiveness beyond efficacy and safety (21–24). As the conceptual, methodologic, and practical barriers to the use of HQL measures are being resolved, their inclusion in clinical trials is increasing (24). In fact, cancer clinical trials now mandate the inclusion of HQL outcome measures (25). In a chronic disease such as IC that affects patients through an array of subjective symptoms, and in which available treatments are not curative, it is important to know whether treatment, e.g., intravesical DMSO with its known side effects such as dysuria and bladder irritation, outweighs the HQL burden of the symptoms associated with the disease itself.

Inclusion of HQL measures in clinical trials of new treatments for IC will inform patients and clinicians about the balance between the efficacy and safety of the investigational therapy from the patients perspective. It also informs policy makers and pharmaceutical manufacturers about the benefits of palliative therapies.

Use of HQL Measures in Individual Patient Care

There is limited information on the effects of routine measurement of HQL in clinical practice. However, the clinical effectiveness of comprehensive geriatric assessments that employ standardized assessment instruments has been documented (26,27). The potential benefits of these assessments include (a) detection of decreased functioning, (b) guidance in management decisions and resource use, and (c) improvement of patient outcomes (28). Thus, HQL measurement in patients with IC could yield similar benefits.

Detection of Decreased Functioning and Well-Being

Standardized HQL questionnaires offer the opportunity to increase the detection of functional limitations and psychological distress. Two-thirds to three-fourths of U.S. adults in a 1990 survey reported that physicians rarely or never ask about the extent of their limitations in performing everyday activities, even in the presence of chronic conditions (28), and numerous studies show that physicians underdetect functional patient disabilities, especially those related to social activities (29,30). Differences in severity of psychological distress are also not apparent to treating physicians (31). Social and role functioning and emotional well-being are highly relevant to IC patients, as many are young, active, and working. Problems in these health domains are likely to be underdetected in IC.

Because of the likelihood of underdetection of HQL problems in IC and the known disparity between physicians' and patients' ratings of their health status (9,32), patient-completed health status information could help clinicians caring for patients with IC to detect limitations or declines in functioning and well-being and could serve as one step in the multistage diagnostic screening process. Longitudinal health status assessment in a dialysis clinic revealed new information rather than merely restating the clinicians' intuition about their patients' functioning and well-being, despite the fact that the dialysis clinicians had regular and frequent contact with their patients (33). Primary care practitioners in small private practices using the Dartmouth COOP Charts indicated that for one of every four patients, the charts uncovered important information about the patient that resulted in specific clinical management actions in 40% of patients (34). In epilepsy, routine assessment of patients HQL using the SF-36 resulted in increased clinicians' knowledge about their patients for more than 60% of the encounters and in changes in management attributed to the availability of the HQL data in 13% (35).

Guidance in Management: Shared Decision Making

According to IC patients, in developing a working relationship, physicians should not diminish the importance of questions and the emotions of their patients. Appreciation is expressed for physicians who take time to listen to IC patients and acknowledge their apprehension and fear as valid concerns. The SF-36 HRL questionnaire could act in tandem with the MD/RN interview in the evaluation, monitoring, and treatment of IC patients.

Frequently, patients can not or will not utilize a support group or have difficulty discussing fears and concerns of living with IC. Some patients report that they "deal with it" better alone. Methods found helpful by patients attempting to find relief and live within the confines of frequency and pain include acupuncture, stress management, behavior modification, and diet control in addition to a support group and more conventional pharmacologic or surgical treatment.

There is a clear need for an age-related support group for newly diagnosed women in their mid- to late teens and early 20s. Questions abound within this age group regarding school, travel, sports involvement, social interactions, uncertainties within a dating relationship, marriage, pregnancy, and hereditary involvement. The uncertainties expressed confirm the need for patient education on both an individual and interactive level.

Investigational therapies, e.g., intravesical BCG and Cystistat, expand the number of therapeutic options for clinicians and patients. As long as there is no cure for IC, the therapeutic goal is to choose from the available treatment options the regimen that provides the most benefits and the least adverse effects for an individual patient.

Clinicians considerations of the outcomes of therapy, however, may be different from the quality-of-life considerations important to patients. The clinician's focus may be on freedom from symptoms, whereas a patient may be more concerned about the actual and potential side effects of the treatment, or the financial burden associated with the therapy. These considerations may influence decision-making and therapeutic strategies. Liang proposes that appropriate health behavior should be thought of as a behavior that meets the person's goals and achieves some mutually definable outcome (36). The HQL measures could provide useful information for the IC patient and the physician to decide on the desired treatment outcomes and to monitor treatment progress.

Clinicians are aware of the considerable variability among patients with respect to preferences in the tradeoffs between symptom control and adverse effects of therapy. For example, intravesical Clorpactin lavage is viewed negatively by many patients because of their concerns about pain and symptom exacerbation posttreatment. As the life situation changes for an individual, so may individual priorities for the goals and the individual evaluation of the outcomes of therapy. Treatment of IC therefore needs to be individualized and tailored to the patient's physical and emotional status and well-being.

Adding to the traditional data base of signs, symptoms, and laboratory data, standardized information about HQL would provide the clinician and the patient with an assessment of the overall effectiveness, current treatment, and permit comparison of the HQL effects of the current treatment to those of previous treatments. By quantifying the patient's subjective experience, HQL assessment makes that experience more accessible to the clinicians who care for the patient. This could result in a more focused and effective clinician-patient interaction and increased patient participation in the decision-making process. In turn, patients' participation may increase their sense of control over their illness, allay anxiety, and improve compliance, clinical outcomes, and satisfaction with care (37).

Guidance in Management: Multidisciplinary Approach

A multidisciplinary approach to assessment and care of the elderly has become a characteristic of geriatric medicine. Standardized assessment of physical, psychological, and social functioning in the elderly population led to the discovery of previously unrecognized, treatable problems (26). Observations and questions presented by IC patients and their families generate discussion explaining methods of pain management and various treatment modalities as well as discussions identifying and developing coping mechanisms for living with chronic pain and the ever present need for treatment. The Multidisciplinary Pain Clinic is an essential vehicle in the care of IC patients. The team, consisting of physician, nurse, psychologist, and physical therapist, collaborating with urology, gynecology, and primary care, is a viable option providing additional information and support for patients and their families.

Although physicians are equipped to act on many of the problems that arise in IC patients, medical and surgical treatment alone may not resolve all IC-related problems (see Chapter 25). Care by a multidisciplinary team is therefore the optimal treatment approach to address the educational, psychiatric, psychological, and social service needs of selected individuals with IC and their families. Within such multidisciplinary treatment programs, HQL measurement could fulfill three potential purposes: screen for patients who would benefit most from multidisciplinary care; communicate among the different providers about patients progress; and measurement of the success of multidisciplinary care.

Improvement of Outcomes: HQL and Satisfaction with Care

Some researchers have started to evaluate whether routine HQL measurement and feedback of the data to clinicians improves patients' perceptions of their functioning and well-being. Although the participating clinicians usually believe that the assessments are useful, a positive effect of routine HQL measurement on patients' functioning and well-being has not been consistently demonstrated (38,39).

After a one-time 2-hour multimedia educational session, Rubenstein and colleagues (38) provided an "experimental subject" group of physicians with their patients' profiles on the Functional Status Questionnaire (FSQ) every 4 months for 1 year. "Control" group physicians did not receive education or their patients' FSQ scores. Almost all clinicians in the experimental group felt that the questionnaire was accurate and useful and that it would improve patients' health and physician–patient communication about functional status. In addition, almost half of the experimental group had used the results of the questionnaire to change therapy. However, no significant differences ($p > 0.05$) in any dimension of function were detected between experimental and control groups. Physicians' unfamiliarity with patients' HQL scale scores, the complexity of the HQL measures used, and the lack of readily available HQL information at the time of the office visit have been thought to be responsible for the failure to demonstrate a beneficial effect of HQL assessment. A more powerful educational intervention would be needed to produce measurable effects of the HQL information on outcomes of care (38,39). When physicians received management and resource suggestions in addition to patients' FSQ profiles, as well as continued educational interventions, experimental patients' mental health ($p < 0.02$) and social functioning ($p < 0.01$) scores were significantly better than those of control group patients (40).

Patients with IC continually seek reassurance that research is ongoing, anxiously awaiting a cure as well as an explanation for the cause of disease. Concerns are also voiced pertaining to the inability or potential inability of the IC sufferer to execute professional responsibilities. Physical and emotional limitations may result in loss of work days leading to financial hardship. These issues increasingly involve health care providers with written and telephone correspondence with attorneys, insurance companies, and pharmaceutical companies as patients seek information regarding social security disability, financial assistance with medications, and eligibility regarding handicapped rights and options. The Interstitial Cystitis Association and its local support groups can be invaluable resources to patients and their families as they seek information/support/assistance in managing the physical and psychological adjustments in living with a chronic disease.

It has been suggested that assessment of functioning and well-being is associated with increased patient satisfaction with care (28). Patients whose physicians underestimated their level of limitations in activities caused by their disease are more likely to report dissatisfaction with their treatment. At least 60% of respondents in a national survey wanted their physicians to ask about their physical functioning and emotional well-being or both, and more than half were willing to fill out a questionnaire concerning these aspects of HQL, indicating patients' preference for comprehensive health care (28). These perceptions are most certainly shared by patients with IC. Combined with diagnosis and treatment concerns, financial burdens are the realities of daily living. The IC impacts every aspect of life: intimacy and physical relationships, social interaction, caring for family and home, pregnancy, diet, exercise, travel and education. Personal experiences in conducting HQL research with people with IC indicate that patients welcome the interest demonstrated in how their IC and its treatment affect their lives. However, to date there are no data to support the routine use of HQL measurements relative to improving IC patients' HQL and their satisfaction with care.

Future Research Issues

Advances in Measurement

A modular approach to health status assessment has been advocated to increase the comprehensiveness and specificity of patient-completed health status questionnaires (6,14). Currently, there is no health status questionnaire that specifically addresses problems faced by IC patients. Such a questionnaire could be developed with the help of patient and care provider focus groups and will need to undergo testing of its practicality, reliability, and validity. It then can be added to core measures of general health. A symptom index for IC (41) has recently been described (see Chapter 34).

Measurement Application in Clinical Trials

Well-tested general as well as IC-specific questionnaires should be included in clinical trials of pharmacologic, surgical, and psychological treatments of IC. Several issues related to the clinical trials of use of HQL measures have been raised as subjects for future investigation (42). For IC research, the questions to be answered include how HQL variables are related to other clinical variables such as urinary frequency, urgency, or pain or to the pathophysiological markers of the disease. Another issue is how to summarize the HQL effects of a treatment, especially when multiple HQL dimensions are assessed and the treatment has differential or opposite effects on different HQL domains and/or on HQL domains and clinical variables. Furthermore, the question remains how to interpret HQL differences between alternative treatments, and what difference is meaningful to patients and clinicians that would warrant the choice of one treatment over another.

Measurement Application in Clinical Practice

Most patients like to share with their clinicians how they feel and function in their daily lives (28). To incorporate routine HQL assessment in clinical practice, some technical and educational barriers have to be overcome (43). However, the ability to measure general health status does not necessarily translate into the ability to treat problems and improve general health status (38,39). To facilitate implementation, to make interpretation of the information possible, and to allow management decisions to incorporate the data, clinicians need to know what the causal pathways are that link clinical and health status concepts (44,45). Advances in computerized medicine and the advent of electronic medical records will facilitate the creation of data bases that include both HQL and clinical data as well as treatment information and laboratory testing.

CONCLUSIONS

No urology textbook teaches clinicians how to interpret general health status scale scores. Education of clinicians in the meaning of these scores is needed, as well as further research to interpret IC patients' results on general and disease-specific questionnaires. Linking health status data to familiar clinical information is crucial to the identification of management steps in response to the information. Furthermore, this synthesis will facilitate clinicians' familiarization with HQL measurement instruments and their use in clinical practice.

The aim of medical care is to prolong life, eliminate or reduce deviations in biological functioning, relieve pain and suffering, ease fear and anxiety through compassionate interactions and acts of caring, and improve general functioning and well-being (46). Ultimately, for HQL data to be considered important enough to be implemented in routine care, their benefit has to be demonstrated to clinicians and payers. We hypothesize that having patient-completed assessments of their functioning and well-being available at the clinic visit will allow a more systematic focus on quality-of-life issues. The demonstration that standardized health status measures contribute to improving the outcomes of our care for IC patients is a challenge to clinicians and researchers in the field of interstitial cystitis.

REFERENCES

1. Ratner V, Slade D, Greene G. Interstitial cystitis: a patient's perspective. *Urol Clin North Am* 1994;21(1):1–5.
2. Webster DC, Brennan T. Use and effectiveness of psychological self-care strategies for interstitial cystitis. *Health Care Women Int* 1995; 16(5):463–475.
3. Ellwood PM. Outcomes management: a technology of patient experience. *N Engl J Med* 1988;318:1549–1556.
4. Sigerest HE. *Medicine and Human Welfare.* New Haven, CT: Yale University Press, 1941;100.
5. World Health Organization. *Basic Documents: WHO Constitution.* Geneva: WHO, 1948.
6. Ware JE. Measuring functioning, well-being, and other generic health concepts. In: Osoba D, ed. *Effect of Cancer on Quality of Life.* Boca Raton: CRC Press, 1991;7–23.
7. Lembke PA. Measuring the quality of medical care through vital statistics based on hospital service areas: 1. Comparative study of appendectomy rates. *Am J Public Health* 1952;42:276–286.
8. Ware JE. The status of health assessment 1994. *Annu Rev Public Health* 1995;16:327–354.
9. Slevin ML, Plant H, Lynch D, Drinkwater J, Gregory WM. Who should measure quality of life, the doctor or the patient? *Br J Cancer* 1988; 57:109–112.
10. Stewart AL, Ware JE, eds. *Measuring Functioning and Well-Being. The Medical Outcomes Study Approach.* Durham, NC: Duke University Press, 1992.
11. Wilkin D, Hallam L, Doggett MA. *Measures of Need and Outcome for Primary Health Care.* Oxford: Oxford University Press, 1992.
12. Temkin NR, Dikmen S, Machamer J, et al. General versus disease-specific measures: further work on the Sickness Impact Profile for head injury. *Med Care* 1992;27:S44–S53.
13. Kantz ME, Harris WJ, Levitsky K, et al. Methods for assessing condition specific and generic functional status outcomes after total knee replacement. *Med Care* 1992;30:MS240–MS252.
14. Patrick DL, Deyo RA. Generic and disease-specific measures in assessing health status and quality of life. *Med Care* 1989;27: S217–S232.
15. Ware JE, Sherbourne CD. The MOS 36-Item Short-Form Health Survey (SF-36): I. Conceptual framework and item selection. *Med Care* 1992;30:473–483.
16. Ware JE, Snow KK, Kosinsky M, Gandek B. *SF-36 Health Survey. Manual and Interpretation Guide.* Boston: New England Medical Center, 1993.
17. Ware JE. The SF-36 Health Survey. In: Spilker B, ed. *Quality of Life and Pharmacoeconomics in Clinical Trials,* 2nd ed. Philadelphia: Lippincott-Raven, 1996:337–345.
18. Ware JE, Kosinski M, Keller SD. *SF-36 Physical and Mental Health Summary Scales: A User's Manual.* Boston: The Health Institute, New England Medical Center, 1994.
19. Taylov AR, Ware JE, Greenfield S, Nelson EC, Perrin E, Zubkoff M. The Medical Outcomes Study. An application of methods for monitoring the results of medical care. *JAMA* 1989;262:925–930.
20. Schweitzer R, Kelly B, Foran A, et al. Quality of life in chronic fatigue syndrome. *Soc Sci Med* 1995;41(10):1367–1372.

21. Deyo RA. Measuring functional outcomes in therapeutic trials for chronic disease. *Control Clin Trials* 1984;5:223–240.
22. Deyo RA, Patrick DL. Barriers to the use of health status measures in clinical investigation, patient care, and policy research. *Med Care* 1989; 27:S254–S268.
23. Osoba D. The Quality of Life Committee of the Clinical Trials Group of the National Cancer Institute of Canada: organization and functions. *Qual Life Res* 1992;1:211–218.
24. Editorial. Quality of life and clinical trials. *Lancet* 1995;346:1–2.
25. Gotay CC, Korn EL, McCabe MS, et al. Quality of life assessment in cancer treatment protocols: research issues in protocol development. *J Natl Cancer Inst* 1992;84:575–579.
26. Rubenstein L. The clinical effectiveness of multidisciplinary geriatric assessment. *J Am Geriatr Soc* 1983;31:758–762.
27. Almy TP. Comprehensive functional assessment for elderly patients. *Ann Intern Med* 1988;10:70–72.
28. Schor EL, Lerner DJ, Malspeis S. Physicians assessment of functional health status and well-being. The patient's perspective. *Arch Intern Med* 1995;155:309–314.
29. Wartman SA, Morlock LL, Malitz FE, Palm E. Impact of divergent evaluations of physicians and patients and patients complaints. *Public Health Rep* 1983;98:141–145.
30. Calkins DR, Rubenstein LV, Cleary PD, et al. Failure of physicians to recognize functional disability in ambulatory patients. *Ann Intern Med* 1991;114:451–454.
31. Wells KB, Hays RD, Burnam MA, et al. Detection of depressive disorders for patients receiving prepaid of fee-for-service care: Results from the Medical Outcomes Study. *JAMA* 1989;262: 3298–3302.
32. Nerenz DR, Repasky DP, Whitehouse FW, Kahkonen DM. Ongoing assessment of health status in patients with diabetes mellitus. *Med Care* 1992;30:MS112–MS124.
33. Meyer KB, Espindle DM, DeGiacomo JM, et al. Monitoring dialysis patients health status. *Am J Kidney Dis* 1994;24:267–279.
34. Nelson ED, Landgraf JM, Hays RD, Wasson JH, Kirk JW. The functional status of patients. How can it be measuresd in physicians offices? *Med Care* 1990;28:1111–1126.
35. Wagner AK, Vickery BG. The routine use of health-related quality of life measures in the care of patients with epilepsy: rationale and research agenda. *Qual Life Res* 1995;4:169–177.
36. Liang MH. Compliance and quality of life: Confessions of a difficult patient. *Arthritis Care Res* 1989;2:S71–S74.
37. Brody D. The patient's role in clinical decision making. *Ann Intern Med* 1980;93:718–722.
38. Rubenstein LV, Calkins DR, Young RT, Cleary PD, Fink A, Kosekoff J, Jette AM, Davies AR, Delbanco TL, Brook R. Improving patient function: a randomized trial of functional disability screening. *Ann Intern Med* 1989;111:836–842.
39. Kazis LE, Callaghan LF, Meenan RF, Pincus T. Health status reports in the care of patients with rheumatoid arthritis. *J Clin Epidemiol* 1990; 43:1243–1253.
40. Rubenstein LV, McCoy JM, Cope DW, Barrett PA, Hirsch SH, Messer KS, Young RT. Improving patient functional status: a randomized trial of computer-generated resource and management suggestions. *Clin Res* 1989;37:801A.
41. O'Leary MP, Sant GR, Whitmore KE, et al. The interstitial cystitis symptom index. *J Urol* 1996;155(5, Suppl):439A.
42. Cleary PD. Future directions of quality of life research. In: Spilker B. *Quality of Life and Pharmacoeconomics in Clinical Trials.* Philadelphia: Lippincott-Raven Publishers, 1996;73–78.
43. Wasson J, Keller A, Rubenstein L, et al. Benefits and obstacles of health status assessment in ambulatory settings. The clinician's point of view. *Med Care* 1992;30:MS42–MS49.
44. Wilson IB, Cleary PD. Linking clinical variables with health-related quality of life: a conceptual model of patient outcomes. *JAMA* 1995; 273:59–65.
45 Wilson IB, Kaplan S. Clinical practice and patients health status. How are the two related? *Med Care* 1995;33:AS209–AS214.
46. Faden R, Leplege A. Assessing quality of life: moral implications for clinical practice. *Med Care* 1992;30:MS166–MS175.

Interstitial Cystitis, edited by Grannum R. Sant.
Lippincott–Raven Publishers, Philadelphia ©1997.

CHAPTER 34

The Interstitial Cystitis Symptom and Problem Indices: Rationale, Development, and Application

Michael P. O'Leary and Grannum R. Sant

Interstitial cystitis (IC) is commonly referred to as the painful bladder syndrome because of the constellation of symptoms with which it is associated, including irritative voiding symptoms and chronic pelvic or lower abdominal pain. Despite increased research interest, the basic cause of IC and its true incidence are not known (1,2). Furthermore, there is no agreement regarding clinical, endoscopic, or histologic features, and unfortunately, many clinicians do not recognize its features and therefore fail to diagnose it. For those who do, evaluation of the symptom complex of urinary frequency, urgency, suprapubic discomfort, suprapubic, pelvic, or perineal pain, and dyspareunia is difficult and frequently unrewarding. Improved knowledge of the symptoms of IC and an accurate and reproducible way to evaluate them are clearly needed (3).

Health-care decisions faced by patients, physicians, researchers, and policy makers frequently extend far beyond the traditional domains of biological and physiological outcomes. It is now widely accepted that maximization of a patient's health-related quality of life is an overriding goal of modern medical care, especially for chronic diseases for which neither a cure nor impending death is a likely outcome. Interstitial cystitis is such a disease in which survival is not an adequate outcome measure. The prevalence of IC appears to be increasing, but the lack of specific histologic/biochemical disease markers in this condition (2–4) means that disease monitoring and treatment outcomes relate to symptoms, health-related quality of life, and physical and emotional well-being of affected patients.

Interstitial cystitis is a disease or syndrome characterized by irritative voiding symptoms (frequency, urgency, nocturia) and pain (pelvic, suprapubic, vaginal, perineal, etc.). Apart from global assessments of well-being, until recently there were no validated, generally accepted symptom indices or questionnaires for interstitial cystitis. Thus, to appropriately diagnose and treat IC, we need to better understand patients' perceptions of their disease. Scientifically validated methods to obtain this type of information have recently been applied to patients with urologic disease (5). In order to better recognize and treat IC, it is critical for clinicians to have a uniform and reproducible method of assessing symptoms in patients with IC. The authors felt the need to develop an IC Symptom Index using accepted techniques of health status and outcomes measurement, i.e., validity, reliability, responsiveness to change. Such an index could be of invaluable use to clinicians and researchers involved in IC patient care and research. Apart from its adjunct role in clinical decision making, a symptom index will be of particular utility to research endeavors such as the National IC Data Base Project, the NIDDK-supported effort to collect longitudinal data on patients with IC.

Furthermore, assessing the impact of IC on physical, mental, and psychosocial functioning should be an essential element in clinical diagnosis and a major determinant of therapeutic choice. Instruments to assess symptoms and functional status in patients with IC will allow significant improvement in understanding the treated and untreated natural history of IC. Symptom-based measures would ideally complement the functional and

M. P. O'Leary: Division of Urology, Brigham and Women's Hospital, Boston, Massachusetts 02115.

G. R. Sant: Department of Urology and Interstitial Cystitis Clinic, New England Medical Center and Tufts University School of Medicine, Boston, Massachusetts 02111.

health-related generic quality-of-life measures assessed by the SF-36 questionnaire (see Chapter 33). A suitably validated instrument will be particularly useful in clinical trials of new therapies, where it is vital to have reliable and reproducible outcome measures in order to make meaningful comparisons across studies. In this chapter, we describe our recent work to develop and psychometrically validate a self-administered symptom index that we believe will be a useful tool for both clinicians and researchers involved with IC patients.

BACKGROUND

Interstitial cystitis is a urologic condition of unknown etiology that predominantly affects young and middle-aged females and for which there is no universally effective therapy. The investigation of IC is hampered by nonuniform diagnostic criteria, the existence of two clinical forms of the disease (early, nonulcerative versus classic ulcerative), and the possibility that IC is a bladder reflection of a systemic disease or a response to diverse, heterogeneous stimuli (2–4). Interstitial cystitis is characterized by irritative voiding symptoms (frequency, nocturia) and suprapubic or pelvic pain related to and relieved by voiding. The majority of patients with IC are young and middle-aged women (90%), although men and children can be affected, with a possible prevalence of at least 18 per 100,000 women (4). The more common form of the disease is the early variety with normal bladder capacity and an absence of ulcers. Symptoms of IC are usually present for many (3 to 12) years before diagnosis, and spontaneous improvement occurs in about 10% of patients, whereas few patients deteriorate or progress from the early to the late variety of IC. The diagnosis of IC depends on (a) the characteristic complex of voiding symptoms and pain, (b) the typical cystoscopic appearance under regional or general anesthesia, and (c) the absence of objective evidence of other specific bladder disease. Biochemical assays of urinary substances such as eosinophil cationic protein (ECP), histamine metabolites, epidermal growth factor (EGF), and bladder glycosaminoglycan components are all investigational at present and not clinically useful.

Therefore, the diagnosis of this disease depends largely on the recognition and evaluation of symptoms. Furthermore, a variety of different therapies, both pharmacologic and surgical have been advocated for the treatment of IC. However, comparisons of treatment efficacy are difficult if not impossible without reliable and valid outcome measures, in particular with regard to symptoms. A number of questionnaires have been developed and used by investigators in studies of patients with IC, but none has been formally validated. A model for symptom indices that is now familiar to most urologists is the American Urological Association (AUA) Symptom Index for Benign Prostatic Hyperplasia (BPH) (6). This condition is similar to IC in that it is a disease whose morbidity is largely related to symptoms, and one with a plethora of competing therapies (surgical, pharmacologic, minimally invasive, etc.). The BPH Symptom Index was developed because of the need for a reliable and valid instrument to measure symptoms as an integral component in any outcomes study evaluating treatment of BPH (6).

Chronic conditions such as IC almost certainly impact on patients' functional status. Unfortunately, such data are relatively sparse in IC. Held et al. have examined quality of life in patients with IC compared to those on chronic renal dialysis (7). Using crude Likert scales, they concluded that IC patients had much poorer quality of life than those on renal dialysis. Although this is an intuitively attractive hypothesis, comparing scores of health indices may lead to incorrect conclusions (8). There are a number of evaluative instruments that measure elements of functional status such as physical performance, mental health, social and role functioning, and general well-being (9). What do we mean when we use these terms?

FUNCTIONAL STATUS MEASUREMENT

The systematic assessment of function dates from the 1940's, when indices combining various dimensions of function were created to provide coarse ratings among patients with specific diseases (e.g., Karnofsky Index for cancer patients and the New York Heart Association Functional Classes for heart patients) (10). In the 1950's the move toward more refined unidimensional measures of function began. Rehabilitation medicine developed tools to assess physical function, such as the Index of Activities of Daily Living (11). These were followed closely by the development of measures of cognitive and emotional function, primarily by psychiatrists (12,13). Measures of social function were also developed, but they are not as well refined because of conceptual and measurement difficulties.

For clinicians, comprehensive functional assessment can be used to facilitate screening, diagnosis, assessment of disease severity, therapeutic goal setting, choosing treatment, and monitoring patients' clinical courses (14,15). In the realm of health services research, the multidimensional assessment of health, sometimes referred to as health-related quality of life, is increasingly being recognized as a key outcome of medical care (Table 1). In part, this is because improvements in physiological and organ functioning are frequently not paralleled by improvements in symptoms and function. Multidimensional measures are now being used in studies of drug efficacy and will become increasingly more important in studies of quality of care, particularly care of patients with chronic diseases.

TABLE 1. *Disease outcomes measures*

Mortality
Morbidity
Biological measures
Physiological measures
Health status
Quality of life (QOL)
Generic
Disease-specific
Patient-specific
Symptom indices

Both clinical and research measures can be divided into single-domain and multidimensional instruments. A recent review by Applegate and colleagues summarizes the range of single-domain instruments with respect to sensitivity to clinical change, mode of administration, strengths, and weaknesses (16). These instruments have been used both clinically and in research and perform reasonably well, provided their strengths and weaknesses are recognized. The major problems for either use are (a) the time required when they are used in combination and (b) poor sensitivity and specificity.

Multidimensional instruments are of the long and short varieties, the latter often having been derived from the former. Examples of the more lengthy instruments include (a) the Older Americans Research and Service Center Instrument (the OARS) and (b) the Sickness Impact Profile (the SIP). The OARS relies on ratings based on the judgment of trained interviewers and yields information in five function domains: social resources, economic resources, mental health, physical health, and the physical function. In contrast, the SIP, which is completed by the patient and takes at least 30 min to complete, provides information in 14 categories that cover a broader range of issues than the OARS in some areas (e.g., communication and recreation) but a more restricted range in others (e.g., mental health).

Disease-specific measures of quality of life assess particular diagnostic or patient groups for responsiveness or clinically significant change, have adequate content validity because individuals completing the measures are likely to perceive the items as relevant, are more sensitive to change than generic measures, are easier to interpret because the instruments are more restricted, and are more closely associated with changes in clinical disease activity (17,18). Furthermore, disease-specific measures identify important concerns of patients with a particular disease, e.g., IC, and are useful for measuring small, clinically important changes from different treatments. Disease-specific measures have been introduced for a variety of chronic conditions including benign prostatic hyperplasia (BPH), chronic lung disease, low back pain, rheumatoid arthritis, and impotence (5,6,17,19).

Quality-of-life measures have a number of utilities in medicine (Table 2), particularly in the management of chronic illness such as IC and determination of treatment choices when there is no cure or gold-standard of treatment. Condition- or disease-specific quality-of-life measures are becoming more popular, and they are more sensitive to change in a patient's health than generic measures. Recently, patient-specific measures have been introduced in which the patients themselves choose dimensions of concern (e.g., for AIDS, HIV infection) and the weighting of these dimensions.

A number of shorter self-administered instruments have been recently developed. These include the Duke-UNC Profile (20), Dartmouth Coop Charts (21), and the Medical Outcomes Study Short Form 36 (SF-36) (9,18). All can be completed in a fairly brief period of time (15 min or less) by the patients themselves. Of the three, the former two were developed primarily for use in primary care clinical practice. The Duke-UNC Profile has 63 items that measure four dimensions: symptoms status, physical function, emotional function, and social function. It has been shown to be reliable and valid and to be sensitive to various levels of health in a cross-sectional study of family practice patients (40% 18 to 20 years: 7% ≥65 years). However, it measures only four dimensions of health, and its performance over time and among sicker patients has not been studied. The use of SF-36 HQL questionnaire is fully described in Chapter 33. Any of these instruments can be used in studies in patients with IC. Our goal, however, has been to develop a disease-specific instrument, and we have incorporated functional status and quality of life measures into our instrument rather than measure them separately.

TABLE 2. *Quality-of-life measures: Applications*

Population surveys
Medical audit
Clinical trials
Outcomes measures in health services research
Clinical encounters
Cost utility/resource allocation

PRELIMINARY STUDIES

The investigators reviewed the literature on the evaluation of symptoms in IC. Multiple indices have been proposed, but none, to our knowledge, has been formally validated. The steps in the development of the symptom index are outlined in Table 3. We initially designed a preliminary instrument that was evaluated in patient focus groups. This is the first step in any validation study

TABLE 3. *Quality-of-life measurement: The basics*

Multidimensional construct
Validity
Face, content, construct
Criterion
Reliability
Test–retest
Internal
Sensitivity to change
Appropriateness
Practical utility

because the goal is to better understand the illness experience from the patient's perspective. Based on input from patients, a careful review of the literature, and experience with over 400 patients over a 10-year experience at the Interstitial Cystitis Clinic at the New England Medical Center, a preliminary IC Symptom Index was developed. Seventy-three questions covered the following domains: urinary symptoms, pain symptoms, sexual function, menstrual cycle syndrome variability, general health status, and functional status. Urinary symptoms predominate, with 13 questions relating to different aspects of voiding function. Because of what was learned from focus groups where patients had a great deal of input, specific questions were included regarding sexual function and the relationship of symptoms to the menstrual cycle. The questionnaire was designed for self-administration to avoid the bias of interviewers and/or the judgment of physicians or nurses.

FORMAL VALIDATION PROCESS

Based on what we learned from the initial pilot studies using a longer and purposefully redundant instrument, a formal validation process (Table 3) was instituted using a more parsimonious index (22). This includes eight questions on urinary symptoms, three on pain symptoms, three on sexual function, three on general health, three on overall quality of life, and eight demographic questions. The study population included 45 patients with newly diagnosed and endoscopically proven interstitial cystitis. Sixty-seven healthy age-matched women without any urinary symptoms who presented for routine care to a gynecology clinic served as controls (22).

Study subjects and controls were similar in age and socioeconomic status. Patients in both groups had the opportunity to discuss the questionnaire with a nurse or research assistant after completing it to provide feedback on any questions found difficult or confusing. An identical questionnaire was mailed to the patient 1 week after the first completion to examine short-term test–retest reliability.

Data were compiled and analyzed using Pearson product-moment correlation coefficients to examine associations among variables (23). Interclass correlation coefficients were calculated to assess test–retest reliabilities (17,19), and Cronbach's α statistic (24) was used to evaluate internal consistency among the items in individual domains. Finally, cross-tabulations were examined to determine if there were inconsistencies within domains and to assess subjects' range of responses. Using both urinary symptoms and pain symptoms, various ways of constructing a multiitem index were explored. The goal of the analysis was to identify the fewest questions that would reliably and validly describe the illness experience of those with IC and, if possible, distinguish them from those without it.

The seven concepts that appear to best describe the symptoms of IC are burning, urgency, frequency, nocturia, bladder pain, suprapubic or abdominal pain, and back pain. Urgency and pain, however, seem to be defining characteristics of IC. Questions on urgency characterize nearly 90% of study subjects and are highly intercorrelated and discriminate between cases and controls. Daytime frequency is reported by 70% of study subjects and only 16% of controls, but nocturia (at least twice nightly) seems to discriminate better, with over 80% of respondents reporting this and only 10% of controls. Discomfort, pressure, or pain is reported by 96% of study subjects, whereas only 27% of controls report occasional bladder pressure, and fewer than 15% pain. In describing how much of a problem various symptoms are for respondents, frequency and pain are virtually never a problem for control patients!

Because urgency, frequency, nocturia, and pain appear to be defining characteristics of patients with IC, the questions that best describe these symptoms and had the highest intercorrelation with questions in the same domains were combined in an IC Symptom Index (Appendix 1). The symptom index correlates well with a summary index symptom impact on subjects' daily living activities as well as on how problematic (The IC Problem Index) they find their symptoms (Appendix 2). The indices combine well ($\alpha = 0.90$ and 0.94), and test–retest reliability is excellent (0.90 and 0.91). In questions 1, 2, and 3, there are six response options, which can be scored from 0 to 5. Question 4, however, was designed with only five response frames. Both the Symptom Index and the Problem Index strongly discriminate (discriminant validity) IC patients from controls (22).

CONCLUSIONS

The IC Symptom Index and the IC Problem Index were designed to capture the most important voiding and pain symptoms and to assess how problematic patients find them in the clearest and most concise manner possible.

Both instruments have been designed and validated for self-administration to avoid interviewer bias. They are intended for complementary use because measures of symptom severity alone may not adequately capture the significance of the problem from the patient's perspective. In fact, in conditions that result in lower urinary tract symptoms such as benign prostatic hyperplasia, the degree to which patients are bothered may be one of the most important predictors of disease progression.

The indices are not intended as screening tools even though they appear to discriminate between patients with and without IC. Rather, they should be used as an adjunct in diagnosis and should be useful to clinicians and researchers in the evaluation and management of patients with IC.

Our preliminary studies have confirmed the attributes of reliability and validity. The clinical utility of the IC Symptom Index and IC Problem Index is now being tested in an effort to confirm that it is more responsive to change than generic measures such as the SF-36. Its use to monitor patients' symptoms (similar to AUA BPH Symptoms Score) (3,25), response to therapeutic interventions (e.g., DMSO, Elmiron), and the natural history of IC is being assessed. It is important to emphasize the preliminary nature of these analyses. The process of instrument development is iterative and time consuming. However, at the conclusion of these studies, the resulting psychometrically validated instrument should be useful to both clinicians and researchers.

It is our hope that the IC Symptom and Problem instruments will become a standard measure that is used as part of the patient profile, helps in disease management, and becomes part of the outcomes assessment in clinical trials involving IC patients. Uniform, widespread use of these indices in clinical, research, pharmacologic, and quality-of-life studies of IC would be a step forward. This would allow comparisons across different groups of patients and researchers and would standardize the reporting of treatment outcomes, disease natural history, and clinical monitoring of IC patients.

APPENDIX 1. INTERSTITIAL CYSTITIS SYMPTOM INDEX

Score

1. During the past month, how often have you felt the strong need to urinate with little or no warning?
   - [ ] Not at all 0
   - [ ] Less than one time in five 1
   - [ ] Less than half the time 2
   - [ ] About half the time 3
   - [ ] More than half the time 4
   - [ ] Almost always 5
2. During the past month, have you had to urinate less than 2 hr after you have finished urinating?
   - [ ] Not at all 0
   - [ ] Less than one time in five 1
   - [ ] Less than half the time 2
   - [ ] About half the time 3
   - [ ] More than half the time 4
   - [ ] Almost always 5
3. During the past month, how often did you most typically get up at night to urinate?
   - [ ] None 0
   - [ ] Once 1
   - [ ] Two times 2
   - [ ] Three times 3
   - [ ] Four times 4
   - [ ] Five or more times 5
4. During the past month, have you experienced pain or burning in your bladder?
   - [ ] Not at all 0
   - [ ] A few times 2
   - [ ] Fairly often 3
   - [ ] Usually 4
   - [ ] Almost always 5

Total Score: __________

APPENDIX 2. INTERSTITIAL CYSTITIS PROBLEM INDEX

During the past month, how much has each of the following been a problem for you?

Score

1. Frequent urination during the day?
   - [ ] No problem 0
   - [ ] Very small problem 1
   - [ ] Small problem 2
   - [ ] Medium problem 3
   - [ ] Big problem 4
2. Getting up at night to urinate?
   - [ ] No problem 0
   - [ ] Very small problem 1
   - [ ] Small problem 2
   - [ ] Medium problem 3
   - [ ] Big problem 4
3. Need to urinate with little warning?
   - [ ] No problem 0
   - [ ] Very small problem 1
   - [ ] Small problem 2
   - [ ] Medium problem 3
   - [ ] Big problem 4
4. Burning, pain, discomfort, or pressure in your bladder
   - [ ] No problem 0
   - [ ] Very small problem 1
   - [ ] Small problem 2
   - [ ] Medium problem 3
   - [ ] Big problem 4

Total Score: __________

REFERENCES

1. Parivar F, Bradbrook RA. Interstitial cystitis. *Br J Urol* 1986; 58:239–244.
2. Fall M, Johansson SL, Aldernborg F. Chronic interstitial cystitis: a heterogeneous syndrome. *J Urol* 1987;137:35–38.
3. Sant GR. Interstitial cystitis. pathogenesis, evaluation and treatment. *Urol Ann* 1989;3:171–196.
4. Oravisto KJ. Epidemiology of interstitial cystitis. *Ann Chir Gynaecol Finn* 1975;64:75–77.
5. O'Leary MP, Barry MJ, Fowler FJ Jr. Hard measures of subjective outcomes: validating symptom indexes in urology. *J Urol* 1992;148:1546.
6. Barry MJ, Fowler FJ, O'Leary MP, et al. The American Urological Association symptom index for benign prostatic hyperplasia. *J Urol* 1992;148:1549–1557.
7. Held PJ, Hanno PM, Wein AJ, et al. Epidemiology of interstitial cystitis. In: Hanno PM, Staskin DR, Krane RJ, Wein AJ, eds. *Interstitial Cystitis*. New York: Springer-Verlag, 1990;29–48.
8. McDowell I, Newell C. *Measuring Health*. New York: Oxford University Press, 1987.
9. Ware JE. Standards for validating health measures: definition and content. *J Chron Dis* 1987;40:473–476.
10. Deyo RA. The quality of life, research and care. *Ann Intern Med* 1991; 114:695–697.
11. Katz S, Ford AB, Moskowitz RW, et al. Studies of illness in the aged: the index of ADL, a standardized measure of biological and psychosocial function. *JAMA* 1963;185:914–916.
12. Zung WWK. A self-rating depression scale. *Arch Gen Psychiatry* 1965; 12:63–67.
13. Folstein MF, Folstein S, McHugh PR. Mini-mental state: a practical method for grading the cognitive state of patients for the clinician. *J Psychiatr Res* 1975;12:189–198.
14. Rubenstein LV, Calkins DR, Greenfield S, et al. Health status assessment of elderly patients. Report of the Society of General International Medicine Task Force on Health Assessment. *J Am Geriatr Soc* 1989; 37:562–569.
15. Fretwell MD. Comprehensive functional assessment (CFA) in everyday practice. In: Hazard WR, Andres R, Bierman EL, Blass JP, eds. *Principles of Geriatric Medicine in Gerontology.* New York: McGraw-Hill, 1990;218–223.
16. Applegate WB, Blass JP, Williams TF. Instruments for the functional assessment of older patients. *N Engl J Med* 1990;322:1207–1214.
17. Patrick DL, Deyo RA. Generic and disease-specific measures in assessing health status and quality of life. *Med Care* 1989;27(Suppl 3):S17–S32.
18. Guyatt GH, Feeny DH, Patrick DL. Measuring health-related quality of life. *Ann Intern Med* 1993;118:622–629.
19. Tsevat J, Weeks JC, Guadagnoli E, et al. Using health-related quality of life information. clinical encounters, clinical trials and health policy. *J Gen Intern Med* 1994;9:576–582.
20. Parkerson GRJ, Gehlbach SH, Wagner EH, et al. The Duke–UNC Health Profile. An adult health status instrument for primary care. *Med Care* 1981;18:806–828.
21. Nelson EC, Landgraf JM, Hays RD, et al. The functional status of patients. How can it be measures in physicians offices? *Med Care* 1990;28:1111–1126.
22. O'Leary MP, Sant GR, Whitmore KE, et al. The interstitial cystitis symptom index. *J Urol* 1996;155(5 Suppl):439A.
23. Kleinbaum DG, Kupper LL, Morgenstern H. *Epidemiologic Research. Principles and Quantitative Methods.* New York: Lifetime Learning Publications, 1982.
24. Cronbach LJ. Coefficient alpha and internal structure of tests. *Psychometrika* 1951;16:297.
25. Litwin MS, Hays RD, Fink A, et al. Quality of life outcomes in men treated for localized prostate cancer. *JAMA* 1995;273:129–135.

Subject Index